Allergic Mechanisms and Immunotherapeutic Strategies

Allergic Mechanisms and Immunotherapeutic Strategies

Edited by

ANGELA M. ROBERTS and MATTHEW R. WALKER
Wolfson Research Laboratories, University of Birmingham, UK

JOHN WILEY & SONS
Chichester · New York · Weinheim · Brisbane · Singapore · Toronto

National 01243 779777
International (+44) 1243 779777
e-mail (for orders and customer service enquiries): cs-books@wiley.co.uk
Visit our Home Page on http://www.wiley.co.uk
or http://www.wiley.com

Other Wiley Editorial Offices

John Wiley & Sons, Inc., 605 Third Avenue,
New York, NY 10158–0012, USA

VCH Verlagsgesellschaft mbH, Pappelallee 3,
D-69469 Weinheim, Germany

Jacaranda Wiley Ltd, 33 Park Road, Milton,
Queensland 4064, Australia

John Wiley & Sons (Asia) Pte Ltd, 2 Clementi Loop #02–01,
Jin Xing Distripark, Singapore 129809

John Wiley & Sons (Canada) Ltd, 22 Worcester Road,
Rexdale, Ontario M9W 1L1, Canada

Library of Congress Cataloging-in-Publication Data

Allergic mechanisms and immunotherapeutic strategies / edited by
Angela M. Roberts and Matthew R. Walker.
p. cm.
Includes bibliographical references and index.
ISBN 0–471–96999–0 (hbk : alk. paper)
1. Allergy. 2. Allergy–Immunotherapy. I. Walker, Matthew R.
II. Roberts, Angela M.
[DNLM: 1. Hypersensitivity, Immediate–immunology.
2. Hypersensitivity, Immediate–therapy. 3. IgE–immunology.
4. Desensitization, Immunologic. QW 900 A4336 1997]
QR188.A45 1997
616.97–dc20
DNLM/DLC
for Library of Congress 96–35332
CIP

British Library Cataloguing in Publication Data

A catalogue record for this book is available from the British Library
ISBN 0–471–96999–0
Typeset in 10/12pt Palatino by Vision Typesetting, Manchester
Printed and bound in Great Britain by Biddles Ltd, Guildford
This book is printed on acid-free paper responsibly manufactured from sustainable forestation, for which at least two trees are planted for each one used for paper production.

Contents

List of Contributors

Aftab A. Ansari
National Institute of Arthritis and Musculoskeletal and Skin Diseases, National Institutes of Health, Natcher Building – Room 5AS25S, 45 Center Drive, Bethesda MD 20892–6500, USA

Jean-Pierre Aubry
Immunology Department, Glaxo Institute for Molecular Biology SA, 14 chemin des Aulx, Plan-des-Ouates, 1228 Geneva, Switzerland

Lalit M. Bahuguna
Pathology Department, KG Medical College, Lucknow, India

Andrew J. Beavil
The Randall Institute, King's College London, Division of Biomedical Sciences, 26–29 Drury Lane, London WC2B 5RL UK

Rebecca L. Beavil
The Randall Institute, King's College London, Division of Biomedical Sciences, 26–29 Drury Lane, London WC2B 5RL, UK

Jean Yves Bonnefoy
Immunology Department, Glaxo Institute for Molecular Biology, 14 chemin des Aulx, Plan-des-Ouates, 1228 Geneva, Switzerland

Jean Bousquet
Services des Maladies Respiratoires, Hopital Arnaud de Villeneuve, 34295 Montpellier CEDEX, France

Anne Des Roches
Services des Maladies Respiratoires, Hopital Arnaud de Villeneuve, 34295 Montpellier CEDEX, France

Henriette Dhivert
Services des Maladies Respiratoires, Hopital Arnaud de Villeneuve, 34295 Montpellier CEDEX, France

Mark A. Exley
ImmuLogic Pharmaceutical Corporation, 610 Lincoln Street, Waltham MA 02154, USA. Present address: Department of Hematology/Oncology, Beth Israel Deaconess Medical Center, Harvard Medical School, Boston, MA 02215, USA

Leopoldo Flores-Romo
Immunology Department, Glaxo Institute for Molecular Biology SA, 14 chemin des Aulx, Plan-des-Ouates, 1228 Geneva, Switzerland

Jean François Gauchat
Immunology Department, Glaxo Institute for Molecular Biology SA, 14 chemin des Aulx, Plan-des-Ouates, 1228 Geneva, Switzerland

Hannah J. Gould
The Randall Institute, King's College London, Division of Biomedical Sciences, 26–29 Drury Lane, London WC2B 5RL, UK

Pierre Graber
Immunology Department, Glaxo Institute for Molecular Biology SA, 14 chemin des Aulx, Plan-des-Ouates, 1228 Geneva, Switzerland

Irwin J. Griffith
ImmuLogic Pharmaceutical Corporation, 610 Lincoln Street, Waltham MA 02154, USA

Adnan Hejjaoui
Services des Maladies Respiratoires, Hopital Arnaud de Villeneuve, 34295 Montpellier CEDEX, France

Birgit A. Helm
Department of Biochemistry and Molecular Biology, Krebs Institute for Biomolecular Research, The University of Sheffield, Sheffield S10 2UH, UK

Catharien M. U. Hilkens
Laboratory of Cell Biology and Histology, University of Amsterdam, Academisch Medisch Centrum, Meibergdreef 15, 1105 AZ Amsterdam, The Netherlands

Koji Ito
Department of Medicine and Physical Therapy, Faculty of Medicine, University of Tokyo, 7–3–1 Hongo, Bunkyo-ku, Tokyo 113, Japan

Martien L. Kapsenberg
Laboratory of Cell Biology and Histology, University of Amsterdam, Academisch Medisch Centrum, Meibergdreef 15, 1105 AZ Amsterdam, The Netherlands

Jalel Knani
Services des Maladies Respiratoires, Hopital Arnaud de Villeneuve, 34295 Montpellier CEDEX, France

R. Bruce Knox
Pollen and Allergen Research Group, School of Botany, The University of Melbourne, Grattan Street, Parkville VIC 3052, Australia

Dietrich Kraft
Institute of General and Experimental Pathology, AKH University of Vienna, Währingergürtel 18–20, A–1090 Vienna, Austria

Enrico Maggi
Clinical Immunology Department, Institute of Internal Medicine and Immunoallergology, Policlinico di Carreggi, Viale Morgagni 85, 50134 Firenze, Italy

Jean Louis Ménardo
Services des Maladies Respiratoires, Hopital Arnaud de Villeneuve, 34295 Montpellier CEDEX, France

François-B. Michel
Services des Maladies Respiratoires, Hopital Arnaud de Villeneuve, 34295 Montpellier CEDEX, France

Terumasa Miyamoto
Department of Medicine and Physical Therapy, Faculty of Medicine, University of Tokyo, 7–3–1 Hongo, Bunkyo-ku, Tokyo 113, Japan

Masaharu Muranaka
Department of Medicine and Physical Therapy, Faculty of Medicine, University of Tokyo, 7–3–1 Hongo, Bunkyo-ku, Tokyo 113, Japan

Susanne Natter
Institute of General and Experimental Pathology, AKH University of Vienna, Währingergürtel 18–20, A–1090 Vienna, Austria

Eng K. Ong
Pollen and Allergen Research Group, School of Botany, The University of Melbourne, Grattan Street, Parkville VIC 3052, Australia

Eduardo A. Padlan
Laboratory of Molecular Biology, National Institute of Diabetes and Digestive and Kidney Diseases, National Institutes of Health, Building 5 – Room 303, Bethesda MD 20892, USA

Paola Parronchi
Clinical Immunology Department, Institute of Internal Medicine and Immunoallergology, Policlinico di Carreggi, Viale Morgagni 85, 51034 Firenze, Italy

Jérome Pène
Services des Maladies Respiratoires, Hopital Arnaud de Villeneuve, 34295 Montpellier CEDEX, France

Bruce L. Rogers
ImmuLogic Pharmaceutical Corporation, 610 Lincoln Street, Waltham MA 02154, USA

Susanne Seiberler
Institute of General and Experimental Pathology, AKH University of Vienna, Währingergürtel 18–20, A–1090 Vienna, Austria

Mohan B. Singh
Department of Agriculture and Resource Management, The University of Melbourne, Grattan Street, Parkville VIC 3052, Australia

Alies Snijders
Laboratory of Cell Biology and Histology, University of Amsterdam, Academisch Medisch Centrum, Meibergdreef 15, 1105 AZ Amsterdam, The Netherlands

Frank G. M. Snijdewint
Laboratory of Cell Biology and Histology, University of Amsterdam, Academisch Medisch Centrum, Meibergdreef 15, 1105 AZ Amsterdam, The Netherlands

Wolfgang R. Sperr
Department of Haematology and Haemostaseology, AKH University of Vienna, Währingergürtel 18–20, A–1090 Vienna, Austria

Cenk Suphioglu
Pollen and Allergen Research Group, School of Botany, The University of Melbourne, Grattan Street, Parkville VIC 3052, Australia

Brian J. Sutton
The Randall Institute, King's College London, Division of Biomedical Sciences, 26–29 Drury Lane, London WC2B 5RL, UK

Shuji Suzuki
Department of Medicine and Physical Therapy, Faculty of Medicine, University of Tokyo, 7–3–1 Hongo, Bunkyo-ku, Tokyo 113, Japan

Zsolt Szepfalusi
Institute of General and Experimental Pathology, AKH University of Vienna, Währingergürtel 18–20, A–1090 Vienna, Austria

Shigeru Takafuji
Department of Medicine and Physical Therapy, Faculty of Medicine, University of Tokyo, 7–3–1 Hongo, Bunkyo-ku, Tokyo 113, Japan

Wayne R. Thomas
Division of Molecular Biology, Institute for Child Health Research, PO Box 855, West Perth WA 6872, Australia

Peter Valent
Department of Haematology and Haemostaseology, AKH University of Vienna, Währingergürtel 18–20, A–1090 Vienna, Austria

Rudolf Valenta
Institute of General and Experimental Pathology, AKH University of Vienna, Währingergürtel 18–20, A–1090 Vienna, Austria

Frans L. van der Heijden
Laboratory of Cell Biology and Histology, University of Amsterdam, Academisch Medisch Centrum, Meibergdreef 15, 1105 AZ Amsterdam, The Netherlands

R. J. Joost van Neerven
Laboratory of Cell Biology, and Histology, University of Amsterdam, Academisch Medisch Centrum, Meibergdreef 15, 1105 AZ Amsterdam, The Netherlands

Eddy A. Wierenga
Laboratory of Cell Biology and Histology, University of Amsterdam, Academisch Medisch Centrum, Meibergdreef 15, 1105 AZ Amsterdam, The Netherlands

Robert J. Young
The Randall Institute, King's College London, Division of Biomedical Sciences, 26–29 Drury Lane, London WC2B 5RL, UK

Preface

There is now considerable evidence that environmental and social changes, including increased urbanization, industrialization, air pollution and large-scale arable monoculture, have combined to produce an increase in the incidence of allergic individuals. It is currently estimated that greater than 1 in 10 individuals are afflicted with some form of allergy, which although generally not life threatening, causes varying forms of discomfort or debilitation leading to lost work and/or decreased performance. IgE-mediated hypersensitivities such as seasonal allergic rhinitis (hayfever), eczema, urticaria and asthma consequently represent considerable medical and socio-economic problems.

Delineating the primary immunological and biochemical bases of allergic symptoms (i.e. the interaction of cell surface bound IgE with allergenic substances eliciting the cascade production of inflammatory mediators by mast cells and basophils) has allowed the symptoms associated with many forms of allergies to be reasonably controlled. Current approaches to the clinical management of allergy largely rely either upon allergen avoidance and/or the long-term use of pharmacological agents (e.g. steroids and anti-histamines). These are designed to counteract the effects of the inflammatory agents released as a consequence of the binding of allergens to IgE molecules. Although these may be reasonably effective they are no longer wholly acceptable on practical and intellectual grounds. This is especially the case given that molecular and cellular immunobiology research has provided many insights into the precise mechanisms determining IgE production. These afford the opportunity to develop of a range of novel, and potentially curative, immunotherapies for IgE-mediated hypersensitivities.

Drawing contributions from many of the pioneering research groups, this book summarizes some of the most pertinent discoveries, and how they may be exploited for the development of immunotherapeutic strategies based upon modulating IgE production. The next decade looks set to be one of excitement and anticipation for both researcher and allergic sufferer, during which it will become clear which of these potential therapeutic avenues will lead to the successful development of effective and long-lasting desensitization strategies. Indeed, it is increasingly likely that the dilemma facing clinical allergologists by the next century will be which of the available treatments to use.

*Angela M. Roberts**
Matthew R. Walker
Wolfson Research Laboratories, University of Birmingham, UK
*Present address: Worcester Royal Infirmary NHS Trust, UK

1 Development of Structural Models for a Study of the Interaction of Human IgE with Class-specific Fc-receptors

EDUARDO A. PADLAN and BIRGIT A. HELM*

*Laboratory of Molecular Biology, NIDDKD, National Institutes of Health, Bethesda, USA; and *Department of Biochemistry and Molecular Biology, Krebs Institute for Biomolecular Research, The University of Sheffield, Sheffield, UK*

INTRODUCTION

The persistent interest in antibodies of the immunoglobulin (Ig)E isotype following the discovery of this novel Ig class in 1966 by Ishizaka *et al.* [1] stems primarily from their demonstration of its role as the mediator of type I hypersensitivity disorders. Although IgE antibodies may play an important role in host defence to parasites and oncogenic viruses [2], this beneficial effect is generally considered of limited value in countries that enjoy high standards of hygiene and where the synthesis of an antibody of the IgE isotype is regarded as an unwanted immune response linked to the development of allergy and asthma. Allergic reactions are rarely fatal, but with the recent alarming increase in IgE-mediated atopies in response to airborne and food-associated allergens [3] the development of effective treatments in atopic disease, still outstanding after many years of intensive research, is of considerable social, medical and industrial importance.

A better understanding of the key events, components and their interaction in the regulatory circuits that operate in allergic disease is crucial for the development of rational therapeutic interventions in allergy. During the past decade, immuno-allergology has progressed from a phenomenological division of medicine to a molecular science. Many significant advances have been achieved culminating in the cloning and expression of the principal proteins involved in the allergic response including the ligand, its receptors, allergens, interleukins, and interferons [4].

Our own work has concentrated on the interaction of IgE with class-specific Fc-receptors. IgE antibodies are made up of two light chains (κ or λ isotype) which combine with two ε-chain to form the variable region involved in

Allergic Mechanisms and Immunotherapeutic Strategies. Edited by A.M. Roberts and M.R. Walker.

antigen recognition. The ε-chain is a five domain glycoprotein which forms a covalent homodimer via two cystine residues linking opposite Cε2 domains. In normal individuals, the plasma levels of this antibody are lower than those of any other class; their synthesis is thought to be tightly controlled by a network of B and T lymphocytes. IgE has not only the lowest levels but also the shortest serum half-life of all classes of immunoglobulins. The majority of IgE molecules are found bound, through residues located in the Fc portion of the molecule, to mast cells, basophils and dendritic cells which express high-affinity receptors (FcεRI) [5]; low-affinity receptors (FcεRII/CD23) are expressed on a diverse population of white blood cells collectively known as inflammatory cells, on some T cells and dendritic cells [6]. Cross-linking by cognate antigen/allergen of cellular receptors occupied by IgE results in the release of the pharmacologically active agents that cause the clinical symptoms of allergy or confer protective immunity to parasites and some viral infections [7].

The initial binding of IgE to FcεRI, although of very high affinity (nmolar range), is a reversible process. It sensitizes, but does not activate target cell degranulation unless the ligand is aggregated, and there is no evidence from *in vitro* studies that two soluble α-chain molecules can engage IgE-Fc [8]. This 'safety lock' probably results from the bent conformation of IgE [9]. An identification of the complementary sites and their modes of interaction should make an important contribution towards the design of rational therapeutic interventions in allergy.

The FcεRI complex from several species has been cloned [10] and current evidence indicates that FcεRI is a multi-subunit receptor composed of a single α-chain, a β-subunit, and two disulphide-linked γ-chains. Hydropathy plots indicate that the complete tetramer contains seven transmembrane helices [10]. The extracellular portion of the α-subunit has two Ig-like domains which comprise the IgE binding site. Although both IgE and its receptors are heavily glycosylated, it is known that carbohydrate does not contribute to the complementary interaction. Recent evidence suggests that three independent regions in the second Ig-like domain are involved in the binding of the ligand to the receptor, and there is also evidence that the first Ig-like domain of the α-chain is required to confer high-affinity binding for the ligand [11,12].

The second receptor for IgE binds the ligand with low affinity (mmolar range) and is a single chain transmembrane glycoprotein; it is not a member of the Ig superfamily, but belongs to a class of calcium-dependent (C-type) carbohydrate-binding proteins [13].

Currently, no high-resolution structure determinations exist for IgE or its receptors and the outcome of attempts to grow ordered crystals or to generate materials suitable for nuclear magnetic resonance analysis remains uncertain. In the absence of such information, we have developed models which are based on sequence similarity with known structures, complemented by data obtained from protein engineering studies for the ligand [14,15] and its receptors [16,17], to gain information regarding the location of those regions in the molecules which are involved in the complementary interaction. The coordinates of the interaction might form the starting point for the development of rational anti-allergic drugs. Structural predictions made by the models will be used to guide future protein engineering experiments and these in turn may yield additional information to stimulate further analysis and subsequent refinement of the projected structures.

MODELLING OF THE HUMAN IgE MOLECULE

The earliest crystallographic analyses of antibody structures showed that antibody domains have the same basic fold [18,19]. Each domain consists of two sheets of anti-parallel β-strands, the sheets being linked by a disulphide bond. The variable domains of the light and heavy chains are similar to each other in three-dimensional structure, as are the constant domains. Homologous domains from different species are very similar and are essentially superposable.

The structural similarity of homologous domains has encouraged us to attempt to model the structure of the constant domains of IgE on the basis of sequence similarity with the domains of IgG_1, for which three-dimensional structures are available [20,21]. A sequence alignment of the domains in the Fc of IgE and IgG_1 is presented in Table 1.1. It is found that $C\varepsilon3$ is more similar to $C\gamma2$ (32% identity), $C\varepsilon4$ to $C\gamma3$ (32% identity), and $C\varepsilon2$ to $C\gamma3$ (20% identity). In IgG_1, the $C\gamma3$ domains were found to be in close association, whereas the $C\gamma2$ domains are far apart, with the carbohydrate moieties attached to Asn297 lying between the two $C\gamma2$ domains [21]. A comparison of the sequences, especially of the residues involved in the inter-domain interactions, suggests that the mode of association of the two $C\varepsilon2$ and of the two $C\varepsilon4$ would be like that found for the $C\gamma3$ domains, and, in view of the probable glycosylation of Asn394, that the $C\varepsilon3$ domains would be far apart and separated by carbohydrate also.

Based on the demonstration of the parallel nature of the inter-ε-chain disulphide bonds [15] formed by the cystines at positions 241 and 328 (Table 1.1), we proposed a model structure which projects an extended segment of seven residues spanning the inter-domain region between $C\varepsilon2$ and $C\varepsilon3$, which is probably deformable. This heptapeptide would be analogous to the hinge peptide in IgG_1 (Table 1.1), which has been shown to be flexible [20]. The site in human IgE, which interacts with FcεRI, has been mapped to the segment between residues 343 and 353 in the $C\varepsilon3$ domain [22]. In our model structure of IgE-Fc this segment is proposed to form a loop which is homologous to the A loop in $C\gamma2$ which binds to the rat neonatal Fcγ receptor (FcγRn) [23]. A possible structure for IgE with this segment highlighted is presented in Figure 1.1.

Table 1.1. Sequence alignment of the domains in the Fc of human IgE and IgG1

```
           230       240       250  a     260       270
Cε2     SRDFTPPTVKILQSSCDGGGHFPPTIQLLCLVSGYTPGTINITWLEDGQVMDV
               .....             ...........   ......
Cγ3     -GQPREPQVYTLPPSREE--MTKNQVSLTCLVKGFYPSDIAVEWESNGQPENN

         280       290       300       310       320
Cε2     DLSTASTTQEGELASTQSELTLSQKHWLSDRTYTCQVTYQGHTFEDSTKK
        ...   ..     ..........*****   ........       ....
Cγ3     YKTTPPVLDSDGSFFLYSKLTVDKSRWQQGNVFSCSVMHEALHNHYTQKS

                       330
ε hinge      --------C-ADSNPRG
              ****
γ1 hinge     DKTHTCPPCPAPELLGG

           340        350       360       370       380
Cε3     VSAYLSRPSPFD-LFIRKSPTITCLVVDLAPSKGTVNLTWSRASGKPVNHSTR
         .....   *****       .......        ......  ..
Cγ2     PSVFLFPPKPKDTLMISRTPEVTCVVVDVSHEDPEVKFNWYVDGVEVHNAKTK

         390       400       410       420       430
Cε3     KEEKQRNGTLTVTSTLPVGTRDWIEGETYQCRVTHPHLPRALMRSTTKTS
          ....  .........  *****     ......      .....
Cγ2     PREEQYNSTYRVVSVLTVLHQDWLNGKEYKCKVSNKALPAPIEKTISKAK

         440       450       460       470       480       490
Cε4     GPRAAPEVYAFATPEWPGSRDKRTLACLIQNFMPEDISVQWLHNEVQLPDARHST
              .....          ...........    ......        ...
Cγ3     GQPREPQVYTLPPSREEMTKNQVSLTCLVKGFYPSDIAVEWESNGQPENNYKTTP

              500       510       520       530       540
Cε4     TQPRKTKGSGFFVFSRLEVTRAEWEQKDEFICRAVHEAASPSQTVQRAVSVNPGK
         ..       ..........*****   ........        ......
Cγ3     PVLDSD--GSFFLYSKLTVDKSRWQQGNVFSCSVMHEAL-HNHYTQKSLSLSPGK
```

The residues which are in β-strands are indicated by dots above them. those in α-helices by asterisks. Secondary structure designations were obtained with program DSSP [37] on Protein Data Bank Entries: 2IG2 and 1FC1.

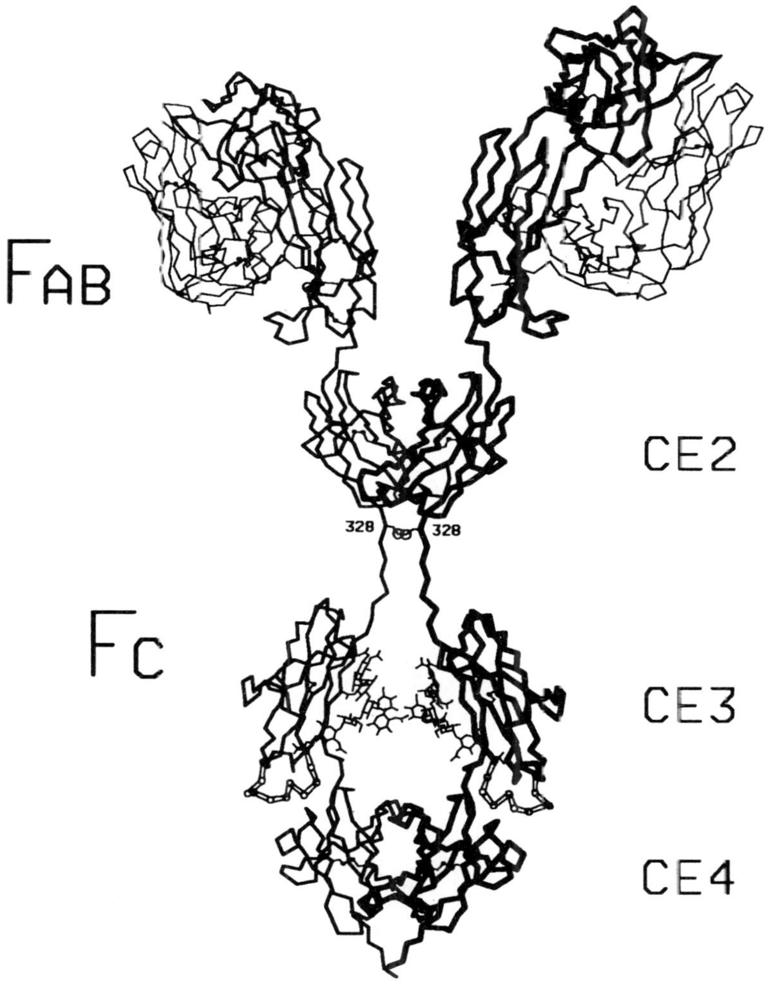

Figure 1.1. α-carbon trace of a possible structure of human IgE with various fragments and domains indicated. The light chains are drawn with thin lines and the heavy chains with thick lines, one thicker than the other. The inter-ε-chain cystine at position 328 is labelled. The segment, 343–353, which is involved in the binding to FcεRI [22] is drawn with bigger circles and wide, empty bonds in both heavy chains

The sites in IgE that interact with FcεRII/CD23 are also located in the Cε3 domain between residues 340 and 440. Deletion of the Cε4 domain results in loss of FcεRII/CD23, but not FcεRI binding, and studies indicate that C-terminal truncation of the ε-chain inhibits dimerization of the molecule [24,25]. Cε4 specific residues are, however, not essential for the binding to either receptor since ε/γ chimaerae where Cε4 has been replaced by Cγ3 engage both receptors, although with a 10-fold reduced affinity [25,26]. Collectively, these data indicate that dimerization is essential for the interaction of IgE with FcεRII/CD23, but that a single ε-chain can form the site of attachment for FcεRI.

Energy transfer measurements [9] suggest that the Fc and Fab fragments of IgE are not coplanar, rather that the molecule is bent. We propose that the bending is made possible by the hinge segment between Cε2 and Cε3. The presence of proline at position 333 (the fifth residue in the hinge heptapeptide) may induce the bending. A bent model of IgE is readily constructed (Figure 1.2).

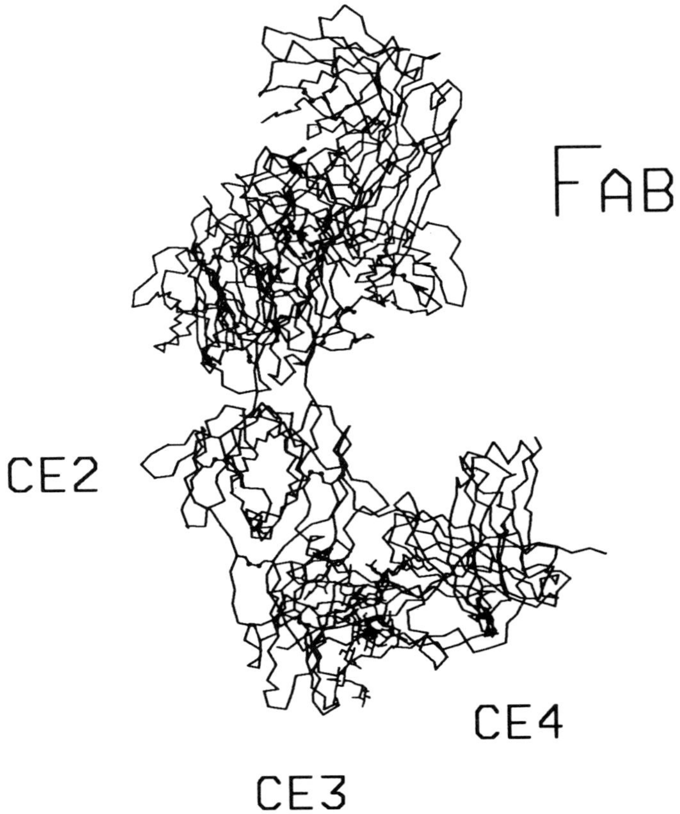

Figure 1.2. Stereodrawing of the α-carbon trace of a possible structure of human IgE, bent at the hinge segment spanning the interdomain region between Cε2 and Cε3

MODELLING OF THE EXTRACELLULAR DOMAIN OF THE α-SUBUNIT OF FcεRI

The two Ig-like domains of the α-subunit are homologous (Table 1.2), with 22 identities, and both would be classified as belonging to the C-2 set of Ig domains [27]. We have built models of these two Ig-like domains on the basis of sequence similarity with antibody domains [16]. An alignment of the sequences of the first Ig-like domain of the α-subunit and of antibody domains of known three-dimensional structure is presented in Table 1.3. A model of the first domain was built by piecing together four segments from the listed antibody domains which are the most similar in amino acid sequence to the corresponding regions in the α-subunit (Table 1.3); the CL domain of a murine κ-light chain served as the template for the composite structure. The second Ig-like domain of the α-subunit was then modelled after the first. The relative association between the two Ig-like domains, which are both required for high-affinity IgE binding [11], is uncertain. One possible mode of association [16] is shown in Figure 1.3.

THE INTERACTION BETWEEN IgE AND FcεRIα

An attempt to localize the IgE binding site on FcεRI has been made [12] by the use of monoclonal antibodies specific for the α-subunit. Some of the antibodies inhibited IgE binding and some did not. A study of the binding of these antibodies to a set of overlapping synthetic peptides spanning the entire extracellular portion of the α-subunit identified the segment 100–115 (Table 1.2) as probably involved in the binding to IgE. More recent studies have employed homologue-graft scanning [11] and the outcome of those observations demonstrated that at least three independent IgE binding regions are located in the second Ig-like domain of FcεRIα. Those regions are found between residues Trp87 to Lys128 (which contains the segment 100–115 mentioned above), Tyr129 to Asp145, and Ser146 to Val169 [11], and together encompass nearly the whole second domain (Table 1.2). We have marked the boundaries of these segments in Figure 1.3, where the segment 100–115 is also shown. In the homologous receptor, FcγRII, the residue at position 131 was found to be critical for the binding to IgG_2 [28]; the location of residue 131 is indicated also in Figure 1.3.

As mentioned above, the complementary site in IgE, which interacts with FcεRIα, has been mapped to a segment in the N-terminal region of the Cε3 domain [22] which is homologous to the site where IgG binds to FcγRn. In contrast, however, to the interaction of IgG with FcγRn, where two receptor molecules bind a single IgG-Fc region both in solution and in the co-crystals [23], IgE-Fc only binds to one α-chain [7]. A detailed understanding of the bent conformation of the IgE molecule, which is thought to render one of the

Table 1.2. Alignment of the amino acid sequences of the two immunoglobulin-like domains of the human FcεRI α-subunit

10 20 30 40

V P Q K P K V S **L** N P P W N R I F K **G** E N V T **L** T **C** N **G** N N F F E **V** S S T K W F H N **G** S L S E E T

90 100 110 120 130

W L L **L** Q A S A E V V M E **G** Q P L F **L** R **C** H **G** W R N W D **V** Y K V I Y Y K D **G** E A L K Y W Y E

50 60 70 80

N S S L N **I** V **N A** K F **E D S G** E **Y** K **C** Q H Q Q V N **E S E P** V Y L E **V** F S D

140 150 160 170

N H N I S **I** T **N A** T V **E D S G** T **Y** Y **C** T G K V W Q L D Y **E S E P** L N I T **V** I K A

Identical residues are shown in bold letters.

Table 1.3. Alignment of the amino acid sequence of the first immunoglobulin-like domain of the human FcεRI α-subunit and of antibody domains of known three-dimensional structure

	10	20 … 30	40
1.*	V **P** Q K **P** K **V S L** N **P P**	W N R I F K **G** E N **V T L T C** N G **N N F F**	E V S S T **K W** F H **N G S** L **S** E E
2.	R A D A A **P** T **V S** I F **P P**	S S E Q L T S G G A S V V **C** F L **N N F** Y P K D	I N V **K W** K I D **G S** E R Q N G V L N S W T
3.	Q P K A N **P** T **V** T **L** F **P P**	S S E E L Q A N K A **T L** V **C** L I S D **F** Y P G A	V T V A **W** K A D **G S** P V K A G V E T T K P
4.	E S A R N **P** T I Y P L T	L P P A L S S D P **V** I I G **C** L I H D Y **F** P S G	T M N V T **W** G K S **G** K D I T T V N F P P
5.	A S T K G **P** S **V** F P L A **P**	S S K S T S **G** G T A A **L** G **C** L V K D Y **F** P Q P	V T V S **W** N S G A L T **S** G V H T F P A
6.	**P** S **V** F **L** F **P P**	K P K D T L M I S R T P E V **T C** V V V D V S H E D P Q V K F N	**W** Y V D **G** V Q V H N A K T K P
7.	G Q **P** R E **P** Q **V** Y T L **P P**	S R E E M T K N Q **V** S **L T C** L V K G **F** Y P S D	I A V E **W** E S **N G** Q P E N N Y K T T P

	50 … 60 … 70	80
1.	T N **S** S **L** N I V N A K F **E D** S G **E Y K C Q** H **Q** Q V	N E **S** E **P V** Y L E **V** F S D
2.	D Q D S K D S T Y S M S **S** T **L** T L T K D E Y **E** R H N S **Y** T **C** E A T H K	T S T S **P** I V K S F N R N E C
3.	S K Q S N N K Y A A S **S** Y **L** S L T P E Q W K S H R S **Y** S **C Q** V T H E	G S T **V** E K T **V** A P T E C S
4.	A L A S G G R Y T M S N Q **L** T L P A V E C P E G E S V **K C** S V **Q** H D	**S** N **P V** Q E L D V N C S G
5.	V L Q S S G L Y S L S **S** V V T V P S S S L G T Q T **Y** I **C** N V N H K	P S N T K **V** D K R **V** E P K S C
6.	R E Q Q Y N S T Y R V V **S** V **L** T V L H Q N W L **D** G K **E Y K C** K V S N K	A L P A **P** I E K T I S K A K
7.	P V L D S D G S F F L Y **S** K **L** T V D K S R W Q Q G N V F S **C** S V M H E	A L H N H Y T Q K S L S L

1. first domain of the human FcεRI α-subunit, 2. murine J539 CL, 3. human Kol CL, 4. murine J539 CH1, 5. human Kol CH1, 6. human IgG_1 CH2, and 7. human IgG_1 CH3. The residues, which are identical to those in the FcεRI domain, are shown in bold letters. The segments, which were pieced together to generate the composite domain structure, are indicated by dots above the appropriate sequences.

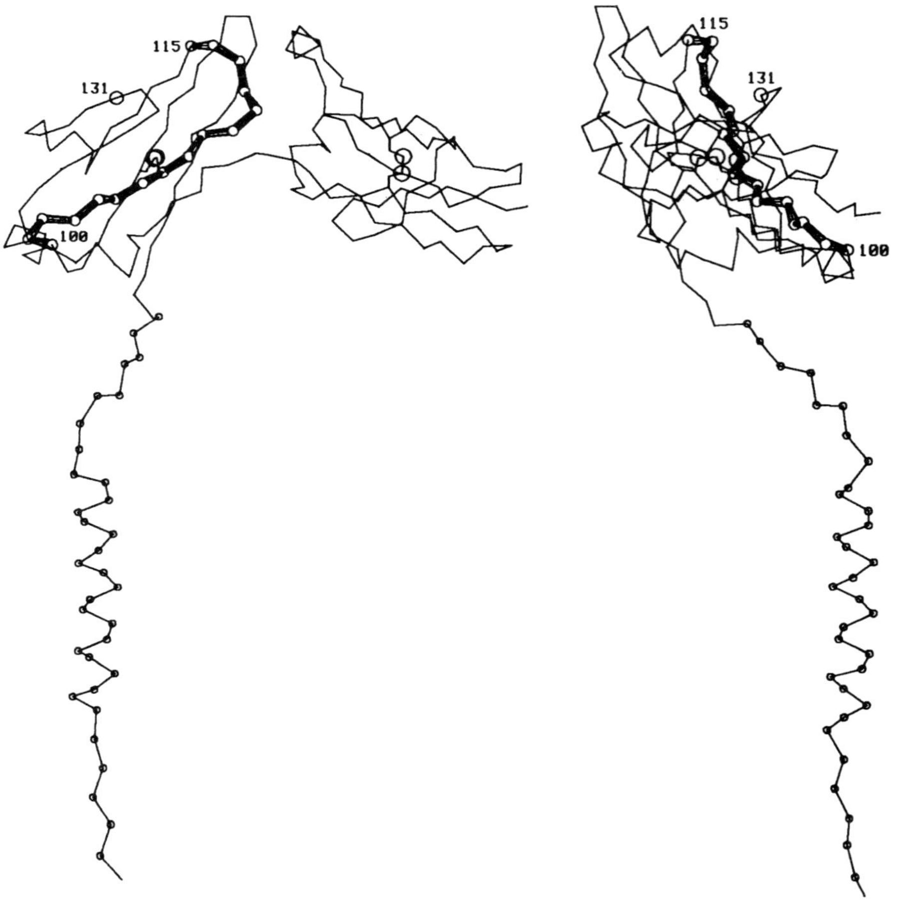

Figure 1.3. Two views of the α-carbon trace of a possible structure for human FcεRIα. The segment 100–115, which is probably involved in the binding to IgE [12], is drawn with big circles and wide, filled bonds; position 131, which in the homologous receptor, FcγRII, has been found to be critical for the binding to IgG_2 [28], is indicated by an open circle. The additional residues of FcεRIα have been added for completeness and are indicated with filled circles; the putative transmembrane region was built as an α-helix

ε-chains inaccessible to another molecule of the receptor or to antibodies directed against the receptor binding site in IgE, will have important consequences for the design of anti-allergic vaccines. Several murine monoclonal and human anti-IgE antibodies have already been described [29–31] that recognize epitopes in IgE which are inaccessible following IgE/receptor interaction. The identification of such epitopes therefore has tremendous

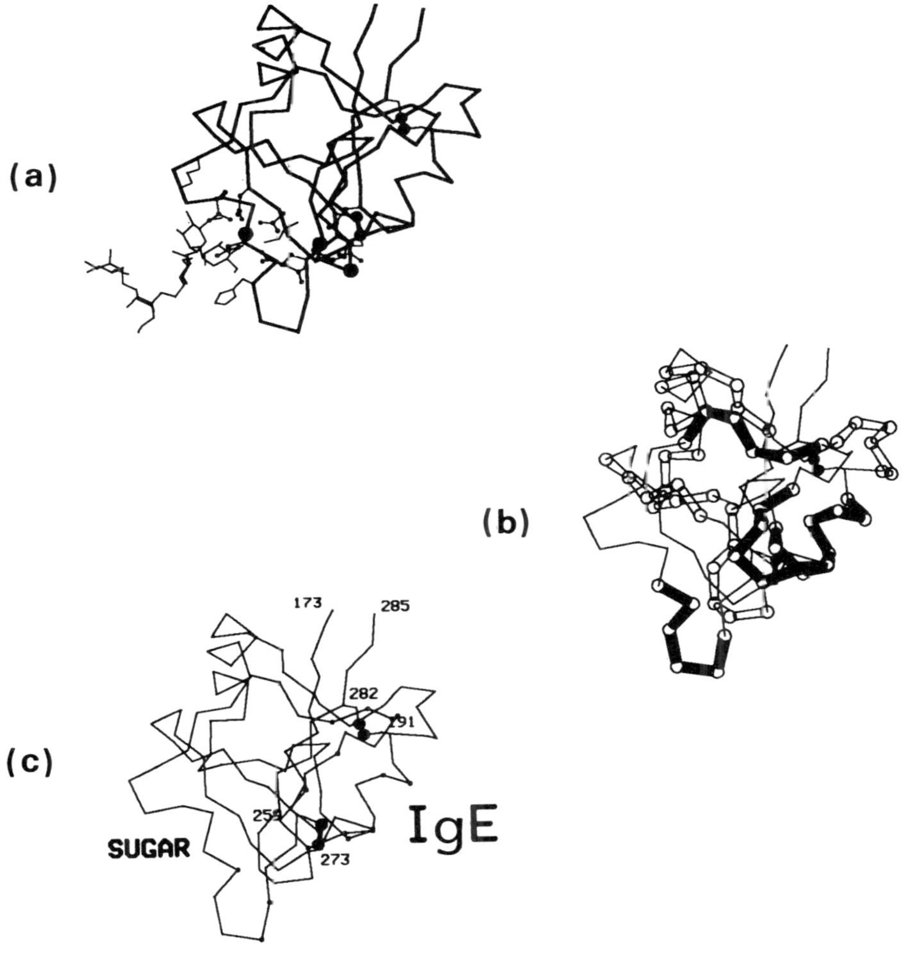

Figure 1.4. (a) The α-carbon trace of the rat mannose binding protein [33,34]. The side chains of the cystines, which form disulphide bridges (the $S\gamma$ are drawn with filled circles), and of the residues, which contact the calcium atoms and the carbohydrate, are included in the drawing. The three calcium atoms in the structure are drawn with large, dark circles and the side chain atoms of the ligands to the calciums are indicated by small, filled circles. The $Man_6GlcNac_2Asn$ asparaginyl-oligosaccharide, which was bound to the protein in the crystal structure, is drawn with thin lines, as are the protein side chains in contact with this ligand. (b) The α-carbon trace of the modelled FcεRII/CD23 lectin-homology domain [17] showing the peptides, which were found [35] to be crucial to IgE binding (indicated by the thick, filled bonds), and those which are probably not involved in IgE binding (indicated by the empty bonds). (c) The α-carbon trace of the modelled FcεRII/CD23 lectin-homology domain, with the proposed IgE and carbohydrate binding sites indicated [17]. The termini and the cystines are labelled

Table 1.4. Alignment of the lectin homology regions of human and murine FcεRII/CD23 and rat mannose-binding protein

```
                  180       190       200       210       220
                   |         |         |         |         |
hu CD23     KCYYFGKGTKQWVHARYACDDMEGQLVSIHSPEEQDFLTKHASHTGSWIGLRNLDLK
mu CD23     KCYYFGKGSKQWIQARFACSDLQGRLVSIHSQKEQDFLMQHINKKDSWIGLQDLNME

             sssssssss hhhhhhhhhh   ss     hhhhhhhhhhh    ssssss
rat MBP     KFFVTNHERMPFSKVKALCSELRGTVAIPRNAEENKAIQEVAK TSAFLGITDEVTE
            |         |       @ |         |         |          |
           110       120       130       140       150        160


           230       240       250       260       270       280
            |         |         |         |         |         |
hu CD23     GEFIWVDGSHVDYSNWAPGEPTSRSQGEDCVMMRGSGRWNDAFCDRKLGAWVCDRL
mu CD23     GEFVWSDGSPVGYSNWNPGEPNNGGQGEDCVMMRGSGQWNDAFCRSYLDAWVCEQL

               ss                        ssss     ssss      sssssss
rat MBP     GQFMYVTGGRLTYSNWKKDEPNDHGSGEDCVTIVDNGLWNDISCQ ASHTAVCEFP
                |         |         |    #    |        #|       @  |
               170       180       190       200       210        220
```

ssss, hhhh β-sheet and α-helical regions, respectively, in the rat mannose binding protein (PDB Entry 2MSB) as identified by program DSSP [37]. @, # Cystine residues which are disulfide-linked to each other in the rat MBP [33].

implications for the development of vaccines suitable for the treatment of all IgE-mediated allergies.

MODELLING OF FcεRII/CD23

The three-dimensional structure of one member of the family of C-type carbohydrate-binding proteins, the rat mannose-binding protein (MBP), has been determined crystallographically [33,34] (Figure 1.4a). The rat MBP shows significant sequence similarity to the lectin-homology region of human and murine FcεRII/CD23 and has analogous disulphide bridges (Table 1.4). These molecules are very similar even in length with only two one-residue gaps needed for optimal alignment of the sequences. We have built models of the lectin-homology domains of human and murine FcεRII/CD23 based on sequence similarity with rat MBP [17].

The site in CD23 which interacts with IgE has been mapped by homologue-scanning mutagenesis by Bettler *et al.* [35] who found six peptide segments in human FcεRII/CD23 to be critical for activity; six other segments were considered unlikely to contribute to IgE binding. (The loss of IgE binding activity upon replacement of two segments appears to be primarily due to a resultant change in the global structure of the molecule, as demonstrated by altered binding by conformation-sensitive antibodies.) The location of the four segments, which are probably directly involved in IgE binding, and of the six nonessential peptides in our modelled FcεRII/CD23 is shown in Figure 1.4b. There is a region to which all the critical segments, and only the critical segments, contribute and we propose this as the site for IgE binding (Figure 1.4c).

The site of interaction between FcεRII/CD23 and CD21/CR2 has been shown to be calcium dependent and to be inhibited by fucose-1-phosphate, and has been predicted to map to the lectin-homology domain and to a site that is close, but not identical, to the IgE binding site [36]. This site seems very likely to be analogous to the carbohydrate binding site of the rat MBP (Figure 1.4a) and which, in our modelling, would be located on the other side of the FcεRII/CD23 molecule relative to the IgE binding site (Figure 1.4c).

CONCLUSION

The models which we have developed for IgE and its receptors can only be correct in general terms. Nonetheless, they can serve as guides in the design of protein engineering experiments to pinpoint more closely the structural variables and residues which contribute to the complementary interaction. In addition, these models may lend themselves as possible probes in crystallographic analyses by molecular replacement techniques, should these molecules yield crystals suitable for crystallographic study.

ACKNOWLEDGEMENTS

This work was supported in part by a NATO Collaborative Research Grant and by a grant from the Science and Engineering Research Council and EU grant PL 931184 to BAH.

REFERENCES

1 Ishizaka K, Ishizaka T, Hornbrook MM. Physicochemical properties of human reaginic antibody. *J Immunol* 1966; **97**: 840–847
2 Helm BA. The interaction of human IgE with class-specific Fc-receptors. In Merret T, El Shami AL (eds) *Advances in the Biosciences*, vol 74. London: Pergamon Press, 1989; 83–91.
3 Kraft D, Sehon A. *Molecular Biology and Immunology of Allergens*. Boca Raton: CRC Press, 1992.
4 Helm BA, Ling Y, Rhodes N, Padlan EA. Can structural and functional studies on components of the immunoglobulin E receptor/effector system assist the design of rational IgE antagonists? In: Miyamato T, Okuda M (eds) *Progress in Allergy and*

Clinical Immunology 2: Impact of Biotechnology on Allergy Research. Seattle: Hogrefe and Huber, 1992; 589–599.

5 Metzger H. Transmembrane signaling: The joy of aggregation. *J Immunol* 1992; **149**: 1477–1487.

6 Mossalay MD, Debre P. CD23: a cytokine with dual membrane and soluble forms. *Res Immunol* 1992; **143**: 421–464.

7 Nagy E, Berczi I, Sehon AH. Growth inhibition of murine mammary carcinoma by monoclonal IgE antibodies specific for the mammary tumor virus. *Cancer Immunol Immunother* 1991; **34**: 63–69.

8 Yagi S, Yanagida M, Tanida I, Hasegawa A, Okumura K, Ra C. High-level expression of the truncated alpha chain of human high-affinity receptor for IgE as a soluble form by baculovirus-infected insect cells. Biochemical characterization of the recombinant product. *Eur J Biochem* 1994; **220**: 593–598.

9 Zheng Y, Shopes B, Holowka D, Baird B. Conformation of IgE bound to receptor and in solution. *Biochemistry* 1991; **30**: 9125–9132.

10 Blank U, Ra C, Miller L, White K, Metzger H, Kinet J-P. Complete structure and expression in transfected cells of high affinity IgE receptor. *Nature* 1989; **337**: 187–189.

11 Hulett MD, McKenzie IFC, Hogarth PM. Chimeric Fc receptors identify immunoglobulin-binding regions in human FcγRII and FcεRI. *Eur J Immunol* 1993; **23**: 640–645.

12 Riske F, Hakimi J, Mallamaci M, Griffin M, Pilson B, Tobkes N, Lin P, Danho W, Kochan J, Chizzonite R. High affinity human IgE receptor (FcεRI). *J Biol Chem* 1991; **266**: 11245–11251.

13 Richards ML, Katz DH. Biology and chemistry of the low affinity IgE receptor. *Crit Rev Immunol* 1991; **11**: 65–86.

14 Padlan EA, Davies DR. A model of the Fc of immunoglobulin E. *Mol Immunol* 1986; **23**: 1063–1075.

15 Helm BA, Ling Y, Teale C, Padlan EA, Brueggemann M. The nature and biological importance of the inter-ε chain disulfide bonds in human IgE. *Eur J Immunol* 1991; **21**: 1543–1548.

16 Padlan EA, Helm BA. A modeling study of the α-subunit of human high-affinity receptor for immunoglobulin-E. *Receptor* 1992; **2**: 129–144.

17 Padlan EA, Helm BA. Modeling of the lectin-homology domains of the human and murine low-affinity Fcε receptor (FcεRII/CD23). *Receptor* 1993; **3**: 325–341.

18 Poljak RJ, Amzel LM, Avey HP, Chen BL, Phizackerley RP, Saul F. Three-dimensional structure of the Fab′ fragment of a human immunoglobulin at 2.8-Å resolution. *Proc Natl Acad Sci USA* 1973; **70**: 3305–3310.

19 Schiffer M, Girling RL, Ely KR, Edmundson AB. Structure of a λ-type Bence-Jones protein at 3.5-Å resolution. *Biochemistry* 1973; **12**: 4620–4631.

20 Marquart M, Deisenhofer J, Huber R, Palm W. Crystallographic refinement and atomic models of the intact immunoglobulin molecule Kol and its antigen-binding fragment at 3.0 Å and 1.9Å resolution. *Mol Biol* 1980; **141**: 369–391.

21 Deisenhofer J. Crystallographic refinement and atomic models of a human Fc fragment and its complex with fragment B of protein A from *Staphylococcus aureus* at 2.9- and 2.8-Å resolution. *Biochemistry* 1981; **20**: 2361–2369.

22 Helm BA, Sayers I, Higginbottom A, Machado DC, Ling Y, Ahmad K, Padlan EA, Wilson APM. Identification of the high-affinity receptor binding region in human immunoglobulin E. *J Biol Chem* 1996; **271**: 7494–7500.

23 Burmeister WP, Huber AH, Bjorkmann PJ. Crystal structure of the complex of rat neonatal Fc receptor with Fc. *Nature* 1994; **372**: 379–383.

24 Helm B, Marsh P, Vercelli D, Padlan E, Gould H, Geha R. The mast cell binding site

on human immunoglobulin E. *Nature* 1988; **331**: 180–183.

25 Vercelli D, Helm B, Marsh P, Padlan E, Geha RS, Gould H. The B cell binding site on human immunoglobulin E. *Nature* 1989; **338**: 649–650.

26 Weetall M, Shopes B, Holowka D, Baird B. Mapping the site of interaction between murine IgE and its high affinity receptor with chimeric Ig. *J Immunol* 1990; **145**: 3849–3854.

27 Williams AF, Barclay AN. The immunoglobulin superfamily – domains for cell surface recognition. *Ann Rev Immunol* 1988; **6**: 381–405.

28 Warmerdam PAM, van der Winkel JGJ, Vlug A, Westerdaal NAC, Capel PJA. A single amino acid in the second Ig-like domain of the human Fcg receptor II is critical for human IgG_2 binding. *J Immunol* 1991; **147**: 1338–1343.

29 Davis FM, Gossett LA, Pinkston KL, Liu RS, Sun LK, Kim YW, Chang NT, Chang TW, Wagner K, Bews J, Brinkmann V, Towbin H, Subramanian N, Heuser C. Can anti-IgE be used to treat allergy? *Springer Seminars Immunopathol* 1993; **15**: 51–73.

30 Robertson MW, Liu FT. IgE structure function relationship defined by sequence directed antibodies induced by synthetic peptides. *Mol Immunol* 1988; **25**: 103–107.

31 Kitani S, Kraft D, Fischer C, Mergenhagen SE, Siraganian RP. Inhibition of allergic reactions with monoclonal antibodies directed against the high affinity IgE receptor. *J Immunol* 1988; **140**: 2585–2588.

32 Presta LG, Lahr SJ, Shields RL, Porter JP, Gorman C, Fendly BM, Jardieu PM. Humanization of an antibody directed against human IgE. *J Immunol* 1993; **151**: 2623–2628.

33 Weis WI, Kahn R, Fourme R, Drickamer K, Hendrickson WA. Structure of the calcium-dependent lectin domain from a rat mannose-binding protein determined by MAD phasing. *Science* 1991; **254**: 1608–1615.

34 Weis WI, Drickamer K, Hendrickson WA. Structure of a C-type mannose-binding protein complexed with an oligosaccharide. *Nature* 1992; **360**: 127–134.

35 Bettler B, Texido G, Raggini S, Ruegg D, Hofstetter H. Immunoglobulin E-binding site in Fcε receptor (FcεRII/CD23) identified by homolog-scanning mutagenesis. *J Biol Chem* 1992; **267**: 185–191.

36 Pochon S, Graber P, Yaeger M, Jansen K, Bernard A, Aubry JP, Bonnefoy JY. Demonstration of a second ligand for the low affinity receptor for immunoglobulin E (CD23) using recombinant CD23 constituted into fluorescent liposomes. *J Exp Med* 1992; **176**: 389–397.

37 Kabsch W, Sanders C. Dictionary of protein secondary structure: Pattern recognition of hydrogen-bonded and geometrical features. *Biopolymers* 1983; **22**: 2577–2637.

2 The Structural Basis of IgE-receptor Interactions in the Allergic Response

BRIAN J. SUTTON, REBECCA L. BEAVIL, ANDREW J. BEAVIL, ROBERT J. YOUNG and HANNAH J. GOULD
The Randall Institute, King's College London, UK

INTRODUCTION

The important role played by antibodies of the immunoglobulin E (IgE) class in allergy has long been recognized [1], but only during the past few years have we come to understand as much about the nature of the molecules with which IgE interacts. Two cell surface receptors for IgE are now well characterized, a 'high-affinity' receptor ($K_a \approx 10^{10}$ M^{-1}), and a 'low affinity' receptor ($K_a \approx 10^7$ M^{-1}); both interact with the Fc region of IgE (see below) and are therefore termed FcεRI and FcεRII respectively. FcεRI is found principally on mast cells and basophils, and it is the binding of IgE to this receptor which sensitizes these cells to degranulation and release of mediators of the type I hypersensitivity reaction, upon contact with multivalent allergen [2]. FcεRII, now known to be identical to the surface antigen CD23, was first identified on B cells, but it has since been found on a variety of inflammatory cells (including macrophages and eosinophils), follicular dendritic cells (FDC), Langerhans cells, and T cells [3]. It has been implicated in a variety of different functions such as the presentation of IgE-antigen complexes by B cells, and IgE-dependent cytotoxic activities of inflammatory cells, but the recent identification of a counter-structure for FcεRII other than IgE, namely the B-cell antigen CD21 [4], considerably broadens the scope for involvement of FcεRII in the allergic response and the immune system in general. FcεRII/CD23 and CD21 may constitute an adhesion pair to enhance B-cell–T-cell interaction, and facilitate B-cell maturation in germinal centres of lymph nodes through interaction with FDCs [5]. FcεRII exhibits yet further versatility, for soluble fragments of FcεRII (sFcεRII) derived by proteolysis of the cell surface molecule stimulate the growth and differentiation of antibody-producing plasma cell precursors, and enhance IgE synthesis in particular [4].

Allergic Mechanisms and Immunotherapeutic Strategies. Edited by A.M. Roberts and M.R. Walker.

Proteolysis of FcεRII is inhibited by the binding of IgE to the intact receptor however, and thus negative feedback control can be exerted by IgE-antigen complexes within this network of molecular interactions [6].

Further discoveries continue to be made concerning the cellular localization of these receptors. FcεRI has been found on both Langerhans cells [7,8], which may therefore serve locally in antigen presentation, and also on eosinophils [9]. CD40-ligand (CD40-L), a T-cell surface molecule, has also been found on mast cells [10], and since mast cells also secrete IL-4, they appear to be able to substitute for T cells in tissue such as the skin, lungs and gut [10]. Thus all the necessary molecular signals for IgE expression and up-regulation (IL-4, CD40-L and FcεRII) are available locally at the site of allergenic challenge.

Other molecules are undoubtedly also involved in this network, such as the IgE-binding protein (εBP) which may enhance IgE-mediated activation of mast cells by interaction with IgE and/or FcεRI [11,12]. Yet despite this complexity, it is clear that recent advances in our understanding of the molecular interactions that underlie the allergic response offer real prospects for therapeutic intervention at the site of the allergenic challenge. If such intervention is to involve the design of novel therapeutic agents, it demands knowledge at the level of detailed three-dimensional structure, and it is this information which we shall review in this Chapter, concentrating on the three molecules IgE, FcεRI and FcεRII.

IMMUNOGLOBULIN E

The IgE molecule consists of two identical heavy (ε) chains, and two identical light (κ or λ) chains, folded into domains as depicted in Figure 2.1. The Fc region, which can be released by limited proteolysis, retains full binding activity for both receptors [13,14] and consists of the disulphide-linked Cε2–Cε3–Cε4 domains of the two heavy chains. No crystal structure is available for IgE-Fc, but models have been proposed [15,16; see Chapter 1] based upon homology with IgG-Fc, the structure of which is known [17]. Unfortunately there is no exact homologue for the $(C\varepsilon 2)_2$ domain pair which in IgG is replaced by the hinge region, but the Cε3 and Cε4 domains may be modelled with considerable confidence, and these are shown in Figure 2.2. Also shown are the carbohydrate chains attached to Asn394 in each chain, which are homologous to those in the Cγ2 domains of IgG (at Asn297) and also conserved in antibodies of other classes. IgE-Fc contains two additional glycosylation sites, one in Cε2 (Asn265) and another in Cε3 (Asn371, see Figure 2.2), and these have been shown to modulate receptor binding affinity, at least for FcεRII [18]. Glycosylation at these IgE-specific sites is incomplete [18]; it has been postulated that heterogeneity in IgE glycosylation may be related to atopy, and particular glycoforms are certainly recognized by IgE

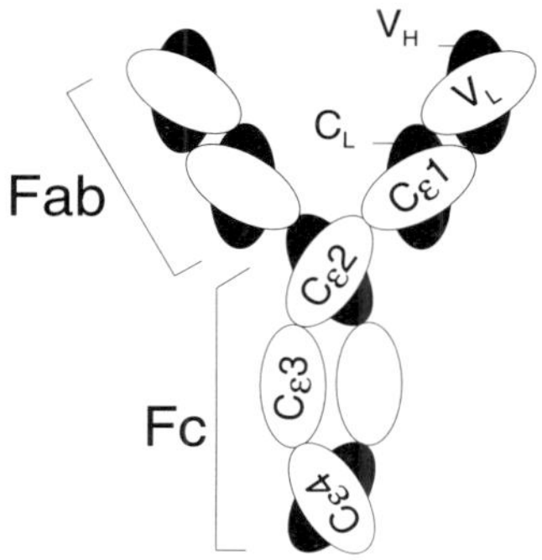

Figure 2.1. Schematic domain structure of IgE

binding factors [19,20] that may enhance FcεRI binding activity (as described below).

In order to locate the binding site for FcεRI within IgE-Fc, recombinant ε-chain peptides have been expressed in *Escherichia coli* [21,22] or mammalian cells [23], and chimaeric IgE molecules generated with individual domains substituted by their counterparts from mouse IgE or IgG sequences [24–27]. These studies led to the conclusion that the site lies within Cε3, and implicated involvement of the segment between residues 330 (the start of the Cε3 exon) and 361 [reviewed, 28]. Only two parts of this segment are exposed in the three-dimensional structure, namely 330–335 at the N-terminus of the domain (shown in Figure 2.2), and the loop region 342–354 close to the interface with Cε4. The latter region has been implicated in studies with a synthetic peptide consisting of residues 345–352 which, at relatively high concentrations, inhibited passive sensitization of human basophils [29]. Other evidence supports the former region at the N-terminus of Cε3. Early studies indicated that the tryptic digestion site in the Cε2–Cε3 link region of rat IgE is protected in the receptor complex [30], and this residue, Arg334, is also contained within the original pentapeptide sequence (330–334) identified by Hamburger [31] from Ig sequence comparisons (and initially reported to inhibit the Prausnitz–Küstner reaction). This region is also structurally homologous to residues in IgG that have been shown to contribute to the binding site for FcγRI and II [32,33]. For this reason Pro333, structurally homologous to the critical residue Leu234 in the lower hinge region of IgG, was targetted; mutation to Glu was found to reduce the affinity for receptor by a factor of five [34]. It appears therefore that the IgG-FcγRI/II and IgE-FcεRI interactions may be structurally homologous, and this is further supported by more recent mutagenesis studies that implicate involvement of other adjacent regions of the surface of Cγ2 in IgG [35,36], and Cε3 in IgE [37], such as the hinge proximal loop between the final two β-strands of these domains (Figure 2.2).

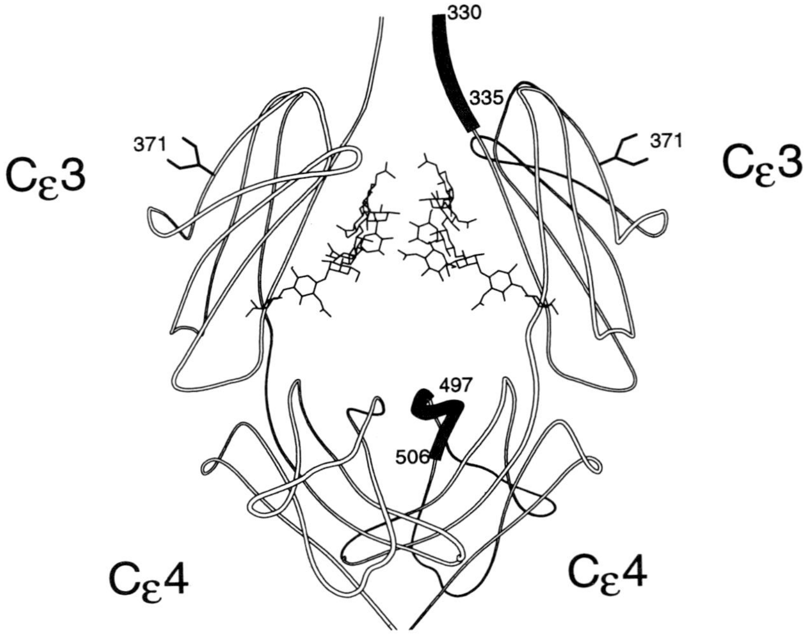

Figure 2.2. The fold of the polypeptide chain within the Cε3 and Cε4 domains of IgE-Fc, together with the Asn394 N-linked oligosaccharide chains. The glycosylation sites at Asn371 are also shown. The segments 330–335 (part of the putative IgE binding site) and 497–506 (potential vaccine peptide) are discussed in the text

The location of the binding site for FcεRII is not so well defined, but it too lies within Cε3, and is probably close to the ε-specific glycosylation site at Asn371 [27,38,39] (see Figure 2.2). However, the carbohydrate is not directly involved in either FcεRII [38] or FcεRI [21] binding.

The FcεRI binding site is at a particularly interesting location within the IgE molecule for it includes the only solvent-accessible site in the Fc region at which identical segments of the two heavy chains come close together (Figure 2.2). Binding to one chain would therefore very likely prevent binding to the other on steric grounds, rendering IgE incapable of binding more than one receptor molecule. It is clearly important that free IgE cannot crosslink two receptors and trigger mast cell degranulation. The fact of this 1:1 stoichiometry, which has been observed experimentally both for IgE [40] and for IgE-Fc [41], is further reinforced by the discovery that the IgE molecule adopts a bent structure both in solution and when bound to its receptor [42]. The distance between the Fab arms and the C-terminus of the Fc is considerably shorter (6.9 nm) than that expected for an extended, planar Y-shaped IgE (17.5 nm) and thus, as shown in Figure 2.3, a receptor binding site in the N-terminal linker region of Cε3 is expected to be exposed on the

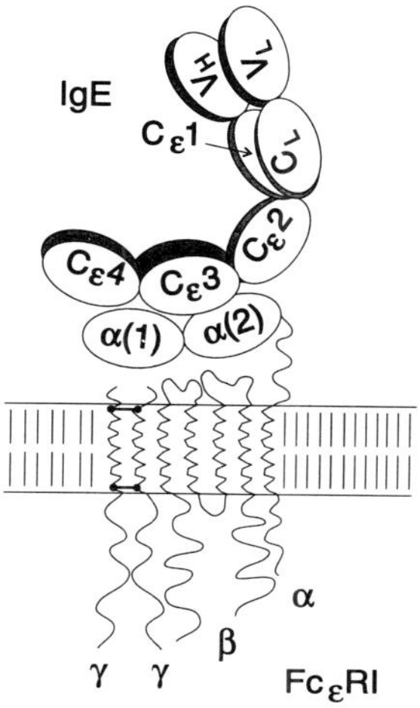

Figure 2.3. Schematic interaction between IgE and the two extracellular domains of the α-chain of FcεRI. Molecules and membrane are drawn to scale. (Alternative models in which the IgE is rotated relative to the α-chain about an axis perpendicular to the membrane and passing through the site of interaction are also compatible with the data)

'convex' side of the molecule, but not on the 'concave' side. This also explains why anti-IgE antibodies that recognize certain IgE epitopes are capable of blocking receptor binding, yet do not bind to receptor-bound IgE or degranulate mast cells. Such antibodies have therapeutic potential.

THE HIGH AFFINITY RECEPTOR FcεRI

This receptor consists of four polypeptide chains, $\alpha\beta\gamma_2$, which form a complex in the membrane with seven transmembrane hydrophobic segments, as shown schematically in Figure 2.3. The α-chain has the most substantial extracellular region, and is entirely responsible for IgE binding; the β and γ chains are required for assembly of the complex and for signal transduction following receptor crosslinking by IgE-antigen complexes [2, for review]. The sequence of the extracellular region of the α-chain indicates that it consists of two domains that belong to the immunoglobulin superfamily, indicated as α(1) and α(2) in Figure 2.3. These domains have very similar sequences to the extracellular domains of the IgG-binding polypeptides of the various FcγR molecules, but as a group they are clearly distinct from the V and C type domains found in the immunoglobulins. Rather, they belong to an intermediate type known as C2 [43]. A model of the structure of these domains has been generated based principally upon immunoglobulin C

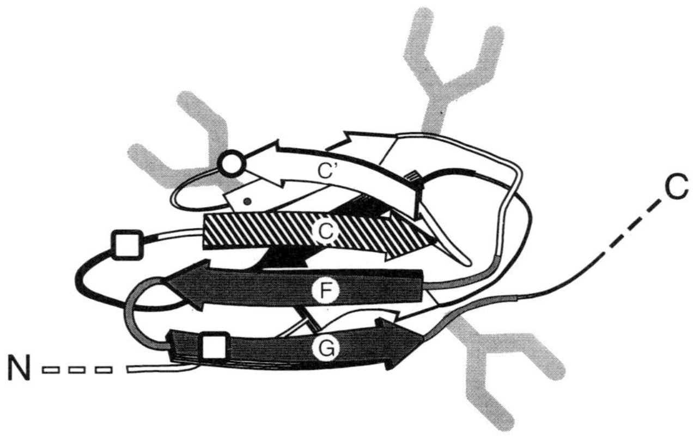

Figure 2.4. The predicted fold of the polypeptide chain within the α(2) domain of FcεRIα; β-strands are represented by the broad arrows. The hatched, shaded and black segments, and individual residue positions (circle and squares) are discussed in the text. The three potential N-linked oligosaccharide moieties are also shown

domain structures [44]. However, the recent crystal structure determinations of the cell surface antigens CD4 and in particular CD2 [45], the second domain of which has been classified as C2-type, are also helpful for modelling α(1) and α(2) [34].

The IgE binding site has been shown to reside principally in α(2), by phage display of individual domains [40,46], and by expression of chimaeric α-chain [47,48]. A schematic representation of the structure of the α(2) domain is shown in Figure 2.4, based upon homology modelling with the CD2 structure as the principal template [34]. The four β-strands that constitute one face of the domain (C′CFG) are indicated in the figure, together with the three glycosylation sites that are present in the human α(2) domain sequence. A number of pieces of evidence point to the importance of this face in the interaction with IgE. A stretch of seven residues is conserved between human and rat sequences, but not in the IgG receptors, and this corresponds to strand C (cross-hatched in Figure 2.4) [49]; the binding site for IgG in the homologous domain of FcγRII involves residues of strands F and G and the intervening loop (stippled in Figure 2.4) [48,50,51]. Furthermore, polymorphic substitutions that affect IgG binding to the homologous FcγRII [50] are located on this face of the domain (as indicated by the circle and squares in Figure 2.4). IgE binding is blocked, however, by an antibody to a peptide [52] that corresponds to strand B on the opposite face of the domain and the BC loop (indicated in black in Figure 2.4). Much of strand B will be occluded by the glycosylation site on the adjacent strand, and the BC loop region may therefore be the segment recognized by the antibody; certainly the four-strand face is free from glycosylation, which is not involved in IgE binding.

The topology of the interaction between IgE and the α-chain of FcεRI may therefore be depicted as in Figure 2.3, in which the orientation of the IgE molecule with respect to the membrane is determined by the resonance energy transfer data for receptor-bound IgE [42]. This model, and the delineated regions of interaction on both Cε3 of IgE and α(2) of FcεRI, now provide a basis for the design of site-directed mutagenesis experiments, and synthesis of peptides as potential inhibitors of the interaction.

THE LOW AFFINITY RECEPTOR FcεRII/CD23

FcεRII is a type-II integral membrane protein, i.e. it is oriented in the membrane with a cytoplasmic N-terminus. Near the extracellular C-terminus there is a domain that is homologous to members of the C-type lectin superfamily, a group that includes molecules such as the asialoglycoprotein receptor (AsgpR), another type-II membrane protein, and the selectins. Between the lectin domain and the single transmembrane region lies a segment in which a repeating sequence pattern has been observed, and this pattern of heptads, with hydrophobic residues at the first and fourth positions, has been predicted to adopt an α-helical coiled-coil structure [53,54]. Such a structure leads to the prediction that the receptor will form either dimers or trimers in the membrane, and oligomerization of both murine [55] and human membrane-bound FcεRII [56] to trimers has now been observed in crosslinking studies. AsgpR contains a similar heptad repeat pattern and has been shown by crosslinking studies in the membrane to form trimers, and thus the overall architecture of FcεRII, AsgpR, and other members of this family, is expected to be very similar [54]. This is the structure shown in Figure 2.5. The coiled-coil region is expected to form a 'stalk' of approximately 15 nm in length, acting as a spacer between the lectin domain and the membrane. The significance of this oligomeric structure will be discussed below.

Attached to the C-terminal side of the C-type lectin domain is an apparently unstructured 'tail' containing a reverse RGD (Arg–Gly–Asp) sequence; this may play a role in adhesion interactions but as yet no counter-structure has been identified for this motif. At the cytoplasmic N-terminus, two forms of the protein that differ in the first 6/7 amino acids have been characterized [reviewed in 3,57]. Critical residues in the cytoplasmic sequences of these two isoforms have been identified as responsible for the alternative functions of endocytosis, mediated by FcεRIIa, and phagocytosis, mediated by FcεRIIb [58]. This functional distinction correlates with their cellular expression: FcεRIIa is constitutively expressed on B cells, whereas FcεRIIb is dependent upon IL-4 for expression on a variety of cell types, including the monocytes and eosinophils involved in IgE-dependent immunity.

The soluble fragments of FcεRII (sFcεRII) are released from the membrane-bound molecule by proteolysis in the stalk region. The first cut occurs close to

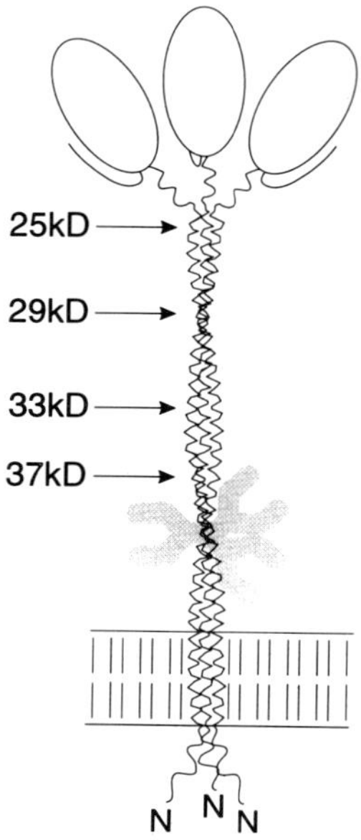

Figure 2.5. Schematic representation of the predicted trimeric structure of human FcεRII; the C-type lectin domain with C-terminal tail is separated from the membrane by a region of α-helical coiled-coil structure. Sites of proteolytic cleavage are indicated, together with the sizes of the soluble fragments released; the single glycosylation site in each chain is also shown. Molecule and membrane are drawn to scale

the sole glycosylation site in each chain, to release a 37 kDa fragment, and then further proteolysis occurs to generate the relatively stable 25 kDa fragment consisting of the lectin domain and C-terminal tail (see Figure 2.5) [3,57]. A smaller, 16 kDa fragment lacking the tail has also been characterized. All of these fragments retain binding activity for IgE, the site for which clearly resides in the lectin domain. However, they exhibit different functional activities; for example the larger sFcεRII species promote IgE synthesis, while the 16 kDa fragment is inhibitory [3,4,57,59].

The recent crystal structure determinations of the mannose binding protein (MBP) [60–62] and E-selectin [63] have provided a model for the three-dimensional structure of the homologous lectin domain of FcεRII, which is shown schematically in Figure 2.6. Of the two Ca^{2+} ions in MBP, only the site marked Ca2 in Figure 2.6 is conserved in human FcεRII; IgE binding is Ca^{2+}-dependent, and since loops close to the Ca^{2+} ions (shaded in Figure 2.6) have also been identified as potential IgE binding regions [64], it appears that the IgE binding site is distant from both the stalk and the DGR-containing tail. The Ca2 site in MBP is also the oligosaccharide binding site [65], and thus in FcεRII it may also mark the site of the interaction with

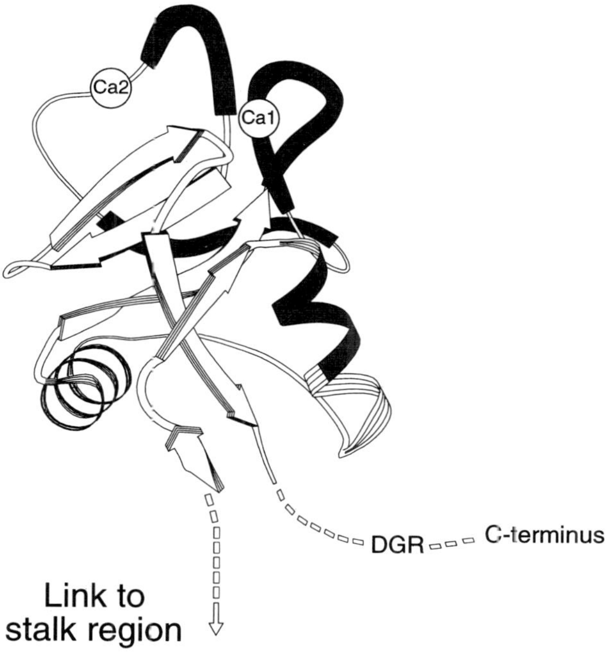

Figure 2.6. The fold of the polypeptide chain within the C-type lectin domain of FcεRII, modelled on the crystal structures of mannose-binding protein (MBP, see text). Of the two Ca^{2+} sites in MBP, Ca2 is conserved in human FcεRII. Putative IgE binding regions are shaded, and the reverse RGD (Arg–Gly–Asp) sequence in the tail peptide is shown

CD21, since this interaction is known to involve oligosaccharide moieties on CD21 [66]. Thus the IgE and CD21 binding sites in FcεRII almost certainly overlap; this also accounts for the observation that although recognition of IgE by FcεRII does not involve carbohydrate [38], binding is inhibitable by certain sugars [3].

The binding of IgE to FcεRII may thus occur as shown in Figure 2.7a. The oligomeric structure of the receptor may be critical for its ability to engage IgE and IgE-antigen complexes for internalization, enhancing the relatively low affinity between a single lectin head domain and IgE (cf. AsgpR in the clearance of glycoproteins). IgE binding also inhibits the release of sFcεRII from the membrane, but it is clear from this model that simple steric blocking of the primary site of proteolysis near the base of the stalk cannot occur. We have thus proposed an allosteric mechanism, in which IgE binding stabilizes the coiled-coil structure and enhances its resistance to proteolysis [53]. The coiled-coil structure also predicts that the larger soluble

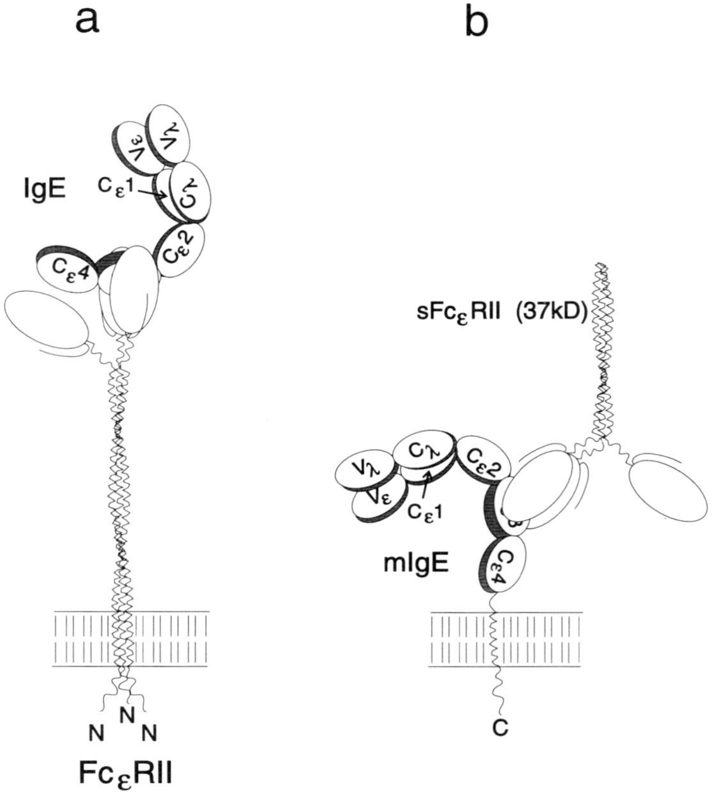

Figure 2.7. Schematic representations of (a) the interaction between IgE and membrane-bound FcεRII, and (b) trimeric soluble FcεRII and membrane-bound IgE (see text). Molecules and membrane are drawn to scale

fragments may remain as oligomers, whereas the smaller fragments may be monomeric. Thus the 37 kDa sFcεRII (Figure 2.7b) could crosslink membrane-bound molecules such as mIgE or CD21 on B cells, promoting IgE synthesis, whereas the smaller monomeric sFcεRII would be inhibitory, as is observed [59]. The coiled-coil structure is clearly critical for the remarkable diversity in FcεRII function.

OTHER COMPONENTS OF THE IgE NETWORK

CD21 is now clearly established as an important component, acting as a counter-structure for FcεRII, and involved in the regulation of IgE production

[4] and as an adhesion pair on B cells [67]. While the polypeptide part of this protein consists of a tandem array of domains of known structure (the short consensus repeat domain common to many complement proteins; see [6] for review), it is the structure of the relevant oligosaccharides which must now be determined. FcεRII has recently been found to exhibit a specificity for terminal galactose residues [68].

Considerable progress has also been made concerning the nature of the IgE-binding protein (εBP, also known as Mac-2), which can bind to both IgE and FcεRI on mast cells, and modulate their interactions at the cell surface [11,12]. The molecule consists of a C-terminal S-type lectin domain, and an extensive proline-rich, tandemly repeated N-terminal region, which may mediate oligomerization [11,19]. εBP recognizes oligosaccharide moieties on IgE and FcεRI and, if oligomeric, would be able to enhance crosslinking of these components at the mast cell surface; various models for these interactions have been proposed [12]. One potentially very important property of εBP is its ability to recognize particular glycoforms of IgE [19,20], and this may relate to an individual's susceptibility to hypersensitivity.

IMPLICATIONS FOR THERAPY

Our understanding of the structure and interactions of IgE and its receptors has reached a stage at which a number of targets for intervention can be identified. The best characterized is undoubtedly the IgE–FcεRI interaction, and knowledge of the asymmetrically bent structure of IgE, and the receptor site, can be used to target blocking antibodies or design smaller inhibitory compounds. The anti-IgE approach, including humanized versions of the antibodies, is being pursued by a number of groups [69–72]. Soluble FcεRIα is also being developed as a blocking agent [73,74]. Another approach has been to identify a peptide that can act as a vaccine to raise blocking antibodies [75,76]; the location of one such peptide (residues 497–506 [75]) is indicated in Figure 2.1. These and other strategies will be discussed elsewhere in this volume. However, the recent discoveries concerning the oligosaccharide binding functions of the C-type lectin FcεRII (with CD21) and the S-type lectin εBP (with IgE and FcεRI) suggests that the development of carbohydrate-based compounds to interfere with these interactions will be a major focus for future studies.

ACKNOWLEDGEMENTS

The authors wish to thank the Medical Research Council and the National Asthma Campaign for their support, and The Nuffield Foundation for the award of a Research Fellowship (BJS).

REFERENCES

1 Ishizaka K, Ishizaka T. Identification of γE-antibodies as a carrier of reaginic activity. *J Immunol* 1967; **99**: 1187–1198.
2 Metzger H. The receptor with high affinity for IgE. *Immunol Rev* 1992; **125**: 37–48.
3 Delespesse G, Sarfati M, Wu CY *et al*. The low-affinity receptor for IgE. *Immunol Rev* 1992; **125**: 77–97.
4 Aubry J-P, Pochon S, Graber P *et al*. CD21 is a ligand for CD23 and regulates IgE production. *Nature* 1992; **358**: 505–507.
5 Bonnefoy J-Y, Pochon S, Aubry J-P *et al*. A new pair of surface molecules involved in human IgE regulation. *Immunol Today* 1993; **14**: 1–2.
6 Sutton BJ, Gould HJ. The human IgE network. *Nature* 1993; **366**: 421–428.
7 Wang B, Rieger A, Kilgus O *et al*. Epidermal Langerhans cells from normal human skin bind monomeric IgE via FcεRI. *J Exp Med* 1992; **175**: 1353–1358.
8 Bieber T. FcεRI on human Langerhans cells: a receptor in search of new functions. *Immunol Today* 1994; **15**: 52–53.
9 Gounni AS, Lamkhioued B, Ochiai K *et al*. High-affinity IgE receptor on eosinophils is involved in defence against parasites. *Nature* 1994; **367**: 183–186.
10 Gauchat J-F, Henchoz S, Mazzei G *et al*. Induction of human IgE synthesis in B cells by mast cells and basophils. *Nature* 1993; **365**: 340–343.
11 Liu FT. S-type mammalian lectins in allergic inflammation. *Immunol Today* 1993; **14**: 486–490.
12 Liu F-T, Frigeri LG, Gritzmacher CA *et al*. Expression and function of an IgE-binding animal lectin (εBP) in mast cells. *Immunopharmacology* 1993; **26**: 187–195.
13 Stanworth DR, Humphrey JH, Bennich H *et al*. Inhibition of Prausnitz–Küstner reaction by proteolytic-cleavage fragments of a human myeloma protein of immunoglobulin E class. *Lancet* 1968; **ii**: 17–18.
14 Ishizaka K, Ishizaka T, Lee EH. Biologic function of the Fc fragments of E myeloma protein. *Immunochemistry* 1970; **7**: 687–702.
15 Padlan EA, Davies DR. A model of the Fc of immunoglobulin E. *Mol Immunol* 1986; **23**: 1063–1075.
16 Helm BA, Ling Y, Teale C *et al*. The nature and importance of the inter-ε chain disulfide bonds in human IgE. *Eur J Immunol* 1991; **21**: 1543–1548.
17 Deisenhofer J. Crystallographic refinement and atomic models of a human Fc fragment and its complex with fragment B of protein A from *Staphylococcus aureus* at 2.9 and 2.8 Å resolution. *Biochemistry* 1981; **20**: 2361–2370.
18 Young RJ, Owens RJ, Mackay GA *et al*. Secretion of recombinant human IgE-Fc by mammalian cells and biological activity of glycosylation site mutants. *Prot Eng* 1995; **8**: 193–199.
19 Robertson MW, Albrandt K, Keller D *et al*. Human IgE-binding protein: A soluble lectin exhibiting a highly conserved interspecies sequence and differential recognition of IgE glycoforms. *Biochemistry* 1990; **29**: 8093–8100.
20 Robertson MW, Liu F-T. Heterogeneous IgE glycoforms characterized by differential recognition of an endogenous lectin (IgE-binding protein) *J Immunol* 1991; **147**: 3024–3030.
21 Helm BA, Marsh P, Vercelli D *et al*. The mast cell binding site on human immunoglobulin E. *Nature* 1988; **331**: 180–183.
22 Helm BA, Kebo D, Vercelli D *et al*. Blocking of passive sensitization of human mast cells and basophil granulocytes with IgE antibodies by a recombinant human ε-chain fragment of 76 amino acids. *Proc Natl Acad Sci USA* 1989; **88**: 9465–9469.

23 Basu M, Hakimi J, Dharm E *et al.* Purification and characterization of human recombinant IgE-Fc fragments that bind to the human high affinity IgE receptor. *J Biol Chem* 1993; **269**: 13118–13127.
24 Weetall M, Shopes B, Holowka D *et al.* Mapping the site of interaction between murine IgE and its high affinity receptor with chimeric Ig. *J Immunol* 1990; **145**: 3849–3854.
25 Nissim A, Jouvin M-H, Eshhar Z. Mapping of the high affinity Fcε receptor binding site to the third constant region domain of IgE. *EMBO J* 1991; **10**: 101–107.
26 Nissim A, Ashhar Z. The human mast cell receptor binding site maps to the third constant domain of immunoglobulin E. *Mol Immunol* 1992; **29**: 1065–1072.
27 Nissim A, Schwarzbaum S, Siraganian R *et al.* Fine specificity of the IgE interaction with the low and high affinity Fc receptor. *J Immunol* 1993: **150**: 1365–1374.
28 Gould HJ. The interaction between immunoglobulin E and its high-affinity receptor. In: Holgate ST, Church MK (eds) *Genetics of Asthma*. London: Gower, 1992; 293–304.
29 Nio N, Seguro K, Ariyoshi Y *et al.* Inhibition of passive sensitization of human peripheral basophils by synthetic human immunoglobulin E peptide fragments. *FEBS Lett* 1993; **319**: 225–228.
30 Perez-Montfort R, Metzger H. Proteolysis of soluble IgE-receptor complexes: localization of sites on IgE which interact with the Fc receptor. *Mol Immunol* 1982; **19**: 1113–1125.
31 Hamburger RN. Peptide inhibition of the Prausnitz–Küstner reaction. *Science* 1975; **189**: 389–390.
32 Duncan AR, Woof JM, Partride LJ *et al.* Localization of the binding site for the human high-affinity Fc receptor on IgG. *Nature* 1988; **332**: 563–564.
33 Lund J, Winter G, Jones PT *et al.* Human FcγRI and FcγRII interact with distinct but overlapping sites on human IgG. *J Immunol* 1991; **147**: 2657–2662.
34 Beavil AJ, Beavil RL, Chan CMW *et al.* Structural basis of the IgE-FcεRI interaction. *Biochem Soc Trans* 1993; **21**: 968–972.
35 Canfield SM, Morrison SL. The binding affinity of human IgG for its high affinity Fc receptor is determined by multiple amino acids in the C_H2 domain and is modulated by the hinge region. *J Exp Med* 1991; **173**: 1483–1491.
36 Lund J, Pound JD, Jones PT *et al.* Multiple binding sites on the C_H2 domain of IgG for mouse FcγRII. *Mol Immunol* 1992; **29**: 53–59.
37 Presta L, Shields R, O'Connell L *et al.* The binding site on human immunoglobulin E for its high affinity receptor. *J Biol Chem* 1994; **269**: 26368–26373.
38 Vercelli D. Helm BA, Marsh P *et al.* The B-cell binding site on human immunoglobulin E. *Nature* 1989; **338**: 649–651.
39 Ghaderi AA, Stanworth DR. Epitope mapping of the site(s) of binding of FcγRII/CD23 within human IgE. *Mol Immunol* 1993; **30**: 1655–1663.
40 Robertson MW. Phage and *Escherichia coli* expression of the human high affinity immunoglobulin E receptor α-subunit ectodomain. *J Biol Chem* 1993; **268**: 12736–12743.
41 Keown MB, Ghirlando R, Young RJ *et al.* Hydrodynamic studies of a complex between the Fc fragment of human IgE and a soluble fragment of the FcεRI α chain. *Proc Natl Acad Sci USA* 1995; **92**: 1841–1845.
42 Zheng Y, Shopes B, Holowka D *et al.* Conformations of IgE bound to its receptor FcεRI and in solution. *Biochemistry* 1991; **30**: 9125–9132.
43 Williams AF, Barclay AN. The immunoglobulin superfamily – domains for cell surface recognition. *Ann Rev Immuncol* 1988; **6**: 381–405.
44 Padlan EA, Helm BA. A modelling study of the α-subunit of human high-affinity receptor for immunoglobulin E. *Receptor* 1992; **3**: 129–142.

45 Jones EY, Davis SJ, Williams AF *et al.* Crystal structure at 2.8 Å resolution of a soluble form of the cell adhesion molecule CD2. *Nature* 1992; **360**: 232–239.
46 Scarselli E, Esposito G, Traboni C. Display of functional domains of the human high affinity IgE receptor on the M13 phage surface. *FEBS Lett* 1993; **329**: 223–226.
47 Mallamaci MA, Chizzonite R, Griffin M *et al.* Identification of sites on the human FcεRIα subunit which are involved in binding human and rat IgE. *J Biol Chem* 1993; **268**: 22076–22083.
48 Hulett MD, McKenzie, Hogarth PM. Chimeric Fc receptors identify immunoglobulin binding regions in human Fc[g]RII and Fc[e]RI. *Eur J Immunol* 1993; **23**: 640–645.
49 Shimizu A, Tepler I, Benfey PN *et al.* Human and rat mast cell high affinity immunoglobulin E receptors: characterization of putative α-chain gene products. *Proc Natl Acad Sci USA* 1988; **85**: 1907–1911.
50 Hogarth PM, Hulett MD, Ierino FL *et al.* Identification of the immunoglobulin binding regions (IBR) of FcγRII and FcεRI. *Immunol Rev* 1992; **125**: 21–35.
51 Hulett MD, Witort E, Brinkworth RI *et al.* Identification of the IgG binding site of the human low affinity receptor for IgG FcγRII. *J Biol Chem* 1994; **269**: 15287–15293.
52 Riske F, Hakimi J, Mallamaci M *et al.* High affinity human IgE receptor (FcεRI). Analysis of functional domains of the α-subunit with monoclonal antibodies. *J Biol Chem* 1991; **266**: 11245–11251.
53 Gould HJ, Sutton BJ, Edmeades R *et al.* CD23/FcεRII: C-type lectin membrane protein with a split personality? *Monogr Allergy* 1991; **39**: 28–49.
54 Beavil AJ, Edmeades RL, Gould HL *et al.* α-helical coiled-coil stalks in the low-affinity receptor for IgE (FεRII/CD23) and related C-type lectins. *Proc Natl Acad Sci USA* 1992; **89**: 753–757.
55 Dierks SE, Bartlett WC, Edmeades RL *et al.* The oligomeric nature of the murine FcεRII/CD23. *J Immunol* 1993; **150**: 2372–2382.
56 Beavil RL, Graber P, Aubonney N *et al.* CD23/FcεRII and its soluble fragments can form oligomers on the cell surface and in solution. *Immunology* 1995; **84**: 202–206.
57 Conrad DH, Campbell KA, Bartlett WC *et al.* Structure and functions of the low affinity IgE receptor. *Adv Exp Med Biol* 1994; **347**: 17–30.
58 Yokata A, Yukawa K, Yamamoto A *et al.* Two forms of the low-affinity Fc receptor for IgE differentially mediate endoctosis and phagocytosis: identification of the critical cytoplasmic domains. *Proc Natl Acad Sci USA* 1992; **89**: 5030–5034.
59 Sarfati M, Bettler B, Letellier M *et al.* Native and recombinant soluble CD23 fragments with IgE suppressive activity. *Immunology* 1992; **76**: 662–667.
60 Weis WI, Kahn R, Fourme R *et al.* Structure of the calcium-dependent lectin domain from a rat mannose-binding protein determined by MAD phasing. *Science* 1991; **254**: 1608–1615.
61 Weis WI, Drickamer K. Trimeric structure of a C-type mannose-binding protein. *Structure* 1994; **2**: 1227–1240.
62 Sheriff S, Chang CY, Ezekowitz AB. Human mannose-binding protein carbohydrate recognition domain trimerizes through a triple α-helical coiled-coil. *Nature Struct Biol* 1994; **1**: 789–794.
63 Graves BJ, Crowther RL, Chandran C *et al.* Insight into E-selectin/ligand interaction from the crystal structure and mutagenesis of the lec/EGF domains. *Nature* 1994; **367**: 532–538.
64 Bettler B, Texido G, Raggini S *et al.* Immunoglobulin E-binding site in Fcε receptor (FcεRII/CD23) identified by homolog-scanning mutagenesis. *J Biol Chem* 1992; **267**: 185–191.
65 Weis WI, Drickamer K, Hendrickson WA. Structure of a C-type mannose-binding protein complexed with an oligosaccharide. *Nature* 1992; **360**: 127–134.

66 Aubry J-P, Pochon S, Gauchat J-F *et al.* CD23 interacts with a new functional extracytoplasmic domain involving N-linked oligosaccharides on CD21. *J Immunol* 1994; **152**: 5806–5813.
67 Björck P, Elenström-Magnusson C, Rosén A *et al.* CD23 and CD21 function as adhesion molecules in homotypic aggregation of human B lymphocytes. *Eur J Immunol* 1993; **23**: 1771–1775.
68 Kijimoto-Ochiai S, Horimoto E, Uede T. Demonstration of the interaction between the CD23 molecule and the galactose residue of glycoproteins. *Immunol Lett* 1994; **40**: 49–53.
69 Davis FM, Gossett LA, Pinkston KL *et al.* Can anti-IgE be used to treat allergy? *Springer Semin Immunopathol* 1993; **15**: 51–73.
70 Kolbinger F, Saldanha J, Hardman N *et al.* Humanization of a mouse anti-human IgE antibody: a potential therapeutic for IgE-mediated allergies. *Prot Eng* 1993; **6**: 971–980.
71 Presta LG, Lahr SJ, Shields RL *et al.* Humanization of an antibody directed against IgE. *J Immunol* 1993; **151**: 2623–2632.
72 Saban R, Haak-Frendscho M, Zine M *et al.* Human FcεRI-IgG and humanized anti-IgE monoclonal antibody MaE11 block passive sensitization of human and rhesus monkey lung. *J Allergy Clin Immunol* 1994; **94**: 836–843.
73 Ra C, Kuromitsu S, Hirose T *et al.* Soluble human high-affinity receptor for IgE abrogates the IgE-mediated allergic reaction. *Int Immunol* 1993; **5**: 47–54.
74 Haak-Frendscho M, Ridgway J, Shields R *et al.* Human IgE receptor α-chain IgE chimera blocks passive cutaneous anaphylaxis reaction *in vivo*. *J Immunol* 1993; **151**: 351–358.
75 Stanworth DR, Jones VM, Lewin IV *et al.* Allergy treatment with a peptide vaccine. *Lancet* 1990; **336**: 1279–1281.
76 Hellman L. Profound reduction in allergen sensitivity following treatment with a novel allergy vaccine. *Eur J Immunol* 1994; **24**: 415–420.

3 The Role of Surface Molecules in the Control of Human IgE Synthesis

LEOPOLDO FLORES-ROMO, JEAN FRANÇOIS GAUCHAT, PIERRE GRABER, JEAN-PIERRE AUBRY and JEAN YVES BONNEFOY

Immunology Department, Glaxo Institute for Molecular Biology, Geneva, Switzerland

INTRODUCTION

The traditional view concerning IgE synthesis has been that of soluble regulatory factors, the lymphokines, keeping IgE secretion in balance; with interleukins, IL-4 and IL-13, inducing and interferons (IFN) suppressing isotype production by B lymphocytes. Disturbances of this cytokine equilibrium by stimulation of Th2-type cells (as seems to occur in some parasitoses, for example) results in upregulation of IgE production. However, this scheme has been challenged in recent years. Evidence is emerging that other factors and cells also play a crucial role in modulating IgE synthesis.

Therapeutic approaches have focused mostly on the effector phase of allergy, searching for drugs that prevent the release and the activities of allergy mediators. Unravelling the primary events that trigger high IgE production will no doubt increase the chances of finding more efficacious therapeutic strategies. Few attempts exist in determining early events of the IgE production cascade. Targeting IL-4 *in vivo* and *in vitro* by using antibodies [1], gene deletion [2], and soluble receptors [3] is still a promising approach. However, recent studies suggest that regulation in the IgE system is strongly dependent on cell contact-mediated events occurring during the initial phases of the immune response. Here, we discuss two pairs of surface molecules which appear to have a pivotal role in regulating human IgE synthesis (see Figure 3.1).

Allergic Mechanisms and Immunotherapeutic Strategies. Edited by A.M. Roberts and M.R. Walker.

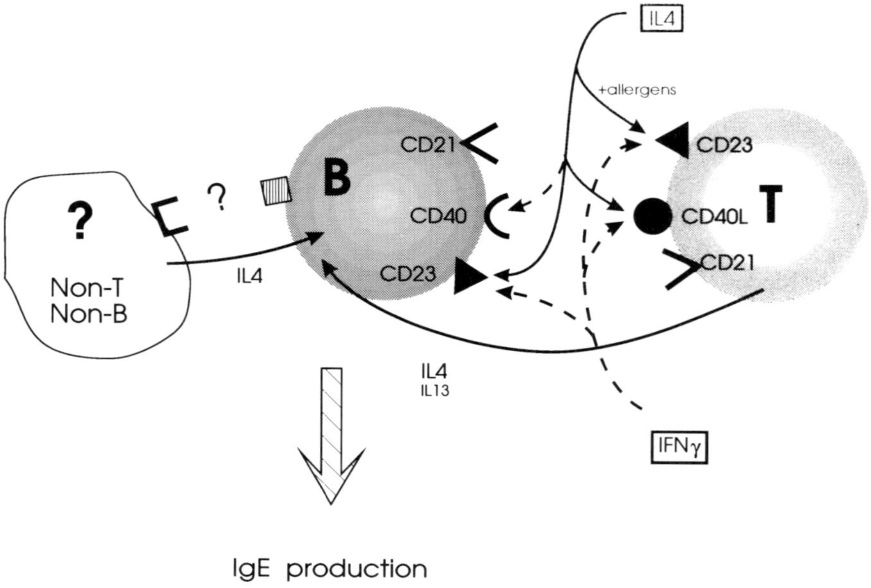

Figure 3.1. IgE production. Minimal interactions of surface molecules: CD21–CD23 and CD40–CD40 ligand. IgE production is dependent on two sets of signals, one of them being provided by IL-4 and the other, to a lesser extent, by IL-13. The other signal is strictly dependent on cell-to-cell physical interactions. An example of the latter is the occupancy of B cell-CD40 antigen, whose ligand (CD40L) is on T cells, and is regulated by IL-4 and IFNγ. However, cognate T–B interactions are not essential to produce IgE. Furthermore, certain non-T, non-B cells can also produce IL-4 and drive B cells to IgE production, but the surface molecules participating on these cells have not yet been established. CD23 is also regulated by IL-4 and IFNγ and it is assumed that CD23 antibodies preventing IgE production *in vitro* might be acting on B cells, probably interfering with certain cell–cell interactions. B-cell CD21 has recently been identified as a functional ligand for CD23: its engagement on B lymphocytes by either anti-CD21 antibodies, or by recombinant CD23, upregulates IgE synthesis *in vitro*. These findings have raised the possibility that CD23-bearing cells might interact with CD21 on B cells to regulate IgE production. In this regard, CD23 has been detected on T cells and its expression shown to be upregulated by IL-4 and allergen exposure. Thus, it is possible that (allergen/IL-4-upregulated) CD23 on T cells may interact with CD21 on B cells, leading the latter to secrete IgE. There is little information concerning CD21 in T lymphocytes, and its contribution to IgE regulation through a putative interaction with B-cell CD23 still remains to be elucidated. IFNγ downregulates the expression of the surface molecules indicated, usually counteracting and balancing IL-4 activities

CD23-CD21 AND IgE

It has been said that FcεRII/CD23 was discovered twice [4], once as a low affinity IgE receptor on B lymphocytes in the mid-1970s [5], and again as a B-cell marker associated with activation and Epstein–Barr Virus (EBV) infection [6,7] in the early 1980s. It was not until 1987 that it was found that both these independently-described molecules were one and the same [8,9]. CD23, a type II glycoprotein of the C-type lectins, shows some evolutionary divergence to its ligand. CD23 is the only Fc receptor with a different chromosomal location, and is the only one that does not belong to the immunoglobulin superfamily [10]. Two molecular forms of CD23 have been described, which differ in their intracytoplasmic region [11].

The possibility that CD23 plays a role in IgE synthesis emerged after the discovery of IgE and simultaneously with the discovery of CD23, as an IgE receptor on B lymphocytes that differed from that known in mast cells and basophils. That possibility, however, did not begin to crystallize until the early work of Delespesse's group, who showed that soluble IgE-binding factors obtained from human B-cell lines had the ability to potentiate IgE synthesis by B cells from normal and atopic donors [12,13]. *In vivo*, the findings of high cell-surface expression as well as of elevated serum CD23 levels in hyper-IgE syndrome and various allergic and parasitic diseases [14–16], provided circumstantial evidence for CD23 involvement in IgE production. This was later substantiated by another correlative finding *in vivo*, that peak levels of serum CD23 in patients from autologous bone marrow transplantation anticipated the rise in IgE levels observed in these patients [17].

Several groups have shown, *in vitro*, that IL-4 and IL-13 upregulate CD23 [18,19] as well as IgE production [19,20], and it has been suggested that the latter phenomenon is somewhat dependent on the former. This idea has been reinforced by reports of antibodies to CD23 inhibiting the IL-4-induced IgE production in an isotype-selective manner [13,21–23]. These findings suggested that inhibitory antibodies were either blocking a CD23 activity that was needed in the IL-4-permissive system, and/or interfering with certain cell–cell interactions that were essential for IgE production. The latter possibility was further substantiated by experiments in which cell–cell interactions in a mixed lymphocyte reaction were also inhibited by antibodies to CD23 [24]. Moreover, CD23 was localized specifically in the areas of cell-to-cell contact *in situ* [24]. In keeping with this, strong cell aggregates were reported upon transfection of EBV genes inducing CD23 expression [25]. Conversely, antibodies to CD23 were shown as efficient as anti-LFA-1 antibodies in preventing B-cell aggregation [26].

This notion is also in line with previous observations in which inhibition of T cell–B cell physical contact also prevented the synthesis of IgE, even though IL-4 was present in the system [27]. These important findings strongly argued for the essential role of direct cell–cell contact for the B cells to produce IgE. Interestingly, the CD23 antibodies inhibiting IgE production [20–22], and the homotypic [26] and heterotypic [23,28] cell–cell interactions, map to the lectin domain of CD23. This region shares homology with certain well-known adhesion molecules such as ELAM-1, MEL-14 and GMP-140 [29], and also embodies the IgE binding activity [10,30]. Only recently it was found that this domain encompasses the binding to CD21 [31], which (unlike the IgE binding) is carbohydrate-dependent [32]. This finally disclosed the other, IgE-independent function of the CD23 lectin domain.

Several roles have been ascribed to CD23 *in vitro*, such as IgE regulatory functions [13,21], rescue of B cells from apoptosis and growth promoting activity [4,33], maturation of thymocytes [34] and myeloid precursors [35], protective immunity [36], and antigen presentation [23,37–39].

Recently CD23-deficient and overexpressing transgenic mice have been generated. Overexpression of either membrane CD23 or soluble CD23 (38 kDa) did not alter lymphoid cell maturation [40]. The CD23 deficient mice do not display IgE-dependent augmentation of an immune response [41]. Another report indicates that focusing of antigen onto CD23 and sIg can simultaneously give a tolerogenic signal [42]. Inactivation of the CD23 gene does not modify the capacity of mice to develop an IgE response to *Nippostrongylus brasiliensis* [41,43,44]. This result is in line with previous findings using a rat anti-mouse CD23 antibody. Moreover, membrane CD23 transgenic mice showed an impairment of IgE responses. In contrast, soluble CD23 transgenic mice behaved like non-transgenic mice regarding IgE production [40], suggesting that in the mouse system at least, the soluble form of CD23 does not exhibit the same activity as the membrane form. Immunization of CD23 knock-out mice with thymus-dependent antigen resulted in an increase of IgE production, which was interpreted as evidence for CD23 providing a negative feedback regulation for IgE synthesis [44].

Polyclonal antibodies raised to the human CD23 lectin domain, highly conserved between murine and human CD23 [10,45], were shown to recognize a surface molecule on rat B lymphocytes that have been stimulated *in vivo* with homologous IgE. This process has been previously shown to upregulate the rat lymphocyte IgE receptor and widely used to study the rat FcεRII [46]. Intact anti-CD23 antibodies or their Fab fragments were found to be highly efficient in diminishing the IgE response induced by pertussis toxin (PT) + ovalbumin (OVA) in this animal model [47]. Moreover, expression of rat B cell FcεRII showed a clear correlation to serum IgE levels, as it has been described for human CD23 in subjects with high IgE levels [14–16]. Cloning of rat CD23 revealed a high degree of protein homology to murine and human CD23. The sequence also revealed that rat CD23, in a similar fashion to its murine homologue, but unlike the human counterpart, lacks the inverted RGD sequence close to the extracellular carboxy-terminus [47]. This *in vivo* model does not exclude the possibility of CD23 also acting through soluble forms. However, the fact that CD23 has indeed been shown to participate in several cell–cell interactions including T–B cell conjugate formation [28], antigen presentation [24,37–39], B cell homotypic adhesion [25,26], and given its physical association to MHC Class II [24,48], indicates that cell-associated CD23 is likely to play a major role in IgE regulation.

The pleiotropic and non-IgE-related activities described for CD23 [4], and the finding that CD23 epitopes involved in cytokine activities are distinct from those for IgE binding [49], suggested that this molecule was probably interacting with more than one ligand. To test this possibility, fluorescent liposomes incorporated with either glycophorin or recombinant full-length CD23 were assessed for binding to different cell types. Several antibodies were tested in this model to look for inhibition of CD23-liposome binding. A myeloma cell line, RPMI-8226, showed a strong binding of CD23 liposomes, and this binding was abolished by monoclonal antibodies to CD21. This was confirmed by CD23-liposome binding to CD21 transfectants [31]. These results identified CD21, the EBV- and complement receptor-2 (CR2), as a second ligand for CD23. Functionally, this was corroborated by the fact that engagement of B-cell CD21 by either anti-CD21 antibodies or by recombinant CD23 leads to increased IgE production in the presence of IL-4 [31]. The findings also revealed that the IgE promoting effects of CD23 were most probably exerted through CD21. These results are in keeping with previous reports that EBV can substitute the co-stimulatory signal required in the IL-4-permissive system to induce IgE secretion by human B lymphocytes [50].

Structurally, CD21 consists of 15–16 short consensus repeats of 60–75 amino acids (SCRs) followed by a transmembrane domain and an intracytoplasmic region. The sites of interaction of CD23 on CD21 were determined using purified recombinant CD23 incorporated into fluorescent liposomes and CD21 mutants bearing various deletions of extracytoplasmic SCRs. The sites of interaction of CD23 on CD21 are on SCRs 5–8 and 1–2. The first site is involved in a lectin–sugar type of interaction and the second site in a protein–protein interaction. By mutating, together or individually, the three asparagines present in SCRs 5–8, Asn370 and 295 (but not Asn492) were shown to be critically involved in the binding of CD23 [51]. SCRs 5–8 therefore represent a novel functional domain on the CD21 molecule and is the first demonstration of an activity in an extracytoplasmic region of CD21 outside of SCRs 1–4.

Amongst the other ligands for CD21 (EBV, C3d,g and IFNα), only EBV virus which binds to SCR 2 can inhibit the binding of CD23 to CD21. Furthermore, even a peptide from gp350/220 of EBV that is known to bind to CD21 is able to decrease CD23 binding to CD21 [52]. Monoclonal antibodies which map in SCRs 5–8 inhibit the most CD23 binding to CD21 and mimic the most CD23 activities [51]. Interestingly, the EBV-peptide which inhibited CD23 binding to CD21 also inhibited IgE and IgG_4 production induced by

IL-4. The two other CD21 ligands, C3 and IFNα, did not affect binding of CD23 to CD21 nor the production of IgE and IgG_4 [52].

Clinical data support the role of CD23–CD21 in human IgE-mediated diseases. Allergen induces CD23 expression on CD4-positive T cells and CD21 expression on B cells in patients with allergic asthma [53]. Moreover, CD23 expression on lymphocytes is decreased in allergic children undergoing hyposensitization [54].

On the other hand, the finding that CD21 is a ligand for CD23, bringing together these two important molecules for B (and probably T) lymphocytes, opens new avenues of research in both directions. The notion of certain controversial activities described for CD23, such as autocrine B-cell growth [55], could well be explained through interaction with CD21. Conversely, it is also possible that some activities of EBV on B cells may be related to its ability to increase the expression and release of CD23, which may act through CD21. Whether C3 and CD23 are functionally linked to each other, or whether the two molecules fortuitously share a common ligand, remains to be explored, especially since complement components themselves have been implicated in B-cell growth and activation [56].

Although CD23 was originally described as a B-cell restricted molecule in humans, and its presence in T cells considered negative, convincing evidence has been presented that CD23 is also expressed in T lymphocytes. Low T cell-CD23 expression has been reported in nonatopic subjects and elevated in certain atopic and hyper IgE syndrome patients [15,57,58] although others did not find this increment [59]. T cell CD23 is upregulated in activated tonsil, but not peripheral blood T cells from nonatopic individuals [60], and seems to convey similar functions as in B cells. It is involved in T-cell proliferation as assessed by co-stimulation assays with anti-CD23 antibodies, suggesting that CD23 engagement in T cells may have some role in T-cell activation, and during cell–cell interactions [60]. It is worth noting that CD23 expression on T cells has been shown to be specifically upregulated upon exposure to allergens [61,62]. The cloning of human T cell FcεRII revealed that it was restricted to the FcεRIIb form [63]. T cell-IgE receptors have also been described in rat [57] and mouse [45].

Another CD23-positive cell type, crucially involved in the generation and the maintenance of immune responses is the follicular dendritic cell (FDC). These cells, located exclusively in the germinal centres of secondary lymphoid tissues, are strong expressors of CD23 both in humans [4] and mice [64], and their expression varies according to the area of the follicle under scrutiny [4]. The function, however, of these high levels of CD23 on FDC is still unknown. It is probably involved in B-cell rescue, activation, and growth during germinal centre reactions [4,33]. CD23 is one of the signals that can rescue germinal centre B cells (GCC) from apoptosis [33], and this is mirrored by anti-CD21 antibodies [65], thus suggesting that CD23 on FDC may affect B-cell development in germinal centres by acting through CD21. In mice,

FDC-CD23 is upregulated upon exposure to parasites, and clearly involved in the capture and retention of IgE-immune complexes [64]. Interestingly, both CD23 and IgE have been found strongly upregulated on FDC from patients bearing high levels of serum IgE [66]. These observations open the possibility that immune complexes consisting of IgE and allergen, and retained (probably for long periods) on FDC through CD23, might be relevant in the maintenance of long-term IgE responses and in the generation of IgE-memory B cells; an exciting topic not yet explored for IgE.

CD40–CD40 LIGAND AND IgE

That T lymphocytes have a major role in the IgE system was highlighted in the early 1970s in animals rendered incapable of developing IgE responses upon thymectomy [67]. Likewise, the abnormal levels of IgE observed in patients with certain T cell-related disorders [68], suggested the regulatory influences of T cells on IgE. Later, it was shown *in vitro* that human normal B cells could be induced to IgE secretion by T-cell clones, irrespective of whether the clones were derived from atopic or nonatopic, or from the same or different individuals, as the source of the B cells [69], thus pointing against the need for cognate interactions. The search for T-cell regulatory factors controlling IgE production established IL-4 and IL-13 as the soluble factors inducing IgE production in an isotype-selective manner [19,70]. This IgE-inducing activity of IL-4 was shown to be reciprocally regulated by IFNγ and susceptible to modulation by other factors [22,23,70]. Later studies unambiguously demonstrated that cytokines alone were not capable of driving purified B cells to synthesize IgE, the presence of T cells was an essential prerequisite [22,27,71]. By using membranes to separate the cells allowing soluble factors to diffuse, it was established that in order to produce IgE, the B cells needed not only IL-4, but also a strict physical interaction with T cells was essential [27]. This contact-mediated signal was also shown with membrane preparations of activated but no resting CD4+T cells [72]. Disrupting this direct T–B contact by using antibodies to adhesion or accessory surface molecules such as CD2, CD3, CD4, LFA-1, or MHC Class II, strongly inhibited IgE production. Thus it was clear that IgE synthesis was dependent on at least two sets of signals, one provided by soluble factor IL-4 and IL-13, and the other one by physical, but not necessarily cognate, interaction with T lymphocytes.

Studies were then undertaken to investigate which B-cell surface molecules could be involved in the T–B interactions leading to IgE synthesis. Triggering of the B-cell molecule CD40 was thus identified as a potent stimulus of IgE synthesis in the absence of T lymphocytes [74,73].

The CD40 molecule, a type I glycoprotein of 50 kD, belongs to a growing family of cytokine receptors, including tumour necrosis factor receptor (TNFR) and nerve growth factor receptor (NGFR), among others [75].

Although CD40 was originally described as a bladder carcinoma-associated marker [76], it soon developed a prominent role in immune regulation. The variety of striking effects revealed with anti-CD40 antibodies anticipated its relevance: as a very potent activator of B lymphocytes [77], inducing both homotypic [26,77,78] and heterotypic [79] adhesion, in preventing germinal centre B-cell apoptosis [80], as the only (non-EBV) means to sustain long-term human B-cell growth *in vitro* [81], and later, as a potent inducer of IgE production in conjunction with IL-4 [73,74]. This latter activity of CD40 has been characterized at the molecular level demonstrating germ-line ε transcription and switch recombination [82,83] during the process of IgE production. This provided some indication as to the nature of the second set of signals required for IgE production.

The race to identify the CD40 counterpart, CD40L (ligand), initially thought to be a potent soluble lymphokine, provided unexpected results. Although CD40L was first cloned from mouse thymoma cells EL-4 [84], it was able to activate human B lymphocytes and drive IgE production in the presence of IL-4 [84], thus confirming previous observations made with CD40 ('agonistic') antibodies. The human CD40L however, was cloned later on [85–88], having 78% protein homology to its murine counterpart. The regulation of the surface expression of CD40L in T-cell subsets has been analysed during a construct of CD40L-Fc and various stimuli. Surface CD40L expression was stronger in CD4+ than in CD8+ T cells, and this correlated also with CD40L mRNA levels. CD40L expression, however, was not different between CD45RA and CD45RO T lymphocytes [88]. Treatment of PBL T cells with PMA-ionomycin strongly upregulated both CD40L expression and CD40L mRNA. Interestingly, treatment of T cells with factors controlling IgE synthesis, such as IL-4 and IFNγ, was also shown to reciprocally affect CD40L expression. In fact, the mRNA levels of CD40L were highly upregulated after seven days of treatment of PBL T cells with IL-4, and this effect was clearly inhibited by simultaneous treatment with IFNγ [88]. This strongly suggests that CD40L belongs to the group of molecules regulated in a co-ordinated manner by IL-4 and IFNγ.

The prominent role exhibited by the CD40 molecule in B-cell physiology led researchers to investigate its counterpart in some patients presenting low to absent levels of most immunoglobulins, except IgM. Previous reports had shown that B cells from these patients were able to re-acquire immunoglobulin switching capacity if cultured with T cells [89], thus precluding an intrinsic B-cell defect. It was soon found that naturally occurring mutations in the T cell CD40L were responsible for certain immunodeficiencies, characterized by normal to high levels of IgM but absence (or low levels) of all the other isotypes [90–94]. This unfortunate natural CD40L knock-out model revealed that integrity of CD40L on T cells is essential for B cells to achieve Ig class switching, including IgE.

To identify new cellular mechanisms for the control of IgE production, we tested the ability of mast (HMC-1) and basophilic (KU-812) cell lines to induce IgE synthesis in purified B cells stimulated with IL-4 in the absence of T cells [95]. Induction of IgE production and an increase in IgG synthesis was observed when B cells were incubated with HMC-1 or KU-812 cells. IgE production was preceded by a marked increase in IL-4-induced germline ε RNA synthesis. The induction of IgE and the increase in IgG synthesis brought about by HMC-1 or KU-812 cells in the presence of IL-4 was inhibited by competition with a chimaeric recombinant fusion protein consisting of the extracellular domain of human CD40 fused to a murine IgG constant region (CD40-Fc). These results indicated that mast or basophilic cell lines could replace T cells to provide the contact-mediated signal that is required, in conjunction with IL-4, for the induction of IgE production. Inhibition of this production by CD40-Fc indicated an involvement of CD40L.

Normal purified lung mast cells and blood basophils were also able to support IgE production by B cells, in the absence of T cells [95]. In contrast to mast cells, basophils were able to induce IgE synthesis even in the absence of exogenous IL-4. Therefore IgE synthesis can be induced by the interaction of B cells with mast cells and basophils in the presence of IL-4. Mast cells and basophils can express CD40L which is known to be able to provide, in conjunction with IL-4, the minimal signals required to induce IgE production. This suggests that mast cells and basophils are likely to play an important role in the induction and maintenance of allergic reactions. Thus, Ig switching previously thought to take place only in lymph node germinal centres may also occur in peripheral organs such as the lung or the skin.

Eosinophils were also found to express CD40L. In contrast to T cells, mast cells and basophils, eosinophils were unable to induce IgE switching from B cells [96]. The CD40L expressed on activated eosinophils is nevertheless functional. Fixed eosinophils can trigger B cell proliferation in the presence of IL-4. Inhibition of this proliferation by CD40-Fc indicated an involvement of CD40L. Those differences regarding IgE switching capability between eosinophils and T cells or basophils could be due to different levels of CD40L expression.

CONCLUDING REMARKS

The sequelae of clinical manifestations triggered by minute quantities of IgE in allergic reactions make this immunoglobulin a very potent pharmacological agent, whose balanced production has to be under tight and probably redundant control. IgE synthesis is a complex event requiring the involvement of not only soluble factors for promoting and suppressing its production, since it is also strictly dependent on certain contact-mediated mechanisms. The IgE-inducing lymphokine, IL-4, was initially thought to be produced exclusively by defined T-cell subsets. Recent studies however, have shown that certain non-T, non-B cells, basophils and mast cells can also produce this cytokine [97–99] and drive activated B cells to IgE production [95,100], indicating further levels of complexity and control for IgE. Moreover, IL-13 has recently been shown to induce IgE and CD23, independent of IL-4 [19]. Studies on the contact-dependent events revealed that whereas ubiquitous cell adhesion molecules can participate during cell interactions needed for IgE production, their effects are not restricted to this isotype. At least two pairs of complementary surface molecules, CD23–CD21 and CD40–CD40L, are clearly implicated in regulating this isotype. Studies with antibodies [13,21–23,31] or the ligands [31,87] for these molecules have highlighted their role in IgE regulation. These findings certainly complicate the initial picture of IgE synthesis depending exclusively on one soluble factor, IL-4, and one main regulatory cell type, the CD4+ Th2-type lymphocyte. However, this also opens new possibilities for potential therapeutic interventions. Antibodies to IL-4 and to CD23 have proven useful in reducing IgE levels *in vitro* and *in vivo*. The relative contributions of each of the factors so far known to participate in the IgE system remain to be established. CD23–CD21 and CD40–CD40L interactions are clearly relevant, and more *in vivo* models are still required to validate the *in vitro* findings, and to explore alternative therapeutic approaches.

ACKNOWLEDGEMENTS

The authors wish to thank K Hardy and J Knowles for reviewing the manuscript and for support, and S Henchoz and T Jomotte for their contribution to this work.

REFERENCES

1 Finkelman FD, Katona IM, Urban JF, *et al*. Suppression of *in vivo* polyclonal IgE responses by monoclonal antibody to the lymphokine B-cell stimulatory factor 1. *Proc Natl Acad Sci USA* 1986; **83**: 9675–9678.
2 Kuhn R, Rajewsky K, Muller W. Generation and analysis of interleukin-4 deficient mice. *Nature* 1991; **254**: 707–710.
3 Sato TA, Widmer MB, Finkelman FD, *et al*. Recombinant soluble murine IL-4 receptor can inhibit or enhance IgE responses *in vivo*. *J Immunol* 1993; **150**: 2717–2723.
4 Gordon J, Flores-Romo L, Cairns J, *et al*. CD23: A multi-functional receptor/lymphokine? *Immunol Today* 1989; **10**: 153–157.
5 Gonzalez-Molina A, Spiegelberg HL. Binding of IgE myeloma proteins to human cultured lymphoblastoid cell lines. *J Immunol* 1976; **117**: 1838–1845.
6 Kintner C, Sudgen B. Identification of antigenic determinants unique to surfaces of cells transformed by Epstein-Barr virus. *Nature* 1981; **294**: 458–460.
7 Thorley-Lawson DA, Nadler LM, Bahn AK, *et al*. Blast-2 (EBVCS), an early cell

surface marker of human B cell activation, is superinduced by Epstein–Barr virus. *J Immunol* 1985; **143**: 3007–3012.

8 Yukawa K, Kikutani H, Howaki H, *et al.* A B cell-specific differentiation antigen CD23, is a receptor for IgE (FcεR) on lymphocytes. *J Immunol* 1987; **138**: 2576–2580.

9 Bonnefoy JY, Aubry JP, Peronne C, *et al.* Production and characterization of a monoclonal antibody specific for the human lymphocyte low affinity receptor for IgE: CD23 is a low affinity receptor for IgE. *J Immunol* 1987; **138**: 2970–2978.

10 Gould H, Sutton B, Edmeades R, *et al.* CD23/FcεRII: C-type lectin membrane protein with a split personality? In: Gordon J (ed) *CD23: A Novel Multifunctional Regulator of the Immune System that Binds IgE. Monogr Allergy*. Basel: Karger, 1991; **29**: 28–49.

11 Yokota A, Kikutani H, Tanaka T, *et al.* Two species of human FcεRII (CD23): tissue-specific and IL-4-specific regulation of gene expression. *Cell* 1988; **55**: 611–618.

12 Sarfati M, Rector E, Wong K, *et al.* *In vitro* synthesis of IgE by human B lymphocytes. II. Enhancement of the spontaneous IgE synthesis by IgE-binding factors secreted by RPMI 8866 lymphoblastoid B cells. *Immunology* 1984; **53**: 197–214.

13 Sarfati M, Delespese G. Possible role of human lymphocyte receptor for IgE (CD23) or its soluble fragments in the *in vitro* synthesis of human IgE. *J Immunology* 1988; **141**: 2195–2199.

14 Thompson LF, Spiegelberg HL, Buckley RH. IgE-Fc receptor positive T and B lymphocytes in patients with the hyper IgE syndrome. *Clin Exp Immunol* 1985; **59**: 77–84.

15 Nagai T, Adachi M, Noro N, *et al.* T and B lymphocytes with immunoglobulin E Fc receptors (FcεR) in patients with nonallergic hyperimmunoglobulinemia E: Demonstration using a monoclonal antibody against FcεR-associated antigen. *Clin Immunol Immunopathol* 1985; **35**: 261–275.

16 Yanagihara Y, Sarfati M, Marsh D, *et al.* Serum levels of IgE-binding factor (soluble CD23) in diseases associated with elevated IgE. *Clin Exp Allergy* 1990; **20**: 395–401.

17 Bengtsson M, Gordon J, Flores-Romo L, *et al.* B cell reconstitution after autologous bone marrow transplantation: Increase in serum CD23 precedes IgE and B cell regeneration. *Blood* 1989; **73**: 2139–2144.

18 DeFrance T, Aubry JP, Rousset F, *et al.* Human recombinant interleukin 4 induces FcεR (CD23) on normal B lymphocytes. *J Exp Med* 1987; **165**: 1459–1467.

19 Lebman D, Cofman RL. Interleukin 4 causes isotype switching to IgE in T cell-stimulated clonal B cell cultures. *J Exp Med* 1988; **168**: 853–862.

20 Punnonen J, Aversa G, Cocks BG, *et al.* Interleukin 13 induces interleukin 4-independent IgG_4 and IgE synthesis and CD23 expression by human B cells. *Proc Natl Acad Sci USA* 1993; **90**: 3730–3734.

21 Bonnefoy JY, Mermod JJ, Shields J. Inhibition of human IL-4-induced IgE synthesis by a subset of anti-CD23/FcεRII monoclonal antibodies. *Eur J Immunol* 1990; **20**: 139–144.

22 Pene J, Rousset F, Briere F, *et al.* IgE production by normal human lymphocytes is induced by interleukin 4 and suppressed by intereferons γ and α and prostaglandin E_2. *Proc Natl Acad Sci USA* 1988; **85**: 6880–6884.

23 Pene J, Rouseet F, Briere F, *et al.* Interleukin 5 enhances interleukin 4-induced IgE production by normal human B cells. The role of soluble CD23 antigen. *Eur J Immunol* 1988; **18**: 929–935.

24 Flores-Romo L, Johnson GD, Veronesi A, *et al.* Functional implication for the topographical association between MHC Class II and the low affinity receptor for IgE: occupancy of CD23 blocks the ability of B cells to present alloantigen to T cells. *Eur J Immunol* 1990; **20**: 2465–2469.

25 Wang F, Gregory CD, Rowe M, *et al.* Epstein–Barr virus nuclear antigen-2 specifically induces expression of the B cell activation antigen CD23. *Proc Natl Acad Sci USA* 1987; **84**: 3452–3456.
26 Bjorck P, Elenstrom-Magnusson C, Rosen A, *et al.* CD23 and CD21 function as adhesion molecules in homotypic aggregation of human B lymphocytes. *Eur J Immunol* 1993; **23**: 1771–1775.
27 Vercelli D, Jabara HH, Arai KI, *et al.* Induction of human IgE synthesis requires interleukin 4 and T/B cell interactions involving the T cell receptor/CD3 complex and MHC Class II antigens. *J Exp Med* 1989; **169**: 1295–1307.
28 Aubry JP, Shields JG, Jansen KU, Bonnefoy JY. A multiparameter flow cytometric method to study surface molecules involved in interactions between subpopulations of cells. *J Immunol Methods* 1993; **159**: 161–171.
29 Bevilacqua MP, Stengelin S, Gimbrone MA, *et al.* Endothelial leukocyte adhesion molecule 1: an inducible receptor for neutrophils related to complement regulatory proteins and lectins. *Science* 1989; **243**: 1160–1165.
30 Bettler B, Maier R, Ruegg D, *et al.* Binding site for IgE of the human low affinity receptor (FcεRII/CD23) is confined to the domain homologous with animal lectins. *Proc Natl Acad Sci USA* 1989; **86**: 7118–7122.
31 Aubry JP, Pochon S, Graber P, *et al.* CD21 is a ligand for CD23 and regulates IgE production. *Nature* 1992; **353**: 505–507.
32 Pochon S, Graber P, Yaeger M, *et al.* Demonstration of a second ligand for the low affinity receptor for IgE (CD23) using recombinant CD23 reconstituted into fluorescent liposomes. *J Exp Med* 1992; **176**: 389–397.
33 Liu YJ, Cairns JA, Holder M, *et al.* Recombinant 25 KDa CD23 and interleukin-1 promote the survival of germinal center B cells: evidence for bifurcation in the development of centrocytes rescued from apoptosis. *Eur J Immunol* 1991; **21**: 1107–1114.
34 Mossalayi MD, Arock MM, Bertho JM, *et al.* Soluble CD23 (FcεRII) and interleukin-1 synergistically induce early human thymocyte maturation. *J Exp Med* 1990; **171**: 959–964.
35 Mossalayi MD, Arock M, Bertho JM, *et al.* Proliferation of early human myeloid precursors induced by interleukin-1 and recombinant soluble CD23. *Blood* 1990; **75**: 1924–1927.
36 Capron A, Dessaint JP, Capron M, *et al.* From parasites to allergy: a second receptor for IgE. *Immunol Today* 1986; **7**: 15–18.
37 Kehry MR, Yamashita LC. FcεRII (CD23) function on mouse B cells: role in IgE dependent antigen focusing. *Proc Natl Acad Sci USA* 1989; **86**: 7556–7560.
38 Pirron U, Schlunch T, Prinz JC, *et al.* IgE-dependent antigen focusing by human B lymphocytes is mediated by the low affinity receptor for IgE. *Eur J Immunol* 1990; **20**: 1547–1551.
39 Grosjean I, Lachaux A, Bella C, *et al.* CD23/CD21 interaction is required for presentation of soluble protein antigen by lymphoblastoid B cell lines to specific CD4+ T cell clones. *Eur J Immunol* 1994; **24**: 2982–2986.
40 Texido G, Eibel H, Le Gros G, van der Putten H. Transgene CD23 expression on lymphoid cells modulates IgE and IgG_1 responses. *J Immunol* 1994; **153**: 3028–3042.
41 Fujiwara H, Kikutani H, Suematsu S, Naka T, Yoshida K, Tanaka T, Suemura M, Matsumoto N, Kojima S. The absence of IgE antibody-mediated augmentation of immune responses in CD23-deficient mice. *Proc Natl Acad Sci USA* 1994; **91**: 6835–6839.
42 Morris SC, Lees A, Holmes JM, Jeffries RD, Finkelman FD. Induction of B cell and T cell tolerance *in vivo* by anti-CD23 mAb. *J Immunol* 1994; **152**: 3768–3776.
43 Stief A, Texido G, Sansig G, Eibel H, Le Gros G, van der Putten H. Mice deficient in

CD23 reveal its modulatory rule in IgE production but no role in T and B cell development. *J Immunol* 1994; **152**: 3378–3390.
44 Yu P, Kosco-Vilbois M, Richards M, Kohler G, Lamers MC. Negative feedback regulation of IgE synthesis by murine CD23. *Nature* 1994; **369**: 753–756.
45 Conrad DH. FcεRII/CD23: the low affinity receptor for IgE. *Ann Rev Immunol* 1990; **8**: 623–645.
46 Yodoi J, Ishizaka T, Ishizaka K. Lymphocytes bearing receptors for IgE. II. Induction of Fcε-receptor bearing rat lymphocytes by IgE. *J Immunol* 1979; **123**: 455–462.
47 Flores-Romo L, Shields J, Humbert Y, Graber P, Aubry JP, Gauchat JF, Ayala G, Allet B, Chavez M, Bazin H. Inhibition of an *in vivo* antigen-specific IgE response by antibodies to CD23. *Science* 1993; **261**: 1038–1041.
48 Bonnefoy JY, Guillot O, Spits H, *et al.* The low affinity receptor for IgE (CD23) on B lymphocytes is spatially associated with HLA-DR antigens. *J Exp Med* 1988; **167**: 57–72.
49 Mossalayi DM, Arock M, Delespesse G, *et al.* Cytokine effects of CD23 are mediated by an epitope distinct from the IgE binding site. *EMBO J* 1992; **11**: 4323–4328.
50 Thyphronitis G, Tsokos GC, June C, *et al.* IgE secretion by Epstein–Barr virus-infected purified human B lymphocytes is stimulated by interleukin 4 and suppressed by interferon γ. *Proc Natl Acad Sci USA* 1989; **86**: 5580–5584.
51 Aubry JP, Pochon S, Gauchat JF, Nueda-Marin A, Holers VM, Graber P, Siegfried C, Bonnefoy JY. CD23 interacts with a new functional extracytoplasmic domain involving N-linked oligosaccharides on CD21. *J Immunol* 1994; **152**: 5806–5813.
52 Henchoz-Lecoanet S, Jeannin P, Aubry, JP, Graber P, Bradshaw CG, Pochon S, Bonnefoy JY. The Epstein–Barr virus-binding site on CD21 is involved in CD23 binding and IL-4-induced IgE and IgG_4 production by human B cells. *Immunol* 1996; **88**: 35–39.
53 Gagro A, Rabatic S. Allergen-induced CD23 on CD4+ T lymphocytes and CD21 on B lymphocytes in patients with allergic asthma: evidence and regulation. *Eur J Immunol* 1994; **24**: 1109–1114.
54 Gagro A, Rabatic S, Trescec A, Dekaris D, Medar-Lasic M. Expression of lymphocytes FcεRII/CD23 in allergic children undergoing hyposensitization. *Int Arch Allergy Appl Immunol* 1993; **101**: 203–208.
55 Swendeman S, Thorley-Lawson DA. The activation antigen BLAST-2, when shed, is an autocrine BCGF for normal and transformed B cells. *EMBO J* 1987; **6**: 1637–1642.
56 Hearn JM, Fearon DT. Structure and function of the complement receptors CR1 (CD35) and CR2 (CD21). *Adv Immunol* 1989; **46**: 183–219
57 Yodi J, Ishizaka K. Lymphocytes bearing Fc receptors for IgE. I. Presence of human and rat T lymphocytes with Fcε receptors. *J Immunol* 1979; **122**: 2577–2583.
58 Takigawa M, Tamamori T, Horiguchi D, *et al.* FcεRII/CD23 positive lymphocytes in atopic dermatitis. I. The proportion of FcεRII+lymphocytes correlates with the extent of skin lesion. *Clin Exp Immunol* 1991; **84**: 275–282.
59 Thompson LF, Mellon MH, Zeiger RS, *et al.* Characterization with monoclonal antibodies of T lymphocytes bearing Fc receptors for IgE and IgG in atopic patients. *J Immunol* 1983; **131**: 2772–2776.
60 Armitage RJ, Goff LK, Beverley PCL. Expression and functional role of CD23 on T cells. *Eur J Immunol* 1989; **19**: 31–35.
61 Prinz JC, Baur X, Mazur G, *et al.* Allergen-directed expression of Fc recetors for IgE (CD23) on human T lymphocytes is modulated by interleukin 4 and interferon γ. *Eur J Immunol* 1990; **20**: 1259–1264.
62 Yamaoka KA, Tsukidate S, Higaki M, *et al.* Induction of FcεRII/CD23 on human T

cells by excretory and secretory antigen of *Dirofilaria immitis*. *Int Arch Allergy Appl Immunol* 1991; **95**: 92–93.
63 Nonaka M, Hsu DK, Hanson CM, *et al*. Cloning of cDNA coding for low-afinity Fc receptors for IgE on human T lymphocytes. *Int Immunol* 1989; **1**: 254–259.
64 Maeda K, Burton GF, Padgett DA, *et al*. Murine follicular dendritic cells and low affinity Fc receptors for IgE (FcεRII). *J Immunol* 1992; **148**: 2340–2347.
65 Bonnefoy JY, Henchoz S, Hardie D, *et al*. A subset of anti-CD21 antibodies promote the rescue of germinal center B cells from apoptosis. *Eur J Immunol* 1993; **23**: 969–972.
66 Mitani S, Takagi K, Oka T, *et al*. Increased immunoglobulin ε Fc receptor bearing cells in germinal centers of hyperimmunoglobulinemia ε patients. *Int Arch Allergy Appl Immunol* 1988; **87**: 63–69.
67 Okumura K, Tada T. Regulation of homocytotropic antibody formation in the rat. III. Effect of thymectomy and splenectomy. *J Immunol* 1971; **106**: 1019–1025.
68 Buckley RH, Fiscus SA. Serum IgD and IgE concentrations in immunodeficiency diseases. *J Clin Invest* 1975; **55**: 157–165.
69 Romagnani S. Regulation and deregulation of human IgE synthesis. *Immunol Today* 1990; **11**: 316–321.
70 Coffman RL, Carty J. A T cell activity that enhances polyclonal IgE production and its inhibition by interferon g. *J Immunol* 1986; **136**: 949–954.
71 Del Prete GF, Maggi E, Parronchi P, *et al*. IL-4 is an essential factor for the IgE synthesis induced *in vitro* by human T cell clones and their supernatants. *J Immunol* 1988; **140**: 4193–4198.
72 Gascan H, Aversa GH, Gauchat JF, *et al*. Membranes of activated CD4+ T cells expressing T cell receptor (TcR) $\alpha\beta$ or TcR $\gamma\delta$ induce IgE synthesis by human B cells in the presence of interleukin 4. *Eur J Immunol* 1992; **22**: 1133–1141.
73 Jabara HH, Fu SM, Geha RS, *et al*. CD40 and IgE: synergism between anti-CD40 monoclonal antibody and interleukin 4 in the induction of IgE synthesis by highly purified human B cells. *J Exp Med* 1990; **172**: 1861–1864.
74 Rousset F, Garcia E, Banchereau J. Cytokine-induced proliferation and immunoglobulin production of human B lymphocytes triggered through their CD40 antigen. *J Exp Med* 1991; **173**: 705–710.
75 Stamenkovic I, Clark EA, Seed B. A B lymphocyte activation molecule related to nerve growth factor receptor and induced by cytokines. *EMBO J* 1989; **8**: 1403–1410.
76 Paulie S, Ehlin-Henriksson B, Mellstedt H, *et al*. A p50 surface antigen restricted to human urinary bladder carcinomas and B lymphocytes. *Cancer Immunol Immunother* 1985; **20**: 23–28.
77 Gordon J, Millsum MJ, Guy GR, *et al*. Resting B lymphocytes can be triggered directly through the CDW40 (Bp50) antigen. *J Immunol* 1988; **140**: 1425–1430.
78 Barrett TB, Shu G, Clark EA. CD40 signalling activates CD11a/CD18 (LFA-1)-mediated adhesion in B cells. *J Immunol* 1991; **146**: 1722–1729.
79 Flores-Romo L, Estoppey D, Bacon KB. Anti-CD40 antibody stimulates the VLA-4-dependent adhesion of normal and LFA-1-deficient B cells to endothelium. *Immunology* 1993; **79**: 445–451.
80 Liu YJ, Joshua DE, Williams GT, *et al*. Mechanism of antigen-driven selection in germinal centers. *Nature* 1989; **342**: 929–931.
81 Banchereau J, de Paoli P, Valle A, *et al*. Long-term growth of human B cell lines dependent on interleukin 4 and antibody to CD40. *Science* 1991; **251**: 70–72.
82 Shapira SK, Vercelli D, Jabara HH, *et al*. Molecular analysis of the induction of immunoglobulin IgE synthesis in human B cells by interleukin 4 and engagement of CD40 antigen. *J Exp Med* 1992; **175**: 289–292.

83 Gauchat JF, Aversa G, Gascan H, *et al*. Modulation of IL-4 induced germline RNA synthesis in human B cells by tumor necrosis factor α, anti-CD40 monoclonal antibodies or transforming growth factor b correlates with levels of IgE production. *Int Immunol* 1992; **4**: 397–406.
84 Armitage RJ, Fanslow WC, STrockbine L, *et al*. Molecular and biological characterization of a murine ligand for CD40. *Nature* 1992; **357**: 80–82.
85 Hollenbaugh D, Grosmaire LS, Kullas CD, *et al*. The human T cell antigen gp39, a member of the TNF gene family, is a ligand for the CD40 receptor: expression of a soluble form of gp39 with B cell co-stimulatory activity. *EMBO J* 1992; **12**: 4313–4321.
86 Graf D, Korthauer U, Mages HW, *et al*. Cloning of TRAP, a ligand for CD40 on human T cells. *Eur J Immunol* 1992; **22**: 3191–3194.
87 Spriggs MK, Armitage RJ, Strockbone L, *et al*. Recombinant human CD40 ligand stimulates B cell proliferation and immunoglobulin E secretion. *J Exp Med* 1992; **176**: 1543–1550.
88 Gauchat JF, Aubry JP, Mazzei G, *et al*. Human CD40-ligand: molecular cloning, cellular distribution and regulation of expression by factors controlling IgE production. *FEBS Lett* 1993; **315**: 259–266.
89 Hill A, Chapel H. X-linked immunodeficiency. The fruits of cooperation. *Nature* 1993; **361**: 11.
90 DiSanto JP, Bonnefoy JY, Gauchat JF, *et al*. CD40 ligand mutations in X-linked immunodeficiency with hyper-IgM. *Nature* 1993; **361**: 541–543.
91 Korthauer U, Graf D, Mages HW, *et al*. Defective expression of T-cell CD40 ligand causes X-linked immunodeficiency with hyper-IgM. *Nature* 1993; **361**: 539–541.
92 Aruffo A, Farrington M, Hollenbaugh D, *et al*. The CD40 ligand, gp39, is defective in activated T cells from patients with X-linked hyper-IgM syndrome. *Cell* 1993; **72**: 291–300.
93 Allen RC, Armitage RJ, Conley, ME, *et al*. CD40 ligand defects responsible for X-linked hyper-IgM syndrome. *Science* 1993; **259**: 990–993
94 Fuleihan R, Ramesh N, Loh R, *et al*. Defective expression of the CD40 ligand in X chromosome-linked immunoglobulin deficiency with normal or elevated IgM. *Proc Natl Acad Sci USA* 1993; **90**: 2170–2173.
95 Gauchat J-F, Henchoz S, Mazzei G, Aubry J-P, Brunner T, Blasey H, Life P, Talabot D, Flores-Roma L, Thompson J, Kishi K, Butterfield J, Dahinden C, Bonnefoy J-Y. Induction of human IgE synthesis in B cells by mast cells and basophils. *Nature* 1993; **365**: 340–343.
96 Gauchat JF, Hencoz S, Fattah D, *et al*. CD40 ligand is functionally expressed on human eosinophils. *Eur J Immunol* 1995; **25**: 863–865.
97 Piccinni MP, Macchia D, Parronchi P, *et al*. Human bone marrow non-B, non-T cells produce interleukin 4 in response to cross-linkage of Fcε and Fcγ receptors. *Proc Natl Acad Sci USA* 1991; **88**: 8656–8660.
98 Brunner T, Heusser CH, Dahinden CA. Human peripheral blood basophils primed by interleukin 3 (IL-3) produce IL-4 in response to immunoglobulin E receptor stimulation. *J Exp Med* 1993; **177**: 605–611.
99 Brown MA, Pierce JH, Watson CJ, Falco J, Ihle JN, Paul WE. B cell stimulatory factor-1/interleukin-4 mRNA is expressed by normal and transformed mast cells. *Cell* 1987; **50**: 809–818.
100 Lederman F, Heusser C, Schlienger C, *et al*. Interleukin 3-treated non-B, non-T cells switch activated B cells to IgG_1/IgE synthesis. *Eur J Immunol* 1992; **22**: 2783–2787.

4 T-cell Epitopes: Is there Immunodominance?

AFTAB A. ANSARI and LALIT M. BAHUGUNA*
NIAMSD, National Institutes of Health, Bethesda, Maryland, USA; and
**Pathology Department, KG Medical College, Lucknow, India*

An epitope is that part of an antigen molecule that is recognized by the immune system, and thus results in an immune response. A B-cell epitope binds to B cells and antibodies, while a T-cell epitope binds to T cells. A protein antigen usually contains multiple B- and T-cell epitopes, which may be overlapping, adjacent, or distant to each other. Based on several studies, including those on sperm whale myoglobin [1,2], pertussis toxin [3], bovine ribonuclease [4], hen egg-white lysozyme [5,6], staphylococcal nuclease [7], influenza haemagglutinin [8,9], ragweed allergen Ra3 [10], bacteriophage λ repressor protein cl [11], and hen ovalbumin [12], it appears that T-cell responses to native antigens are limited to one or a limited number of T-cell epitopes, irrespective of the major histocompatibility complex (MHC) haplotype. Thus, it is usually believed that, of the multiple possible epitopes in an antigen, a few are 'immunodominant' in that either they stimulate the highest immune response and/or they are recognized by most members of a species. The immunodominant epitopes are potentially powerful tools for peptide vaccination/immunotherapy of infectious, allergic, and autoimmune diseases. The T-cell epitope has been the subject of considerable investigation for about two decades. A commonly employed procedure for T-cell epitope mapping involves generating T-cell clones in response to the whole antigen, and then investigating the responses of the individual clones to short, overlapping synthetic peptides encompassing the entire antigen molecule. Since a T-cell clone represents only one T cell of the individual, the information thus obtained using a limited number of clones may not be applicable to the individual or species as a whole. It is therefore not surprising that studies using T-cell clones have led to the belief that the T-cell responses to many antigens are limited to one or a few epitopes. It remains to be investigated whether a few T-cell clones from an individual represent the whole T-cell repertoire and response to the specific antigen.

Allergic Mechanisms and Immunotherapeutic Strategies. Edited by A.M. Roberts and M.R. Walker.

In view of this limitation we developed an epitope mapping procedure that relates to the whole individual as opposed to a few cells from the individual. We applied this procedure to the T-cell epitope mapping of an allergen Lol p 3 from ryegrass.

Ryegrass, *Lolium perenne* (Lol p), is one of the major grass species causing pollen allergy in humans. Several proteins, including Lol p 3, from the grass pollen have been isolated, characterized, and sequenced [13–15]. Lol p 3 is a 97 amino acid residue long protein allergen which contains no cysteine residues [14].

SYNTHETIC PEPTIDES

Overlapping peptides corresponding to the complete 97 residue long sequence of Lol p 3 were synthesized at a core facility of the Johns Hopkins University. Nine peptides were synthesized, which each had 10 residue overlaps and were 20 residues long, except the C-terminal peptide which was 17 residues long (Figure 4.1).

ISOLATION OF PERIPHERAL BLOOD MONONUCLEAR CELLS (PBMC)

Human peripheral blood mononuclear cells (PBMC) were isolated from heparinized blood by gradient centrifugation on Histopaque-1077 (Sigma Chemical Company, St. Louis, MO) following the manufacturer's instructions. The PBMC were isolated from grass-allergic subjects as well as from non-allergic subjects. Short-term T-cell lines (STTCL) were obtained from the PBMC as follows.

GENERATION OF STTCL

PBMC were washed three times with Dulbecco's phosphate buffer saline (pH 7.2) and then resuspended to a concentration of 50×10^6 cells/ml in RPMI 1640 supplemented with 5% heat inactivated human AB + serum, 2 mM L-glutamine, 25 mM HEPES, 100 U/ml penicillin, 100 μg/ml streptomycin, 10 μg/ml gentamicin (GIBCO, Grand Island, NY), and 5×10^{-5} M 2-mercaptoethanol (Sigma Chemical Co, St. Louis, MO). The PBMC suspension was stimulated with the purified antigen Lol p 3 at a final concentration of 5 μg/ml. The cells were then transferred to a 25 ml tissue culture flask and incubated at 37°C with 5% CO_2 in air for six days. The second stimulation of PBMC was performed by replacing the medium from each flask with fresh complete medium containing human recombinant interleukin-2 (rIL-2) at a concentration of 25 U/ml. Four days later, the medium was replaced with

Lol p 3 Major

1 10 20 30 40 50 60 70 80 90 97
TKVDLTVEKG SDAKTLVLNI KYTRPGDTLA EVELRQHGSE EWEPMTKKGN LWEVKSAKPL TGPMNFRFLS KGGMKNVFDE VIPTAFTVGK TYTPEYN

#1 #3 #5 #7 #9

#2 #4 #6 #8

Figure 4.1. Amino acid sequence of Lol p 3 showing the overlapping peptides used in this study. The sequence is from reference [14]

another dose of rIL-2 at the same concentration in order to expand the proliferating cells. On day 14 or 15, the cells were washed three times with DPBS to remove free rIL-2, and the cells were used in proliferation assays.

PROLIFERATION ASSAYS

Two proliferation assays were performed, one using whole PBMC, and the other using the STTCL. All assays were done in triplicate in 96-well microtitre plates in 200 μl volumes. For the assays using PBMC, 5×10^5 PBMC were cultured in the presence of 1.2 μg/ml of one of the nine peptides or in the absence of the peptides (controls) at 37°C with 5% CO_2 in air for 4 days. For the assays using STTCL, 2×10^4 cells per well from the T-cell line were cultured in absence or presence of different concentrations of the synthetic peptides together with irradiated (5000 rad) autologous PBMC (T-cell:PMBC ratio, 1:20). After four days, the cultures were pulsed with tritiated thymidine for about 15 h, after which the cells were harvested for determining radioactivity incorporated in DNA. The peptide dose-response curves were different for different subjects, with most peptides exhibiting maximum response at the concentration of 1.2 μg/ml when assayed in the dose range of 0.24 μg/ml to 30 μg/ml.

DOSE RESPONSE

For each of the nine peptides, dose-response curves were obtained in the peptide concentration range of 0.24–30 μg/ml, for PBMC and T-cell lines from 10 different human subjects. Most subjects exhibited maximum thymidine incorporation at 1.2 μg/ml for most of the peptides. At a fixed peptide concentration of 1.2 μg/ml, proliferative responses were studied in three, four, and five-day cultures (prior to pulsing with tritiated thymidine). Results shown are the maximum responses observed; this was usually in four-day cultures. Compared to other allergens like mite allergens, Lol p 3 does not induce high proliferation *in vitro*.

COMPARED TO PBMC, STIMULATED STTCL IDENTIFY MORE EPITOPES

Typical responses of one (JH) grass-allergic subject's PBMC (dotted bars) and T-cell line (hatched bars) to the nine peptides are shown in Figure 4.2, along with the responses to buffer control. The counts per minute (CPM) values shown are not subtracted from the control CPM values. For this subject as well as others, the control CPM values were generally lower, whereas ΔCPM values and stimulation indices were higher for the T-cell lines than those for PBMC. In this subject, the PBMC showed no prolif-

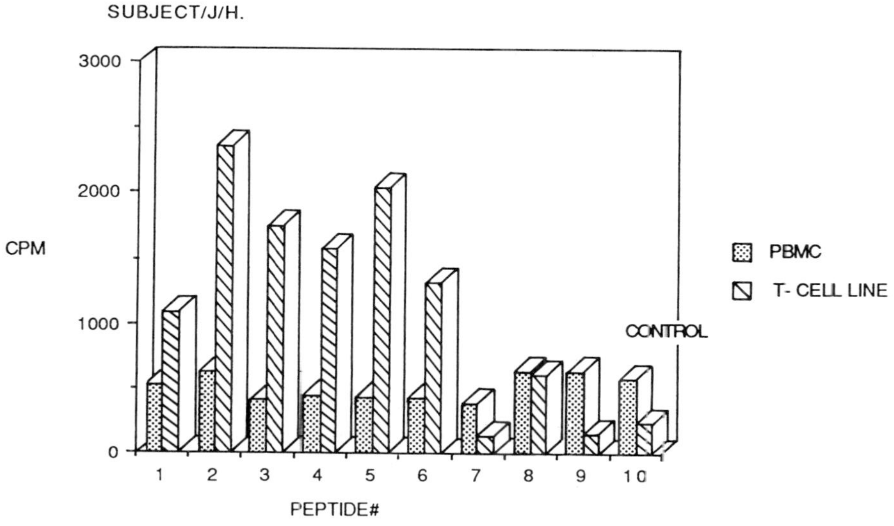

Figure 4.2. *In vitro* response of PBMC (dotted bars) and STTCL (hatched bars), from a subject JH, to the nine peptides (1–9) and buffer control (10). Experimental conditions are described in the text

erative response to any of the nine peptides above the control level, whereas the T-cell line showed appreciable responses to seven peptides, with peptides 2 and 5 being the most stimulatory. Peptides 7 and 9 were not stimulatory for this subject.

Figure 4.3 shows the responses of PBMC and T-cell lines from another grass allergic individual (MLE). In this case, proliferative response was detectable even using PBMC, although the response is much enhanced with the T-cell line. In the T-cell lines, four peptides (2,6,7, and 8) stimulated responses, whereas in PBMC only two of them (peptides 7 and 8) were stimulatory above the control levels.

COMPARED TO PBMC, STTCL GIVE HIGHER STIMULATION INDEX

As can be seen in Figure 4.3, stimulation indices (test CPM in presence of peptide divided by control CPM in absence of peptide) were higher with the T-cell line than those with PBMC. This is not only because the denominator (control value) for the T-cell line is lower, but also because the numerator (test CPM value) for the T-cell line is higher compared to those for PBMC. This was the general trend with most subjects. This observation is not unexpected

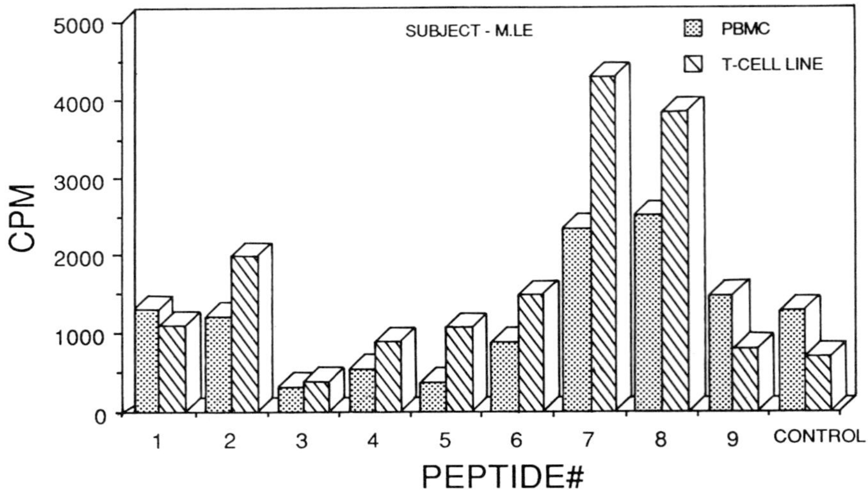

Figure 4.3. *In vitro* response of PBMC (dotted bars) and STTCL (hatched bars), from a subject MLE, to the nine peptides and buffer control. Experimental conditions are described in the text

considering that the T-cell lines are somewhat enriched in the antigen-specific cell population.

EACH SUBJECT RESPONDS TO MULTIPLE EPITOPES

There was no subject whose cells responded to all the nine peptides. Two subjects (JPT and JUL) responded to one peptide each, while others responded to two or more peptides (Table 4.1). Each subject or group of subjects recognized a different set of the peptides.

ALL PEPTIDES ENCOMPASSING THE ENTIRE ANTIGEN MOLECULE STIMULATE T CELLS

There was no peptide to which cells from all the subjects responded (Table 4.1). Peptide 2 may perhaps be referred to as the immunodominant peptide as it elicited response in the largest number of subjects (8/10) in this small group. More important, each of the nine peptides was 'antigenic' in that it elicited appreciable responses in T-cell lines from several subjects. Since the T-cell lines were derived by stimulation of PBMC with the whole antigen and not with the specific peptides, one would not necessarily expect all the

Table 4.1. Summary of human T-cell response to the nine synthetic overlapping peptides of Lol p 3. The first three patients (JPT, CTH, and JUL) were non-atopic, while the remaining seven were grass-allergic. *In vitro* T-cell proliferative responses to the peptides were determined using T-cell lines and PBMC as described in the text

	Peptide number									
Subject-ID	1	2	3	4	5	6	7	8	9	Total
JPT					+					1(0)
CTH	+	+=			+			+		4(1)
JUL			+							1(0)
KGU	+	+=								2(1)
JDE		+=	+	+=	+	+=	+	+=	+	8(4)
JH	+	+	+	+	+	+		+		7(0)
DMD	+=	+=	+=	+=			+=	+=	+=	7(7)
BHA	+	+		=	+	+	=	=	+	5(3)
MLE		+				+	+=	+=		4(2)
LBS	+	+	+				+		+	5(0)
TOTAL	6	8	5	4	5	4	5	6	4	

Positive immune response of T-cell line (+) or PBMC (=)

peptides encompassing the antigen to be stimulatory in the proliferation assay.

ALLERGIC VS. NON-ALLERGIC SUBJECTS

Of the 10 subjects studied, three (JPT, CTH, and JUL) were non-atopic, and seven were grass-allergic (Table 4.1). Generally, the magnitude of proliferation in response to the peptides was lower in the PBMC and T-cell lines obtained from the non-allergic subjects compared to the allergic subjects. In addition, the grass-allergic subjects each responded to multiple Lol p peptides, whereas only one of the non-allergic subjects responded to more than one peptide.

IMPLICATIONS

The short-term T-cell lines were generated by *in vitro* stimulation of PBMC, first with the whole antigen for six days (in absence of IL-2), followed by propagation of the stimulated cells with IL-2 for eight to nine days. During the initial six-day period, T cells that are responsive to the antigen would be stimulated and would express on their surface IL-2 receptor (IL-2R), while other T cells in absence of antigen-stimulation would not express IL-2R. In the second phase of the culture with IL-2, the antigen-stimulated IL-2R+ cells would proliferate, while the unstimulated cells would gradually start to die. Thus, the procedure used in this study is expected to produce a T-cell line that is enriched with most of the T cells of the study subject that are capable of antigenic stimulation with any processed part of the antigen used in the initial stimulation. This short-term T-cell line is expected to be a fair representation of the subject's T-cell repertoire to the specific antigen. The procedure described here is also a part of many T-cell cloning protocols. For T-cell cloning, the short-term T-cell line obtained as above may be further propagated and then cloned in microtitre plates at one cell per well. Thus, each T-cell clone represents one cell of the subject; the short-term T-cell line generated as above, on the contrary, probably represents a majority of the antigen-specific repertoire of the subject.

A true T-cell clone, by definition, is homogeneous, and therefore an extremely valuable resource for studies that require such homogeneity, such as the studies of MHC restriction, T-cell receptor, antigen presentation, etc. In proliferation assays, T-cell clones generally yield clean data with low control values and high stimulation indices. However, concern is raised about using the individual clones for T-cell epitope mapping. Each clone is usually specific for a particular epitope of the antigen. Using a limited number of antigen-specific clones for T-cell epitope mapping might lead to a skewed result. The problem may be further compounded because we do not know how many individual distinct clones are enough for such studies, and also because unless detailed characterization has been carried out, we are not sure whether each clone being used is a distinct clone, or a sister of another clone. Moreover, during the cloning procedure only the 'strong' clones may have survived, while the 'weak' ones, which may have been specific for other epitopes of the antigen, may not have survived, leading to further skewing of the mapping data.

Whole PBMC would be a more complete representation of the subject's T-cell repertoire to a specific antigen. However, for obvious reasons, PBMC usually give very low signal to noise ratios in proliferation assays, although they have been successfully used with a few highly potent antigens [16].

The 'short-term T-cell line' (STTCL, for the lack of a better terminology) used in this study is expected to be enriched with antigen-specific T cells and also to be a fair representation of the subject's T-cell repertoire to the antigen. Using STTCL from 10 subjects we demonstrated that each subject or group of subjects responds to a different set of Lol p 3 epitopes, and that T-cell epitopes are distributed across the entire antigen molecule. Thus, although the response of an individual T cell or T-cell clone may be limited to *one* epitope, and that of STTCL (or of a person) may be limited to a *few* epitopes, the response of a species as a whole is *not limited* to a few epitopes of the antigen. This phenomenon may be important for the survival of the species through various epidemic diseases.

We cannot offer any explanation for the previous observations that have clearly shown for several antigens that T-cell response to an antigen is generally restricted to a limited number of epitopes [1–12]. An explanation may perhaps be obtained by performing the epitope mapping studies using STTCL or a comprehensive set of T-cell lines, clones, or hybridomas. The T-cell response to hen ovalbumin was earlier believed to be restricted to one or a few peptide regions [12], but studies using mouse T–T hybridomas identifed at least nine different peptide regions of the protein that were recognized by one or more of the hybridomas [17]. It is possible that additional regions of the protein might be recognized as containing T-cell epitopes by using STTCL.

In the present study we have demonstrated that T-cell epitopes are distributed throughout the length of the Lol p 3 molecule, and that, although T-cell response of an individual subject may or may not be restricted to a few epitopes, the response of the human species is *not* limited to a few epitopes. Nevertheless, a limited number of these regions (peptide 2 in this study) appears to be immunodominant in that it elicits a response in the majority of the subjects. Thus, two phenomena, unlimited T-cell epitopes in a given antigen, and immunodominance, appear to be exhibited by this antigen side by side. This may be a more general phenomenon than is usually recognized.

ACKNOWLEDGEMENTS

We thank all volunteers involved in the study for their co-operation and interest. We also thank the Hazleton Biotechnologies, Vienna, VA, USA, and the Biological Response Modifiers Program, National Cancer Institute, USA, for the generous gift of human recombinant IL-2. This work was performed at the Johns Hopkins Asthma and Allergy Center, Department of Medicine, Baltimore, MD, and was supported by the following grants to AAA: AI-25372 from the NIH, and PP0200 from the National Multiple Sclerosis Society.

REFERENCES

1 Kurata A, Berzofsky JA. Analysis of peptide residues interacting with MHC molecule or T-cell receptor: can a peptide bind in more than one way to the same MHC molecule. *J Immunol* 1990; **144**: 4526–4535.
2 Brett SJ, Cease KB, Ouyang CS, Berzofsky JA. Fine specificity of T-cell recognition of the same peptide in association with different I-a molecules. *J Immunol* 1989; **143**: 771–779.
3 Kim KJ, McKinness S, Manclark CR. Determination of T-cell epitopes on the S1 subunit of pertussis toxin. *J Immunol* 1990; **144**: 3529–3534.
4 Lorenz RG, Tyler AN, Allen PM. T-cell recognition of bovine ribonuclease: self/non-self discrimination at the level of binding to the IA^K molecule. *J Immunol* 1988; **141**: 4124–4128.

5 Gammon G, Geysen HM, Apple RJ, *et al.* T-cell determinant structure: cores and determinant envelops in three mouse major histocompatibility complex haplotypes. *J Exp Med* 1991; **173**: 609–617.

6 Adorini L, Appella E, Doria G, Nagy ZA. Mechanisms influencing the immunodominance of T-cell determinants. *J Exp Med* 1988; **168**: 2091–2104.

7 Shaeffer EB, Sette A, Johnson DJ, *et al.* Relative contribution of 'determinant selection' and 'holes in the T-cell repertoire' to T-cell responses. *Proc Natl Acad Sci USA* 1989; **86**: 4649–4653.

8 Burt DS, Mills KHG, Skehel JJ, Thomas DB. Diversity of the class II (I-A^k/1E^k)-restricted T-cell repertoire for influenza hemagglutinin and antigenic drift: six non-overlapping epitopes on the HA1 subunit are defined by synthetic peptides. *J Exp Med* 1989; **170**: 383–397.

9 Barnett BC, Burt DS, Graham CM, *et al.* I-A^d restricted T-cell recognition of influenza hemagglutinin: synthetic peptides identify multiple epitopes corresponding to antibody-binding regions of the HA1 subunit. *J Immunol* 1989; **143**: 2663–2669.

10 Kurisaki JI, Atassi H, Atassi MZ. T-cell recognition of ragweed allergen Ra3: localization of the full T-cell recognition profile by synthetic overlapping peptides representing the entire protein chain. *Eur J Immunol* 1986; **16**: 236–240.

11 Roy S, Scherer MT, Briner TJ, *et al.* Murine MHC polymorphism and T-cell specificities. *Science* 1989; **244**: 572–575.

12 Shimonkevitz R, Colon S, Kappler J, *et al.* Antigen recognition by H-2 restricted T cells: a tryptic ovalbumin peptide that substitutes for processed antigen. *J Immunol* 1984; **133**: 2067–2074.

13 Ansari AA, Kihara TK, Marsh DG. Immunological studies of *Lolium perenne* (rye grass) pollen allergens, Lol p I, II and III. *J Immunol* 1987; **139**: 4034–4041.

14 Ansari AA, Shenbagamurthi P, Marsh DG. Complete primary structure of a *Lolium perenne* (perennial rye grass) pollen allergen, Lol p III: comparison with known Lol p I and II sequences. *Biochemistry* 1989; **28**: 8665–8670.

15 Ansari AA, Shinomiya N, Zwollo P, Marsh DG. HLA-D gene studies in relation to immune responsiveness to a grass allergen Lol p III. *Immunogenetics* 1991; **33**: 24–32.

16 O'Hehir RE, Lamb JR. From epitopes to immunotherapy. In: Druce HM, Bousquet JB (co-chairs) Proceedings of a Symposium. Paris: *Histamine and Beyond – Directions in Allergy and Respiratory Medicine*, 1992: 24–26.

17 Vidard L, Rock KL, Benacerraff B. Diversity in MHC class II ovalbumin T-cell epitopes generated by distinct proteases. *J Immunol* 1992; **149**: 498–504.

5 The Role of Th1 and Th2 Subsets in Atopic Allergy

EDDY A. WIERENGA, R.J. JOOST VAN NEERVEN, FRANS L. VAN DER HEIJDEN, CATHARIEN M.U. HILKENS, ALIES SNIJDERS, FRANK G.M. SNIJDEWINT and MARTIEN L. KAPSENBERG

Laboratory of Cell Biology and Histology, University of Amsterdam, The Netherlands

INTRODUCTION

ATOPIC ALLERGY

Atopic allergy is a genetically determined immune syndrome with variable clinical manifestations, including allergic rhinitis, allergic asthma, constitutional eczema, conjunctivitis, or combinations of these and other disorders. Typical pathophysiologic characteristics, common to all types of atopy, are elevated serum levels of allergen-specific IgE and systemic and local tissue eosinophilia. Inhalation allergens frequently involved in atopic allergy include proteins derived from house dust mites, domestic animals and several grass and tree pollen species. In sensitized atopic individuals, repeated challenges with such allergens may lead to production of allergen-specific IgE and, consequently, to immediate (type I) hypersensitivity. Allergen-specific IgE can readily be detected in the serum of atopic patients by radio allergosorbent tests (RAST) and immediate hypersensitivity can be monitored within minutes after intracutaneous prick tests.

In addition to the immediate response, a late phase response to the same allergen(s) is also frequently observed six to 24 hours after allergen exposure. The late phase response is characterized by intense, local perivascular cell infiltrations, comprising activated CD4+ T helper (Th) lymphocytes and several types of inflammatory cells, typically including high numbers of activated eosinophils. Continuous late phase responses to ubiquitous allergens may lead to serious tissue damage, causing chronic hypersensitivity of the airways in allergic asthma and skin lesions in atopic dermatitis.

Allergic Mechanisms and Immunotherapeutic Strategies. Edited by A.M. Roberts and M.R. Walker.

CYTOKINES IN ATOPIC ALLERGY

The course of an antigen-specific immune response is largely determined by a complex network of interactions between soluble cytokines and specific cytokine receptors on select sets of immune cells. Cytokines derived from CD4+ Th cells have an important role in this cytokine network. The encoding genes of at least 20 different Th cell-derived cytokines have been cloned, and in most cases the biological effects of the recombinant and natural cytokine proteins have been studied extensively. Of particular relevance for this chapter are the cytokines regulating IgE synthesis by B lymphocytes and the ones acting on eosinophils. IgE synthesis is induced by interleukin (IL)-4, and interferon (IFN)-γ suppresses this effect [1]. In addition to IL-4, the later described T cell-derived cytokine IL-13 also is able to induce IgE synthesis [2]. Major eosinophilotrophic cytokines are IL-5, IL-3 and granulocyte/macrophage colony-stimulating factor (GM-CSF). Various effects on eosinophils in different compartments of the body are controlled by these three cytokines. IL-5 in particular seems to be crucial for the development of eosinophilia [3].

SUBSETS OF CD4+ T LYMPHOCYTES

Many Th cells do not produce the complete set of known cytokines. Analysis of large panels of T-lymphocyte clones (TLC) randomly generated from murine spleen tissue indicated that murine Th cells fall into distinct subsets with respect to their cytokine secretion profile and hence to their function [4,5]. All Th cells produce certain cytokines in common (e.g. tumour necrosis factor (TNF)-α, GM-CSF and IL-3), but many T cells selectively produce either IL-2, IFN-γ and TNF-β (Th1 cells), or IL-4, IL-5, IL-6 and IL-10 (Th2 cells). Further studies in the mouse identified an additional subset of Th0 cells that produce most, if not all, cytokines simultaneously [6,7]. This intermediate subset may comprise precursor cells for the Th1 and Th2 subsets as well as fully mature effector cells.

Th0 responses are observed in reaction with various antigens. In response to intracellular micro-organisms, however, Th-cell responses are biased to high levels of IFN-γ and IL-2 and low levels of IL-4 and IL-5 (Th1 responses). These Th1 responses are protective, because IFN-γ effectively stimulates the intracellular killing of microbes in phagocytic cells. In contrast, in response to certain helminth species, Th-cell responses are biased to Th2 responses with low secretion of IFN-γ and IL-2 and high secretion of IL-4 and IL-5. In such cases Th2 responses are protective, because IL-4 induces IgE production and IL-5 promotes the production of eosinophils, both of which are considered to contribute to the expelling of the helminths.

Several immune diseases in the mouse and the human result from selective activation of T cells with an aberrant, non-protective cytokine secretion profile [8,9]. Comparative *in vitro* studies with human allergen-specific TLC from atopic and nonatopic individuals showed that eosinophilia and elevated serum levels of allergen-specific IgE are causally related with the predominant occurrence and activation of allergen-specific Th2 cells. In this chapter the functional properties of these cells and their role in the pathophysiology of atopic disease will be discussed.

ALLERGEN-SPECIFIC Th1 AND Th2 CELLS

ALLERGEN-SPECIFIC T-CELL CLONES

Allergen-induced proliferative responses can readily be monitored in peripheral blood mononuclear cells (PBMC) of atopic individuals, implicating the presence of allergen-specific T cells in the peripheral blood and, therefore, the possibility of cloning them from this compartment. Although such allergen-specific responses in PBMC of nonatopic control individuals with negative RAST scores for inhalation and food allergens are normally significantly lower [10], it also proved to be possible to clone allergen-specific T cells from these individuals [11].

Allergen-specific TLC from atopic and nonatopic individuals express identical levels of CD2, CD3-TCRα/β complex, CD4, CD11a, CD25, CD26, CD27, CD29 and CD45RA [12,13], both on rested and on stimulated cells. Comparing two-weeks-rested cells, the patients' TLC express higher levels of CD28 [13], a membrane-bound glycoprotein mediating an important co-stimulatory signal thought to prevent T-cell anergy [14]. Upon restimulation, however, TLC from both sources increase CD28 expression to comparable levels, suggesting that the transient difference on rested cells reflects different activation states rather than a property based on which T cells from atopics and nonatopics can be distinguished.

DIVERSITY OF ALLEGEN-SPECIFIC T-CELL RESPONSES

Dissection of the specificity of the T-cell response to complex allergenic entities such as house dust mite *Dermatophagoides pteronyssinus* (Dp), a ubiquitous source of indoor inhalation allergens, suggests that these T-cell responses are quite diverse, because of the variety of potential allergenic Dp proteins. Binding studies with large panels of sera from Dp-allergic patients identified at least seven major Dp allergens [15], Der p 1 to 7, to which more than 40% of the Dp allergic patients produce IgE, but several other Dp proteins may be recognized as well. Both in atopic and control individuals, a similar diversity is observed in the specific T-cell reactivity with Dp, in most cases including substantial reactivity with the major allergens Der p 1 and 2 [11,16–20].

Current studies in several laboratories are directed at the definition of the precise T-cell epitopes of allergenic proteins, which may be important for the design of novel forms of immunotherapy in which, to prevent cross-linking of

IgE on mast cells and basophils, synthetic peptides are used instead of native allergens. Studies on various allergens, including Der p 1 [18] and Der p 2 [19,20], have indicated that in most cases the allergen contains multiple T-cell epitopes that are dispersed throughout the molecule. Polyclonal T-cell responses to panels of overlapping synthetic peptides showed for instance that in individual donors up to six different epitopes can be distinguished within the Der p 2 molecule [19].

Adding to the diversity of Dp-specific T cells is their genetic restriction of antigen recognition, which may be in association with HLA-DR- [11,19,20], as well as HLA-DP- [21] and HLA-DQ-encoded molecules [22,23]. Due to the diversity in the protein and peptide specificities and the variable HLA-restriction patterns of allergen-reactive T cells, a clear association between allergy and a particular HLA haplotype is an exception rather than a rule.

ATOPIC PATIENTS HAVE ALLERGEN-SPECIFIC Th2 CELLS

Allergen (Dp)-specific TLC generated from the peripheral blood of atopic Dp-allergic (asthma or eczema) patients with high serum levels of Dp-specific IgE proved to be Th2 cells that, upon antigen-specific or mitogenic stimulation, produce high amounts of IL-4 and IL-5 but low levels of IFN-γ and IL-2 [12,13]. Despite the enormous diversity in the fine specificity of these Dp-specific TLC, their cytokine secretion profile and consequent function are strikingly similar. More recent studies in atopic patients have now confirmed the predominance of Th2 cells in responses to several inhalation allergens, including Dp [24], Dp major allergen Der p 1 [18], ryegrass (*Lolium perennes*) pollen [24,25], and domestic cat [23]. Dp-specific TLC from non-atopic control individuals, on the other hand, are Th1-like cells that produce high levels of IFN-γ and IL-2 without substantial IL-4 and IL-5 [12]. Allergen-specific Th1 and Th2 cells produce comparable amounts of GM-CSF, IL-3, IL-6 and TNF-α.

TLC specific for *Candida albicans* (CA) or tetanus toxoid (TT), generated either from Dp-allergic patients without CA- or TT-specific IgE or from non-allergic control, donors have an intermediate Th0 cytokine secretion profile [12]. Therefore, Th2 cells in atopics seem to be compartmentalized within the population of allergen-specific T cells.

REGULATION OF IgE SYNTHESIS BY Th1 AND Th2 CELLS

Th cells have to meet several functional conditions to be efficient helper cells for the induction and support of IgE synthesis by B cells. These conditions include a favourable cytokine secretion profile to induce the production of germline ε transcripts, the ability to provide an additional co-stimulatory signal via CD40 on the B-cell membrane to accomplish the actual isotype switch to IgE, and the lack of cytotoxicity towards antigen-presenting B cells. Only Th2 cells have all these properties.

CYTOKINE SECRETION PROFILES AND INDUCTION OF IgE SYNTHESIS

The function of an individual T-cell clone in a biological process can be related to the secretion level of a responsible cytokine (e.g. IL-2 in a T-cell proliferation assay) or to the secretion ratio of different cytokines if antagonizing cytokines are involved simultaneously. A relevant example is the induction of IgE synthesis by IL-4 and its inhibition by IFN-γ [26]. IL-4 induces the production of germline ε transcripts in B cells [27,28], which is a first critical step in the isotype switch to IgE [29]. IFN-γ downregulates IL-4-induced production of germline ε transcripts in PBMC, but not in highly purified B cells [30], implicating an indirect inhibitory effect requiring accessory cells or factors produced by these cells.

As a consequence of the high IL-4/IFN-γ secretion ratios of allergen-specific Th2 clones of atopic patients, supernatants of such clones were able to induce IgE synthesis in cultures of B-cell-enriched (50–70%) PBMC of non-atopic control individuals [12,13]. Supernatants of Th1 clones did not induce IgE synthesis and even inhibited the IgE-inducing properties of Th2 supernatants if added to the B cells simultaneously. Similar results were reported for supernatants of randomly cloned T cells [31,32] and allospecific TLC [26] with high and low IL-4/IFN-γ ratios. The recently described cytokine IL-13 is produced both by Th1 and Th2 cells and can, like IL-4, induce germline ε transcripts in purified B cells and IgE synthesis in PBMC [2]. However, the almost complete inhibition of IL-4-induced IgE synthesis by anti-IL-4 antibody [12,26], even in the presence of exogenous IL-13, and the finding that IL-4 knockout mice are not able to produce IgE [33], poses a question as to the relative contribution of IL-13 to the regulation of IgE production.

A CONTACT-MEDIATED SECOND SIGNAL IS REQUIRED FOR IL-4-INDUCED IgE SYNTHESIS

If highly purified B cells are cultured in the presence of IL-4, germline ε transcripts can be detected but not the mature full length IgE heavy chain transcripts [27] nor, of course, secreted IgE. Only after reconstitution of the cultures with T cells can IL-4-induced IgE synthesis be restored [1]. No known soluble cytokine or combination of cytokines can replace this T-cell function. The additional signal required to support IL-4-induced IgE synthesis is provided by CD4+ T cells via an MHC-unrestricted physical T/B cell contact. This was made particularly clear by the demonstration that T and B cells do not have to be histocompatible to mediate the signal [34], and that separation of T and B cells by a semipermeable membrane abolishes

IL-4-induced IgE production [30,34]. Mimicking the supportive effect of CD4+ T cells are certain monoclonal antibodies to CD40 antigen [35,36], a glycoprotein expressed on the B-cell membrane. The finding that isolated membranes of stimulated CD4+ T cells were still able to support IL-4-induced IgE synthesis [37] suggested the inducible expression of a CD40 ligand on CD4+ T cells. Indeed, this ligand was recently identified and described as TNF-related activation protein (TRAP) [38] or CD40 ligand (CD40L) [39]. It appears to be a transmembrane protein required for immunoglobulin class switching in general, rather than being specific for the isotype switch to IgE. It was shown that patients suffering from X chromosome-linked hyper-IgM immunodeficiency have deletions or point mutations in the CD40L-encoding mRNA, clustered in the part encoding the extracellular domain [38,39]. The consequent expression of an abnormal CD40L molecule is that B cells of these patients are not able to switch from IgM to other isotypes. It may be speculated that triggering of CD40 activates isotype non-specific DNA recombination, which in the presence of IL-4 is directed to IgE.

In principle, activated Th1 and Th2 cells can both efficiently trigger CD40 on B lymphocytes and support exogenous IL-4-induced IgE synthesis. In the case of Th1 cells, however, this helper function is evident only if the T cells are pre-activated separately from the B cells. If the T cells are activated in the presence of the B cells, for instance with immobilized anti-CD3 antibody in cultures with normal B cells or with specific antigen presented by autologous Epstein–Barr virus (EBV)-transformed B cells, the co-stimulatory effect of Th1 cells is masked to a considerable extent, due to their cytolytic potential [40].

CYTOLYTIC ACTIVITY OF Th1 CELLS TOWARDS AUTOLOGOUS APC

Classically, CD4+ T cells were considered to be helper T cells for Ig production after MHC class II-restricted antigen recognition on antigen-presenting B cells, and CD8+ T cells were defined as being cytotoxic for target cells presenting viral or other endogenous peptides in association with MHC class I molecules. However, the functional distinction of CD4+ and CD8+ T cells as based on these parameters is far from absolute: CD8+ T cells may secrete cytokines such as IL-2 and IL-4 [9,31] which are important in the regulation of Ig production and, on the other hand, subsets of CD4+ T cells have cytolytic potentials towards APC upon MHC class II-restricted antigen recognition. In the mouse [41,42] and later in the human [13,43], cytotoxic CD4+ T cells were found to be restricted to the Th1 subset. Within the panels of allergen (Dp)-specific TLC, the Th1 clones showed strong cytolytic activities towards peripheral blood monocytes and EBV-transformed B cells upon antigen-specific or anti-CD3-mediated stimulation [13,40]. As a result of this lytic activity, total Ig secretion by the EBV-B cells was strongly decreased. Comparable results were found for all individual isotypes, including IgE. Strikingly, none of the Dp-specific Th2 clones from the atopic patients were cytotoxic and, instead, increased Ig production by EBV-B cells.

The present data indicate that the synthesis of IgE by B cells is controlled by a complex combination of signals and that CD4+ T cells play a central regulatory role in this process. In this respect, allergen-specific Th2 cells of atopic patients differ from allergen-specific Th1 cells of healthy control individuals in that they efficiently induce and support Ig synthesis in general and IgE synthesis in particular. These properties follow from their lack of cytotoxicity towards antigen-presenting B cells and their capacity to provide co-stimulation via CD40. In addition, their high IL-4/IFN-γ secretion ratios favour isotype switch to IgE. Selective activation of allergen-specific Th2 cells in atopic patients is therefore considered to be causally related with the elevated serum levels of allergen-specific IgE.

Th1 AND Th2 CELLS IN THE INFLAMMATORY LATE PHASE RESPONSE

As discussed above, allergen-specific Th2 cells have a major role in the regulation of IgE synthesis. However, increased production of allergen-specific IgE and the consequent immediate hypersensitivity to these allergens are only part of the pathophysiology of atopic disease. Normally, the immediate allergic response is followed by an inflammatory late phase response, 6–24 h after allergen exposure. Frequent or continuous allergen encounters may lead to chronically inflammed tissue lesions. Different lines of evidence suggest an important regulatory role of Th2 cells in the late phase response, as well.

HIGH NUMBERS OF ALLERGEN-SPECIFIC Th2 CELLS IN AFFECTED TISSUES

The histological appearance of atopic lesional skin is characterized by perivascular cellular infiltrates in the dermis, mainly consisting of CD4+ T cells [44,45]. The additional accumulation of potential antigen-presenting cells and the high expression of HLA-DR on the infiltrating CD4+ T cells [46] indicate an active local T-cell reactivity in the lesional areas. It should be mentioned that dermal infiltrates hardly contain any B cells, suggesting that IgE synthesis does not occur locally in the skin.

These histological features lead to the assumption that skin lesions in atopic dermatitis, as induced by exposure to certain allergens, are associated with local intradermal reactivity of CD4+ T cells that specifically react with these particular allergens. This hypothesis was confirmed by the analysis of the frequency of allergen-specific T cells in panels of randomly generated TLC from lesional skin biopsies, applying a high-efficiency cloning protocol. Reactivity was screened with relevant allergens, as selected on the basis of high RAST scores (i.e. high levels of specific IgE) in the serum of the patients concerned. Studies with house dust mite [47] and ryegrass pollen (*Lolium perennes*) allergens [25] indicated increased frequencies (up to 47%) of specific TLC in panels from inflamed skin, compared to autologous blood (3% or less). Many of the allergen-specific TLC both from the peripheral blood and the skin lesions were Th2 cells with high IL-4/IFN-γ secretion ratios. These findings suggest the accumulation of allergen-specific Th2 cells in lesional skin areas, which is in agreement with the demonstration in atopic patients of selective mRNA expression of the Th2-associated gene cluster IL-3, IL-4, IL-5 and GM-CSF in skin biopsies, 24 h after intradermal allergen (*Phleum pratense*) challenge [48]. Applying *in situ* mRNA hybridization techniques, increased frequencies of Th2 cells could also be detected in bronchoalveolar lavage material from atopic asthma patients [49]. Although in the latter case the specificity of the Th2 cells is unknown, it is tempting to speculate on an active role of allergen-specific Th2 cells in the allergic inflamation in atopic skin and lung tissue.

An unanswered question is whether the high frequencies of allergen-specific Th2 cells at the sites of inflammation are due to selective homing or to selective local activation and expansion. Although regulation on the level of T-cell homing cannot be excluded, indirect evidence suggests that local presentation of allergens is largely facilitated by trapping of circulating allergen-IgE immune complexes by the low-affinity IgE-Fc receptor (FcεRII=CD23), expressed on local APC.

IgE-FACILITATED ALLERGEN PRESENTATION (FAP) IN ATOPIC PATIENTS

The efficiency of antigen presentation to T cells can be strongly increased by Fc receptor (FcR)-mediated trapping and endocytosis of circulating immune-complexed antigen by the APC. FcγR-focused uptake of IgG-complexed antigen and its subsequent presentation to T cells has been described *in vitro* for antigen-presenting B cells [50,51] and more professional types of APC [52]. Compared to random fluid phase endocytosis, this mechanism of facilitated antigen presentation (FAP) was shown to lower the minimally required antigen dose for efficient T-cell activation 100–1000-fold.

The uptake and presentation of IgE-complexed allergens by APC can be focused in a similar way via CD23 [53,54]. CD23 expression on various types of APC, including monocytes [55] and Langerhans cells [56], is upregulated by IL-4. Consequently, IL-4-containing supernatants of activated allergen-specific Th2 clones readily increase CD23 expression, even on the normally low CD23-expressing monocytic cell line U937 [47]. It is therefore plausible to assume that the high IL-4 levels of allergen-specific Th2 cells contribute to the increased expression of CD23 on APC in atopic patients [57].

Functional *in vitro* experiments using a model with CD23-expressing EBV-B cells indicated highly efficient FAP of allergens after preincubation of the allergens in serum of atopic patients with a corresponding allergy [58]. Serum from Der p 2- or cat-allergic patients with high serum titres of specific IgE was preincubated with low doses of the respective allergen, to allow the formation of allergen-IgE complexes. Subsequently, the pretreated serum was incubated with the EBV-B cells to allow trapping of the allergen-IgE complexes. Cells were then washed thoroughly to remove unbound allergen, and co-cultured with allergen-specific autologous T cells. FAP was made evident by the capacity of these conditioned APC to induce T-cell proliferation using a 1000-fold lower allergen concentration than normally needed in a standard T-cell proliferation assay in which T cells, APC and allergen are brought together without pretreatments. Additional experiments confirmed the involvement of IgE and CD23 in the FAP effect:

1 Serum of nonatopic control individuals without specific IgE was ineffective.
2. Pretreatment of the atopic serum with anti-IgE antibody completely abrogated FAP, whereas anti-IgG antibody did not.
3. Pretreatment of the APC with anti-CD23 antibody inhibited FAP significantly and an isotype-matched control antibody did not.
4. FAP still occurred if the APC were pre-incubated with complexed serum at 4°C, not allowing random fluid phase internalization of free antigens.

Although the cascade of events in the ongoing T-cell reactivity in chronically inflamed atopic tissue remains enigmatic, some speculations can be made based on the above-described observations. The proposed mechanism (Figure 5.1) completely depends on the presence of allergens. It is unclear, so far, how and where allergens enter the system, but they may penetrate via the intestines or via lesional areas in the skin or the lungs where the epithelium is damaged. Upon entry they will be complexed by circulating allergen-specific IgE, produced in the draining lymphoid tissues. The allergen-IgE complexes are easily trapped by CD23-expressing APC, for instance dendritic cells in the dermis. By means of FAP, locally infiltrated allergen-specific Th2 cells are efficiently activated to produce IL-4 which, in turn, further upregulates or maintains CD23 expression on the APC. Minute amounts of allergen would be sufficient to keep this mechanism going. It should be realized that high affinity IgE receptors (FcRεRI) that, in contrast to CD23, are able to bind uncomplexed IgE, may add significantly to the IgE-mediated FAP capacity of APC.

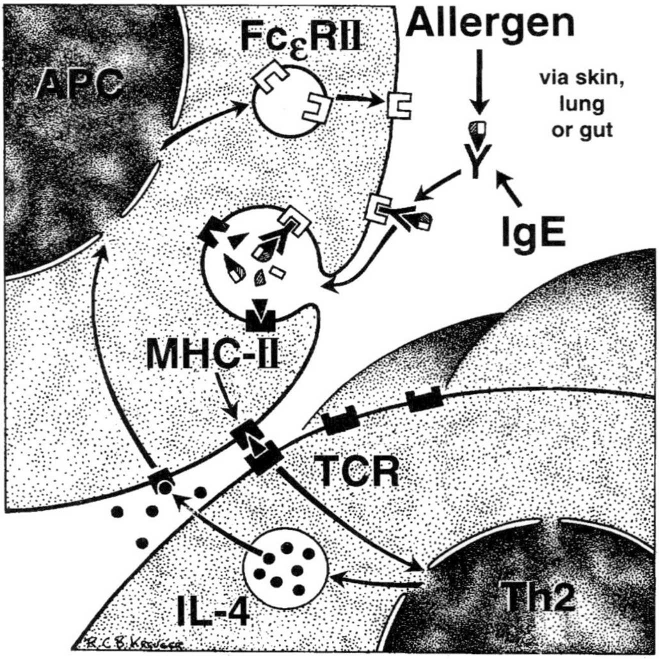

Figure 5.1. Proposed FAP mechanism explaining ongoing reactivity of allergen-specific T cells in atopic lesions (further explained in the text)

Th2 CELL-DERIVED IL-5 IS CRUCIAL FOR DEVELOPMENT OF EOSINOPHILIA

A discussion of the role of Th2 cells in eosinophilia is included in this chapter, because local tissue eosinophilia, as an important component of the late phase allergic response, is IgE-dependent, albeit indirectly. For example, the initial influx of eosinophils is induced by chemotactic mediators released by allergen-triggered IgE-sensitized mast cells and basophils. In chronically inflamed lesions, cytokines secreted by continuously activated Th2 cells will add to the chemotactic signals. Many of the consecutive events in the development of systemic and local tissue eosinophilia are controlled by soluble cytokines. *In vitro* studies with recombinant cytokines have indicated that eosinophil differentiation and proliferation in the bone marrow, the extension of their lifespan in the periphery, their migration into the sites of inflammation, and the activation of their destructive function, in principle, can all be induced by any of the individual Th2-derived cytokines IL-5, GM-CSF and IL-3 [reviewed in 59]. Although GM-CSF and IL-3 are produced in similar amounts by Th1 cells [3], eosinophilia is not a common or pronounced feature of typical Th1-mediated diseases, e.g. contact allergy [60] or tuberculoid leprosy [61], suggesting a critical role for IL-5 in the develoment of eosinophilia. In a study with eosinophils from the bone marrow or the blood of nonatopic donors, supernatants of activated Th1 and Th2 clones and neutralizing anti-cytokine antibodies, the relative contributions of the three individual cytokines were analysed in the regulation of sequential events in the development of eosinophilia [3]. It could be demonstrated that the step critically depending on IL-5 is the expansion of immature committed eosinophils in the bone marrow. Eosinophil expansion was strongly induced by Th2 supernatants but not by Th1 supernatants and it could be blocked completely and selectively by anti-IL-5 antibody. As Th1 and Th2 supernatants were equally chemoattractive for peripheral blood eosinophils, the influx of eosinophils in affected atopic tissues may result from local T-cell activity in general in combination with systemic eosinophilia, rather than from the Th2 cytokine profile of the activated T cells, *per se*. On the other hand, it may be these continuously activated Th2 cells that are the major source of IL-5 required to develop systemic eosinophilia.

INTERVENTION IN Th2 CYTOKINE SECRETION

The causal relation between predominant activation of Th2 cells in response to allergens and the pathophysiology of atopic disease is a generally accepted concept [62,63] and is summarized in Table 5.1. The apparently important, in some cases decisive, effects of Th2-derived cytokines in certain pathological events stress the need for research on possibilities to intervene in their production. Two possible intervention strategies will be discussed briefly.

FUNCTIONAL INACTIVATION OF ALLERGEN-SPECIFIC T CELLS WITH SYNTHETIC PEPTIDES

Current T-cell desensitization protocols with native allergens may give rise to anaphylactic reactions mediated by pre-formed allergen-specific IgE. In contrast, linear peptide fragments of allergens are not readily recognized by allergen-specific IgE [64], but are still able to silence specific T cells in experimental models. Novel desensitization protocols with synthetic allergen peptides may therefore prove to be useful in preventing over-production of Th2 cytokines.

Indeed, animal model studies showed that allergen-specific T-cell responses to native allergens could be downregulated *in vivo* by prior intranasal [65] or subcutaneous [66] administration of epitope-containing peptides of Der p 1 or Fel d 1, respectively. *In vitro* experiments with human cells demonstrated that Der p 1-specific T cells can be made functionally inactive with high doses of synthetic peptides containing the relevant epitope

Table 5.1. Functional subsets of allergen-specific human Th1 and Th2 cells

	Th1 from controls	Th2 from patients
Phenotype		
CD3-TCRα/β	+	+
CD4	+	+
CD8	−	−
Lymphokine profile		
IFN-γ	high	low
IL-2	high	low
IL-4	low	high
IL-5	low	high
IL-6	low	low
GM-CSF	high	high
TNF-α	high	high
IL-3	high	high
Functions		
cytokine-mediated IgE help	−	+
contact-mediated Ig help	+	+
cytolysis of APC	+	−
CD23 upregulation on APC	+	++
eosinophil expansion	−	+

Adapted from Kapsenberg *et al.*, *Eur J Dermatol* 1992; **2**: 601–607

[20,67–69]. Thus anergized T cells show increased CD25 and decreased TCR expression and, interestingly, increased IFN-γ production [69]. Although the diverse specificities of T-cell responses to complex allergenic entities would suggest the need for mixtures of peptides of several proteins to achieve successful desensitization, these exciting results may lead to the development of more efficient protocols for immunotherapy (see Chapter 11).

MODULATION OF CYTOKINE PROFILES BY SOLUBLE STEERING FACTORS

The cytokine secretion profiles of cloned T cells are relatively stable and have properties that are not dictated by the epitope or HLA specificity [70], nor by the Vβ usage of the TCR [18,19]. Compared to antigen-specific stimulation with APC, identical cytokine profiles are found after mitogenic stimulation with lectins or monoclonal antibodies to CD3 or CD2 [13]. These cytokine profiles can be modulated, however, by factors derived from APC and/or accessory cells. For instance, if cloned Th0 cells are stimulated in the presence of prostaglandin (PG)E_2, a factor produced by various cell types including APC, the production of IL-2 and IFN-γ is suppressed, whereas the production of IL-4 and IL-5 is upregulated [71,72], thus giving rise to a Th2-like cytokine profile. The cytokine IL-12, produced by various APC types, strongly increases IFN-γ production by stimulated T cells [73]. In the case of established TLC, such PGE_2- and IL-12-induced effects are only transient, because upon subsequent restimulation in the absence of these factors, the original cytokine profile is observed again [74,75,76]. *In vivo*, on the other hand, modulatory factors may have long-lasting effects. Mouse model experiments showed that the Th2-associated susceptibility of BALB/C mice to *Leishmania major* infection could be overcome by treatment with anti-IL-4 and IL-12, both of which reversed the non-protective Th2 cytokine profile of responding T cells [70,77]. In contrast, treatment of *Leishmania*-resistant mouse strains with anti-IFN-γ resulted in a Th1 to Th2 shift and, thus, susceptibility to infection [79]. Several other soluble factors are known to skew the cytokine profile of activated T cells, including IL-10 [80], hormones [81] and TGF-γ [82].

The precise mechanisms by which these and other factors exert their effects are still the subject of investigation, but the use of such knowledge may be helpful for the design of future therapies for diseases that are causally related to unbalanced cytokine production by T cells.

REFERENCES

1 Pène J, Rousset F, Brière F *et al.* IgE production by normal human lymphocytes is induced by interleukin 4 and suppressed by interferons γ and α and prostaglandin E_2. *Proc Natl Acad Sci USA* 1988; **85**: 6880–6884.

2 Punnonen J, Aversa G, Cocks BG *et al.* Interleukin 13 induces interleukin 4-independent IgG_4 and IgE synthesis and CD23 expression by human B cells. *Proc Natl Acad Sci USA* 1993; **90**: 3730–3734.

3 Wierenga EA, Backx B, Snoek M *et al.* Relative contributions of human types 1 and 2 T helper cell-derived eosinophilotrophic cytokines to development of eosinophilia. *Blood* 1993; **82**: 1471–1479.

4 Mosmann TR, Cherwinski H, Bond MW *et al.* Two types of murine helper T cell clone. I. Definition according to profiles of lymphokine activities and secreted proteins. *J Immunol* 1986; **136**: 2348–2357.

5 Mosmann TR, Moore KW. The role of IL-10 in crossregulation of Th1 and Th2 responses. *Immunoparasitol Today* 1991; A49–A53.

6 Firestein GS, Roeder WD, Laxer JA *et al.* A new murine CD4+ T cell subset with an unrestricted cytokine profile. *J Immunol* 1989; **143**: 518–525.

7 Street NE, Schumacher JH, Fong TAT *et al.* Heterogeneity of mouse helper T cells: Evidence from bulk cultures and limiting dilution cloning for precursors of Th1 and Th2 cells. *J Immunol* 1990; **144**: 1629–1639.

8 Scott P, Kaufmann SHE. The role of T-cell subsets and cytokines in the regulation of infection. *Immunol Today* 1991; **12**: 346–348.

9 Salgame P, Abrams JS, Clayberger C *et al.* Differing lymphokine profiles of functional subsets of human CD4 and CD8 T-cell clones. *Science* 1991; **254**: 279–282.

10 Rawle FC, Mitchell EB, Platts-Mills TAE. T-cell responses to the major allergen from the house dust mite *Dermatophagoides pteronyssinus*, antigen P1: comparison

of patients with asthma, atopic dermatitis, and perennial rhinitis. *J Immunol* 1984; **133**: 195–201.
11 Wierenga EA, Snoek M, Bos JD *et al*. Comparison of diversity and function of house dust mite-specific T-lymphocyte clones from atopic and non-atopic donors. *Eur J Immunol* 1990; **20**: 1519–1526.
12 Wierenga EA, Snoek M, De Groot C *et al*. Evidence for compartmentalization of functional subsets of CD4+ T lymphocytes in atopic patients. *J Immunol* 1990; **144**: 4651–4656.
13 Wierenga EA, Snoek M, Jansen HM *et al*. Human atopen-specific Types 1 and 2 T helper cell clones. *J Immunol* 1991; **147**: 2942–2949.
14 Schwartz RH. Costimulation of T lymphocytes: the role of CD28, CTLA-4 and B7/BB1 in interleukin-2 production and immunotherapy. *Cell* 1992; **71**: 1065–1068.
15 Thomas WR. Mite allergens groups I–VII. A catalogue of enzymes. *Clin Exp Allergy* 1993; **23**: 350–353.
16 O'Hehir RE, Garman RD, Greenstein JL *et al*. The specificity and function of T-cell responsiveness to allergens. *Ann Rev Immunol* 1991; **9**: 67–95.
17 O'Brien RM, Thomas WR, Wootton AM. T-cell responses to the purified allergens from the house dust mite *Dermatophagoides pteronyssinus*. *J Allergy Clin Immunol* 1992; **89**: 1021–1031.
18 Yssel H, Johnson KE, Schneider PV *et al*. T cell activation-inducing epitopes of the house dust mite allergen Der p I. Proliferation and lymphokine production patterns by Der p I-specific CD4+ T cell clones. *J Immunol* 1992; **148**: 738–745.
19 Van Neerven RJJ, Van't Hof W, Ringrose JH *et al*. T-cell epitopes of house dust mite major allergen Der p II. *J Immunol* 1993; **151**: 2326–2335.
20 O'Hehir RE, Verhoef A, Panagiotopoulou E *et al*. Analysis of human T-cell responses to the group II allergen of *Dermatophagoides Spp*. (house dust mite): Localisation of major antigenic sites. *J Allergy Clin Immunol* 1993; **92**: 105–113.
21 Higgins JA, Lamb JR, Marsh SGE *et al*. Peptide-induced nonresponsiveness of HLA-DP restricted human T cells reactive with *Dermatophagoides Spp*. (house dust mite). *J Allergy Clin Immunol* 1992; **90**: 749–756.
22 Verhoef A, Higgins JA, Thorpe CJ *et al*. Clonal analysis of the atopic immune response to the group II allergen of the house dust mite *Dermatophagoides Spp*. (Identification of HLA-DR and DQ restricted T-cell epitopes). *Int Immunol* 1993; **5**: 1589–1597.
23 Van Neerven RJJ, Van de Pol MM, Van Milligen FJ *et al*. Characterization of cat dander-specific T lymphocytes from atopic patients. *J Immunol* 1994; **152**: 4203–4210.
24 Parronchi P, Macchia D, Piccinni MP *et al*. Allergen- and bacterial antigen-specific T-cell clones established from atopic donors show a different profile of cytokine production. *Proc Natl Acad Sci USA* 1991; **88**: 4538–4542.
25 Ramb-Lindhauer Ch, Feldmann A, Rotte M *et al*. Characterization of grass pollen reactive T-cell lines derived from lesional atopic skin. *Arch Dermatol Res* 1991; **283**: 71–76.
26 Pène J, Rousset F, Brière F *et al*. IgE production by normal human B cells induced by alloreactive T-cell clones is mediated by IL-4 and suppressed by IFN-γ. *J Immunol* 1988; **141**: 1218–1224.
27 Jabara HH, Schneider LC, Shapira SK *et al*. Induction of germ-line and mature Cε transcripts in human B cells stimulated with rIL-4 and EBV. *J Immunol* 1990; **145**: 3468–3473.
28 Gauchat JF, Lebman DA, Coffman RL *et al*. Structure and expression of germline ε transcripts in human B cells induced by interleukin 4 to switch to IgE production. *J Exp Med* 1990; **172**: 463–473.
29 Rothman P, Li SC, Alt F. The molecular events in heavy chain class-switching.

Semin Immunol 1989; **1**: 65–77.
30 Gascan H, Gauchat JF, de Waal Malefyt R *et al*. Regulation of human IgE synthesis. *Clin Exp Allergy* 1991; **21** Suppl 1: 162–166.
31 Paliard X, de Waal-Malefijt R, Yssel H *et al*. Simultaneous production of interleukin 2, interleukin 4 and interferon gamma by activated human CD4+ and CD8+ T-cell clones. *J Immunol* 1988; **141**: 849–855.
32 Maggi E, Del Prete G, Macchia D *et al*. Profiles of lymphokine activities and helper function for IgE in human T-cell clones. *Eur J Immunol* 1988; **18**: 1045–1050.
33 Kühn R, Rajewski K, Müller W. Generation and analysis of interleukin 4 deficient mice. *Science* 1991; **254**: 707–710.
34 Parronchi P, Tiri A, Macchia D *et al*. Noncognate contact-dependent B cell activation can promote IL-4-dependent *in vitro* human IgE synthesis. *J Immunol* 1990; **144**: 2102–2108.
35 Jabara HH, Fu SM, Geha RS *et al*. CD40 and IgE: synergism between anti-CD40 monoclonal antibody and interleukin 4 in the induction of IgE synthesis by highly purified human B cells. *J Exp Med* 1990; **172**: 1861–1864.
36 Gascan H, Gauchat JF, Aversa GG *et al*. Anti-CD40 monoclonal antibodies or CD4+ T cell clones and IL-4 induce IgG_4 and IgE switching in purified human B cells via different signalling pathways. *J Immunol* 1991; **147**: 8–13.
37 De Vries JE, Gauchat JF, Aversa GG *et al*. Regulation of IgE synthesis by cytokines. *Curr Opin Immunol* 1991; **3**: 851–858.
38 Korthäuer U, Graf D, Mages HW *et al*. Defective expression of T-cell CD40 ligand causes X-linked immunodeficiency with hyper-IgM. *Nature* 1993; **361**: 539–541.
39 DiSanto JP, Bonnefoy JY, Gauchat JF *et al*. CD40 ligand mutations in X-linked immunodeficiency with hyper-IgM. *Nature* 1993; **361**: 541–543.
40 Wierenga EA, Snoek M, Van der Heijden FL *et al*. Regulation of immunoglobulin E synthesis by T-cell clones. In: Godard Ph, Bousquet J, Michel FB (eds) *Advances in Allergology and Clinical Immunology*. Carnforth: Parthenon Publishing, 1992: 23–31.
41 Tite JP, Janeway CA. Cloned helper T cells can kill B lymphoma cells in the presence of specific antigen: Ia restriction and cognate vs. noncognate interactions in cytolysis. *Eur J Immunol* 1984; **14**: 878–886.
42 Tite JP, Powell MB, Ruddle NH. Protein-antigen specific Ia-restricted cytolytic T cells: analysis of frequency, target cell susceptibility, and mechanism of cytolysis. *J Immunol* 1985; **135**: 25–33.
43 Del Prete GF, de Carli M, Ricci M *et al*. Helper activity for immunoglobulin synthesis of T helper type 1 (Th1) and Th2 human T-cell clones: The help of Th1 clones is limited by their cytotoxic capacity. *J Exp Med* 1991; **174**: 809–813.
44 Zachary CB, MacDonald DM. Quantitative analysis of T lymphocyte subsets in atopic eczema, using monoclonal antibodies and flow cytofluorimetry. *Br J Dermatol* 1983; **108**: 411–422.
45 Sillevis Smitt JH, Bos JD, Hulsebosch HJ *et al*. *In situ* immunophenotyping of antigen presenting cells and T-cell subsets in atopic dermatitis. *Clin Exp Dermatol* 1986; **11**: 159–168.
46 Zachary CB, Allen MH, MacDonald DM. *In situ* quantification of T lymphocyte subsets and Langerhans cells in the inflammatory infiltrate of atopic eczema. *Br J Dermatol* 1985; **112**: 149–156.
47 Van der Heijden FL, Wierenga EA, Bos JD *et al*. High frequency of IL-4-producing CD4+ allergen-specific T lymphocytes in atopic dermatitis lesional skin. *J Invest Dermatol* 1991; **97**: 389–394.
48 Kay AB, Ying S, Varney V *et al*. Messenger RNA expression of the cytokine gene

cluster IL-3, IL-4, IL-5, and GM-CSF in allergen-induced late-phase cutaneous reactions in atopic subjects. *J Exp Med* 1991; **173**: 775–778.

49 Robinson SD, Hamid Q, Ying S *et al.* Predominant Th2-like bronchoalveolar T lymphocyte population in atopic asthma. *N Engl J Med* 1992; **326**: 298–304.

50 Chesnut RW, Grey HM. Studies on the capacity of B cells to serve as antigen-presenting cells. *J Immunol* 1981; **126**: 1075–1079.

51 Rock KL, Benacerraf B, Abbas AK. Antigen presentation by hapten-specific B lymphocytes. *J Exp Med* 1984; **160**: 1102–1113.

52 Celis E, Zurawski VR, Chang TW. Regulation of T-cell function by antibodies: Enhancement of the response of human T-cell clones to hepatitis B surface antigen by antigen-specific monoclonal antibodies. *Proc Natl Acad Sci USA* 1984; **81**: 6846–6850.

53 Kehry MR, Yamashita LC. Low-affinity IgE receptor (CD23) function on mouse B cells: role in IgE-dependent antigen focusing. *Proc Natl Acad Sci USA* 1989; **86**; 7556–7560.

54 Pirron U, Schlunck T, Prinz JC *et al.* IgE-dependent antigen focusing by human B lymphocytes is mediated by the low-affinity receptor for IgE. *Eur J Immunol* 1990; **20**: 1547–1551.

55 Vercelli D, Jabara HH, Lee BW *et al.* Human recombinant interleukin 4 induces FcεR2/CD23 on normal human monocytes. *J Exp Med* 1988; **167**: 1406–1416.

56 Bieber T, Rieger A, Neuchrist C *et al.* Induction of FcεR2/CD23 on human epidermal Langerhans cells by human recombinant interleukin 4 and γ interferon. *J Exp Med* 1989; **170**: 309–314.

57 Borish L, Pellegrini J, Rabson A. Increased expression of low affinity IgE receptors in patients with allergic disorders: Correlation with IgE concentration. *Int J Immunopathol Pharmacol* 1990; **3**: 1–9.

58 Van der Heijden FL, Van Neerven RJJ, Van Katwijk M *et al.* Serum-IgE-facilitated allergen presentation in atopic disease. *J Immunol* 1993; **150**: 3643–3650.

59 Weller PF. Roles of eosinophils in allergy. *Curr Opin Immunol* 1992; **4**: 782–787.

60 Kapsenberg ML, Wierenga EA, Stiekema FEM *et al.* Th1 lymphokine production profiles of nickel-specific CD4+ T lymphocyte clones from nickel contact allergic and non-allergic individuals. *J Invest Dermatol* 1992; **98**: 59–63.

61 Haanen JBAG, de Waal Malefijt R, Res PCM *et al.* Selection of a human T helper type 1-like T cell subset by mycobacteria. *J Exp Med* 1991; **174**: 583–592.

62 Kapsenberg ML, Wierenga EA, Bos JD *et al.* Functional subsets of allergen-reactive human CD4+ T cells. *Immunol Today* 1991; **12**: 392–395.

63 Romagnani S. Lymphokine production by human T cells in disease states. *Ann Rev Immunol* 1994; **12**: 227–257.

64 Van't Hof W, Driedijk PC, Van den Berg M *et al.* Epitope mapping of the *Dermatophagoides pteronyssinus* house dust mite major allergen Der p II using overlapping synthetic peptides. *Mol Immunol* 1991; **28**: 1225–1232.

65 Hoyne GF, O'Hehir RE, Wraith DC *et al.* Inhibition of T cell and antibody response to house dust mite allergen by inhalation of the dominant T-cell epitope in naive and sensitized mice. *J Exp Med* 1993; **178**: 1783–1788.

66 Briner TJ, Kuo MC, Keating KM *et al.* Peripheral T-cell tolerance induced in naive and primed mice by sucutaneous injection of peptides from the major cat allergen Fel d I. *Proc Natl Acad Sci USA* 1993; **90**: 7608–7612.

67 O'Hehir RE, Aguilar BA, Schmidt TJ *et al.* Functional inactivation of *Dermatophagoides spp*. (house dust mite) reactive human T-cell clones. *Clin Exp Allergy* 1991; **21**: 209–215.

68 O'Hehir RE, Busch R, Rothbard JB *et al.* An *in vitro* model of peptide-mediated immunomodulation of the human T-cell response to *Dermatophagoides spp* (house

dust mite). *J Allergy Clin Immunol* 1991; **87**: 1120–1127.
69 O'Hehir RE, Yssel H, Verma S *et al.* Clonal analysis of differential lymphokine production in peptide and superantigen-induced T-cell anergy. *Int Immunol* 1991; **3**: 819–826.
70 Van Neerven RJJ, Van de Pol MM, Wierenga EA *et al.* Peptide specificity and HLA restriction do not dictate lymphokine production by allergen-specific T lymphocyte clones. *Immunology* 1994; **82**: 351–356.
71 Snijdewint FGM, Kalinski P, Wierenga EA *et al.* Prostaglandin E_2 differentially modulates cytokine secretion profiles of human T helper lymphocytes. *J Immunol* 1993; **150**: 5321–5329.
72 Hilkens CMU, Vermeulen H, Van Neerven RJJ *et al.* Differential modulation of T helper type 1 (Th1) and T helper type 2 (Th2) cytokine secretion by prostaglandin E_2 critically depends on interleukin 2. *Eur J Immunol* 1995; **25**: 59–63.
73 Trinchieri G. Interleukin-12 and its role in the generation of Th1 cells. *Immunol Today* 1993; **14**: 335–338.
74 Manetti R, Gerosa F, Giudizi MG *et al.* Interleukin 12 induces stable priming for interferon γ (IFN-γ) production during differentiation of human T helper (Th) cells and transient IFN-γ production in established Th2 cell clones. *J Exp Med* 1994; **179**: 1273–1283.
75 Yssel H, Fasler S, de Vries JE *et al.* IL-12 transiently induces IFN-γ transcription and protein synthesis in human CD4+ allergen-specific Th2 T cell clones. *Int Immunol* 1994; **6**: 1091–1096.
76 Hilkens CMU, Snijders A, Snijdewint FGM *et al.* Modulation of T-cell cytokine secretion by accessory cell-derived products. *Eur Respir J* 1996; **9**: Suppl. 27: 90s–94s.
77 Sypeck JP, Chung CL, Mayor SEH *et al.* Resolution of cutaneous Leishmaniasis: interleukin 12 initiates a protective T helper type 1 immune response. *J Exp Med* 1993; **177**: 1797–1802.
78 Sadick MD, Heinzel BJ, Holaday RT *et al.* Cure of murine Leishmaniasis with anti-IL-4 monoclonal antibody. Evidence for a interferon γ-independent mechanism. *J Exp Med* 1990; **171**: 115–127.
79 Belosevic M, Finbloom DS, van der Meide PH *et al.* Administration of monoclonal anti-IFN-γ antibodies *in vivo* abrogates natural resistance of C3H/HeN mice to infection with *Leishmania major*. *J Immunol* 1989; **143**: 266–274.
80 Sher A, Gazeeinelli RT, Oswald I *et al.* Role of T-cell derived cytokines in the down regulation of immune responses in parasitic and retroviral infection. *Immunol Rev* 1992; **127**: 183–204.
81 Daynes RA, Araneo BA, Dowell TA *et al.* Regulation of murine lymphokine production *in vivo*. III The lymphoid tissue microenvironment exerts regulatory influences over T helper cell function. *J Immunol* 1990; **171**: 979–996.
82 Swain SL, Huston G, Tonkonogy S *et al.* TGF-β and IL-4 cause helper T cell precursors to develop into distinct effector helper T cells that differ in lymphokine secretion pattern and cell surface phenotype. *J Immunol* 1991; **147**: 2991–3000.

6 Molecular Analysis of House Dust Mite Allergens

WAYNE R. THOMAS
Institute For Child Health Research, West Perth, Australia

SCOPE OF HOUSE DUST MITE ALLERGY

INTRODUCTION

House dust mites are prevalent in all but the driest of environments. About 10–15% of the population is allergic to mites and the allergy is strongly associated with asthma, allergic rhinitis and eczema [1–3]. Mite exposure has also been associated with chronic rhinosinusitis, where interestingly the immunological correlation is stronger with IgG antibody than IgE [4]. In this respect it must be remembered that although the interaction of IgE on mast cells and allergen releases inflammatory mediators, allergic inflammation may be induced independently by lymphokines released from T cells [5]. Similarly, desensitization produced from the injection of increasing doses of antigens can be achieved independent of alterations in antibody [6,7]. Hence clinical improvement occurs after a few months while IgE antibody first increases and then declines slowly over a period of years. IgG antibody is induced by immunotherapy but does not always correlate with clinical improvement when individual patients are considered. The immune response to allergens thus poses some intriguing questions into the nature of the inflammation, the different manifestations of disease, the mechanisms of desensitization and why only a minority of the population is affected. Fundamental to answering these questions and developing more informative diagnostics and safe and effective immunotherapeutics is the characterization of the allergens.

IMPORTANCE OF DIFFERENT SPECIES

The most abundant species found in house dust are from the family Pyroglyphidae [3,8,9]. *Dermatophagoides pteronyssinus* is found world-wide and because of its predilection for a humid climate is almost the sole member of the genus *Dermatophagoides* reported in some countries such as the UK [10,11] and Australia [12,13]. *Dermatophagoides farinae* prefers a drier

Allergic Mechanisms and Immunotherapeutic Strategies. Edited by A.M. Roberts and M.R. Walker.

climate and is found in most European countries [14,15], the USA [16] and Japan [17]. *D. microcerus*, a sibling species to *D. farinae*, is also found in much of Europe [14,18]. A list of countries reported to have these mites has been presented by Platts-Mills and de Weck [3] although this could now be updated. Another pyroglyphid *Euroglyphus maynei*, although not as abundant as the *Dermatophagoides*, is found quite widely in the USA, Europe and Australia [11,18–22]. In Australia [20], *E. maynei* was present in levels identified as at-risk for the development of allergy in 25% of homes and was the predominant species in 10%. Further evidence for its importance is the finding of IgE reactive with *E. maynei* on western blotting and crossed radioimmunoelectrophoresis [21–23]. One further species of mite found in house dust and in grain stores and documented to be of significance to allergic disease is *Blomia tropicalis* from the family Glycophidae, characterized by many long setae covering the body. As listed by Arruda and Chapman [24] they are widely distributed in tropical and subtropical regions: Brazil, Venezuela, Hong Kong, Taiwan, Surinam, India, Spain, Egypt, Nigeria and the USA. In the USA it is found in high levels in Florida [16,24]. Sera from patients in Brazil and the USA have high levels of *Blomia*-specific antibodies which cannot be absorbed with *Dermatophagoides* spp. extracts [24] and *Blomia*-specific allergens have been detected by crossed radioimmunoelectrophoresis [25]. It will be important to consider species variations for research and clinical investigation and treatment. It is difficult to see how genetic studies on immune responses can be conducted in areas where multiple species exist with varying levels of cross reactivity at the T- and B-cell level. Cross reactivity in the B-cell compartment would have no relationship to the recognition of T-cell epitopes determining immune responsiveness. Likewise if T-cell modulation is the key to immunotherapy then the one or more species causing the sensitization must be determined, not antibody cross reactivities. As discussed below, the serological cross reactivity between *D. farinae* and *D. pteronyssinus* is variable and not necessarily large, making the quantitation of antibody difficult. Importantly, several species frequently cohabit the same house at levels sufficient to cause sensitization [14,16,20].

RANGE OF ALLERGENS

The number of significant allergens produced by house dust mites is a difficult question. The first analysis using crossed radioimmunoelectrophoresis by Lind and Lowenstein [26] identified 18 different allergens, two of which gave strong binding in almost all positive patients. A further three reacted with over 25%, while binding by other components was sporadic and usually weak. Most patients recognize between four and eight allergens. In a second report by the same authors, they identified two major allergens [27]. A similar analysis by Krilis *et al.* [28] identified 11 IgE binding components, two of which bound IgE from 80% of allergic sera, two with 40–50% binding, three with 22–26% and the remaining four with 9–13%. In their first report on western blotting, Tovey and Baldo [29] found patients had one to seven well-defined IgE binding components in a heterogeneous pattern. Only one out of seven sera bound an allergen equivalent to Der p 1 although four had a band equivalent to Der p 2. Bengtsson and colleagues [30] reported western profiles showing strong reactivity to one to three bands especially with a 14–15 K Mr, possibly Der p 2. In a large study, Tovey, Ford and Baldo [31,32] compiled reactivities of 96 high RAST-allergic sera. High frequency IgE binding was identified in fractions of Mr 16 K (88%, Der p 2), a 30/32 K doublet (68%, Der p 3), 15 K (49%, Der p 5), 26 K (50%) and 25 K (43%, Der p 1). Here the brackets contain the frequency of reactivity followed by the possible identity of the allergen in today's nomenclature. Two very high molecular weight bands and a 54/56 K doublet, possibly Der p 4, bound IgE in over 30% while the rest of the 32 different IgE binding components had sporadic reactivity. The number of bands recognized by each patient, 6–10, is at the high end of the spectrum as compared to their subsequent report where most patients recognized 2–6 [33]. This may be the result of using high RAST sera. These authors also showed that Der p 1 lost much of its serological reactivity in western blotting explaining their inability to detect high frequency IgE binding. Later they also showed that IgE binding reactivity of Der p 2 was enhanced by the denaturing process used in western blotting [34].

The exact position of the other frequently reacting bands, however, varies from report to report with Lin *et al.* [35] identifying bands at Mr 110, 60, 55, 43, 33, 27, 16 and 14 K, Hill *et al.* [23] bands of Mr 40, 28, 25 and 14 K, and Nakanishi and Shimokata bands of 13, 16, 25, 30, 43 and 60 K [36]. Such variation can be expected from differences in the concentrations of allergens [37] and in molecular weight variations, perhaps by degradation. Three forms of the Der p 3 allergen have been reported which vary from extract to extract [38–40] and the Der p 7 allergen also has three molecular weight forms [41]. There are also differences in the electrophoretic conditions and in patient selection. One study indicated that Der p 1 as estimated by western blotting may be recognized more by asthmatics and Der p 2 more by children with eczema [42], but subsequent investigations have found the allergens are equally recognized by both categories [19,43].

While the scanning electrophoretic techniques attempt to examine all allergens they have limitations, especially in quantitation. Apart from losing or gaining IgE binding capacity on denaturation, dose–response curves for antigen binding can be sharp and the concentration of the allergens can vary in different extracts. The ratio of Der p 1 varies 40-fold [37]. The first house dust mite allergens to be purified were Der p 1 and Der p 2. Chapman and Platts-Mills isolated a 24 kDa protein by monitoring fractions with RAST and skin tests [44]. It gave almost 100% reactivity and, remarkably, absorptions showed that the allergen reacted with 40–70% of the anti-mite IgE. This result was even more remarkable because the anti-mite antibodies themselves constituted 15–60% of total IgE. Der p 1 was subsequently isolated by others and the high reactivity confirmed [45,46]. As well as purifying Der p 1, Lind purified the allergen DpX [46] subsequently shown to be Der p 2. The name DpX did not arise because it was a mystery allergen but because it was one of two components found by Lind and Lowenstein which could not be detected by staining in cross immunoelectrophoresis, but it could be detected when probed with allergic serum and radiolabelled anti-IgE. The other was called DpY. RAST assays comparing Der p 1 and 2 showed both had high reactivity with almost all of the 24 allergic sera tested although Der p 1 was far more potent at inhibiting IgE reactivity to discs coated with mite extract. This would have been, at least in part, due to the higher concentration of Der p 1 in extracts [39]. Quantitative studies have confirmed the high frequency of reactivity of these allergens (80%) and that their combined concentration constitutes over 50% of the reactivities in half the responders [19]. The group 3 allergens were first isolated as Der f 3 [39] and the sequence recognized by Stewart as that of a serine protease [38] who then isolated Der p 3 by benzamidine-Sepharose affinity chromatography indicating it was equivalent to mite trypsin [47]. Der p 4 was similarly isolated as mite amylase by affinity chromatography [48]. Mite chymotrypsin, now designated Der p 6, was isolated by ion exchange and size chromatography and shown by sequence and substrate affinity to be mite chymotrypsin [49]. The allergens now designated by Der p 5 and Der p 7 were both characterized from cDNA clones isolated by screening plaque expression libraries with IgE from allergic patients [41,50]. Each of these purified allergens designated 1–7 react with IgE in at least 40% of allergic sera so, with the exception of the very high molecular weight moieties, they could account for most of the important specificities seen by electrophoresis.

MONOCLONAL ANTIBODIES

Monoclonal antibodies have played a central part in elucidating the structure and immunology of mite allergens. Chapman, Sutherland and Platts-Mills produced monoclonals to Der p 1 in 1984 [51] and this was followed by monoclonals to Der p 1 and Der f 1 [52–54], Der p 2 [54] and Der f 2 and Der p 3 [39] by this and other laboratories. Monoclonals have been invaluable for identifying allergens and the exchange of reagents has permitted a direct comparison of allergens isolated by different groups. They have also facilitated the large scale purification of allergens for biochemical analysis or experiments. Other important uses include their use as probes for monitoring and quantitating the amount of allergen in house dust [55] and for determining antigenic differences in allergens of the different mite species both experimentally [52,53] and for environmental assays. The precision and reproducibility of the monoclonal methods has enabled the identification of levels of environmental allergen predicted to cause allergic sensitization [2,46,57]. Monoclonal antibodies have been used to study the epitopes on allergens and a new use is to isolate and monitor the conformation of allergens produced by recombinant DNA technology [58].

MOLECULAR PROPERTIES OF DEFINED ALLERGENS

GROUP 1 ALLERGENS

Der p 1 was first defined by an estimated molecular weight of 25 kDa, a heterogeneous pI of 4.5–7.2 [44] and reactivity to defined polyclonal and monoclonal antibodies [44,46,55]. Apart from its high frequency IgE binding, Der p 1 has been of special interest because it is a major constituent of the dung ball [10]. These 10–40 μg particles contained 10 mg/ml of the allergen or about 0.1 ng per dung ball, and levels of this allergen found in house dust can be very high – 50 μg per g of dust is not uncommon [59]. The Der f 1 of *D. farinae* was described by several authors [60–62] and the N-terminal sequence determined [60,61] as well as for the closely related Der m 1 [61]. Der f 1 and Der m 1 were identical in 30/31 residues while Der p 1 and Der f 1 were identical in 20/28 residues. cDNA cloning which followed revealed that Der p 1 had a polypeptide of 222 residues, a MW of 25.37 K and was a member of a large family of cysteine proteases which included papain from the papaya, actinidin from the kiwi fruit and mammalian cathepsin D [63,64]. Because the X-ray crystallographic structure of these homologues has been solved [65,66] it is possible to speculate on the structure of the allergen. They consist of two globular domains essentially formed independently by the N- and C-terminal halves of the molecule. The domains are connected by an outside loop formed by the residues in the middle of the linear sequence as well as interactions from the N- and C-terminal regions. A substrate binding cleft with catalytic residues contributed by each domain is formed by the juxtaposition of the domains. Although the overall homology of the group 1 allergens and the other cysteine proteases is only about 25% it is clearly identified by two blocks of highly conserved residues surrounding the active cysteine 34 and the active histidine 171 as well as a further AsnSerTrp190–92 sequence which forms part of the substrate binding site. Importantly for structural predictions it contains 26/29 of the hydrophobic core residues which condense to form the globular domains. Disulphide bonds presumably form between the cysteines 31–71 and 65–71 because these residues are conserved in other cysteine proteases. A third bridge is possible between the final cysteine pair 4 and 117. Like other cysteine proteases of this family, Der p 1 is produced firstly as a preproenzyme containing a 19-residue leader sequence and a 79-residue proenzyme sequence [67,68]. The proenzyme region which may be important for folding is of a similar size to other cysteine protease proenzyme sequences and contains some conserved residues. As a confirmation to sequence analysis both Der p 1 and Der f 1 isolated from mites have been shown to have cysteine protease activity [69,70]. The Der p 1 sequence also contained an N-glycosylation site from residues 53–55 which is consistent with the report of carbohydrates in highly purified preparations of the natural allergen [44]. Further indication of the functional significance of this glycosylation site was obtained from the sequence of Der f 1. Although the AACACGTCT encoding AsnThrSer in Der f 1 was considerably different to the AATCAATCA encoding AsnGlnSer in Der p 1, both retained the motif for glycosylation.

The comparison of Der p 1 and Der f 1 [67] showed an overall homology of 80%. The divergence was largely restricted to the N-terminal residues 1–20 (45%), the C-terminal 201–222 (31%) and a central region of 91–130 (30%). The intervening sequences, 21–90 and 131–200 which formed the two globular domains, showed 6% and 14% divergence respectively. As outlined above, the central and terminal residues form more flexible structures connecting the domains. Thus residues 21–90 and 131–200 contain 24/26 of the conserved hydrophobic core residues. Although 34/41 of the substitutions between Der p 1 and Der f 1 were conservative with respect to their predicted effect on tertiary structure, the influence on T-cell epitopes would be considerable. The regions of divergent sequence correspond to the regions containing the antigenic differences between the allergens [71]. In this analysis, the epitopes recognized by a hyperimmune rabbit antiserum were determined by dot-blot assays with recombinant fusion peptides isolated by screening a random fragment library for immunoreactive clones. Most of the antibody could be accounted for by specificities binding to residues 34–47, 60–72, 82–99, 112–140 and 166–194. The binding shared between Der p 1 and Der f 1 was in 34–47, 60–72 and 166–194, while binding specific for Der p 1 was in 82–99 and 112–140.

The species-specific regions described are therefore in the outside flexible loop in the centre of the molecule connecting the domains and contain considerable sequence variation. The exact nature of this flexible loop has now been documented by the molecular modelling studies of Topham *et al.* [72]. It has also been shown in a similar unpublished analysis that mice immunized with Der p 1 make their most consistent antibody response to determinants in fusion peptide 98–140, consistent with the finding that most mouse monoclonal antibodies produced to Der p 1 have displayed species specificity [51,53]. Cross reactivity of human IgE to Der p 1 and Der f 1 has been studied but not with sera from patients known to be exposed to only one or other of the mite species. Although cross reactivity can readily be demonstrated by absorption [52], quantitative inhibition of an ELISA assay found the cross reactivity was quite variable and often 100–1000-fold more allergen was required for heterologous inhibition [61]. Perhaps unexpectedly the results in this study showed that Der m 1 was usually able to inhibit responses to Der p 1 at a lower concentration than Der f 1, sometimes with a 100-fold difference.

The sequence of most of Eur m 1 from *E. maynei* has been examined using a PCR amplification from DNA [73]. Despite being in a different genera, the 20% sequence divergence from both *Dermatophagoides* sequences was the same as the divergence between the *Dermatophagoides* species. Of the 212 translated amino acid residues, 169 were invariant between Der p 1, Der f 1 and Der m 1, and 14 residues were unique to Der m 1; six were in positions which varied in all the species and eight in positions where the Der p 1 and Der f 1 were the same. In the remaining 30 residues not shared by all the species Eur m 1 had the residue found in Der p 1 in 18 and Der f 1 in 12. With respect to the position of the substitutions, 3/14 of the residues unique to Der m 1 were within residues 1–20 and 7/14 within residues 91–130 in keeping with the position of amino acid variation found between Der p 1 and Der f 1. Indeed, taking all species into the calculation 50% of residues in positions 1–20 show variation and 42% of 91–130 compared to 7% from 21–90 (including some Der p 1 polymorphisms described below) and 14% from 131–200. No *Euroglyphus*-specific residues were found in the C-terminal 201–223 although the sequence only extended to 212. Eur m 1 has also been shown to react with the 4C1 monoclonal antibody which also binds both Der p 1 and Der f 1 [23].

Polymorphism has been found within Der p 1 sequences [68]. All of five cDNA clones constructed from mites obtained from the one source, CSL-Ltd Australia, were different, with each translated sequence varying from the others by one to three residues, usually with conservative changes. Two aspects are noteworthy. Firstly, it is uncommon for genes to exhibit this degree of diversity. The many sequences obtained for example in globin genes testing for mutations have found, with the exception of the allelic polymorphism under investigation, remarkable conservation. A further example has shown that the alcohol dehydrogenase genes from 11 different subspecies of *Drosophila melanogaster* has only one amino acid variation [74]. Secondly, the polymorphisms were the result of different combinations of single substitutions in five positions. Thus position 50 could be Tyr or His, position 81 Glu or Lys, position 124 Ala or Val, position 136 Ser or Thr, and position 215 Glu or Gln. The clones sequenced to date indicate that Der p 1 may have any combination of these substitutions, a possibility supported by the sequence of environmental isolates (unpublished) which have the same variations and the genomic sequence of Kent *et al.* [73] which shows yet another combination. The sequences of three environmental isolates indicate that the polymorphism is largely restricted to that described above for commercial mites. Four-fifths of the substitutions found in the cDNA to sequences found in Der f 1 which, along with the fact that they are found in more than one clone, shows they are not cloning artifacts. Although the substitutions are mostly conservative with respect to the tertiary structure they could be expected to influence T-cell epitopes. Finally, the polymorphisms described have calculated pIs of 5.58–6.06 which is insufficient to account for the range of 4.4–7.1 described for natural Der p 1.

GROUP 2 ALLERGENS

Allergens eventually shown to be the 14 kDa Der p 2 [27,46,75] and Der f 2 [39,62] were identified by their high-frequency IgE binding. They are usually present in higher concentration in body extracts than spent mite medium [39,62] and present at about a five-fold lower concentration than the group 1 allergens. Monoclonal antibodies produced against Der p 2 were important for defining and isolating the allergen [54] and cross reacted with the Der f 2 [1]. Similarly, monoclonal antibodies to Der f 2 have been shown to cross react with Der p 2 [39]. N-terminal amino acid sequences obtained for both allergens showed identity in 4/35 positions, considerably higher than the group 1 allergens [39]. cDNA sequences determined for Der p 2 [76,77] and Der f 2 [78,79] showed this extended over 88% of the whole molecule. Both allergens had 129 residues and a calculated MW of 14 K with no N-glycosylation sites. Unlike the group 1 allergens there are no unequivocal homologues in the data bases. Stewart *et al.*, however, have pointed out that the size of Der p 2, and stability to heat and reduction resemble lysozyme [80]. In addition they found a purified 14 kDa fraction contained lysozyme activity, a protein with the N-terminal sequence of Der p 2 and reactivity with an antiserum raised against recombinant Der p 2 [81]. Definitive evidence would be to demonstrate lysozyme activity in affinity purified or recombinant Der p 2 preparations and reactivity of the lysozyme fraction with monoclonal antibody. More recently it has been pointed out that Der p 2 has significant sequence identity with a human epididymal protein and an almost exact matching of cysteine residues and size [82]. It is intriguing that the group 2 allergens may be a secretion from the male reproductive tract which forms a large part of the mass of male mites. The function of the HE1 protein is unknown and still may have a lysozyme or related function. The group 2 allergens contain six cysteines and Nishiyama *et al.* found the disulphide bonds were between Cys 8–119, Cys 21–27 and Cys 73–78 [83], the N- and C-terminal bonding resembling lysozyme. The two cDNA sequences of Yuuki showed polymorphisms of residue 76, 88, 111 and 125. All were substitutions of small aliphatic residues some of which were in the PCR products reported by Trudinger *et al.* [79] and Thomas *et al.* [40]. Some additional changes were found in the PCR sequences but these may be amplification errors. A study of Der f 2 polymorphism has shown that variants differing by four aliphatic exchanges can be detected in mite extracts and one of these can be distinguished by reactivity with a monoclonal antibody and, more importantly, by its stability [84].

The allergen incorrectly called Lep d 1 from *Lepidoglyphus destructor* has now been fully sequenced and shown to be a group 2 allergen. It has the same cysteine arrangement and 40% sequence identity with Der p 2 and Der f 2 [85].

GROUP 3 ALLERGENS

Der f 3 was first isolated by salt precipitation and size exclusion chromatography by Heymann *et al.* [39] as a 30 kDa IgE binding protein. In a paper entitled *Antigenic and structural analysis of group II allergens* they described the purification, the N-terminal sequence and the production of an anti-Der f 3 monoclonal antibody. Stewart *et al.* recognized the published sequence as that of a serine protease and published a homologous sequence obtained from a 17 kDa fraction of *D. pteronyssinus* [38]. Several related molecules were further indicated by the finding that the monoclonal anti-Der f 3 of Haymann *et al.* could affinity purify components of 30, 28 and 21 kDa from spent mite media [40]. Stewart *et al.* then used benzamidine to affinity purify a 30 kDa IgE binding protein with the same N-terminal sequence as that reported previously showing that Der p 3 is a trypsin-like protein and demonstrated the presence of nine isoforms by isoelectric focusing [47]. The identity of Der p 3 as trypsin has been further shown by substrate specificities [86] although there is some evidence that one of the bands detected by western blotting may be or contain a related enzyme, elastase [87]. It should be noted however that monoclonal anti-Der f 3 purifies a 30/28 kDa doublet [40] but not elastase activity [87].

The cDNA sequence of a Der p 3 clone is now known [88]. The mature enzyme sequence was 233 amino acids with a calculated MW of 25 K. It contained the residues for the catalytic and binding sites for the substrate specificity of trypsins. Additionally its identity to Der p 3 was shown by its complete homology to the 18 N-terminal residues published by Stewart *et al.* [38] and strong homology to two internal peptides sequenced from cyanogen bromide cleavage fragments of Der f 3. The homology of these cleavage fragments (18 and 16 residues) with the Der p 3 sequence was 88% and 63%, more or less in keeping with the overall 80–90% homology found for *Dermatophagoides* group 1 and 2 allergens. The difference in the homologies of the two peptides was also reflected in their homology with bovine trypsin which was 61% and 25%. Perhaps, therefore, regions of increased sequence divergence will be found as for the group 1 allergens. The sequence of the autolytic peptide fragment reported by Stewart *et al.* [47] was present but in a different position to that proposed by these authors. The Der p 3 contained three pairs of disulphide bonds with positions 42–58, 168–182, and 191–220 predicted by the homology to bovine trypsin. The clone contained a Cys15 which is unpaired, perhaps an evolutionary vestige corresponding to a paired cysteine found in this region in other trypsins.

GROUP 4 ALLERGENS

Der p 4 was isolated by the strategy of testing mite enzymes, purified by substrate affinity, for IgE binding activity [48]. Amylase isolated by precipitation with glycogen was found to bind IgE in 46% of adults and 25% of children. It had an Mr of 56–63 K judged by analysis in reducing and non-reducing SDS–PAGE gels run with varying conditions. The 19-residue N-terminal sequence had some homology with other amylases, a finding which has now been confirmed by unpublished DNA sequence data of B.J. Bennett and W.R. Thomas.

GROUP 5 ALLERGENS

Tovey *et al.* [50] used IgE plaque immunoassay to isolate a cDNA clone which reacted with IgE in 40% of allergic sera. IgE affinity purified from the recombinant protein was then used to probe mite extracts by western blotting and reacted with an Mr 14 K band. The sequence published from the clone encoded a 17 kDa polypeptide with no N-glycosylation sites and no cysteines which was being produced as fusion with the β-galactosidase in the vector. In the absence of flanking sequence, no further analysis could be made until Lin *et al.* [89] isolated cDNA clones encoding the same allergen which contained 5′ and 3′ flanking regions. It was possible to identify the starting codon of the allergen and hence a proposed 132 residue polypeptide with the first 19 residues comprising a proposed leader sequence. The mature protein had a calculated molecular weight of 15 K. Recombinant fusion proteins constructed for the mature polypeptide showed IgE binding with 50% of allergic sera as well as positive skin test reactivity. No homologues have been found in the data bases. Following the cDNA analysis, an N-terminal sequence of the protein isolated from mite extracts has been determined which shows the polypeptide has 112 residues beginning at Asp designated residue 2 in the study of Lin *et al.* [90]. The derived molecular weight would then be 13.415 kDa. The group 5 allergen has now been defined in *Blomia tropicalis* in which it may be one of the most important allergens [91] reacting with 70% of sera.

GROUP 6 ALLERGENS

Chymotrypsin has been characterized by Yasueda *et al.* as the group 6 allergens in *D. farinae* and *D. pteronyssinus* [49]. They have an N-terminal amino acid sequence of a serine protease showing 50% homology with mite trypsin. The substrate and inhibitor specificity showed these Mr 25 K enzymes were chymotrypsins and studies with monoclonal and mouse polyclonal antibodies showed they were antigenically unrelated to the group 3 trypsins.

GROUP 7 ALLERGENS

The cDNA defining the group 7 allergens was isolated by IgE-plaque immunoassay. It encoded a 215 residue polypeptide with no cysteines, a single N-glycosylation site and a predicted 17 residue leader peptide. The calculated molecular weight of the 198 residue mature protein was 22 K and no homologues were detected in the data bases [41]. Rabbit antibodies affinity purified from the clone, however, showed reactivity with components of Mr 29, 27 and 24 K by western blotting (30,31) and 26 K in a subsequent study [92]. About 40% of patients react to the allergen as determined by skin-test and blotting. Absorption studies showed there was IgE reactivity at least to the 29 and 27 K moieties and possibly to the 13 and 11 K bands. The reactivity of IgE purified from Der p 7 to multiple bands is very interesting and it has been shown that the 31 and 30 kDa reduce to a band of 27 kDa leaving the 26 kDa band which is still considerably higher than the 22 kDa estimate for the polypeptide. (The estimated size of Der p 7 bands differs slightly in each study due to the different SDS–PAGE conditions.) It has not been possible to detect the allergen in spent mite media indicating that it may be labile. The Der f 7 has now been examined and shown to be 86% identical [93].

UNDESIGNATED ALLERGENS

The allergens listed above were characterized in time to be included in the 1994 revision of the allergen nomenclature [94]. Several other allergens have now been reported, some as significant as the named allergens. A cDNA clone encoding a 39 kDa polypeptide which reacted with IgE in 13/43 patients has now been described [95] for *D. farinae* as well as a cDNA clone producing heat shock protein, hsp70, reacting with four out of 41 patients [96]. Both were obtained by screening cDNA expression libraries with IgE. An allergen similarly isolated from *D. pteronyssinus* and found to react with IgE in 77/193 sera (40%) was identified as a 26 kDa glutathione transferase [97]. It showed 50% homology with mammalian glutathione transferases and was identicial in the residues conserved in these enzymes. Since glutathione transferases are a large family of proteins there may be interesting cross reactivities. A final allergen studied by Stewart *et al.* [87] is another serine protease, elastase, which is approximately 30 kDa and has a high frequency of reactivity with allergic sera (80–90%).

IMMUNE RESPONSES TO MITE ALLERGENS

RANK ORDER

The importance of Der p 1 was established by Chapman and Platts-Mills. Nearly all (90%) of the patients responded to this allergen *in vitro* or on skin test and absorption showed that half of the anti-mite IgE antibodies were directed to this allergen [44]. The frequency and degree of reactivity was confirmed by others including the quantitative studies of Van der Zee *et al.* which showed 80% binding [54]. Lind *et al.* showed a lower molecular weight allergen had an IgE binding frequency similar to Der p 1 [27] which has been shown for Der p 2 [54]. Der p 2 appears as the stronger staining allergen by western blotting but this is probably because its reactivity increases after incubation in detergent [32,34]. RAST inhibition studies showed Der p 1 was far more reactive [27] although it could be biased by having more Der p 1 in extracts. The quantitative report of Van der Zee *et al.* [54] also showed that Der p 1 usually bound two to three times the amount of IgE as Der p 2 but subsequent data from the same group [19] have shown a more even reactivity. Quantitative intradermal skin tests have shown that Der p 1 and Der p 2 have a similar end point titration [39]. Meyer *et al.* [98] report that 80% of patients recognized Der p 1 or Der p 2, with Der p 1 exclusive reactivity being more frequent, and that positive sera absorbed with these allergens showed little reactivity with the other components of mite extracts.

Some recent data may indicate that the degree of reactivity may depend on the type of patient [43]. Sera from children attending an allergy clinic had reactivity concentrated on Der p 1 and 2 and a high molecular weight component of 90–100 K, but in a direct comparison, IgE from most of the adults who, in this study being diagnosed for allergy for the first time, had no or only weak reactivity to Der p 1 and 2. Correspondingly, they had a different pattern of allergen binding by western blotting. It must be emphasized that the adults here were distinct from volunteers who have had long-standing allergy from childhood. Such volunteers usually have IgE with high binding activity for Der p 1 and 2 as well as many other components. The report of low reactivity to Der p 1 and 2 reported by White *et al.* may be from a similar selection of patients [99]. Shibasaki and colleagues [100] have reported a similar phenomenon in infants in whom, during the first three years, the western blotting pattern is largely restricted to Der p 2 (Der p 1 does not blot well), and then the response becomes more heterogeneous.

Western blotting has shown a high frequency of IgE reactive bands at Mr 30 K or as a 28/30 K doublet [31,32] which has been thought to be Der p 3. This differed from the initial report of Heymann *et al.* [39] where only 16% reactivity by fluid phase radioimmune assay was found, but subsequent reports with solid phase assays confirmed the high frequency reactivity [40,47,49,86]. The amount of anti-group 3 IgE in sera has been consistently shown to be less than that to Der p 1 [47] or to both Der p 1 and 2 [49]. Recently Farris, Platts-Mills, Chapman and Heymann have used RAST to show that although 64% of the patients had IgE to Der f 3 the levels were low and did not correlate well with anti-whole mite titres [100a]. The report of Ando *et al.* [86], shows a similar rank of binding although some high binding of Der f 3 was apparent. The elastase allergen [87] has a similar binding frequency.

Quantitative data have been reported for the group 6 allergens. Yasueda *et al.* [49] presented RAST data which showed that Der p 6 and Der f 6 bound IgE in about 40% of mite-allergic subjects and, when positive like the group 3, were at a considerably lower level than the group 1 and 2 allergens. The RAST results correlated well with skin tests. No quantitative information is available for the group 4 and 5 allergens but these each react with IgE in about 40% of allergic sera and the indications are that it may be strong, even though at a lower frequency. The group 7 allergens have recently been found to have the same IgE binding capacity as the group 2 allergens in 50% of responders (data in preparation, cited in [93]). It may therefore be very important.

T-CELL RESPONSES TO PURIFIED ALLERGENS

T cells reactive to purified allergens can be detected in allergic [101–106] and non-allergic [102–104,106] individuals. The allergic patients usually have a higher level of stimulation as well as lymphokine production favouring IgE synthesis [103,107]. The data of some authors has shown a correlation of the magnitude of Der p 1 and/or 2 reactivity with disease [101,105]. It is however clear that large T-cell proliferation responses can be stimulated by purified allergens in the absence of IgE. This is shown definitively by O'Brien and Thomas [43] where antibody and T-cell responses to Der p 1 and 2 were compared. A correlation has however been reported between the TH1 and TH2 type interleukins and diseases. Patients who mainly produced interferon-γ mRNA after polyclonal stimulation with Der p 2 had mild disease, while patients with severe disease produced only IL-4. Intermediate patients produced a mixture [108].

Few studies have compared the ability of different allergens from mite extracts to stimulate T cells. The results of Okano *et al.* [109] and O'Hehir *et al.* [110] show that T cells respond to a range of allergens. O'Hehir *et al.* found a predominance of reactivity to the group 2 allergens in a limited number of patients while Okana *et al.* found the major reactivity was in higher molecular weight fractions and, in the one patient tested, the T cells produced IL-4. In the direct comparisons of Der p 1 and Der p 2 polyclonal proliferative responses, both allergens stimulated to the same degree which correlated in most patients [43,105].

EPITOPES

Immune responses to mites are induced by protracted low-dose exposure to the antigen and are therefore different to infections or injections. IgE responses are in themselves quite unusual because the level of this immunoglobulin is usually low and the allergen-specific IgE can be high [44]. The potential therefore exists for the expansion and selection of a restricted repertoire which could be reflected in the epitopes recognized.

Early studies with group 1 allergens firmly established that the IgE recognition was dependent on the intact tertiary structure as shown by acid hydrolysis of disulphide bonds and heat sensitivity [61,111]. The IgE binding determinants were spread over at least four sites as shown by competition with different monoclonal antibodies [52,61]. Recombinant fusion peptides [112,113] and synthetic peptides [114] were shown to retain some IgE binding which for the fusion peptides was dependent on conformation and usually required about 30 residues. The fusion peptides which had the most consistent binding were 53–99 and 98–140 [112], which contain the flexible loop and a high sequence divergence between species. Binding was however obtained across the whole molecule in a unique pattern for all seven patients examined. The pattern of binding of IgE and IgG [112] was usually the same, but in some patients IgG bound peptides which bound little or no IgE.

The IgE binding activity of Der p 2 was very sensitive to reduction and alkylation and although resistant to heat [111], synthetic peptides [116–118] and fusion [115] had poor IgE binding activity compared to the whole molecule. Even large fusion peptides had little binding although these experiments did not take into account the interaction between the N- and C-terminus which are linked by a disulphide bond. This is reflected in the experiments of Oshika *et al.* [119] who found binding activity in a cleavage fragment 13–129 but not 39–129. They also found binding activity in fragment 1–76. The experiments of Van't Hof, Aalberse and colleagues, who measured the ability of IgE from different individuals to recognize different modifications of a peptide, indicated that the response was heterogeneous [117].

There are no comprehensive studies on T-cell epitopes recognized by populations of mite-sensitive patients. T-cell clones from a limited number of patients recognizing peptides 45–67, 94–104, 107–119, 110–109, 110–131, and 117–143 of Der p 1 have been described [104,120–122]. Most of these epitopes are in the central region of the molecule which shows high sequence variation between species. The importance of the region has been further emphasized in studies in an individual where four epitopes restricted by either DR or DCP were found within 101–131 [123]. A study [124] using fusion peptides has, however, shown that T-cell epitopes are distributed throughout the molecule indicating the data with synthetic peptides may reflect the small sample examined. Like other antigens the epitopes vary presumably with the major histocompatibility molecule serving as the restriction element. T-cell epitopes for Der p 2 have been described in a more systematic fashion. Atopic and non-atopic people responded to epitopes from across the molecule but the authors were able to point to regions which contained at least one epitope for most people. Thus either 61–86 or 78–104 were recognized by 16/17 individuals [106] and the inclusion of a third peptide, e.g. 105–129, would produce a cocktail in which all responders recognized at least one and, more often, two epitopes. The studies of van Neerven *et al.* [118] found a diverse array of Der p 2 synthetic peptides stimulated responses in five atopic patients and concluded there would be at least 10 epitopes. The peptides used were short and hence epitopes were probably missed including the ones recognized to react at the higher frequency found by O'Hehir. Importantly, the peptides examined, with the exception of a low reactivity to 74–87, did not bind IgE which may be significant for immunotherapy.

A major initiative in allergen research is to develop peptide-based immunotherapy which is directed at modifying T-cell activity. The most practical scheme would be to redirect the allergic response by re-educating T-cell clones or inducing new clones to anti-inflammatory cytokines which work in trans and modify responses to all specificities. This has clearly been shown to be possible in mouse experiments where the administration of a peptide containing one epitope of Der p 1 could inhibit the response of the whole molecule, which included responses to other T-cell epitopes [125,126] and importantly could inhibit responses in sensitized animals. Clearly for this strategy, the ability of patients to recognize a number of epitopes is a distinct advantage and in this respect there may be a use for cryptic epitopes which are not usually recognized during sensitization to the whole allergen [126,127].

REFERENCES

1 Platts-Mills TAE, Chapman MD. Dust mites: immunology, allergic disease, and environmental control. *J Allergy Clin Immunol* 1987; **80**: 755–775.
2 Platts-Mills TAE, Thomas WR, Aalberse RC, Vervloet D, Chapman MD. Dust mite allergens and asthma: report of a second international workshop. *J Allergy Clin Immunol* 1992; **89**: 1046–1060.
3 Platts-Mills TAE, de Weck AL. Dust mite allergens and asthma – a world wide problem. *J Allergy Clin Immunol* 1989; **83**: 416–427.
4 Armenaka MC, Grizzanti JN, Obriel B, Rosenstreich DL. Increased immune reactivity to house dust mites in adults with chronic rhinosinusitis. *Clin Exp Allergy* 1993; **23**: 669–677.
5 Corrigan CJ, Kay AB. T cells and eosinophils in the pathogenesis of asthma. *Immunol Today* 1992; **13**: 501–504.
6 McHugh SM, Lavelle B, Kemeny DM, Patel S, Ewan PW. A placebo-controlled trial of immunotherapy with two extracts of *D. pteronyssinus* in allergic rhinitis comparing clinical outcome with changes in antigen-specific IgE, IgG and IgG subclasses. *J Allergy Clin Immunol* 1990; **86**: 521–532.
7 Norman PS. An overview of immunotherapy: Implications for the future. *J Allergy Clin Immunol* 1980; **65**: 87–96.
8 Colloff MJ, Speiksma FTM. Pictorial keys for the identification of domestic mites. *Clin Exp Allergy* 1992; **22**: 823–830.
9 Spieksma FTM. Domestic mites: Their role in respiratory allergy. *Clin Exp Allergy* 1991; **21**: 655–660.
10 Tovey ER, Chapman MD, Platts-Mills TA. Mite faeces are a major source of house dust allergens. *Nature* 1981; **289**: 592–593.

11 Hart BJ, Whitehead L. Ecology of house dust mites in Oxfordshire. *Clin Exp Allergy* 1990; **20**: 203–209.

12 King K, England JF. The house dust mite *D. farinae* in Australia. *Med J Aust* 1983; **2**: 259–260.

13 Green WF, Woolcock AJ, Stuckey M, Sedgwick C, Leeder SR. House dust mites and skin tests in different Australian localities. *Aust NZ J Med* 1986; **16**: 639–643.

14 Lind P. Enzyme-linked immunosorbent assay for determination of major excrement allergens of house dust mite species *D. pteronyssinus, D. farinae*, and *D. microceras*. *Allergy* 1986; **41**: 442–451.

15 Lind P, Ingemann L, Brouvez M. Demonstration of species-specific sensitisation to major allergens of *Dermatophagoides spp.* by solid phase absorption of human IgE antibodies. *Scand J Immunol* 1987; **25**: 1–10.

16 Arlian LG, Bernstein D, Bernstein IL, Friedman S, Grant A, Lieberman P, Lopez M, Metzger J, Platts MT, Schatz M, *et al*. Prevalence of dust mites in the homes of people with asthma living in eight different geographic areas of the United States. *J Allergy Clin Immunol* 1992; **90**: 292–300.

17 Sakaguchi M, Inouye S, Yasueda H, Irie T, Yoshizawa S, Shida T. Measurement of allergens associated with dust mite allergy. II. Concentrations of airborne mite allergens (Der I and Der II) in the house. *Int Arch Allergy Appl Immunol* 1989; **90**: 190–193.

18 Cunnington AM, Lind P, Spieksma FTM. Taxonomic and immunochemical identification of two house dust mites *Dermatophagoides farinae* and *Dermatophagoides microceras*. *J Allergy Clin Immunol* 1987; **79**: 410–411.

19 Calkhoven PG, Aalbers M, Schilte PP, Yntema BJ, Griffioen RW, van Nierop JC, Oranje AP, Aalberse RC. Newly generated IgE antibodies to *Dermatophagoides pteronyssinus* in children are directed against components distinct from Der p I and Der p II. *J Allergy Clin Immunol* 1991; **88**: 265–271.

20 Colloff MJ, Stewart GA, Thompson PJ. House dust mite acarofauna and Der p I equivalent in Australia: the relative importance of *Dermatophagoides pteronyssinus* and *Euroglyphus maynei*. *Clin Exp Allergy* 1991; **21**: 225–230.

21 Colloff MJ. A review of biology and allergenicity of the house dust mite *Euroglyphus maynei* (Acari: Pyroglyphidae). *Exp Appl Acarol* 1991; **11**: 177–198.

22 Arlian LG, Rapp CM, Fernandez-Caldas E. Allergenicity of *Euroglyphus maynei* and its cross-reactivity with *Dermatophagoides* species. *J Allergy Clin Immunol* 1993; **91**: 1051–1058.

23 Hill MR, Newton MR, Hart BJ. Comparative IgE responses to extracts of five species of house dust mite using western blotting. *Clin Exp Allergy* 1993; **23**: 110–116.

24 Arruda LK, Chapman MD. A review of recent immunochemical studies of *Blomia tropicalis* and *Euroglyphus maynei* allergens. *Exp Appl Acarol* 1992; **16**: 129–140.

25 Arlian LG, Vyszenski-Moher DL, Fernandez-Caldas E. Allergenicity of the mite, *Blomia tropicalis*. *J Allergy Clin Immunol* 1993; **91**: 1042–1050.

26 Lind P, Lowenstein H. Identification of allergens in *Dermatophagoides pteronyssinus* mite body extract by crossed radioimmunoelectrophoresis with two different rabbit antibody pools. *Scand J Immunol* 1983; **17**: 263–273.

27 Lind P, Weeke B, Lowenstein H. A reference allergen preparation of the house dust mite *D. pteronyssinus*, produced from whole mite culture – a part of the DAS 76 study. Comparison with allergen preparations from other raw materials. *Allergy* 1984; **39**: 259–274.

28 Krilis S, Baldo BA, Basten A. Antigens and allergens from the common house dust mite *Dermatophagoides pteronyssinus*. Part II. Identification of the major IgE-binding antigens by crossed radioimmunoelectrophoresis. *J Allergy Clin Immunol* 1984; **74**: 142–146.

29 Tovey ER, Baldo BA. Detection of house dust mite allergens and frequency of IgE binding following electroblotting and enzyme immunoassay. *Int Arch Allergy Appl Immunol* 1985; **76**: 82–85.
30 Bengtsson A, Karlsson A, Rolfsen W, Einarsson R. Detection of allergens in mould and mite preparations by a nitrocellulose electroblotting technique. *Int Arch Allergy Appl Immunol* 1986; **80**: 383–390.
31 Tovey ER, Baldo BA. Comparison by electroblotting of IgE-binding components in extracts of house dust mite bodies and spent mite culture. *J Allergy Clin Immunol* 1987; **79**: 93–102.
32 Baldo BA, Ford SA, Tovey ER. Toward a definition of the complete spectrum and rank order of importance of allergens from the house dust mite: *Dermatophagoides pteronyssinus. Adv Biosci* 1989; **74**: 13–31.
33 Ford SA, Tovey ER, Baldo BA. The spectrum of low molecular weight house dust mite (*Dermatophagoides pteronyssinus*) allergens with emphasis on Der p II. *Clin Exp Allergy* 1989; **20**: 27–31.
34 Tovey ER, Ford SA, Baldo BA. Enhanced immunodetection of blotted house dust mite protein allergens on nitrocellulose following blocking with Tween 20. *Electrophoresis* 1989; **10**: 243–249.
35 Lin K-L, Wang S-Y, Hsieh K-H. Analysis of house dust mite – specific IgE, IgG_4, and IgG antibodies during immunotherapy in asthmatic children. *Ann Allergy* 1991; **67**: 63–69.
36 Nakanishi K, Shimokata K. Immunoblot analysis of *Dermatophagoides farinae* antigen. *Ann Allergy* 1990; **64**: 219–231.
37 Ford AW, Rawle FC, Lind P, Spieksma FT, Løwenstein H, Platts-Mills TAE. Standardization of *Dermatophagoides pteronyssinus*: assessment of potency and allergen content in ten coded extracts. *Int Arch Allergy Appl Immunol* 1985; **76**: 58–67.
38 Stewart GA, Thompsom PJ, Simpson RJ. Protease antigens from house dust mite. *Lancet* 1989; **ii**: 462.
39 Heymann PW, Chapman MD, Aalberse RC, Fox JW, Platts-Mills TAE. Antigenic and structural analysis of group II allergens (Der f II and Der p II) from house dust mites (*Dermatophagoides spp*). *J Allergy Clin Immunol* 1989; **83**: 1055–1067.
40 Thomas W, Chua KY, Smith WA. Molecular polymorphisms of house dust mite allergens. *Exp Appl Acarol* 1992; **16**: 153–164.
41 Shen HD, Chua KY, Lin KL, Hsieh KH, Thomas WR. Molecular cloning of a house dust mite allergen with common antibody binding specificities with multiple components in mite extracts. *Clin Exp Allergy* 1993; **23**: 934–940.
42 Thompson SJ, Whitley JH, Naysmith JD, Carswell F. IgE antibodies to *D. pteronyssinus* in atopic patients. *Immunology* 1988; **64**: 311–314.
43 O'Brien RM, Thomas WR. Immune reactivity to Der p I and Der p II in house dust mite sensitive patients attending paediatric and adult allergy clinics. *Clin Exp Allergy* 1994; **24**: 737–742.
44 Chapman MD, Platts-Mills TAE. Purification and characterization of the major allergen from *Dermatophagoides pteronyssinus*-antigen P$_1$. *J Immunol* 1980; **125**: 587–592.
45 Stewart GA. Isolation and characterisation of the allergen Dpt 12 from *Dermatophagoides pteronyssinus* by chromatofocusing. *Int Arch Allergy Appl Immunol* 1982; **69**: 224–230.
46 Lind P. Purification and partial characterization of two major allergens from the house dust mite *Dermatophagoides pteronyssinus. J Allergy Clin Immunol* 1985; **76**: 753–761.
47 Stewart GA, Ward LD, Simpson RJ, Thompson PJ. The group III allergen from the

house dust mite *Dermatophagoides pteronyssinus* is a trypsin-like enzyme. *Immunology* 1992; **75**: 29–35.
48 Lake FR, Ward LD, Simpson RJ, Thompson PJ, Stewart GA. House dust mite-derived amylase: allergenicity and physicochemical characterization. *J Allergy Clin Immunol* 1991; **87**: 1035–1042.
49 Yasueda H, Mita H, Shida T, Ando T, Sugiyama S, Yamakawa H. Allergens from *Dermatophagoides* with chymotryptic activity. *Clin Exp Allergy* 1993; **23**: 384–390.
50 Tovey ER, Johnson MC, Roche AL, Cobon GS, Baldo BA. Cloning and sequencing of a cDNA expressing a recombinant house dust mite protein that binds human IgE and corresponds to an important low molecular weight allergen. (Published erratum appears in *J Exp Med* 1990; **171**: 1387.) *J Exp Med* 1989; **170**: 1457–1462.
51 Chapman MD, Sutherland WM, Platts-Mills TAE. Recognition of two *Dermatophagoides pteronyssinus*-specific epitopes on antigen P1 by using monoclonal antibodies: Binding to each epitope can be inhibited by sera from dust-mite allergic patients. *J Immunol* 1984; **133**: 2488–2495.
52 Chapman MD, Heymann PW, Platts-Mills TAE. Epitope mapping of two major inhalant allergens, Der p I and Der f I, from mites of the genus *Dermatophagoides*. *J Immunol* 1987; **139**: 1479–1484.
53 Horn N, Lind P. Selection and characterisation of monoclonal antibodies against a major allergen in *Dermatophagoides pteronyssinus*. Species-specific and common epitopes. *Int Arch Allergy Appl Immunol* 1987; **83**: 404–409.
54 Van der Zee JS, van Swieten P, Jansen HM, Aalberse RC. Skin tests and histamine release with P1-depleted *Dermatophagoides pteronyssinus* body extracts and purified P1. *J Allergy Clin Immunol* 1988; **81**: 884–895.
55 Chapman MD, Heymann PW, Wilkins SR, Brown MJ, Platts-Mills TAE. Monoclonal immunoassays for major dust mite (*Dermatophagoides*) allergens, Der p I and Der f I, and quantitative analysis of the allergen content of mite and house dust extracts. *J Allergy Clin Immunol* 1987; **80**: 184–194.
56 Pollart SM, Chapman MD, Platts-Mills TAE. Allergen levels inside homes: risk factors for acute asthma attacks. *J Allergy Clin Immunol* 1988; **81**: 242–249.
57 Sporik R, Holgate ST, Platts-Mills TAE. Exposure to house dust mite allergen (Der p I) and the development of asthma in childhood: a prospective study. *N Engl J Med* 1990; **323**: 502–507.
58 Chua KY, Kehal PK, Thomas WR, Vaughan PR, Macreadie IG. High-frequency binding of IgE to the Der p allergen expressed in yeast. *J Allergy Clin Immunol* 1992; **89**: 95–102.
59 Tovey ER, Chapman MD, Wells CW, Platts-Mills TAE. The distribution of dust mite allergen in the houses of patients with asthma. *Am Rev Respir Dis* 1981; **124**: 630.
60 Heymann PWE, Chapman MD, Platts-Mills TAE. Antigen Der f I from the house dust mite *Dermatophagoides farinae*: structural comparison with Der p I from *Dermatophagoides pteronyssinus* and epitope specificity of murine IgG and human IgE antibodies. *J Immunol* 1986; **137**: 2841–2847.
61 Lind, P, Hansen OC, Horn N. The binding of mouse hybridoma and human IgE antibodies to the major fecal allergen, Der p I, of *Dermatophagoides pteronyssinus*. Relative binding site location and species specificity studied by solid-phase inhibition assays with radiolabeled antigen. *J Immunol* 1988; **140**: 4256–4262.
62 Yasueda H, Mita H, Yui Y, Shida T. Isolation and characterization of two allergens from *Dermatophagoides farinae*. *Int Arch Allergy Appl Immunol* 1986; **81**: 214–233.
63 Chua KY, Stewart GA, Thomas WR, Simpson RJ, Dilworth RJ, Plozza IM, Turner KJ. Sequence analysis of cDNA coding for a major house dust mite allergen, Der p I. Homology with cysteine proteases. *J Exp Med* **167**: 175–182.
64 Thomas WR, Stewart GA, Simpson RJ, Chua KY, Plozza TM, Dilworth RJ, Nisbet

A, Turner KJ. Cloning and expression of DNA coding for the major house dust mite allergen Der p I in *Escherichia coli*. *Int Arch Allergy Appl Immunol* 1988; **85**: 127–129.
65 Baker EN. Drenth J. The thiol proteases: structure and mechanism. *Biol Macromol Assemblies* 1987; **3**: 313–368.
66 Musil D, Zucic D, Turk D, Engh RA, Mayr I, Huber R, Popovic T, Turk V, Towatari T, Katunuma N, Bode W. The refined 2.15 Å X-ray crystal structure of human liver cathepsin B: the structural basis for its specificity. *EMBO J* 1991; **10**: 2321–2330.
67 Dilworth RJ, Chua KY, Thomas WR. Sequence analysis of cDNA coding for a major house dust mite allergen, Der f I. *Clin Exp Allergy* 1991; **21**: 25–32.
68 Chua KY, Kehal PK, Thomas WR. Sequence polymorphisms of cDNA clones encoding the mite allergen Der p I. *Int Arch Allergy Appl Immunol* 1993; **101**: 364–368.
69 Stewart GA, Lake FR, Thompson PJ. Faecally derived hydrolytic enzymes from *Dermatophagoides pteronyssinus*: physicochemical characterisation of potential allergens. *Int Arch Allergy Appl Immunol* 1991; **95**: 248–256.
70 Ando T, Ino Y, Haida M, Honma R, Maeda H, Yamakawa H, Iwaki M, Okudairo H. Isolation of cystein protease in the crude extract, *Dermatophagoides farinae*. *Int Arch Allergy Appl Immunol* 1991; **96**: 199–205.
71 Greene WK, Chua KY, Stewart GA, Thomas WR. Antigenic analysis of group I house dust mite allergens using random fragments of Der p I expressed by recombinant DNA libraries. *Int Arch Allergy Appl Immunol* 1990; **92**: 30–38.
72 Topham CM, Srinivasan N, Thorpe CJ, Overington H, Kalsheker NA. Comparative modelling of major house dust mite allergen Der p I: structure validation using an extended environmental amino acid propensity table. *Pro Eng* 1994; **7**: 869–894.
73 Kent NA, Hill MR, Keen JN, Holland PWH, Hart BJ. Molecular characterisation of group I allergen Eur m I from house dust mite *Euroglyphus maynei*. *Int Arch Allergy Appl Immunol* 1992; **99**: 150–152.
74 Kreitman M. Nucleotide polymorphism at the alcohol dehydrogenase locus of *Drosophila melanogaster*. *Nature* 1983; **304**: 412–417.
75 Abe T, Ishii A. Comparison of *Dermatophagoides pteronyssinus* allergens from culture medium extract and whole body extract by using the same probe of pooled human serum. *Allergy* 1987; **42**: 352–358.
76 Thomas WR, Chua KY, Stewart GA, Doyle CR, Turner KJ, Simpson RJ, Dilworth RJ. Analysis and expression of cDNA clones coding for house dust mite allergens. *Adv Biosci* 1989; **74**: 139–147.
77 Chua KY, Doyle CR, Simpson RJ, Turner KJ, Stewart GA, Thomas WR. Isolation of cDNA coding for the major mite allergen Der p II by IgE plaque immunoassay. *Int Arch Allergy Appl Immunol* 1990; **91**: 118–123.
78 Yuuki T, Okumura Y, Ando T, Yamakawa H, Suko M, Haida M, Okudaira H. Cloning and sequencing of cDNAs corresponding to mite major allergen Der f II. *Arerugi* 1990; **39**: 557–561.
79 Trudinger M, Chua KY, Thomas WR. cDNA encoding the major mite allergen Der f II. *Clin Exp Allergy* 1991; **21**: 33–37.
80 Stewart GA, Bird CH, Thompson PJ. Do the group II allergens correspond to lysozyme? *J Allergy Clin Immunol* 1992; **90**: 141–142.
81 Stewart GA, Bird CH, Thompson PJ, Ward LD, Simpson RJ. Similarity between a lysozyme-like enzyme from the house dust mite and the group II allergens. *J Allergy Clin Immunol* 1993; **91**: 356.
82 Thomas WR, Chua K-Y. The major mite allergen Der p 2 – a secretion of the male mite reproductive tract. *Clin Exp Allergy* 1996; **25**: 667–669.
83 Nishiyama C, Yuuki T, Takai T, Okumura Y, Okudaira H. Determination of three

disulfide bonds in a major house dust mite allergen, Der f II. *Int Arch Allergy Appl Immunol* 1993; **101**: 159–166.
84 Nishiyama C, Yuuki T, Usui Y, Iwamoto N, Okumura Y, Okudaira H. Effects of amino acid variations in recombinant Der f II on its human IgE and mouse IgG recognition. *Int Arch Allergy Appl Immunol* 1994; **105**: 62–69.
85 Varela J, Ventas P, Carreira J, Barbas JA, Gimenez-Gallego G, Polo F. Primary structure of Lep d I, the main *Lepidoglyphus destructor* allergen. *Eur J Biochem* 1994; **225**: 93–98.
86 Ando T, Homma R, Ino Y, Ito G, Miyahara A, Yanagihara T, Kimura H, Ikeda S, Yamakawa H, Iwaki M, Okumura Y, Suko M, Haida M, Okudairo H. Trypsin-like protease of mites: purification and characterisation of trypsin-like protease from mite faecal extract *Dermatophagoides farinae*. Relationship between trypsin-like protease and Der f III. *Clin Exp Allergy* 1993; **23**: 777–784.
87 Stewart GA, Kollinger MR, King CM, Thompson PJ. A comparative study of three serine proteases from *Dermatophagoides pteronyssinus* and *D. farinae. Allergy* 1994; **49**: 553–560.
88 Smith W-A, Chua K-Y, Kuo M-C, Rogers BL, Thomas WR. Cloning and sequencing of *Dermatophagoides pteronyssinus* group III allergen Der p III. *Clin Exp Allergy* 1994; **24**: 220–228.
89 Lin KL, Chua KY, Thomas WR, Chiang BL, Hsieh KH. Characterisation of Der p V allergen. cDNA analysis and IgE-mediated reactivity to the recombinant protein. *J Allergy Clin Immunol* 1994; **94**: 989–996.
90 O'Neill GM, Donovan GR, Baldo BA. Sequence analyses of the native form of a major house dust mite allergen and its nascent polypeptide. *Mol Immunol* 1994; **31**: 1447–1448.
91 Arruda LK, Fernandez-Caldas E, Naspitz CK, Montealegre F, Chapman MD. Molecular cloning of *Blomia tropicalis* allergen Blo t 5 and its sequence homology to *D. pteronyssinus* Der p 5. *J Allergy Clin Immunol* 1994; **93**: 205.
92 Shen H-D, Chua K-Y, Lin N-L, Hsieh K-H, Thomas WR. Characterisation of the house dust mite allergen Der p 7 by monoclonal antibodies. *Clin Exp Allergy* 1995; **25**: 416–422.
93 Shen H-D, Chua K-Y, Lin W-L, Hsieh K-H, Thomas WR. Molecular cloning and immunological characterisation of the house dust mite allergen Der f 7. *Clin Exp Allergy* 1995; **25**: 1000–1006.
94 King TP, Hoffman D. Løwenstein H, Marsh DG, Platts-Mills TAE, Thomas WR. Allergen nomenclature. *Int Arch Allergy Appl Immunol* 1994; **105**: 224–233.
95 Aki T, Ono K, Soon-Young P, Wada T, Jyo T, Shigeta S, Murooka Y, Oka S. Cloning and characterization of cDNA coding for a new allergen from the house dust mite, *Dermatophagoides farinae. Int Arch Allergy Appl Immunol* 1994; **103**: 349–356.
96 Aki T, Fujikawa A, Wada T, Jyo T, Shigeta S. Murooka Y, Oka S, Ono K. Cloning and expression of cDNA coding for a new allergen from the house dust mite, *Dermatophagoides farinae*: homology with human heat shock cognate proteins in the heat shock protein 70 family. *J Biochem* 1994; **115**: 435–440.
97 O'Neill G, Donovan GR, Baldo BA. Identification of a major allergen of the house dust mite, *Dermatophagoides pteronyssinus*, homologous with glutathione-S-transferase. *Biochim Biophys Acta* 1994; **1219**: 521–524.
98 Meyer CH, Bond JF, Chen M, Kasaian MT. Comparison of the levels of the major allergens Der p I and Der p II in standardised extract of the house dust mite, *Dermatophagoides pteronyssinus. Clin Exp Allergy* 1994; **24**: 1041–1048.
99 White JM, Hamilton RG, Franklin-Adkidson N, Lichtenstein LM, Kagey-Sobotka A. *Dermatophagoides pteronyssinus* (Dpt). Where is the major allergen? *J Allergy Clin Immunol* 1993; **91**: 355.

100 Shibasaki M, Isoyama S, Takita H. Influence of age on IgE responsiveness to *Dermatophagoides farinae*: An immunoblot study. *Int Arch Allergy Appl Immunol* 1994; **103**: 53–58.

100a Farris H, Flatts-Mills T, Chapman MD *et al*. Immediate hypersensitivity to Der f III in allergic patients. *J Allergy Clin Immunol* 1993; **91**: 374.

101 Rawle FC, Mitchell EB, Platts-Mills TAE. T-cell response to the major allergen from the house dust mite, *Dermatophagoides pteronyssinus*, antigen P1: comparison of patients with asthma, atopic dermatitis and perennial rhinitis. *J Immunol* 1984; **133**: 195–201.

102 Cavaillon JM, Fitting C, Guinnepain MT, Rassemont R, David B. Lymphocyte proliferative responses to the purified *Dermatophagoides farinae* major allergen in untreated and hyposensitized atopic patients. *Allergy* 1988; **43**: 146–151.

103 Wieringa EA, Snoek M, Bos JD, Jansen HM, Kapsenberg ML. Comparison of diversity and function of house dust mite specific T lymphocyte clones from atopic and non-atopic donors. *Eur J Immunol* 1990; **20**: 1519–1526.

104 O'Hehir RE, Garman RD, Greenstein JL, Lamb JR. The specificity and regulation of T-cell responsiveness to allergens. *Ann Rev Immunol* 1991; **9**: 67–95.

105 O'Brien RM, Thomas WR, Wootton AM. T cell responses to the purified major allergens from the house dust mite *Dermatophagoides pteronyssinus*. *J Allergy Clin Immunol* 1992; **89**: 1021–1031.

106 O'Hehir RE, Verhoef A, Panagiotopoulou E, Keswani S, Hayball JD, Thomas WR, Lamb JR. Analysis of human T cell responses to the group II allergen of *Dermatophagoides* species: Localisation of major antigenic sites. *J Allergy Clin Immunol* 1993; **92**: 105–113.

107 O'Hehir RE, Bal V, Quint D, Moqbel R, KAB, Zanders ED, Lamb JR. An *in vitro* model of allergen-dependent IgE synthesis by human B lympocytes: Comparison of the response of an atopic and a non-atopic individual to *Dermatophagoides spp*. (house dust mite). *Immunology* 1989; **66**: 499–504.

108 Byron KA, O'Brien RM, Varigos GA, Wootton AM. *Dermatophagoides pteronyssinus* II – induced interleukin-4 and interferon-γ expression by freshly isolated lymphocytes of atopic individuals. *Clin Exp Allergy* 1994; **24**: 878–883

109 Okana M, Nagano T, Ono T, Masuda Y, Ohta N. Clonal analysis of human T-cell responses to fractionated house dust mite antigens (*Dermatophagoides pteronyssinus*). *Int Arch Allergy Appl Immunol* 1993; **101**: 82–88.

110 O'Hehir RE, Young DB, Kay AB, Lamb JR. Cloned human T lymphocytes reactive with *Dermatophagoides farinae* (house dust mite): a comparison of T- and B-cell antigen recognition. *Immunology* 1987; **62**: 635–640.

111 Lombardero M, Heymann PW, Platts-Mills TAE, Fox JW. Chapman MD. Conformational stability of B cell epitopes on group I and group II *Dermatophagoides spp*. allergens. Effect of thermal and chemical denaturation on the binding of murine IgG and human IgE antibodies. *J Immunol* 1990; **144**: 1353–1360.

112 Greene WK, Cyster JG, Chua KY, O'Brien RM, Thomas WR. IgE and IgG binding of peptides expressed from fragments of cDNA encoding the major house dust mite allergen Der p I. *J Immunol* 1991; **147**: 3768–3773.

113 Greene WK, Thomas WR. IgE binding structures of the major house dust mite allergen Der p I. *Mol Immunol* 1992; **29**: 257–262.

114 Jeannin P, Didierlaurent A, Gras-Masse H, EAA, Delneste Y, Cardot E, Joseph M, Tartar A, Vergoten G, Pestel J. Specific histamine release capacity of peptides selected from the modelized Der p I protein, a major allergen of *Dermatophagoides pteronyssinus*. *Mol Immunol* 1992; **29**: 739–749.

115 Chua, KY, Greene WK, Kehal P, Thomas WR. IgE binding studies with large

peptides expressed from Der p II cDNA constructs. *Clin Exp Allergy* 1991; **21**: 161–166.

116 van't Hof W, Driedijk PC, Van den Berg M, Beck-Sickinger AG, Jung G, Aalberse RC. Epitope mapping of the *Dermatophagoides pteronyssinus* house dust mite major allergen Der p II using overlapping synthetic peptides. *Mol Immunol* 1991; **28**: 1225–1232.

117 van't Hof W, van den Berg M, Driedijk PC, Aalberse RC. Heterogeneity in the IgE binding to a peptide derived from the house dust mite allergen Der p II indicates that the IgE response is highly polyclonal. *Int Arch Allergy Appl Immunol* 1993; **101**: 333–345.

118 Van Neerven RJJ, Van t'Hof W, Ringrose JH, Jansen HM, Aalberse RC, Wierenga EA, Kapsenberg ML. T cell epitopes of house dust mite major allergen Der p II. *J Immunol* 1993; **151**: 2326–2335.

119 Oshika A, Kuroki Y, Sakiyama Y, Matsumoto S, Akino T. A study of the binding of immunoglobulin G and E from children with bronchial asthma to peptides derived from group II antigen of *Dermatophagoides pteronyssinus*. *Pediatr Res* 1993; **33**: 209–213.

120 Yssel H, Johnson, KE, Schneider PV, Wideman J, Terr A, Kastelein R, De Vries JE. T cell activation-inducing epitopes of the house dust mite allergen Der p I. Proliferation and lymphokine production patterns by Der p I-specific CD4+ T cell clones. *J Immunol* 1992; **148**: 738–745.

121 Higgins JA, Lamb JR, Marsh SGE, Tonks S, Hayball JD, Rosen-Bronsens S, Bodmer JJ, O'Hehir RE. Peptide-induced non-responsiveness of HLA-DP restricted human T cells reactive with *Dermatophagoides spp*. (house dust mite). *J Allergy Clin Immunol* 1992; **90**: 749–756.

122 O'Hehir RE, Hoyne GF, Thomas WR, Lamb JR. House dust mite allergy: from T cell epitopes to immunotherapy. *Eur J Clin Invest* 1993; **23**: 763–772.

123 Higgins JE, Thorpe CJ, Hayball RE, Lamb JRJD, O'Hehir RE. Overlapping T-cell epitopes in the group I allergen of *Dermatophagoides* species restricted by HLA-DP and HLA-DR class II molecules. *J Allergy Clin Immunol* 1994; **93**: 891–899.

124 O'Brien RM, Thomas WR, Tait BD. An immunogenetic analysis of T-cell reactive regions on the major allergen from the house dust mite, Der p I, using recombinant truncated fragments. *J Allergy Clin Immunol* 1994; **93**: 628–634.

125 Hoyne GF, O'Hehir RE, Wraith DC, Thomas WR, Lamb JR. Inhibition of T-cell and antibody responses to house dust mite allergen by inhalation of the dominant epitope in naive and sensitised mice. *J Exp Med* 1993; **178**: 1783–1788.

126 Hoyne GF, Callow MG, Kuo M-C, Thomas WR. Inhibition of T-cell responses by feeding peptides containing major and cryptic epitopes: studies with the Der p 1 allergen. *Immunology* 1994; **83**: 190–195.

127 Hoyne GF, Callow MG, Kuo M-C, Thomas WR. Characterisation of T cell responses to the house dust mite allergen Der p II in mice. Evidence for major and cryptic epitopes. *Immunology* 1993; **78**: 65–73.

7 IgE Responses and Pollutant Adjuvants

SHIGERU TAKAFUJI, SHUJI SUZUKI, MASAHARU MURANAKA, TERUMASA MIYAMOTO and KOJI ITO
Faculty of Medicine, University of Tokyo, Japan

Epidemiological studies in some countries show evidence of an increase in the prevalence of atopic diseases during the last decades. In Japan, the incidence of allergic rhinitis caused by Japanese cedar pollens increased from less than 3.8% in 1974 to 16.6% in 1987 in the Nikko district [1]. Inouye *et al.* also compared the IgE antibody-positive rate of sera collected in the early 1970s with that of sera collected in the 1980s using the same method, ELISA [2]. They found a significant increase in the IgE antibody-positive rate in recent years. In Switzerland, the prevalence of hay fever rose from 4.8% in 1958 to 10.0% in 1986 in the city of Zurich [3]. In Sweden, one study in military conscripts demonstrated an increase in allergic rhinitis from 4.9% in 1971 to 8.4% in 1981 [4]. A change in genetic predisposition cannot explain this rapid increase in atopic disease because genetic changes in any population take thousands of years [5]. It is therefore evident that environmental factors are of great importance for the development of atopic disease.

Various environmental factors are thought to have some influence on allergic responses. These include greater exposure to allergens, irritation of the airways, and an enhancement of IgE antibody production. The effect of an increase in exposure to allergens was demonstrated in a study carried out in the highlands of Papua New Guinea [6]. Although asthma was formerly unknown in this region, its incidence induced by house dust mite in persons over 20 years of age increased to 7%. This was in parallel with an increase in house dust mite resulting from a change in life-style (the use of cheap cotton blankets and mattresses). It has also been shown in some developed countries that the prevalence of asthma rose as house dust mites increased in indoor environments [7,8].

It has been reported that air pollutants affect airway reactivity by damaging the epithelium of the respiratory tract. Exposure to ozone resulted in the

Allergic Mechanisms and Immunotherapeutic Strategies. Edited by A.M. Roberts and M.R. Walker.

increase of airway reactivity in humans and animals [9]. Similar effects were shown by exposure to nitrogen dioxide and sulphur dioxide in guinea-pigs [10]. There are some environmental factors which have been reported to enhance IgE antibody production. They include particulate air pollutants, tobacco smoke, metal compounds and plant products. This chapter reviews these environmental factors which affect IgE response as an adjuvant, mainly focusing on particulate air pollutants.

EFFECT OF ENVIRONMENTAL FACTORS OTHER THAN PARTICULATE AIR POLLUTANTS ON IgE PRODUCTION

Clinical and experimental observations indicate that some environmental factors may enhance IgE production and be related to the outbreak of atopic diseases. The relationship between tobacco smoke and IgE production has been reported. In some studies, smokers had higher serum IgE levels and a higher incidence of positive skin tests for environmental allergens than non-smokers [11], although such association was not found by other investigators [12]. Bahna *et al.* demonstrated a characteristic pattern for the influence of cigarette smoking on serum IgE levels [13]. They found that serum IgE levels were highest in smokers who did not actively inhale the smoke or who smoked fewer than 10 cigarettes per day, and was lowest in those who smoked 20 cigarettes or more per day, especially if they actively inhaled the smoke. However, in another report, moderate smokers (those smoking 11–15 cigarettes per day) had the highest IgE levels of those tested [14]. Shirakawa *et al.* demonstrated the combined effect of hard metal exposure and smoking in elevating total IgE [14]. Therefore, they believe that discouragement of smoking or exclusion from employment requiring exposure to hard metal may be of benefit for the improvement of asthma. Kjellman showed that parental smoking had an enhancing effect on serum IgE levels in children at nine and 36 months of age, whereas Ownby and McCullough demonstrated that parental smoking had no effect on total IgE or specific IgE production in children aged 2–17 years [15,16]. In another report, maternal smoking was associated with increased cord IgE levels [17]. A study in rats demonstrated that exposure to tobacco smoke increased serum IgE levels and enhanced specific IgE production, apparently by a local effect on the airways [18]. In mouse experiments, the IgE response was first enhanced and then later suppressed during exposure to cigarette smoke [19].

Mercury is included in some cosmetics, disinfectants and drugs. Effects of mercuric chloride ($HgCl_2$) on IgE production have been reported. In cultures of human peripheral blood mononuclear cells, a combination of pokeweed mitogen (PWM) and $HgCl_2$ increased IgE immunoglobulin-secreting cells (ISC) selectively, although PWM alone produced fewer IgE ISC, and $HgCl_2$ alone induced no significant ISC [20]. A study in rats demonstrated that total IgE levels increased strikingly after injections of $HgCl_2$, and the IgE-specific response to OA was potentiated by injections of $HgCl_2$ in susceptible rats [21]. In studies of metal compounds other than mercury, certain platinum salts, when combined with the adjuvant, were demonstrated to enhance total IgE levels and specific IgE in rats, in comparison with the adjuvant given without platinum salts, although platinum salts alone had no enhancing effect [22].

Inhalation of the dust of castor beans induces persistent IgE responses in atopic and nonatopic humans alike. In a study in rats, Thorpe *et al.* demonstrated that a potent, heat-labile component of castor bean not only induced the IgE response to castor bean protein but also enhanced IgE responses to other antigens such as ovalbumin, and increased total serum IgE but not IgG [23]. They found that the component of castor bean responsible for this effect is the toxin recin. Strannegard showed that birch pollen had an enhancing effect on the production of IgE antibodies to bovine serum albumin in rabbits as well as to bovine γ-globulin in mice [24]. This indicates that birch pollen which exerts a potent allergenicity for man possesses adjuvant activity.

EFFECT OF PARTICULATE AIR POLLUTANTS ON IgE PRODUCTION

Ishizaki *et al.* compared the prevalence of Japanese cedar pollinosis in different areas of the Nikko-Imaichi district and found that the prevalence of Japanese cedar pollinosis was relatively high among residents living beside the intercity main road which had heavy automobile traffic all day long [1]. On the other hand, residents in the cedar forest which had less automobile traffic showed a low prevalence. Since pollen counts in both areas were almost identical, air pollution was considered as a possible enhancing factor. Sulphur oxides (SOx), nitrogen oxides (NOx), carbon monoxide (CO), photochemical oxidant and suspended particulate matter (SPM) are cited as typical air pollutants at present. In Japan, SO_2 and CO have remarkably decreased in the atmosphere and photochemical oxidant has a tendency to decrease in spite of occasional transient increases. However, NO_2 and SPM retain the same level and have not yet decreased. In studies in animals, it has been shown that exposure to SO_2, NO_2 and ozone (the main component of photochemical oxidant) may enhance allergic sensitization [10]. However, the effect of these gaseous pollutants on IgE production has not yet been precisely determined.

EFFECT OF SUSPENDED PARTICULATE MATTER ON IgE PRODUCTION

SPM consists of small particles less than 10 μm in size and originates from various sources such as exhaust particles and soil dust in urban districts of Japan. We collected SPM by a high-volume air sampler and examined the effect of the collected SPM on the IgE antibody production of mice [25]. In our experiment, SPM was collected on four stainless steel collection plates in a high-volume air sampler, which was set up in a polluted district of Tokyo. The full range of SPM was divided into four fractions. The range of particle sizes collected at each stage was as follows: Stage 1, 7.0 μm and larger; Stage 2, 3.3–7.0 μm; Stage 3, 2.0–3.3 μm; and Stage 4, 1.1–2.0 μm. The SPM of Stages 1, 2, 3 or 4 were referred to as SPM-I, SPM-II, SPM-III and SPM-IV, respectively. The samples collected for six consecutive days averaged 105 mg in SPM-I, 30 mg in SPM-II, 11 mg in SPM-III and 14 mg in SPM-IV. The carbon content of the samples was 14.4% in SPM-I, 14.6% in SPM-II, 21.5% in SPM-III and 37.3% in SPM-IV, by mass. Figure 7.1 illustrates the anti-OA IgE antibody responses in mice to intranasal administration of 0.25 μg of OA alone, plus 25 μg of SPM-I, plus 25 μg of SPM-II, plus 25 μg of SPM-III, or plus 25 μg of SPM-IV at three-week intervals. The magnitude of anti-OA IgE antibody responses in mice immunized with OA plus SPM-I, SPM-II, SPM-III or SPM-IV was greater than that in mice immunized with OA alone ($P < 0.01$). There were no significant differences in the IgE antibody responses among mice immunized with OA plus SPM-I, OA plus SPM-II, OA plus SPM-III or OA plus SPM-IV. Figure 7.2 shows the anti-OA IgE antibody responses in mice to intranasal administration of 0.25 μg of OA alone without adjuvant or mixed with small doses of SPM-I, i.e. 0.25 μg of SPM-I or with the same doses of SPM-IV. SPM-I or SPM-IV had an adjuvant effect on the anti-OA IgE antibody production, even in a small dose such as 0.25 μg administered intranasally at three-week intervals. There was no significant difference in the enhancing activity between 0.25 μg of SPM-I and the same dose of SPM-IV. SPM had no significant enhancing effect on the anti-OA haemagglutinating antibody production.

SPM consists mostly of exhaust particles and soil dust in urban districts in Japan [26,27]. In addition, it includes sea salt, tyre wear and secondary particles which have been created by chemical reactions in the atmosphere following emission of gaseous compounds [26]. Exhaust particles are mostly distributed in the fine (<2.5 μm) size fraction [26]. More than 80% of exhaust particles are soot, a large part of which consists of elemental carbon [28]. Soil dust and sea salt are mostly distributed in the coarse (>2.5 μm) size fraction [26]. A large part of soil dust consists of quartz, clay and feldspar. Our analysis revealed that SPM consisted mainly of carbon, quartz, calcite, rock salt, calcium sulphate, mica, chlorite, cristobalite and feldspar (Table 7.1). The particles contained more carbon as the size of the

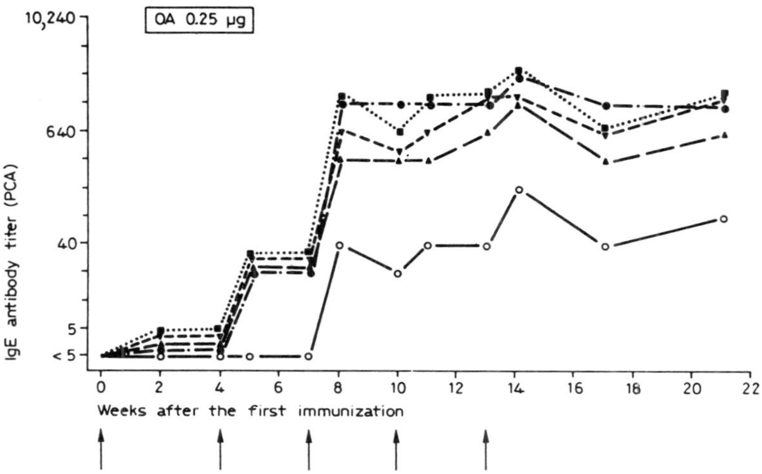

Figure 7.1. Anti-OA IgE antibody production in mice in response to intranasal administration of 0.25 μg of OA alone (○), 0.25 μg of OA plus 25 μg of SPM-I (●), 0.25 μg of OA plus 25 μg of SPM-II (▲) 0.25 μg of OA plus 25 μg of SPM-III (▼), or 0.25 μg of OA plus 25 μg of SPM-IV (■) at three-week intervals. Arrows indicate times of immunization. IgE antibodies in pooled sera from five mice in each group were measured by the PCA assay in rats

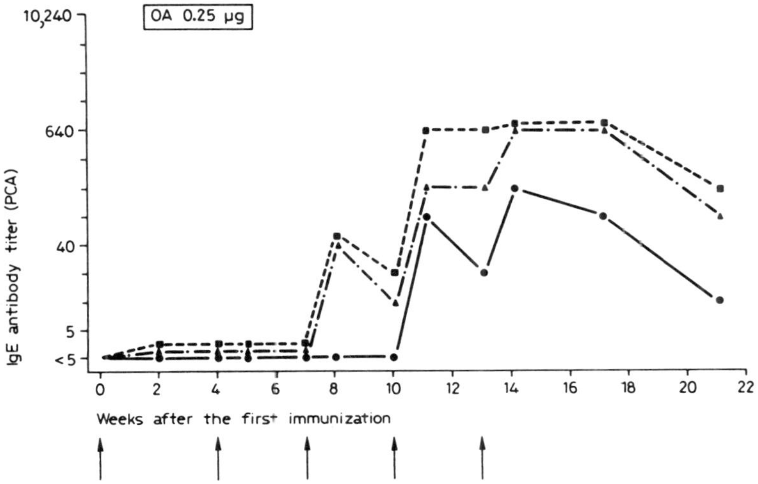

Figure 7.2. Anti-OA IgE antibody production in mice in response to intranasal administration of 0.25 μg of OA alone (●), 0.25 μg of OA plus 0.25 μg of SPM-I (▲), or 0.25 μg of OA plus 0.25 μg of SPM-IV (■) at three-week intervals. Arrows indicate times of immunization. IgE antibodies in pooled sera from five mice in each group were measured by the PCA assay in rats

Table 7.1. Components of SPM

Component	Chemical formula
carbon	C
quartz	SiO_2
calcite	$CaCO_3$
rock salt	NaCl
calcium sulphate	$CaSO_4 \cdot 2H_2O$, $CaSO_4 \cdot 1/2H_2O$
mica	$KAl_2(AlSi_3O_{10})(OH)_2$, $K(Mg,Fe)_3(AlSi_3O_{10})(OH)_2$
chlorite	$(Mg,Fe,Al)_{12}[(Si,Al)_8O_{20}](OH)_{16}$
cristobalite	SiO_2
feldspar	$(K,Na)AlSi_3O_8$, $CaAl_2Si_2O_8$

particles decreased, and more quartz, calcite and rock salt as particle size increased.

In Japan, the concentration of SPM is calculated to be from 40–90 $\mu g/m^3$ of air in general environments of urban districts, and from 200–480 $\mu g/m^3$ of air in locations along busy roads [27]. In the USA, the concentration of SPM in large cities is calculated to be about 100 $\mu g/m^3$ of air [29]. However, the concentration of SPM in more polluted districts may be higher. For example, the concentration of SPM in St. Louis in 1975 was estimated to be 390 $\mu g/m^3$ of air [30], while measurements in Santiago, Chile, in 1981 manifested an average concentration of 575 $\mu g/m^3$ of air [31]. Since SPM has an adjuvant effect on the IgE antibody production in mice even in doses as small as 0.25 μg given at three-week intervals, it is possible the SPM may have some relation to the enhancement of the IgE antibody production in humans.

EFFECT OF DIESEL EXHAUST PARTICULATES ON IgE PRODUCTION

SPM consists of various materials as shown in Table 7.1, but which component has an adjuvant effect on IgE production? We focus on diesel exhaust particulates (DEP) and carbon particles, which form approximately 90% of exhaust particles and are thought to have increased in the atmosphere in Japan.

The number of cars with diesel engines in use has increased in Japan, from 14 897 in 1951 to 5 151 625 in 1983. Particulates emitted from diesel cars weigh 30–100 times more than particulates discharged from catalyst-equipped gasoline-powered cars of corresponding performance [32].

DEP are chain aggregates of very small, spherical primary particles. More than 95% of DEP are smaller than 1 μm; DEP have a mass median diameter of a few tenths of 1 μm [33]. DEP easily remain buoyant in the atmosphere for a long period of time and are undoubtedly inhaled by humans. DEP have a solid carbonaceous core, which has probably formed during the combustion of light fuel oil. A number of hydrocarbon compounds, including some mutagenic substances and other components of exhaust gas, are adsorbed on the surface of carbon particles of large surface area [32].

We examined the effect of DEP administered by intraperitoneal injection or intranasal administration on IgE antibody production [34,35]. Figure 7.3 illustrates IgE antibody responses to repeated intraperitoneal injections of 1 μg or 10 μg of the major allergen of Japanese cedar pollen (JCPA), the most common pollen causing allergic rhinitis in Japan, without adjuvant or mixed with alum or DEP. Mice immunized with 1 μg or 10 μg of JCPA plus 2 mg of DEP developed persistent anti-JCPA IgE antibody responses after the fourth or the second booster injection, respectively. However, the response was not observed in mice immunized with JCPA alone, throughout the period of 24 weeks. Next we administered the antigen and DEP to mice by the intranasal route (the natural mode of entry). Figure 7.4 illustrates the anti-OA IgE antibody responses when mice were administered intranasally with 0.25 μg of OA without adjuvant or mixed with 1 μg, 5 μg or 25 μg of DEP at three-week intervals. DEP had an enhancing effect on the anti-OA IgE antibody production, even in a small dose, such as 1 μg administered by the intranasal route at three-week intervals. As illustrated in Figure 7.5, when mice were given once weekly intranasal 2.5 or 10 μg of JCPA without adjuvant or mixed with 25 μg of DEP, the mice immunized with JCPA plus DEP developed low

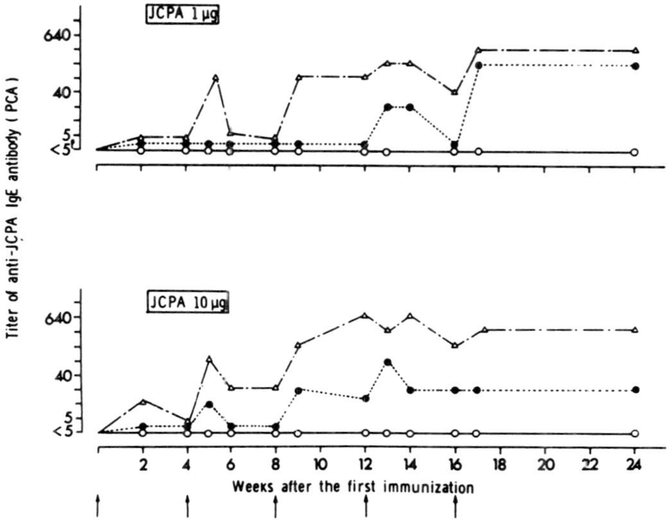

Figure 7.3. Anti-Japanese cedar pollen allergen (JCPA) IgE antibody responses in mice immunized with repeated intraperitoneal injections of JCPA alone (○), JCPA plus 2 mg of alum (△) or JCPA plus 2 mg of DEP (●). Doses of JCPA injected were 1 μg (upper) and 10 μg (lower). Arrows indicate times of immunization. IgE antibodies in pooled sera from five mice in each group were measured by the PCA assay in rats

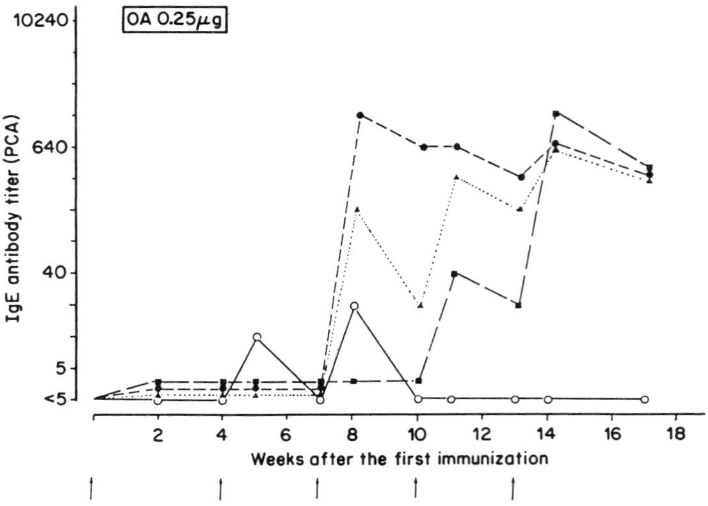

Figure 7.4. Effect of various doses of DEP, administered intranasally, on the induction of anti-OA IgE antibody responses in mice. Mice were inoculated with 0.25 μg of OA alone (○), 0.25 μg of OA plus 1 μg of DEP (▲), 0.25 μg of OA plus 5 μg of DEP (●), or 0.25 μg of OA plus 25 μg of DEP (■) at three-week intervals. Arrows indicate times of immunization. IgE antibodies in pooled sera from five mice in each group were measured by the PCA assay in rats

but persistent IgE antibody responses. However, the response was not observed in mice immunized with JCPA alone.

When the mixture of 500 μg of OA and 10 mg of DEP in 1.5 ml of borate-buffered saline (BBS) was stirred for 1 min, 33.8% (approximately 169 μg) of OA was adsorbed to DEP [34]. In addition, it was demonstrated in our study using intradermal skin testing in four sensitive subjects that the allergenic activity of the JCPA solution (10 μg of JCPA per 1.5 ml of BBS) decreased at least to one-thousandth by stirring the solution with 10 mg of DEP for 1 min. Therefore, as a possible mechanism by which DEP enhance IgE antibody production, depot effects could be considered. Antigens adsorbed to DEP may be released gradually for long periods of time inside the body.

Agarwal *et al.* showed that ragweed antigen activity was present in particles of different size ranges, varying from 0.3 μm to >6 μm [36]. Also Takahashi *et al.* found the existence of exine-free pollen allergen particles together with the intact pollen grains of Japanese cedar in the air during the pollen season [37]. The possibility cannot be excluded that pollen antigens are carried on DEP in the atmosphere. Meanwhile, allergenic substances are readily released from pollen after contact with mucus at the surface of the nasal or upper respiratory mucosa. The allergenic substances thus released may combine with DEP on the mucosal membrane.

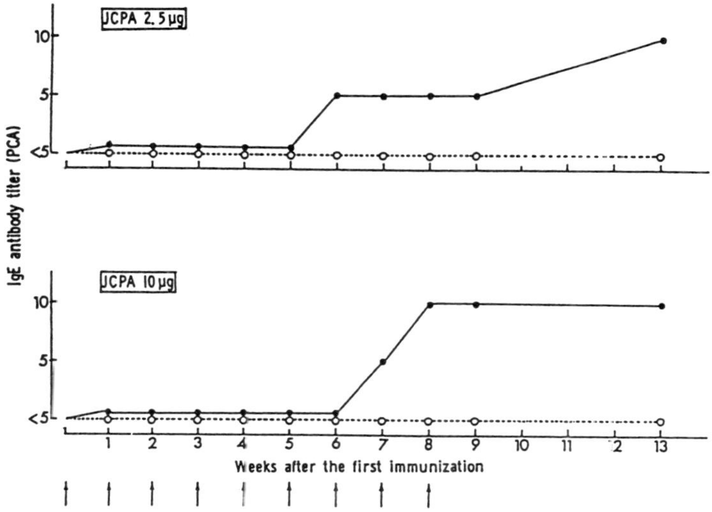

Figure 7.5. Anti-Japanese cedar pollen allergen (JCPA) IgE antibody production in mice in response to weekly intranasal administration of JCPA alone (○) or JCPA plus 25 μg of DEP (●). Doses of JCPA administered were 2.5 μg (upper) and 10 μg (lower). Arrows indicate times of immunization. IgE antibodies in pooled sera from five mice in each group were measured by the PCA assay in rats

A recent study demonstrated that DEP increase local IgE production in humans [38]. A significant rise in nasal IgE but not IgG, IgA or IgM was observed in subjects four days after challenge with 0.3 mg DEP. This increase in IgE occurred by expansion of the local population of IgE-secreting cells and was accompanied by a qualitative change in the pattern of ε mRNA isoforms produced. These results further support the possible contribution of DEP to the increase of respiratory allergic disease.

EFFECT OF CHLORITE ON IgE PRODUCTION

In general, materials capable of adsorbing proteins have adjuvant activities, i.e. alum. Among the components of SPM, we found chlorite as a material capable of adsorbing proteins in addition to DEP [39]. Chlorite $(Mg,Fe,Al)_{12}[(Si,Al)_8O_{20}](OH)_{16}$ is a mineral with layered structure (Figure 7.6) which, as a main constituent of Chinese loess, forms 0.5–1 wt% of SPM. When the mixture of 500 μg of OA and 10 mg of chlorite in 1.5 ml of BBS was stirred for 1 min, 21.0% (approximately 105 μg) of OA was adsorbed to chlorite. We examined the effect of chlorite administered intranasally on IgE production in mice. It has been shown that chlorite has an adjuvant activity for IgE antibody production in mice. Since the amount of chlorite in the

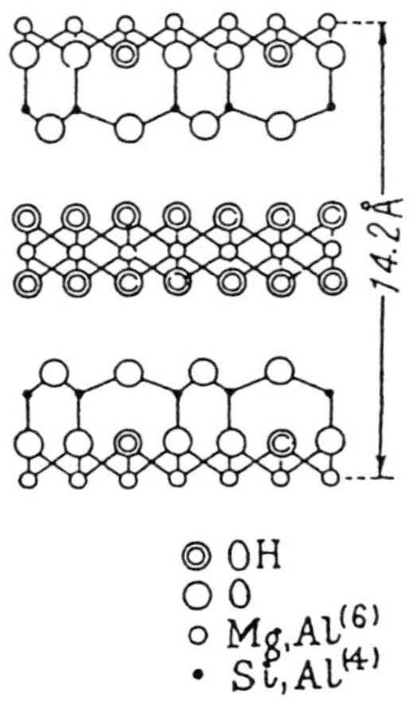

Figure 7.6. Layered structure of chlorite

atmosphere is small, it remains unclear whether chlorite exerts an adjuvant activity in our everyday environment.

EFFECT OF OTHER PARTICULATE MATERIALS ON IgE PRODUCTION

A study in mice has demonstrated the adjuvant activity of fly ash which is the particulate material produced during coal combustion [40]. All particles in fly ash are spheres of largely uniform size. Fly ash consists mostly of Si, Al and contains seven other different atoms (Ca, K, Fe, Zn, Mg, S and Ti) [41]. The difference between DEP or chlorite and fly ash is the capacity to adsorb antigens [34,40]. Fly ash does not adsorb the antigen, whereas DEP and chlorite do. The mechanism of adjuvant activity of fly ash is presently unknown [41]. Studies in mice have also demonstrated the adjuvant activity of manganese and silica which are the main components of various kinds of mineral dust [42,43]. It seems that these particles may exert an effect on IgE production in some labourers in certain working environments, such as mills, mines or quarries. In fact, it was shown that a high proportion of manganese miners had high serum IgE levels or specific IgE antibodies [42].

CONCLUSION

Epidemiological studies in some countries show evidence of an increase in the prevalence of atopic diseases during the last decades. This increase may be explained by a change in certain environmental factors. Therefore, environmental factors which influence IgE production were discussed. It has been shown that tobacco smoke, some metal compounds and some plant products may enhance IgE production. Among air pollutants, we demonstrated the enhancing effect of SPM, which have not yet decreased in the atmosphere in Japan, on IgE production. DEP, the main component of SPM, also have an adjuvant activity for IgE antibody production and may be related to the increase in prevalence of atopic diseases because DEP seem to have increased in urban environments.

ACKNOWLEDGEMENTS

We thank Dr Kazuhiro Koizumi, Dr Kenji Tadokoro and Mr Haruo Ohhashi for their helpful advice on the experiments. This work was supported in part by a grant from the Manabe Foundation.

REFERENCES

1 Ishizaki T, Koizumi K, Ikemori R *et al*. Studies of prevalence of Japanese cedar pollinosis among the residents in a densely cultivated area. *Ann Allergy* 1987; **58**: 265–270.
2 Inouye S, Sakaguchi M, Mori H *et al*. Seroepidemiology of Sugi (Japanese cedar) pollinosis – increase of IgE antibody positive rate in recent years. *J Clin Exp Med (Igaku No Ayumi)* 1986; **138**: 285–286.
3 Wuthrich B. Epidemiology of the allergic diseases: Are they really on the increase? *Int Arch Allergy Appl Immunol* 1989; **90**: 3–10.
4 Aberg N. Asthma and allergic rhinitis in Swedish conscripts. *Clin Exp Allergy* 1989; **19**: 59–63.
5 Zetterstrom O. The increased prevalence of allergic airway disease. *Allergy* 1988; **43**: 10–11.
6 Dowse GK, Turner KJ, Stewart GA *et al*. The association between *Dermatophagoides* mites and the increasing prevalence of asthma in village communities in the Papua New Guinea highlands. *J Allergy Clin Immunol* 1985; **75**: 78–83.
7 Luoma R. Environmental allergens and morbidity in atopic and non-atopic families. *Acta Paediatr Scand* 1984; **73**: 448–453.
8 Takaoka M. Environment and mite allergen. *Jpn J Allergol* 1987; **36**: 537 (Abstract).
9 Golden JA, Nadel JA, Boushey HA. Bronchial hyper-irritability in healthy subjects after exposure to ozone. *Am Rev Respir Dis* 1978; **118**: 287–294.
10 Matsumura Y. The effect of ozone, nitrogen dioxide, and sulfur dioxide on the experimentally induced allergic respiratory disorder in guinea pigs. *Am Rev Respir Dis* 1970; **102**: 430–437.
11 Zetterstrom O, Osterman K, Machado L *et al*. Another smoking hazard: raised serum IgE concentration and increased risk of occupational allergy. *Br Med J* 1981; **283**: 1215–1217.
12 Gerrard JW, Cockcroft DW, Mink JT *et al*. Increased nonspecific bronchial reactivity in cigarette smokers with normal lung function. *Am Rev Respir Dis* 1980; **122**: 577–581.

13 Bahna SL, Heiner DC, Myhre BA. Immunoglobulin E pattern in cigarette smokers. *Allergy (Copenh)* 1983; **38**: 57–64.
14 Shirakawa T, Kusaka Y, Morimoto K. Combined effect of smoking habits and occupational exposure to hard metal on total IgE antibodies. *Chest* 1992; **101**: 1569–1576.
15 Kjellman NIM. Effect of parental smoking on IgE levels in children. *Lancet* 1981; **1**: 993–994.
16 Ownby DR, McCullough J. Passive exposure to cigarette smoke does not increase allergic sensitization in children. *J Allergy Clin Immunol* 1988; **82**: 634–637.
17 Magnusson CGM. Maternal smoking influences cord serum IgE and IgD levels and increases the risk for subsequent infant allergy. *J Allergy Clin Immunol* 1986; **78**: 898–904.
18 Zetterstrom O, Nordvall SL, Bjorksten B *et al.* Increased IgE antibody responses in rats exposed to tobacco smoke. *J Allergy Clin Immunol* 1985; **75**: 594–598.
19 Thomas W, Holt PG, Keast D. Effect of cigarette smoking on primary and secondary immune response of mice. *Nature* 1973; **243**: 240–241.
20 Kimata H, Shinomiya K, Mikawa H. Selective enhancement of human IgE production *in vitro* by synergy of pokeweed mitogen and mercuric chloride. *Clin Exp Immunol* 1983; **53**: 183–191.
21 Prouvost-Danon A, Abadie A, Sapin C *et al.* Induction of IgE synthesis and potentiation of anti-ovalbumin IgE antibody response by $HgCl_2$ in the rat. *J Immunol* 1981; **126**: 699–702.
22 Murdoch RD, Pepys J. Enhancement of antibody production by mercury and platinum group metal halide salts. Kinetics of total and ovalbumin-specific IgE synthesis. *Int Arch Allergy Appl Immunol* 1986; **80**: 405–411.
23 Thorpe SC, Murdoch RD, Kemeny DM. The effect of the castor bean toxin, recin, on rat IgE and IgG responses. *Immunology* 1989; **86**: 307–311.
24 Strannegard O. Adjuvant effect of birth pollen on antibody production. *Int Arch Allergy* 1974; **47**: 14–22.
25 Takafuji S, Suzuki S, Koizumi K *et al.* Enhancing effect of suspended particulate matter on the IgE antibody production in mice. *Int Arch Allergy Appl Immunol* 1989; **90**: 1–7.
26 Mizohata A, Matsuda Y, Sakamoto K *et al.* Chemical composition of particulate air pollutants. *J Jpn Soc Air Pollut* 1986; **21**: 83–103.
27 Fukuoka S, Iida Y, Funeshima M *et al.* A tendency of the concentration distribution of particulate matter alongside roads. *Annual Report of the Tokyo Metropolitan Research Institute for Environmental Protection* 1985: 11–20.
28 Mizohata A. Motor vehicle contribution in particulate matter pollution. Abstract. 26th Congress of the Japanese Society of Air Pollution. 1985: 133–137.
29 Cuddihy RG, McClellan RO, Griffith WC *et al.* Potential health risks from increased use of diesel light duty vehicles. In Lewtas J (ed) *Toxicological Effects of Emissions from Diesel Engines*. New York: Elsevier Scientific, 1982; 353–367.
30 Whitby KT, Charlson RJ, Baker MB *et al.* Measurements of size distribution and concentration. In Sub-committee on Airborne Particles, Committee on Medical and Biologic Effects of Environmental Pollutants, National Research Council (eds) *Airborne Particles*. Baltimore: University Park Press, 1979; 41–61.
31 Tokiwa H, Kitamori S, Nakagawa R *et al.* Demonstration of a powerful mutagenic dinitropyrene in airborne particulate matter. *Mutat Res* 1983; **121**: 107–116.
32 Vostal JJ. Health aspects of diesel exhaust particulate emissions. *Bull NY Acad Med* 1980; **56**: 914–934.
33 McClellan RO. Health effects of exposure to diesel exhaust particles. *Annu Rev Pharmacol Toxicol* 1987; **27**: 279–300.

34 Muranaka M, Suzuki S, Takafuji S *et al*. Adjuvant activity of diesel-exhaust particulates for the production of IgE antibody in mice. *J Allergy Clin Immunol* 1986; **77**: 616–623.
35 Takafuji S, Suzuki S, Koizumi K *et al*. Diesel-exhaust particulates inoculated by the intranasal route have an adjuvant activity for IgE production in mice. *J Allergy Clin Immunol* 1987; **79**: 639–645.
36 Agarwal MK, Swanson MC, Reed CE *et al*. Airborne ragweed allergens: association with various particle sizes and short ragweed plant parts. *J Allergy Clin Immunol* 1984; **74**: 687–693.
37 Takahashi Y, Sakaguchi M, Inouye S *et al*. Existence of exine-free airborne allergen particles of Japanese cedar (*Cryptomeria japonica*) pollen. *Allergy* 1991; **46**: 588–593.
38 Diaz-Sanchez D, Dotson AR, Takenaka H *et al*. Diesel exhaust particles induce local IgE production *in vivo* and alter the pattern of IgE messenger RNA isoforms. *J Clin Invest* 1994; **94**: 1417–1425.
39 Takafuji S, Nishida M, Ishida F *et al*. Adjuvant activity of chlorite for the production of IgE antibody in mice. *Jpn J Allergol* 1989; **38**: 992 (Abstract).
40 Fujimaki H, Hirano S, Takenaka S *et al*. Enhanced IgE antibody production in mice injected with fly ash. *Int Arch Allergy Appl Immunol* 1986; **80**: 127–131.
41 Fujimaki H, Kawagoe A, Ozawa M *et al*. Effects of instillation of fly ash in the lung: physicochemical properties and immune responses. *Am Rev Respir Dis* 1989; **140**: 525–528.
42 Matsui Y, Kino T, Izumi T *et al*. Clinical and experimental studies on increases of immunoglobulins in patients with pneumoconiosis. *Jpn J Thoracic Dis* 1985; **24**: 361–370.
43 Mancino D, Bevilacqua N. Persistent and boosterable IgE antibody production in mice injected with low doses of ovalbumin and silica. *Int Arch Allergy Appl Immunol* 1987; **57**: 155–158.

8 IgE-autoreactivity: A Pathomechanism of Potential Relevance in Severe Atopic Diseases

RUDOLF VALENTA, SUSANNE NATTER, SUSANNE SEIBERLER, ZSOLT SZEPFALUSI, PETER VALENT*, WOLFGANG R. SPERR* and DIETRICH KRAFT

*Institute of General and Experimental Pathology, *Department of Haematology and Haemostaseology, AKH, University of Vienna, Austria*

INTRODUCTION

We have previously reported an example of a distinct IgE-autoreactivity against a human protein [1,2], and identified this protein as profilin, a ubiquitous cytoskeletal protein which acts as an actin-capping protein and participates in signal transduction via the phosphoinositol pathway [3,4]. Using serum IgE from a birch pollen allergic patient we had isolated a cDNA coding for birch profilin [1]. The ubiquitous distribution of profilins in eukaryotes led us to test whether patients allergic to birch profilin might display IgE-cross-reactivity to human profilin. Despite the extremely low degree of sequence homology between birch and human profilin, IgE-cross-reactivity could be found in profilin-allergic individuals.

To investigate further the potential role of IgE-autoreactivity in atopic diseases, groups of individuals with various immunological disorders and atopic diseases, and healthy controls were tested for IgE-reactivity with human proteins derived from histogenetically different cell types [5]. Among the atopic individuals, we have studied patients suffering from allergic rhinoconjunctivitis on contact with exogenous allergens (plant and indoor allergens, e.g. mites, cat and dog hair dander, and moulds), and a group of patients suffering from severe chronic atopy, among them patients suffering from atopic dermatitis and bronchial asthma. While in the rhinoconjunctivitis group only a few patients showed weak IgE-reactivity with human proteins, a high percentage of the severely atopic patients, in particular patients suffering from atopic dermatitis, displayed strong IgE binding to proteins of different molecular weights derived from various human cell types [5].

Allergic Mechanisms and Immunotherapeutic Strategies. Edited by A.M. Roberts and M.R. Walker.

Although patients suffering from atopic dermatitis and atopic asthma display IgE-reactivity against a number of environmental allergens, chronic symptoms and tissue damage in the target organs (skin and respiratory tract) are not always associated with contact to exogenous allergens. The recent study provided evidence that severe atopics display IgE-reactivity against a variety of human proteins from ectodermal, mesodermal and endodermal tissues, thus suggesting an important role of IgE-autoreactivity in the pathogenesis and maintenance of symptoms in chronic atopic diseases [5].

IgE-reactivity against human proteins has been previously described [6–8], but little information concerning the identity and origin of the IgE-defined autoantigens is available. This chapter summarizes evidence for the role of IgE-autoreactivity in chronic atopic diseases, and illustrates that the technique of IgE-immunoscreening of expression cDNA libraries, which has been successfully applied to obtain a number of recombinant allergens, can also be used to isolate human cDNA clones which code for IgE-autoantigens. The ways in which IgE-autoreactivity may contribute to chronic tissue damage in severe atopic patients are discussed.

ATOPIC DISEASE AND IgE-AUTOREACTIVITY

Patients suffering from severe atopic diseases (atopic dermatitis, atopic asthma) display IgE-reactivity against nitrocellulose blotted human epithelial proteins. To investigate whether IgE-reactivity to human proteins is associated with certain forms of atopy, non-allergic individuals, allergic rhinoconjunctivitis patients and patients suffering from severe chronic atopy (atopic dermatitis, asthma bronchiale) were tested for IgE-reactivity to nitrocellulose blotted epithelial protein extracts derived from the human cell line A431.

Figure 8.1 shows that the most intense IgE-reactivity to human proteins was observed in severe atopic patients (block C) whereas non-allergic individuals (block A) displayed no IgE-reactivity with human proteins. Individuals suffering from allergic rhinoconjunctivitis showed rare and weak IgE-reactivity to human proteins (block B). Serum IgE from the atopic individuals bound to a variety of protein bands of different molecular weights. Although those patients with significant IgE-reactivity to human proteins mostly had highly elevated levels of total serum IgE, high serum IgE levels did not represent a prerequisite for IgE-autoreactivity.

EXPRESSION OF IgE-AUTOANTIGENS IN DIFFERENT CELL SOURCES

Serum IgE from severe atopic patients identifies protein bands of different molecular weight in histogenetically different human cell types. To investi-

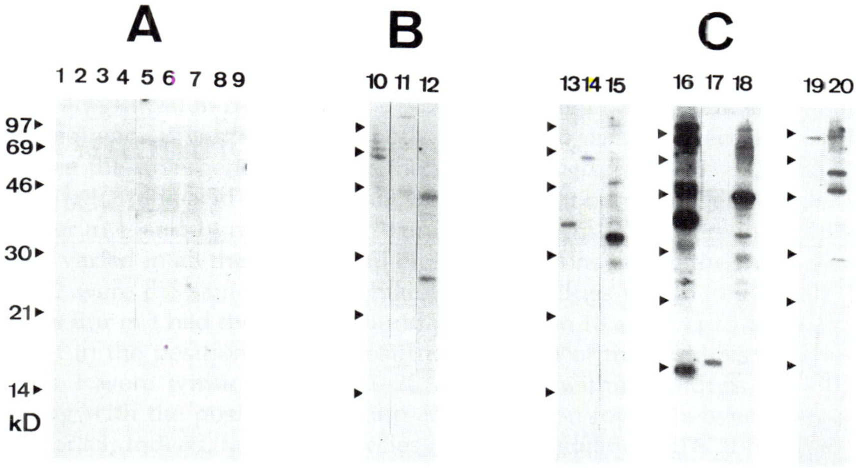

Figure 8.1. IgE-reactivity of different individuals (non-allergic, allergic and atopic individuals) with nitrocellulose blotted human epithelial proteins. A431 proteins were separated by SDS-PAGE, blotted to nitrocellulose and probed with serum IgE from non-allergic individuals and pollen allergic individuals (group A, lanes 1–9). IgE reactivity with human keratinocyte proteins was found in some pollen-allergic patients (group B, lanes 10–12) but was most pronounced in a group of patients suffering from atopic dermatitis (group C, lanes 13–20)

gate whether the IgE-reactivity pattern of atopic individuals varies depending on the cell source used for protein extraction, different cell types were tested (Figure 8.2). Protein extracts were prepared from the epithelial cell line A431 (block K) as well as from primary cultures of human umbilical endothelial cells (block E) and freshly obtained platelets (block T). The three atopic individuals (Figure 8.2, lanes 2–4) showed IgE binding to nitrocellulose blotted proteins from endothelial cells (E), platelets (T) and keratinocytes (K). Protein bands of similar and different molecular weights were detected in the different protein extracts indicating the presence of common and possibly tissue-specific IgE binding determinants. Non-allergic individuals did not display IgE-reactivity to human protein extracts. Further experiments may hence address the question whether there might be a possible association of a certain IgE-autoantigen expression pattern in certain tissues and the manifestation of atopic symptoms in certain organs.

ISOLATION OF cDNAs CODING FOR HUMAN IgE ANTIGENS

In the last years, cDNAs coding for an increasing number of allergens were characterized by molecular biological methods and expressed as recom-

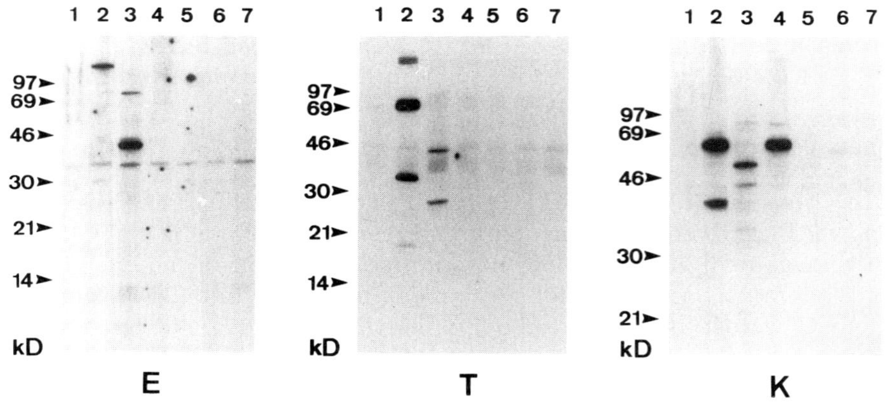

Figure 8.2. IgE-reactivity of individuals with protein extracts from different human cell lines and platelets. Proteins from human endothelial cells (E), human platelets (T) and an epithelial cell line (K) were blotted to nitrocellulose and probed with serum IgE from a non-allergic individual (lane 1), three patients suffering from atopic dermatitis (lanes 2–4), two pollen allergic patients (lanes 5–6) or without addition of serum (buffer control, lane 7)

binant allergens in heterologous expression systems [9,10]. Many of the cDNAs which were isolated by IgE-immunoscreening and expressed as recombinant allergens showed similar immunological properties to the natural allergens. We have therefore chosen the approach of screening human expression cDNA libraries with serum IgE from atopic patients to identify cDNAs coding for IgE autoantigens. A number of phage clones expressing IgE autoantigens could be obtained by this technique and these are currently being characterized by DNA sequencing [11].

Figure 8.3 shows the amplification of three IgE-binding cDNA clones isolated from an expression library prepared from human epithelial cells. Serum IgE from an atopic patient was used to detect filter-immobilized phage-expressing IgE autoantigens. Bound IgE was detected with ^{125}I labelled anti-human IgE antibodies and visualized by autoradiography.

IgE AND IgG BINDING CAPACITY OF RECOMBINANT HUMAN IgE AUTOANTIGENS

The cDNA coding for a human IgE autoantigen designated atopy-related autoantigen 1 (ara-1) [12] was expressed in lysogenic *E. coli* Y1089 as a β-galactosidase fusion protein and purified by affinity chromatography using anti-β-galactosidase antibodies. The purified β-galactosidase fusion protein

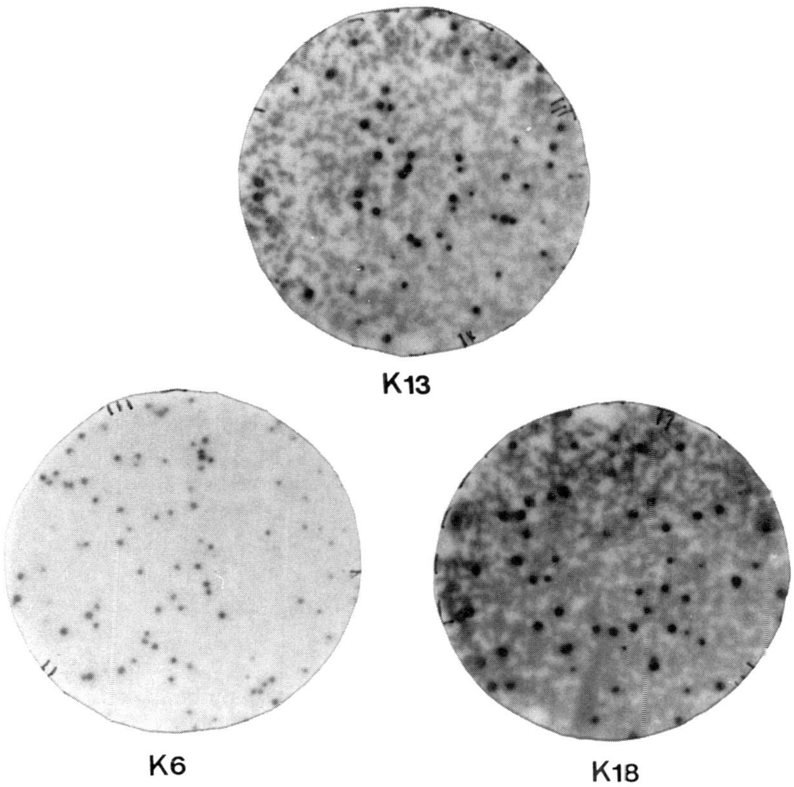

Figure 8.3. Enrichment of IgE binding cDNA clones derived from a keratinocyte expression library by IgE-immunoscreening. Phage clones (K6, K13, K18) were isolated from a human epithelial cDNA library using serum IgE from a patient suffering from atopic dermatitis. The figure shows the first round of enrichment of immunopositive clones. Proteins were transferred to nitrocellulose filters and detected with patient's IgE and ^{125}I labelled anti-human IgE antibodies

was blotted to nitrocellulose and probed with serum IgE and IgG antibodies from two atopic and one nonatopic control individual (Figure 8.4).

Recombinant ara-1 bound IgE from one atopic patient (Figure 8.4, panel 1) with specificity for ara-1 whereas serum IgE from another atopic patient (Figure 8.4, panel 2) with total IgE levels similar to patient 1 but without ara-1 specific IgE antibodies did not react. Serum IgE from a non-allergic individual (Figure 8.4, panel 3) did not bind to recombinant ara-1. Serum from all three individuals contained IgG antibodies specific for ara-1 (Figure 8.4, lanes G). No IgE or IgG reactivity to comparable amounts of nitrocellulose blotted β-galactosidase without the fused ara-1 protein was found with any of the three sera tested (data not shown). The fact that recombinant ara-1 bound IgE

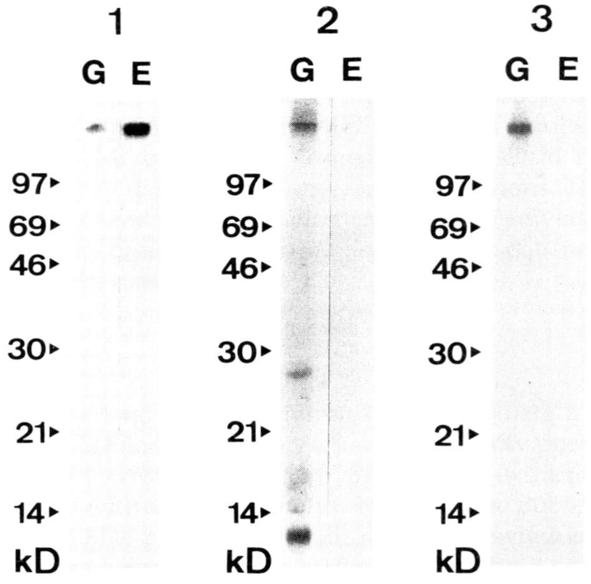

Figure 8.4. IgE and IgG-reactivity of patients with a human recombinant epithelial antigen (ara-1). Sera from three individuals (1–3) were tested for IgE (E) and IgG (G) reactivity with nitrocellulose blotted purified recombinant ara-1 antigen. Ara-1 was expressed as a β-galactosidase fusion protein and therefore migrates at approximately 150 kD. The atopic patient with specificity for ara-1 (1) shows IgE and IgG reactivity to recombinant ara-1 whereas a non-allergic individual (3) and an atopic patient without specificity for ara-1 showed IgG but no IgE reactivity to recombinant ara-1. None of the individuals tested displayed IgE or IgG reactivity to β-galactosidase without fused ara-1

as well as IgG antibodies indicates that the antibody binding requires the Fab portions of the immunoglobulins. It is likely that IgE autoantigens such as ara-1, when complexed to serum IgE, may either be focused via high affinity Fcε receptors on mast cells, basophils or antigen presenting cells, and by this mechanism contribute to chronic inflammation in severe atopic individuals.

CONCLUSION

The research presented here summarizes evidence for a role of IgE autoreactivity in severe chronic atopy. IgE reactivity against human proteins was originally described over 50 years ago [6–8] and the discovery of structural and immunological similarities of exogenous allergens and human proteins [1,13,14] suggested a possible role of autoreactive IgE antibodies in the maintenance of chronic atopic diseases. Using nitrocellulose blotted proteins from histogenetically different human cell lines as well as platelets and MNC from different donors we have demonstrated that patients suffering from severe forms of atopy (atopic dermatits, asthma bronchiale) displayed IgE reactivity against a number of different protein bands. Sera from individuals suffering from other immunological disorders (graft versus host disease, systemic lupus erythematosus and chronic urticaria) did not show IgE-reactivity to the human protein extracts. IgE antibodies from severe atopic patients bound to proteins of similar as well as different molecular weights in extracts from histogenetically different cells [5]. It is hence possible that the expression pattern of certain IgE autoantigens in certain cell types might be linked to the manifestations of symptoms in certain organs (skin, lung). IgE-autoantigens were detected in cultured cells as well as in cells directly obtained from human donors such as platelets and skin (data not shown). Since most of the atopic individuals displayed IgE-reactivity against a number of exogenous antigens it is possible that, as described for profilins, cross-reactivities between exogenous and endogenous antigens might be responsible for IgE-autoreactivity in severe atopics. It is however, also possible that sensitization against IgE antibodies directed primarily against exogenous antigens might lead to tissue damage upon contact with environmental antigens subsequently leading to exposure of endogenous proteins which may then become immunogenic. IgE antibody formation against endogenous antigens would then lead to chronic tissue damage and maintenance of chronic inflammation in severe atopic individuals.

To further characterize IgE autoantigens and to provide information concerning their sequence we have chosen the technique of screening expression cDNA libraries prepared from human cells with serum IgE from atopic individuals. The DNA and deduced amino acid sequence of the isolated IgE autoantigens can then be compared with known protein and DNA sequences to allow their identification. Using serum IgE from a patient suffering from atopic dermatitis we have isolated IgE binding cDNA clones from a human epithelial cell expression cDNA library [11,12]. The IgE autoantigens were expressed in *Escherichia coli* as β-galactosidase fusion proteins and shown also to bind IgG antibodies. The characterization of cDNAs coding for IgE autoantigens will not only provide information concerning the sequence of these proteins but also allow expression of the recombinant IgE autoantigens in heterologous host systems (*Escherichia coli*) for further functional studies which may allow estimation of the pathogenetic role of IgE-autoreactivity in atopy.

ACKNOWLEDGEMENTS

This study was supported by grant P10432, F00501, and F00506 of the Fonds zur Förderung der Wissenschaftlichen Forschung, Vienna, Austria.

REFERENCES

1 Valenta R, Duchêne M, Pettenburger K, Sillaber C, Valent P, Bettelheim P, Breitenbach M, Rumpold H, Kraft D, Scheiner O. Identification of profilin as a novel pollen allergen; IgE autoreactivity in sensitized individuals. *Science* 1991; **253**: 557–560.

2 Valenta R, Duchêne M, Valent P, Sillaber C, Kraft D, Scheiner O. Identification of profilin as novel plant pan-allergen: IgE-autoreactivity in sensitized patients. In: Brown F, Chanock RM, Ginsberg HS, Lerner RA (eds) *Vaccines 92*. New York: Cold Spring Harbor Laboratory Press; 1992: 29.

3 Valenta R, Ferreira F, Grote M, Swoboda I, Vrtala S, Duchêne M, Deviller P, Meagher RB, MacKinney E, Heberle-Bors E, Kraft D, Scheiner O. Identification of profilin as an actin-binding protein in higher plants. *J Biol Chem* 1993; **268**: 22777–22781.

4 Drobak BK, Watkins PAC, Valenta R, Dove SK, Lloyd CW, Staiger CJ. Inhibition of plant plasma membrane phosphoinositide phospholipase C by the actin-binding protein, profilin. *Plant J* 1994; **6**: 389–400.

5 Valenta R, Maurer D, Steiner R, Seiberler S, Sperr WR, Valent P, Spitzauer S, Kapiotis S, Smolen J, Stingl G. Immunoglobulin E response to human proteins in atopic patients. *J Invest Derm* 1996; **107**: 203–208.

6 Simon FA. The allergen of human dander present in the skin of the general body surface. *J Invest Derm* 1947; **9**: 329–332.

7 Hampton SF, Cooke RA. The sensitivity of man to human dander, with particular reference to eczema (allergic dermatitis). *J Allergy* 1941; **13**: 63–76.

8 Simon FA. On the allergen in human dander. *J Allergy* 1944; **15**: 338–345.

9 Scheiner O, Kraft D. Basic and practical aspects of recombinant allergens. *Allergy* 1995; **50**: 384–391.

10 Valenta R, Kraft D. Recombinant allergens for diagnosis and therapy of allergic diseases. *Curr Opin Immunol* 1995; **7**: 751–756.

11 Valenta R, Natter S, Seiberler S *et al.* Identification of a novel human IgE-autoantigen; a link between atopy and autoimmunity. Submitted.

12 Natter S, Seiberler S, Hufnagh *et al.* IgE autoantibodies from atopic dermatitis patients specifically recognise cDNA clones coding for intracellular proteins. Submitted.

13 Spitzauer S, Schweiger C, Sperr WR, Pandjaitan B, Valent P, Mühl S, Ebner C, Scheiner O, Kraft D, Rumpold H, Valenta R. Molecular characterization of dog albumin as a cross-reactive allergen. *J Allergy Clin Immunol* 1994; **93**: 614–627.

14 Spitzauer S, Pandjaitan B, Söregi G, Mühl S, Ebner C, Kraft D, Valenta R, Rumpold H. IgE-crossreactivities against albumins in patients allergic to animals. *J Allergy Clin Immunol* 1995; **96**: 951–959.

9 Specific Immunotherapy

JEAN BOUSQUET, JEAN LOUIS MÉNARDO, ADNAN HEJJAOUI, JALEL KNANI, JÉROME PÈNE, ANNE DES ROCHES, HENRIETTE DHIVERT and FRANÇOIS-B. MICHEL

Arnaud de Villeneuve Hospital, Montpellier, France

Specific immunotherapy (SIT) was introduced in 1911 [1] and for many years remained based on empiricism. Extracts of unknown quality and shelf-life were used and the efficacy of SIT was seriously questioned. The introduction of standardized extracts made it possible to increase the efficacy of immunotherapy and double-blind placebo-controlled studies have demonstrated the efficacy of this form of therapy in rhinitis, asthma and conjunctivitis. However, the increased efficacy of immunotherapy was associated with an increased risk of anaphylactic reactions [2] leading again to question the future of SIT [3]. Most of the studies carried out in our clinic aimed to demonstrate the efficacy of various forms of SIT, to improve the safety of SIT and to characterize which patients should receive SIT to obtain optimal treatment.

VENOM ALLERGY

Allergy to insect venom is a major health problem for a significant number of people. Immunotherapy can reduce the risk of subsequent reaction from about 60% to less than 5%.

EFFICACY

Venom immunotherapy (VIT) with standardized extracts was introduced in the 1970s. Guidelines for treatment were indicated in the late 1970s and it appeared that a monthly dose of 100 μg of venom should protect most patients [4]. However, a small proportion is not completely protected and treatment failures have been reported [5]. It has been proposed that in some patients VIT should be given using a monthly dose of 200 μg in order to protect patients fully.

Allergic Mechanisms and Immunotherapeutic Strategies. Edited by A.M. Roberts and M.R. Walker.

SAFETY

Venoms are potent standardized allergen extracts and systemic reations (SR) are not rare during VIT. Rush protocols may increase the rate of SR and vespid VIT appears to be better tolerated than honey bee venom (HBV) [4].

In order to improve the safety of VIT in honey bee allergic patients, passive immunotherapy was carried out the day before a 1-day rush protocol was administered [6]. A double-blind, placebo-controlled study was carried out to determine whether passive immunization with fractionated IgG from a beekeeper's serum pool was able to protect patients undergoing a rush immunotherapy programme with HBV against untoward systemic reactions, and to observe if the active immunization with HBV could elicit an active IgG immune response towards venom allergens. Hyperimmune IgG was obtained from a pool of sera of beekeepers (Cohn fractions II to III) that was subsequently treated with pepsin for intravenous use. All IgG subclasses were found to be present in the preparation. Twenty-seven patients, highly allergic to HBV, were randomly allocated to two treatment groups. Twenty patients received 10–15 g of fractionated IgG, and seven other patients received saline in a double-blind fashion. The next day, a 3-hour rush protocol attempted to reach a cumulative venom dose of 200 μg; 16 out of the 20 patients who received the fractionated IgG reached this dose without any systemic reaction, whereas none of the seven subjects who received saline could attain it, and all patients had a systemic reaction. The active immunization with HBV elicited a significant increase in venom IgG after 1 week of treatment in the patients who reached the maintenance dose.

We then attempted to find a semi-rush protocol which would lead to a protection within a few days with almost no side effects [7].

DURATION OF VIT

Duration of venom immunotherapy still remains questionable, since some patients outgrow their sensitivity. Two hundred venom-allergic patients (4–82 years; mean±SD, 37.3±14.2 years) who were first observed with systemic reactions (SR) were investigated yearly for up to 3 years [8]. Among these patients, 72 were allergic to honey bee venom, 83 to yellow jacket venom, and 45 to both yellow jacket and Polistes venom. At each visit patients had skin tests and RAST to venom. All patients had the same semi-rush protocol and a monthly maintenance dose of 200 μg. After 1 year of treatment, 19% of bee venom allergic subjects and 35% of vespid venom-allergic individuals had a negative skin test and RAST to the corresponding venom. The percentage of negativation of tests increased after 3 years to 30.5% in bee venom allergic patients and to 54% in vespid venom allergic individuals. This rapid and relatively important negativation of skin tests and RAST may be due to a monthly maintenance dose of 200 μg; 76 patients experienced a field sting without any SR, two patients had a severe SR, and three patients had a mild SR. Although we tried to define parameters that might predict the abolition of venom sensitivity before starting immunotherapy, we could not find any parameter except venom species. Children and adults behave similarly in terms of evolution of venom sensitization. Mean serum venom-specific IgG levels were significantly lower in patients who had lost their sensitivity.

VIT IN BEEKEEPERS

Beekeepers are at a high risk for bee venom allergy. In several studies the prevalence has been estimated to be 15–43% in this group [9,10] as compared to 0.8–5% in the general population [11]. VIT should be offered to all beekepers with recent anaphylaxis who wish to continue beekeeping, and to those with severe anaphylaxis, even when they stop working with bees. A maintenance dose of 200 μg per month is advised because beekeepers are often stung by more than one bee at a time, and it had been shown that this dose gives a higher protection. Moreover, protection should be documented with a sting challenge on the intensive care unit before these patients return to work with bees. Once the sting challenge has been tolerated, protection may be maintained in active beekeepers during the summer months by having them exposed to a bee sting at their own hive every one or two weeks.

POLLEN ALLERGY

EFFICACY AND SAFETY

The efficacy of pollen SIT has been widely documented in optimally designed double-blind placebo-controlled trials performed in rhinitis due to several pollen species. However, this treatment fails completely when inappropriately used [12] and SIT is not equally effective in all patients. There are several parameters which have therefore to be examined, among which the quality of the extracts used, the SIT schedule, cross-reactivities between allergens and the sensitization of patients [13,14] are critical.

Only a few controlled studies have investigated the efficacy of SIT in grass pollen asthma [for review see 15]. Recent studies using aqueous or standardized extracts [12] or formaldehyde-allergoids [16] showed that SIT had a beneficial effect on bronchial symptoms during the pollen season.

Life-threatening reactions may be observed with high quality extracts and, exceptionally, deaths have been reported [15]. The rate of systemic reactions is greater with standardized pollen extracts than with either non-standardized extracts or high molecular weight preparations [17]. However, using

SIT with care, it has been shown that standardized extracts can be used safely [18].

In order to maintain efficacy and to reduce the rate of systemic reactions, several studies were started using allergoids. Specific immunotherapy with unmodified formalinized allergoids is effective in grass pollen allergy, but systemic reactions have been observed [19,20]. A high molecular weight formalinized allergoid (HMW-GOID) was fractionated by gel filtration, retaining molecules of greater than 85 kDa in the expectation of improving safety without sacrificing efficacy. HMW-GOID and unfractionated allergoid (GOID) had a similar allergenic activity assessed by RAST inhibition, but the HMW-GOID preparation was 65 times less reactive when it was tested by skin prick test than the GOID preparation.

A first double-blind, placebo-controlled study was carried out in grass pollen allergic patients with placebo (14 patients), GOID (15 patients), and HMW-GOID (13 patients). An additional group of 18 patients was treated by a rush schedule with a standardized orchard grass pollen extract [16]. A similar mean cumulative dose was administered with both allergoids. The fractionated allergoid only elicited minor systemic reactions similar to reactions elicited by placebo, whereas 20% of patients treated by GOID and 5.5% of patients receiving the standardized extract had a severe systemic reaction. For rhinitis, conjunctivitis, and asthma, the HMW-GOID and the standardized extract had a similar efficacy, significantly greater than placebo. GOID was less effective than the other two active treatments but was significantly more effective than placebo treatment for asthma and conjunctivitis.

A second double-blind, placebo-controlled study was carried out [21]. Eighteen patients received placebo, 19 received the low-dose schedule (maximal dose: 2000 PNU) and 20 received the high-dose schedule (maximal dose: 10000 PNU). Only one patient presented a systemic reaction of moderate severity for a dose of 1200 PNU. Before the onset of the pollen season, patients had a nasal challenge with orchard grass pollen grains, a skin test titration, and the titration of serum-specific IgG. Both groups of patients presented a significant reduction in nasal and skin sensitivities and a significant increase in IgG compared to placebo. Symptoms and medications for rhinitis and asthma were studied during the season, and both groups receiving allergoids had a significant reduction of symptom–medication scores for nasal and bronchial symptoms. There was a highly significant correlation between nasal symptom–medication scores during the season and the results of nasal challenges.

POLYSENSITIZED PATIENTS

The IgE immune response to environmental allergens depends both on genetic and environmental factors and is highly heterogeneous. The IgE response of patients only allergic to grass pollens differs from the response of patients allergic to multiple pollen species [22]. The IgE immunoblots to orchard grass pollens confirmed that polysensitized patients had more proteins revealed than patients only allergic to grass pollens [23]. To determine if both groups of patients present a different response toward specific immunotherapy (IT), a double-blind, placebo-controlled study was performed in 70 patients. Patients receiving the active treatment had a rush IT with either a standardized orchard grass pollen extract or with a standardized mixed pollen extract, prepared depending on the sensitivity of the patients [13]. The maintenance dose was defined as that dose effective in grass pollen IT in previous experiments. The same equipotent maintenance dose was administered for all pollen species. Symptom–medication scores during the pollen season and nasal challenge with orchard grass pollen grains demonstrated that grass pollen allergic patients had a significantly improved efficacy in comparison to placebo treatment, whereas polysensitized patients had a nonsignificant improvement. Serum grass pollen IgG was significantly increased after IT in both treated groups. This study demonstrates that the response toward specific IT differs in patients only allergic to grass pollens in comparison to polysensitized patients. Using a higher allergen dose it might be possible to show efficacy in the polysensitized group, but the rate of systemic reactions using standardized extracts would have been unacceptable.

The reasons explaining the difference in IgE reactivity between mono- and polysensitized patients were examined. Since interleukin-4 (IL-4) and interferon-γ (IFN-γ) regulate human IgE synthesis *in vitro* [24], we determined whether cytokines may be involved in the heterogeneity of atopy by comparing the serum IgE and sCD23 titres to the cytokine profile of T lymphocytes from 44 atopic patients (13 mono- and 31 polysensitized) and seven nonatopic subjects [14]. Monosensitized patients were allergic to grass or cypress pollens or house dust mites, and polysensitized ones to many pollen species or many allergens. Total serum IgE was lower in the control group than in both atopic groups and in the monosensitized group than in the polysensitized one. IgE immunoblots to orchard grass pollen and house dust mites were less heterogeneous in the monosensitized group than in the polysensitized one. IL-4 production by *in vitro* activated peripheral blood mononuclear cells (PBMC) was significantly higher in the polysensitized group than in the monosensitized, and marginal in the control group. In contrast, IFN-γ production was strongly reduced in both atopic groups, and IL-2 production comparable in the three groups. IgE and soluble CD23 (sCD23) release was higher in the atopic groups than in the control, and higher in the polysensitized group than in the monosensitized one. This study shows that PBMC of mono- and polysensitized subjects have a different IL-4 and sCD23 profile and suggests that people may be classified into high and low IgE responders on the basis of IL-4 production.

HOUSE DUST MITE ALLERGY

EFFICACY

Both asthma and rhinitis have been improved with mite SIT, but there are some inconclusive data, and standardized extracts have been used in a few studies only [12].

The candidates for mite SIT in asthma have been studied. A total of 215 patients were enrolled in a controlled trial using a standardized *Dermatophagoides pteronyssinus* extract [25]. They were followed-up for 1 year by means of symptom–medication scores and pulmonary function. Of the total group, 158 received allergen injections and the others were taken as controls. Patients who had other perennial allergies, or aspirin intolerance and/or chronic sinusitis did not improve. Moreover, among the patients allergic only to *Dermatophagoides pteronyssinus*, children presented a significantly greater improvement than adults, and patients with irreversible airflow limitation (FEV_1 under 70% from predicted values after adequate pharmacological treatment) did not benefit from SIT. With tyrosine-adsorbed *Dermatophagoides pteronyssinus* extracts it was noticed that asthmatic children were significantly protected in comparison to placebo [26] whereas results in adults were not always conclusive [27], and the efficacy was only seen after long-term allergen administration.

SAFETY

The safety of mite SIT is critical since many, if not most, patients who die from an allergen injection are asthmatics and, in these patients, death is caused by an irreversible bronchial obstruction [3,15]. Although some investigators suggest that SIT is indicated in severely affected patients, Bousquet *et al.* performed a controlled study in over 1000 patients who received the same maintenance dose using a rush or a step procedure [28,29]. Most patients with FEV_1 under 70% of predicted values developed asthma during SIT, highlighting the importance of avoiding SIT in severe asthmatics. The age of the patient also appears to be of importance. Children under 5 years of age present a significantly greater risk of systemic reaction. The symptoms of the systemic reactions were different in pollen- or mite-allergic individuals [18,29]. In the latter group, as expected, bronchial symptoms were more prevalent than either urticaria or anaphylaxis whereas in pollen allergic individuals asthma was less common. Attempts have been made to reduce systemic reactions, and, as in the case of pollen immunotherapy, it was observed that premedication and exclusion of severe asthmatics lead to an acceptable rate of mild systemic reactions.

DURATION OF EFFICACY AFTER SIT CESSATION

Specific immunotherapy (SIT) using a standardized mite extract is effective and safe when administered under optimal conditions. However, the duration of its effectiveness following cessation of treatment remains unknown. Forty asthmatic subjects who had received SIT with a standardized *Dermatophagoides pteronyssinus* (Der p) extract under the same protocol were studied [30]. All had received SIT for a period of 12–96 months and were not receiving any pharmacological treatment. The FEV_1 was within the normal range in all patients. After cessation of treatment, patients were followed for up to 3 years at 6 monthly intervals. The patient was considered to have relapsed when symptoms of asthma and/or rhinitis occurred and/or when pulmonary function tests were impaired. Skin tests with increasing concentrations of Der p were carried out before and at the end of SIT. Forty five per cent of the patients did not undergo relapse. The duration of efficacy of SIT was related to the duration of SIT itself ($p<0.04$). Most patients who did not relapse had a decrease in skin test reactivity at the end of SIT whereas most patients who relapsed did not show any change ($p<0.003$). The duration of efficacy of SIT after its cessation depends upon the duration of SIT and may be predicted by the effect of SIT on skin tests.

MOULD ALLERGY

Moulds are major allergens in asthma but they often induce polysensitizations and the quality of extracts available in the early 1980s was far from being adequate so that it was proposed to avoid mould SIT. However, efforts have been made to standardize extracts of some moulds such as *Alternaria* and *Cladosporium*, and good quality allergen extracts are now available. A double-blind, placebo-controlled study was performed in 24 patients (5–56 years of age) only allergic to *Alternaria* [31]. The extract was standardized by isoelectric focusing, crossed immunoelectrophoresis, crossed radioimmunoelectrophoresis, RAST inhibition, and skin tests, and contained allergen *Alternaria* major allergen a1 and antigen B. Thirteen patients received the active treatment, and 11 received the placebo. Immunotherapy was started by a 2-day rush protocol; maintenance injections were administered for 1 year. The patient's self-evaluation of the treatment was significantly ($p<0.001$) lower in the placebo-treated group. Global symptom–medication scores, including asthma and rhinoconjunctivitis, were significantly ($p<0.005$) lower in the actively treated group. Nasal challenges with *Alternaria* extract were performed before immunotherapy and after 1 year of treatment. There was no difference in the placebo-treated group and a significantly ($p<0.01$) increased mean provocative dose in the actively treated group. Skin tests were significantly reduced in the actively treated group. Specific IgG increased significantly in the actively treated group and was stable in the placebo-treated group. There was a significant correlation between nasal challenges and nasal symptom–medication scores ($p<0.03$) and the patient's self-evaluation of efficacy ($p<0.05$). This study demonstrated that patients sensitized only to *Alternaria* benefit from specific immunotherapy with a standardized *Alternaria* extract.

REFERENCES

1 Noon L. Prophylactic inoculation against hay fever. *Lancet* 1911; **i**: 1572–1573.
2 Bousquet J, Michel, FB. Safety considerations in assessing the role of immunotherapy in allergic disorders *Drug Safety* 1994; **10(1)**: 5–17.
3 Committee on Safety of Medicines. Desensitising vaccines. *Brit Med J* 1986; **293**: 948.
4 Bousquet J, Muller UR, Dreborg S *et al.* Immunotherapy with *Hymenoptera* venoms. Position paper of the Working Group on Immunotherapy of the European Academy of Allergy and Clinical Immunology. *Allergy* 1987; **42(6)**: 401–413.
5 Bousquet J, Ménardo JL, Velasquez G *et al.* Systemic reactions during maintenance immunotherapy with honey bee venom. *Ann Allergy* **61(1)**: 63–68.
6 Bousquet J, Fontez A, Aznar R *et al.* Combination of passive and active immunization in honeybee venom immunotherapy. *J Allergy Clin Immunol* 1987; **79(6)**: 947–954.
7 Tarhini H, Knani J, Michel FB *et al.* Safety of venom immunotherapy administered by a cluster schedule. *J Allergy Clin Immunol* 1992; **89(6)**: 1198–1199.
8 Bousquet J, Knani J, Velasquez G *et al.* Evolution of sensitivity to *Hymenoptera* venom in 200 allergic patients followed for up to 3 years. *J Allergy Clin Immunol* 1989; **82(3)**: 439–446.
9 Bousquet J, Ménardo JL, Michel FB. Allergy in beekeepers. *Allergol Immunopathol (Madr)* 1982; **10(5)**: 395–398.
10 Bousquet J, Ménardo JL, Aznar R *et al.* Clinical and immunologic survey in beekeepers in relation to their sensitization. *J Allergy Clin Immunol* 1984; **73(3)**: 332–340.
11 Charpin D, Birnbaum, J, Lanteume A *et al.* Prevalence of allergy to *Hymenoptera* stings in different samples of the general population. *J Allergy Clin Immunol* 1992; **90(3)**: 331–334.
12 Bousquet J, Guérin B, Dotte A *et al.* Comparison between rush immunotherapy with a standardised allergen and an alum adjuved pyridine extracted material in grass pollen allergy. *Clin Allergy* 1985; **15(2)**: 179–193.
13 Bousquet J, Becker WM, Hejjaoui A *et al.* Differences in clinical and immunologic reactivity of patients allergic to grass pollens and to multiple-pollen species. *J Allergy Clin Immunol* 1991; **88(1)**: 43–53.
14 Pene J, Rivier A, Lagier B *et al.* Differences in IL-4 release by PBMC are related with heterogeneity of atopy. *Immunology* 1994; **81(1)**: 58–64.
15 Bousquet J, Michel FB. Specific immunotherapy in asthma: is it effective? *J Allergy Clin Immunol* 1994; **94(1)**: 1–11.
16 Bousquet J, Maasch HJ, Hejjaoui A *et al.* Double-blind, placebo-controlled immunotherapy with mixed grass-pollen allergoids. III. Efficacy and safety of unfractionated and high-molecular weight preparations in rhinoconjunctivitis and asthma. *J Allergy Clin Immunol* 1989; **84(4)**: 546–556.
17 Grammer LC, Shaughnessy MA, Finkle SM *et al.* Safety and immunogenicity of immunotherapy with polymerized tree, grass and ragweed in patients with multiple inhalant sensitivities. *J Allergy Clin Immunol* 1986; **77(1)**: 53–58.
18 Hejjaoui A, Ferrando R, Dhivert H *et al.* Systemic reactions occurring during

immunotherapy with standardized pollen extracts. *J Allergy Clin Immunol* 1992; **89(5)**: 925–933.

19 Bousquet J, Hejjaoui A, Skassa-Brociek W *et al*. Double-blind, placebo-controlled immunotherapy with mixed grass-pollen allergoids. I. Rush immunotherapy with allergoids and standardized orchard grass-pollen extract. *J Allergy Clin Immunol* 1987; **80(4)**: 591–598.

20 Bousquet J, Maasch H, Martinot B *et al*. Double-blind, placebo-controlled immunotherapy with mixed grass-pollen allergoids. II. Comparison between parameters assessing the efficacy of immunotherapy. *J Allergy Clin Immunol* 1988; **82(3)**: 439–446.

21 Bousquet J, Hejjaoui A, Soussana M *et al*. Double-blind, placebo-controlled immunotherapy with mixed grass-pollen allergoids. IV. Comparison of the safety and efficacy of two dosages of a high-molecular-weight allergoid. *J Allergy Clin Immunol* 1990; **85(2)**: 490–497.

22 Bousquet J, Coulomb Y, Arrendal H *et al*. Total serum IgE concentrations in adolescents and adults using the phadebas IgE PRIST technique. *Allergy* 1982; **37(6)**: 397–406.

23 Bousquet J, Hejjaoui A, Becker WM *et al*. Clinical and immunologic reactivity of patients allergic to grass pollens and multiple pollen species. I. Clinical and immunologic characteristics. *J Allergy Clin Immunol* 1991; **87(3)**: 737–746.

24 Pene J, Rousset F, Briere F *et al*. IgE production by normal human B cells induced by alloreactive T cell clones is mediated by IL-4 and suppressed by IFN-gamma. *J Immunol* 1988; **141(4)**: 1218–1224.

25 Bousquet J, Hejjaoui A, Clauzel AM *et al*. Specific immunotherapy with a standardized *Dermatophagoides pteronyssinus* extract. II. Prediction of efficacy of immunotherapy. *J Allergy Clin Immunol* 1988; **82(6)**: 971–977.

26 Warner JO, Price JF, Soothill JF *et al*. Controlled trial of hyposensitisation to *Dermatophagoides pteronyssinus* in children with asthma. *Lancet* 1978; **2**: 912–915.

27 Pauli G, Bessot JC, Biggot H *et al*. Clinical and immunologic evaluation of tyrosine-adsorbed *Dermatophagoides pteronyssinus* extract: a double-blind placebo-controlled trial. *J Allergy Clin Immunol* 1984; **74(4)**: 524–535.

28 Bousquet J, Hejjaoui A, Dhivert H *et al*. Immunotherapy with a standardized *Dermatophagoides pteronyssinus* extract. III. Systemic reactions during the rush protocol in patients suffering from asthma. *J Allergy Clin Immunol* 1989; **83(4)**: 797–802.

29 Hejjaoui A, Dhivert H, Michel FB *et al*. Immunotherapy with a standardized *Dermatophagoides pteronyssinus* extract. IV. Systemic reactions according to the immunotherapy schedule. *J Allergy Clin Immunol* 1990; **85(2)**: 473–479.

30 Des Roches A, Paradis L, Knani J *et al*. Immunotherapy with a standardized *Dermatophagoides pteronyssinus* extract. V. Duration of efficacy of immunotherapy after its cessation *Allergy*: In press.

31 Horst M, Hejjaoui A, Horst V *et al*. Double-blind, placebo-controlled rush immunotherapy with a standardized *Alternaria* extract. *J Allergy Clin Immunol* 1990; **85(2)**: 460–472.

10 IgE Recognition of Natural, Recombinant and Chemically Modified Allergens

CENK SUPHIOGLU, ENG K. ONG, R. BRUCE KNOX and MOHAN B. SINGH*

*Pollen and Allergen Research Group, School of Botany, University of Melbourne, Victoria, Australia. *Present address: Department of Agriculture and Resource Management, University of Melbourne, Victoria, Australia*

INTRODUCTION

Allergens are antigens which are capable of eliciting synthesis of IgE antibodies in genetically predisposed individuals following inhalation, ingestion or contact with the skin [1]. In the indoor environment, sources of allergens include house dust mite, moulds (fungal spores), animal dander and certain foods. In the outdoor environment, the principal allergens are pollen grains. Exposure to these allergens leads to:

1. Production of specific IgE antibodies.
2. Binding of allergens to IgE antibodies present on the surface of mast cells and basophils.
3. Release of the mediators of allergic response leading to symptoms of hayfever, allergic asthma and dermatitis [1].

The key factor in allergic diseases is the specific recognition of IgE antibodies by different allergens. Allergens are, effectively, IgE binding proteins [1]. Allergic patients have elevated levels of IgE in their serum [1]. This serum IgE provides a probe for identification of allergens and their cross-reactivity, isolation of genes encoding allergens, determination of their amino acid sequences, and identification of allergenic domains in the molecules.

The identification of allergen molecules has been facilitated by the presence of cross-reactive IgE-binding domains in allergen molecules from different sources. For example, pollen from different genera of grasses contains a number of allergenic proteins, as will be discussed in this chapter, and the serum IgE from an individual sensitized to an allergen from one grass such as

Allergic Mechanisms and Immunotherapeutic Strategies. Edited by A.M. Roberts and M.R. Walker

ryegrass, can recognize cross-reactive allergens in pollen of many other genera of grasses [2].

Recently, this IgE binding property has been utilized to identify cDNA clones in expression libraries. A considerable number of allergen genes have been expressed in bacterial cells. The majority of these retain their IgE binding activities. Fragments of these cDNA clones have been expressed, and synthetic peptides produced which have helped in determining the precise IgE binding domains. In this chapter, we discuss recent advances in our understanding of IgE recognition in the major allergens. Two forms of allergens are now available: allergens isolated from their natural source, and recombinant allergens produced by genetic engineering. The recombinant allergens may have particular relevance in immunodiagnostics and therapy.

NATURAL AND RECOMBINANT ALLERGENS

HOUSE DUST MITE ALLERGENS

House dust mites, *Dermatophagoides pteronyssinus* and *D. farinae*, are the source of the dominant allergens found in the indoor environment. Extracts of *D. pteronyssinus* contain more than 30 proteins that bind IgE from sera of mite-allergic patients [3]. The major allergens, Der p 1 and Der p 2, have been extensively studied [4] and cDNAs encoding them have been cloned [5,6].

Western analysis of extracts of *D. pteronyssinus* shows that 43% of mite-allergic patients possess IgE antibodies that recognize Der p 1, but 88% of the same sample have IgE to Der p 2 [7]. In contrast, purified Der p 1 has been shown by skin test and radioimmunoassay to react with IgE in about 90% of patients allergic to mites [8–10]. Using similar assays, IgE binding to purified Der p 2 has been demonstrated in 92% of patients allergic to mites [11]. IgE specific to Der p 1 comprised over 50% of the total anti-mite IgE antibodies in serum samples [8,12].

Recombinant Der p 1 expressed in *Escherichia coli* reacted with only 50% of the sera which have IgE directed against natural Der p 1 [13]. Absorption analysis showed that recombinant Der p 1 can only inhibit half of the natural Der p 1 reactivity. These results indicate that the expressed protein is not folded into its correct conformation. When yeast was used to express Der p 1 recombinant protein [14], the recombinant protein reacted strongly with IgE, binding to 82% of sera from mite-allergic patients, a similar intensity of binding as obtained with the natural allergen. Recombinant Der p 1 expressed in yeast absorbed out most of the IgE antibodies directed against natural Der p 1 [14]. The recombinant protein expressed in yeast has many of the properties of the natural allergen Der p 1.

Unlike Der p 1, Der p 2 expressed in *E. coli* retained nearly all the IgE binding ability of natural Der p 2. In dot-blot analysis using sera from 12 mite-allergic children and 12 adults, recombinant Der p 2 reacted with IgE from all the adults and 10 out of 12 of the children [15]. The two non-reacting sera showed only weak reactivity to the natural allergen. Recombinant Der p 2 could considerably deplete levels of IgE antibodies in a cross-absorption study to the natural allergen, but could not eliminate them. Thus, the recombinant allergen expressed many but not all of the properties of the natural allergen. A more recent study [16] demonstrated that recombinant Der p 2 was almost as effective as the natural material in stimulating positive immediate hypersensitivity skin test reactions in patients allergic to house dust. Over 60% of the patients, selected for their skin-test reactivity to house dust mite extract and whole mite extract, were skin-test positive to recombinant Der p 2 and 80% contained detectable serum IgE antibody against the recombinant allergen. Thus, recombinant Der p 2 possesses the biological activity equivalent to that of the natural allergen.

Since recombinant Der p 1 and Der p 2 proteins bound IgE, modified peptides corresponding to regions of these allergens were studied for their IgE binding properties. First, peptide fragments were produced by cleaving the cDNA of the allergens randomly or at a specific site and expressing the fragments as fusion proteins with glutathione transferase in pGEX vector. Greene and Thomas [17] used a series of 18 overlapping cDNA fragments covering the entire Der p 1 sequence, and expressed them in pGEX vector to study their IgE binding in a dot-blot radioimmunoassay. Twelve of the peptides reacted positively to IgE antibodies from a patient highly allergic to mites (Figure 10.1). Most IgE antibodies in a cross-absorption study were directed against the N-terminal region of Der p 1 (amino acids 1–116). Peptides from this region could almost completely inhibit IgE binding to the full-length recombinant molecule. In contrast, a peptide of the remainder of the molecules (amino acids 117–222) failed to inhibit IgE binding [17].

In a similar study using seven sera from patients positive to recombinant Der p 1, Greene *et al.* [13] showed that all fragments expressing peptides longer than 30 residues could bind IgE from all patients, whereas those shorter than this reacted selectively (Figure 10.2). Thus, IgE binding to Der p 1 is largely conformational and each serum tested has its own binding pattern.

Second, solid phase overlapping synthetic peptides (octamers) representing the entire sequence of Der p 1 were synthesized for epitope mapping using an ELISA technique [18]. Octapeptides tested with various allergic human sera showed that IgE binding regions centred around amino acids 68, 121 and 151. The intensities of binding were weak compared to that of anti-Der p 1-specific rabbit IgG and human IgG.

In a different approach, Jeannin *et al.* [19] tested the IgE binding ability of four peptides (13–20 mers) by measuring their capacity to induce *in vitro* histamine release. The sequences of these peptides were selected using algorithm predictions and a three-dimensional model of Der p 1 derived from comparison to papain and actinidin (Figure 10.3). In 29 *D. pteronyssinus*-sensitive patients, the selected peptides were able to induce significant

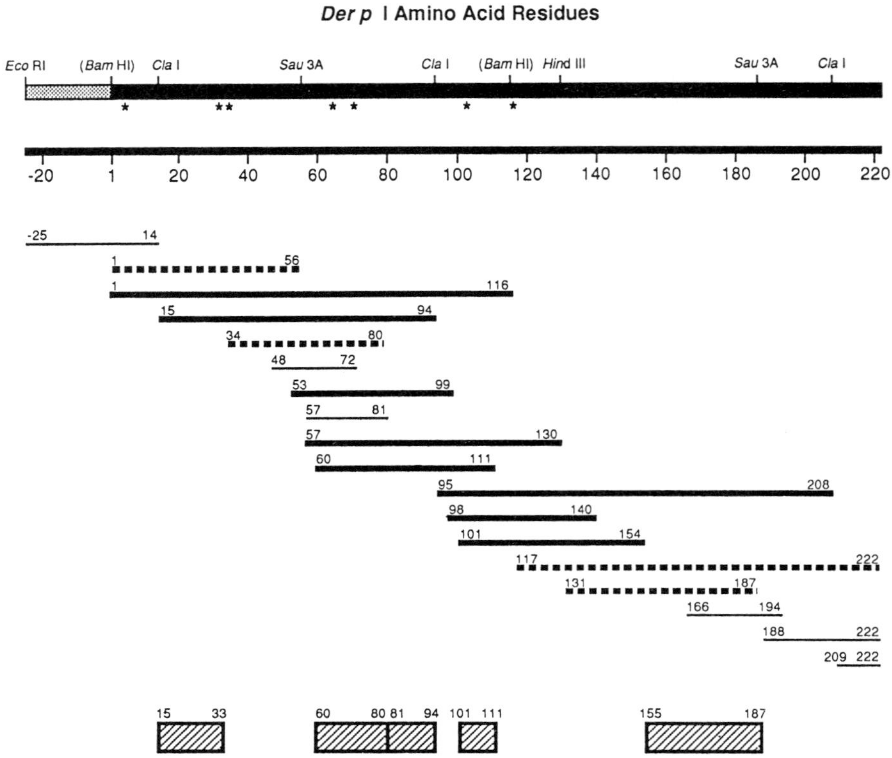

Figure 10.1. Map showing Der p 1 sequence position of the 18 pGEX expression clones which cover the entire mature Der p 1 coding region represented by the solid bar. Peptides with densitometric IgE binding readings of more than 10000 grey scale units are shown in black and readings of less than 500 are shown as lines. Broken bars are those with intermediate readings. Boxes correspond to regions of Der p 1 deduced to account for IgE reactivity. Cysteines at positions 4, 31, 34, 65, 71, 104 and 117 are marked by asterisks. Minus residues are from the proenzyme sequence and are not found in natural Der p 1. [From reference 17]

histamine release [19]. The percentage of release for each peptide differed according to the patients tested and most frequently to peptides corresponding to amino acids 52–71 and 117–133. The results with these synthetic peptides corresponded well with that from the recombinant fragments of Der p 1.

In the case of Der p 2, recombinant fragments coding for peptides up to 93 amino acid residues in length at the N-terminus did not bind IgE [20]. Interestingly, 25% of mite-positive sera had some IgE reactivity with three overlapping recombinant fragments expressing peptides comprising half the linear Der p 2 sequence. IgE binding to the fusion peptides was in all cases

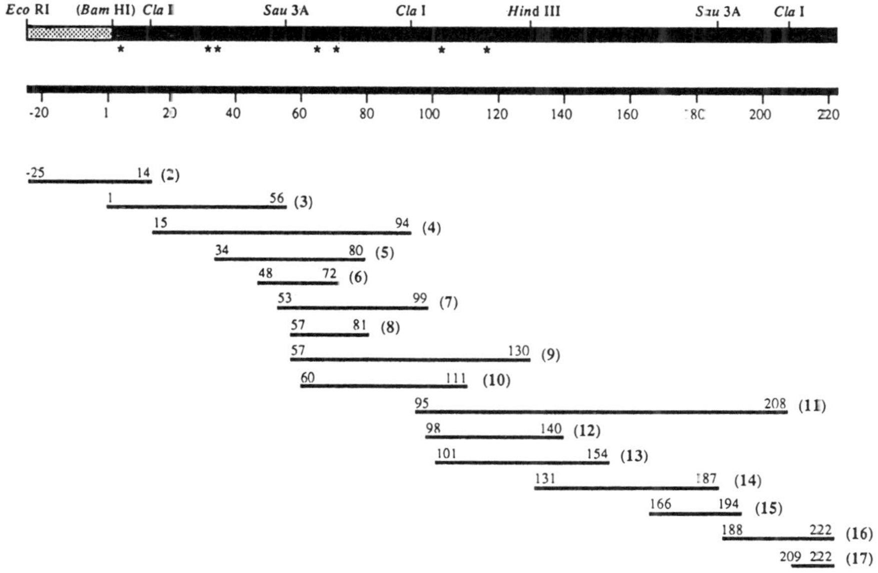

Figure 10.2. Der p 1 cDNA and cDNA fragments used to express fusion peptides. The restriction endonuclease sites used to produce the fragments encoding overlapping peptides are shown on the top, thick bar, where the filled region encodes the mature protein and the open region encodes a truncated proenzyme sequence (−1 to −23). Cysteines at positions 4, 31, 34, 65, 71, 104 and 117 are marked by asterisks. The bar with intermediate thickness shows the amino acid residues of clone 13T and the bar below, the position of the peptide fragments with amino acid residues shown. The numbers in parentheses (2–17) are the peptides. [From reference 13]

weaker than that to the whole molecule. Thus, the IgE recognition sites of Der p 2 are conformational.

However, when sera of a group of atopic dermatitis patients were used, seven out of eight patients had IgE reactive with the peptides suggesting that these patients possess a wider repertoire of anti-Der p 2 IgE antibodies. The intensities of binding compared to that of full-length recombinant Der p 2 were weak [20].

Der p 5 has been cloned from a *D. pteronyssinus* λgt11 cDNA expression library on the basis of strong IgE-reactivity from serum of a house dust mite allergic patient [21]. The cDNA clone encodes a 113-residue mature protein which corresponds to a 14 kDa protein in mite extracts. Recombinant Der p 5 was expressed in a pGEX construct and when tested by western analysis reacted with 50% of sera from house dust mite allergic patients. Moreover, skin-tests with recombinant Der p 5 demonstrated positive reactions in 58% of patients with asthma and 29% with allergic rhinitis alone.

In conclusion, recombinant and modified proteins of house dust mite

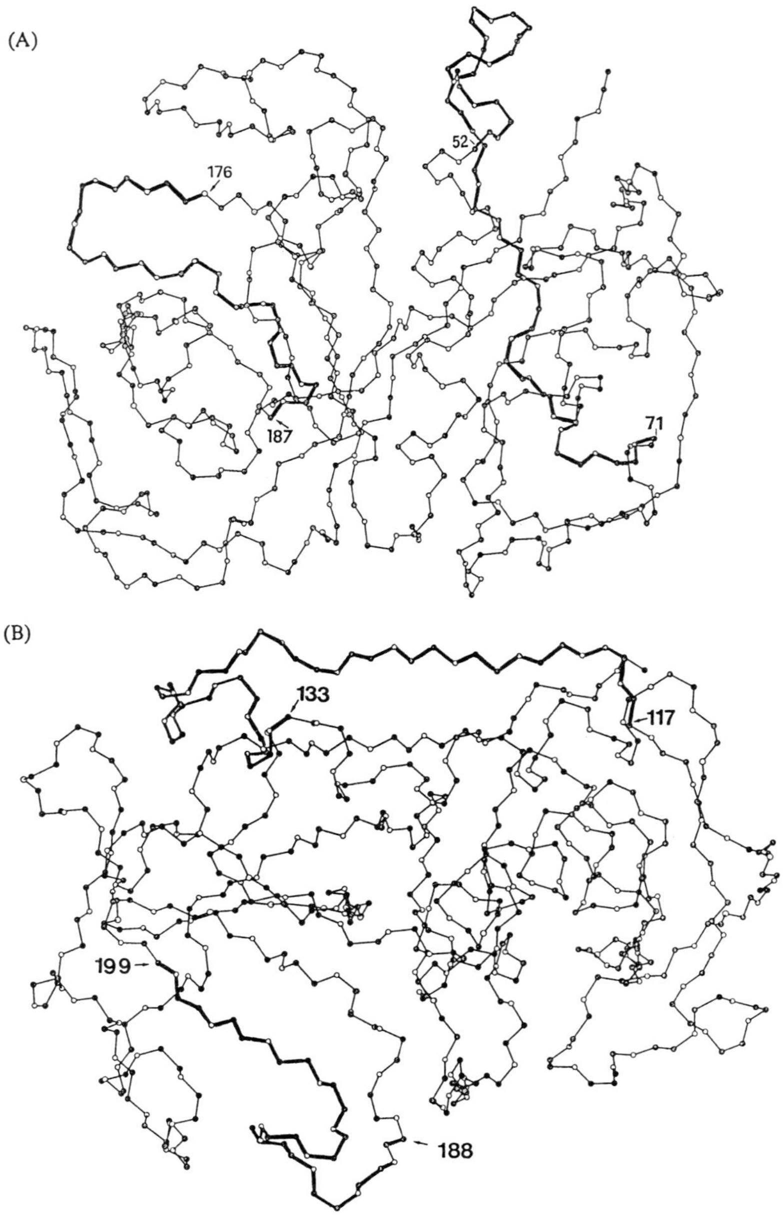

Figure 10.3. Schematic folding of the main chain of the Der p 1 modelized molecule. The N-terminal amino acid is at the left and the C-terminal amino acid is at the right. The peptides 52–71 and 176–187 are indicated in (A); the peptides 117–133 and 188–199 in (B). [From reference 19]

allergens retain the IgE binding properties of their natural counterparts and promise to be useful in future diagnostics.

CAT ALLERGENS

The cat (*Felis domesticus*) is the source of a potent allergen. Immediate hypersensitivity to inhaled allergen produced by the domestic cat has been demonstrated in 20–30% of patients with asthma [22,23]. Most of the IgE in patients allergic to cats is directed against the major cat allergen Fel d 1 [24], although western analysis shows five IgE binding proteins (18, 35, 46, 54 and 66 kDa). The major IgE binding (18 kDa) is to Fel d 1, and 14 out of 15 patients show IgE binding to this allergen [25]. Fel d 1 was first isolated from cat pelt extracts [26], although the main source is in saliva [27]. Fel d 1 is produced by sebaceous cells and stored mainly on the surface of the epidermis and fur [24]. It is a stable 39 kDa glycoprotein [29], consisting of two 18 kDa monomers noncovalently linked to form a dimer [30,31].

As a result of biochemical purification, the N-terminal amino acid sequence of Fel d 1 has been determined [29,30] and together with cDNA cloning resulted in the determination of the complete primary structure of Fel d 1 [31]. PCR cloning shows that Fel d 1 is composed of two mature polypeptides of 70 and 92 amino acids, designated chain 1 and chain 2 respectively [31,32]. A study of pooled sera of cat allergy patients showed that the two purified recombinant proteins corresponding to chains 1 and 2 bind IgE [33]. A range of 30–50% of natural Fel d 1-specific IgE binds to both recombinant chains 1 and 2. However, individual patient's IgE antibodies preferentially bind to either recombinant chain 1 or recombinant chain 2. In a further study, the IgE-reactivity of a set of individual cat allergic patients' sera with purified natural Fel d 1 and *E. coli*-expressed chains 1 and 2 has been compared using both direct binding and competition assays [34]. When examined for direct IgE binding using ELISA, RAST, western blotting and histamine release assays, the natural Fel d 1 and recombinant chain 1 and chain 2, derived from Fel d 1 cDNA, were reactive to IgE from 18 cat allergic patients' sera. On the other hand, both western blot and ELISA competition assays indicated a much higher reactivity to Fel d 1 in solution as compared to the separate recombinant chains, which was also supported by histamine release data. However, the sum of the amount of IgE binding to the recombinant chains was almost similar to the amount of IgE in the sera directed against natural Fel d 1 as assessed by RAST assays. Furthermore, since denaturation of Fel d 1 with alkali conditions was shown to lead to a dramatic decrease in IgE reactivity [34], even though measurable changes to the backbone structure of the protein were minimal, it is suggested that both chains possess a core region determined by their primary structures, and that the major IgE epitopes are dependent on their conformation.

In summary, the determination of the complete primary structure of Fel d 1 should now facilitate the mapping of its antigenic B- and T-cell epitopes and thus lead to a more effective disease management for cat allergic patients.

GRASS POLLEN ALLERGENS

Grass pollen is the source of the dominant allergens found in the outdoor environment. The most important pollen sources are common agricultural pasture grasses that have been widely introduced throughout the world, but vary in temperate and tropical climates. The best characterized are those from cool temperate climates, including Bermuda grass, canary grass, cocksfoot, Kentucky bluegrass, perennial ryegrass, sweet vernal grass, timothy and Yorkshire fog. Apart from Bermuda grass, all these grasses belong to a single sub-family Pooideae. The most comprehensive studies have been made of proteins from ryegrass pollen, and to a lesser extent Kentucky bluegrass, timothy and cocksfoot.

Perennial ryegrass, *Lolium perenne*, pollen extracts contain more than 17 proteins (Figure 10.4) that bind IgE from sera of grass pollen-allergic patients [35]. Although the pattern of allergens appears complex, the immunochemical picture is actually simpler as many of these allergens share cross-reactive epitopes. Out of the 17 IgE binding proteins shown by two-dimensional western analysis, 12 belong to variants of either of two major allergens, Lol p 1 and Lol p 5, which together account for nearly all the IgE binding reactivity of crude ryegrass pollen extract [36]. Lol p 1 was first isolated by Johnson and Marsh [37] and is a 35 kDa glycoprotein, but the carbohydrate moiety (5% of

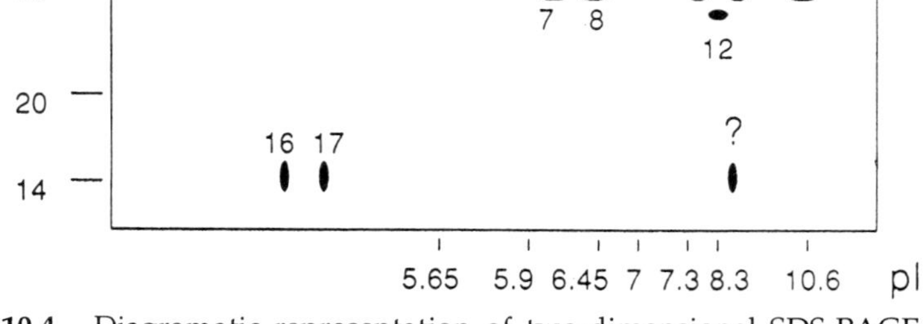

Figure 10.4. Diagramatic representation of two-dimensional SDS-PAGE western analysis of crude ryegrass pollen extract probed with serum IgE from grass pollen allergic individuals. Spot numbers 1–4 refer to group 1 allergens, 5–12 to group 5, 13–15 to group 4, 16–17 to group 2, and ? refers to group 3. [From reference 35]

molecular mass) is not involved in IgE reactivity. Molecular cloning of this allergen has recently been reported [38,39]. There is significant homology between Lol p 1, and the minor allergens Lol p 2 and 3 [39]. The second allergen Lol p 5, a 28–33 kDa protein, has been identified only recently as a result of molecular cloning (initially designated *Lol p* Ib [40]; *Lol p* IX [41]). Its amino acid sequence shows no homology with Lol p 1, but shows significant homology with an allergen cloned from pollen of Kentucky bluegrass [42] and timothy grass [43,44].

At the same time that these allergens were cloned, a timothy grass allergen Phl p 5 was isolated by copper chelate and ion exchange chromatography [45] and members of the same allergen group were identified in other grasses including ryegrass [46]. Eighty five per cent of sera from allergic individuals recognized Lol p 5 while 90% recognized Lol p 1. However, IgE binding appeared to be stronger to Lol p 5 than to the more abundant allergen Lol p 1 [46]. Lol p 5 bound IgE in sera of 17 out of 20 patients. Monoclonal antibodies (mAb) raised against Phl p 5 were subsequently used to isolate Lol p 5 by immunoaffinity purification [47]. The NH_2-terminal of this protein is homologous with the amino sequence of Lol p 5 [40]).

Allergens cross-reactive with Lol p 1 and Lol p 5 have been detected in pollen of other grass genera [43,44,46,48–50]. While Lol p 1 homologues are found in all grass pollens tested, Lol p 5 homologues are apparently confined to the Pooideae group, which includes Kentucky bluegrass, orchard/cocksfoot grass, timothy and Yorkshire fog. For example, Phl p 5 from timothy grass has been isolated from a cDNA expression library using serum IgE from allergic patients and group 5-specific monoclonal and polyclonal antibodies [43]. This allergen bound IgE from about 80% of grass pollen allergic patients. Moreover, recombinant Phl p 5 blocked the binding of patients' IgE to natural group 5 isoallergens on two-dimensional immunoblots and 60% of grass pollen specific IgE from patients sera was preadsorbed with the recombinant allergen. Finally, the purified recombinant Phl p 5 was capable of inducing specific histamine release from blood basophils of grass pollen allergic patients.

More recently, two isoforms of Phl p 5 (Phl p 5A and 5B) have been isolated by immunoscreening of a timothy grass pollen cDNA library with a specific monoclonal antibody and mixed oligonucleotide primed amplification of N-terminal cDNA [44,51]. Phl p 5A revealed a deduced amino acid sequence homology of 81.1% and 86.9% with sequences of Lol p 5 and Poa p 5, respectively [44]. By truncating the allergen from N-terminal and C-terminal ends and expressing the truncated versions in *E. coli,* at least two different IgE epitopes were identified. When tested with sera from 11 grass pollen allergic patients, variable IgE immunoreactivities to both IgE-reactive epitopes were shown. There was also very high homology between the deduced amino acid sequence of Phl p 5B and other group 5 grass pollen allergens [51].

Isoforms of Grass Pollen Allergens

When Lol p 1 was first isolated from ryegrass, the allergen was found to exist as four proteins which differed slightly in their physical characteristics (mobility on starch gels and amino acid composition) but appeared to be immunologically identical [37,52]. These different forms were termed *isoallergens*. Since then several allergens have been shown to exist as a number of forms, differing in physical characteristics [53]. Poa p 1 comprises two isoallergens [54], one being acidic (35.8 kDa, pI 6.4) and the other basic (33 kDa, pI 9.1). Eight isoallergens have been demonstrated by their IgE binding in Phl p 5 [55], four with M_r of 32 and four with M_r of 38, but differing in pI. Smith *et al.* [35] probed two-dimensional western blots of ryegrass pollen proteins with IgE antibodies affinity purified from either recombinant Lol p 1 or Lol p 5. Four isoforms of Lol p 1 were detected differing only in pI, and eight isoforms of Lol p 5, differing in M_r and pI.

Cloning of allergens has also resulted in identification of allergen genes which encode proteins that, despite an overall homology, differ slightly in amino acid sequence (e.g. ragweed, Amb a 1, [56,57] and hornbeam, Car b 1, [58]). These sequence differences may result in differences in reactivity with IgE and IgG antibodies from allergic individuals. For example, the recombinant allergen from ragweed pollen, Amb a 1.1, was recognized by IgE from the sera of more individuals allergic to ragweed than two other forms, Amb a 1.2 and Amb a 1.3 [56]. These allergens, which are not immunologically identical but highly homologous, should be termed *isoforms* or *polymorphic forms* of an allergen. The question needs to be addressed whether all polymorphic forms are capable of eliciting an allergic response in susceptible individuals.

Cloning of cDNAs encoding Lol p 1 [38,39] and Lol p 5 [40,59] has shown that each allergen consists of a family of homologous but distinguishable sequences. Individual cloned members of the Lol p 5 family, i.e. Lol p 5A and Lol p 5B, share amino acid sequence identity exceeding 66%. The differences in sequence between the two polymorphic forms result in differences in their antigenic activity. For example, Lol p 5B is not recognized by mAb FMC-A7, an mAb which binds strongly to Lol p 5A. These differences in antigenic activity suggest that polymorphic form-specific IgE epitopes may exist, and highlight the need to assess the relative potency of all polymorphic forms.

Expression of Cloned Grass Pollen Allergens

Recombinant Lol p 1 and Lol p 5 proteins expressed in bacteria are immunoreactive with IgE antibodies from the sera of allergic individuals. IgE from 90% of patients bound to recombinant Lol p 1, and 80% to Lol p 5 [59]. We have used gene fragmentation [13,60] to examine systematically large numbers of peptides of varying length and position within an antigen.

Random fragment libraries for these major allergens have enabled expressed peptides to be tested for IgE reactivity. With Lol p 5A, a number of peptides ranging in length from 35 to 100 amino acids were found to bind IgE. Although different IgE-reactive epitopes were localized throughout the molecule, the highest frequency and intensity of binding was observed in fragments from the C-terminal half of the molecule. These results confirm our original observations that when two 'half molecules' of Lol p 5A are expressed individually, the majority of the IgE reactive sites occur on the C-terminal half [40].

Thirty-four overlapping peptides (12-mers) based on the amino acid sequence of Lol p 5A have been tested in a solid phase immunoassay for their reactivity with IgE from the sera of individuals allergic to grass pollen. All those with high reactivity with IgE correspond to the C-terminal half of Lol p 5A correlating with results obtained from random fragment libraries. This correlation highlights the usefulness of synthetic peptides in mapping of antigenic sites. For example, overlapping synthetic peptides covering the entire Poa p 5 allergen revealed 10 human IgE-reactive peptides [61]. The majority of the IgE-reactive peptides were confined to the C-terminal region of the molecule.

A recombinant polypeptide fragment that represents the C-terminal amino acid sequence of Poa p 5 has been shown to bind IgE [62]. These similar findings with both ryegrass and Kentucky bluegrass suggest that their IgE epitopes are both in the C-terminal region and are expected to show sequence homology.

Short synthetic peptides can also give important information about conformational epitopes, since all conformational epitopes contain linear segments [63]. Recent studies using peptide-based assays have identified the antigenically important regions of discontinuous sites [64,65], even to the resolution of single critical amino acids within the sites [66]. In future, it will be important to use the synthetic peptide strategy to assess polymorphic form-specific epitopes and relate these epitopes within the context of the folded proteins.

A 25 amino acid synthetic peptide based on the C-terminal region of Lol p 1 has been shown to bind IgE and IgG_4 [67], confirming previous data of Esch and Klapper [68] who first obtained evidence that the C-terminal region contained the major IgE-binding epitope. This binding was inhibited by both Lol p 1 and Lol p 2, demonstrating cross-reactivity between these allergens. Griffith *et al.*, [39] showed that Lol p 2 is homologous with the C-terminal region of Lol p 1, on the basis of its amino acid sequence deduced following cDNA cloning.

It is possible that once the Lol p 1 cDNA is expressed as a non-fusion protein, the folding of the polypeptide chain will more closely resemble that of the natural protein. Expression of other allergen genes in bacteria has proved difficult in some cases, most notably Der p 1 which, when expressed as a fusion protein with glutathione-S-transferase, retained only 50% of the

IgE binding activity of the natural protein and was recognized by IgE from only 50% of individuals allergic to Der p 1 [13]. This protein was difficult to express as a non-fusion protein in bacteria but has since been expressed in yeast at high yield, and the recombinant protein produced reacted with nine out of 11 individuals allergic to Der p 1 [14]. With the ryegrass allergens we have cloned, the recombinant allergens are recognized by more than 75% of ryegrass allergic individuals, however the percentage of IgE reactivity retained by the recombinant allergen has not been determined. Use of different vectors for expression of the recombinant ryegrass allergens may result in increased IgE reactivity and yield of the recombinant protein. With regard to the major Bermuda grass pollen allergen Cyn d 1, we have formerly expressed the allergen in bacteria as a fusion protein with no success of IgE reactivity. However, we have recently expressed the same allergen in the yeast *Pichia pastoris* with good IgE reactivity. This suggests that the post-translational modifications present in yeast (i.e. glycosylation) are important to the IgE reactivity of Cyn d 1. This could also be the case for many more allergens which require the eukaryotic post-translational modifications for correct conformation or epitopic structure.

cDNA clones from cocksfoot [69], Kentucky blue [70,71] and timothy [72] grass pollens have been isolated and sequenced. The cDNA clone of cocksfoot grass pollen was expressed as a 140 kDa β-galactosidase fusion protein containing 24 kDa of cloned allergen protein. Fusion proteins were recognized by IgE antibodies in 75% (6/8) of the atopic sera, but were not detected by non-atopic sera. Furthermore, the reactivity of human IgE antibodies with the fusion protein could be blocked by crude cocksfoot pollen extract.

A recombinant peptide of Kentucky bluegrass (KBG) pollen was synthesized as a fusion protein in *E. coli* [71]. The fusion protein demonstrated binding to IgE antibodies of $> 95\%$ of 55 individual sera tested. A positive correlation ($r=0.90$) was observed between the levels of IgE antibodies corresponding to the fusion protein and natural extracts. Three different protein preparations were compared for IgE binding, namely total KBG pollen proteins, 27–35 kDa gel-purified pollen proteins and the recombinant fusion protein. Results indicated that about 50% of the total IgE-binding of KBG pollen proteins was due to the IgE antibodies specific to the fusion protein. Moreover, the fusion protein supported high proliferation of lymph node cells.

Recombinant fusion proteins of Phl p 1 and Phl p 5 from timothy grass have been used in IgE immunoblots in comparison with natural crude pollen extracts for the diagnosis of grass pollen allergy [72]. Out of the 98 tested grass pollen allergic patients, 97 possessed IgE antibodies which recognized both the fusion and natural proteins. These results are in good agreement with RAST scores and clinical data.

Collectively, the human IgE antibody binding results so far obtained with both recombinant and synthetic peptides suggest that they constitute major allergenic components of grass pollens and thus provide a very assuring promise for the future for their diagnostic and therapeutic value for grass pollen allergy.

OTHER POLLEN AND SPORE ALLERGENS

Birch Pollen Allergens

Birch (*Betula verrucosa*) pollen has three major allergens Bet v 1, Bet v 2 (profilin) and Bet v 3 (Ca^{2+} binding protein). Jarolim *et al.* [73] demonstrated that 56 out of 58 patients with birch pollen allergy showed IgE antibodies to Bet v 1, which has 10 (pH 4.9–5.9) different glycosylated isoforms. Birch pollen allergens share allergenic determinants with other tree pollens (e.g. pollen from hazel or alder [74,75]).

Bet v 1 cDNA clones have been isolated, sequenced [76] and found to be highly homologous to pathogenesis-related plant proteins. cDNA clones encoding Bet v 2 (14 kDa) have been isolated and are highly homologous to profilins from diverse organisms [77]. All 100 patients' sera tested, which reacted with the natural allergens Bet v 1 and 2, showed identical IgE binding pattern to recombinant birch pollen allergens. Another study demonstrated that the recombinant as well as pollen-derived natural Bet v 1 and 2 gave an excellent correlation between allergen-induced histamine release from allergic patients' basophils, and birch pollen RAST [77]. Non-specific histamine release as a result of a cell toxic effect of the allergen preparations was never observed from basophils of donors without birch pollen allergy. More recently, a cDNA coding for a birch pollen allergen, Bet v 3 (23.7 kDa), was isolated from a cDNA expression library using serum IgE from a birch pollen allergic patient and shown to be expressed preferentially in mature pollen [78]. The deduced amino acid sequence of Bet v 3 contained three typical calcium (Ca^{2+}) binding sites and displayed significant homology to Ca^{2+} binding proteins such as calmodulin, troponin and parvalbumin from different eukaryotes. Calmodulins are known to function as Ca^{2+} binding proteins and activators of phosphodiesterase as well as participating in the intracellular transmission of signals involving the phosphatidyl–inositol pathway. Peptides based on the three Ca^{2+} binding sites of Bet v 3 were synthesized and when tested by dot-blots showed to bind ^{45}Ca. Patients' IgE binding to the recombinant Bet v 3 depended on the native protein conformation and protein-bound Ca^{2+} which, upon removal of Ca^{2+}, led to a reversible loss of the IgE binding. Therefore, this represents a conformational IgE epitope which is adopted by a polypeptide upon Ca^{2+} binding.

Oilseed Rape Pollen Allergens

Oilseed rape is a member of the Brassicaceae family and has been introduced to a number of countries and cultivated widely. Brassica vegetables include broccoli, kale, cabbage, mustard and turnip as well as rape, and due to intense commercial interest, this genus is an expanding crop throughout the world [79]. The incidence of rape pollen allergy is very high among occupationally exposed subjects [80]. It is interesting to note that a similar Ca^{2+} binding protein to that of Bet v 3 from birch pollen has been recently isolated from an oilseed rape pollen cDNA expression library using serum IgE from an oilseed rape allergic patient [81]. Moreover, the deducted amino acid sequence of the oilseed rape cDNA clone contained the two typical Ca^{2+} binding sites of Ca^{2+} binding proteins such as calmodulin.

Ragweed Pollen Allergens

Pollen from short ragweed (*Ambrosia artemisifolia*) is one of the major clinical causes of seasonal pollen allergy in North America [82]. Aqueous extracts of short ragweed are highly complex protein mixtures that contain 22 allergens [83]. The two major allergens in the pollen of short ragweed are Amb a 1 (formerly known as antigen E) and Amb a 2 (formerly antigen K). Both of the allergens have been extensively characterized. It has been shown that at least 95% and 50–90% of ragweed pollen allergic patients contain IgE that bind to Amb a 1 and Amb a 2, respectively [82,84].

Early studies using skin tests with Amb a 1-depleted pollen extract led to the estimation that at least 90% of the total allergenic activity in ragweed pollen can be attributed to Amb a 1 [82,85]. Competitive experiments using mAb to inhibit the binding of Amb a 1 by human IgE in ELISA assays have confirmed the early studies that Amb a 1 binds a substantial proportion of human ragweed allergic IgE [86].

A partial sequence of Amb a 1 was obtained by protein sequence analysis and, in conjunction with antibodies raised against the purified natural and denatured Amb a 1, a series of cDNA clones encoding a family of related proteins was identified [87]. The three identified Amb a 1 family members, designated Amb a 1.1, Amb a 1.2 and Amb a 1.3, displayed more than 80% amino acid homology with each other [87]. When the recombinant proteins from each of these clones were expressed in bacteria, all forms were shown to be specifically recognized by pooled ragweed-allergic human IgE on immunoblots [56].

In another study, purified natural Amb a 1 and Amb a 2 and recombinant Amb a 1.1 and Amb a 2, expressed in *E. coli* and purified in their denatured form, were examined by ELISA for their capacity to bind pooled allergic human IgE [88]. Each of these allergens bound a substantial proportion of the IgE as compared with the whole ragweed pollen extract. However, although purified natural Amb a 1 and Amb a 2 were shown to have very similar IgE antibody binding properties, recombinant Amb a 2 had a markedly reduced binding capacity compared with Amb a 1. Furthermore, there was more than 70% reduction in IgE binding to recombinant Amb a 1.1 and more than 80% to recombinant Amb a 2, when compared with IgE binding to their natural equivalents. Since recombinant Amb a 1.1 and Amb a 2, isolated in a denatured form, differ significantly in their IgE binding properties, and natural molecules isolated from pollen do not, IgE antibody binding of Amb a 2 may be largely conformational. Moreover, even though there is detectable sequence identity between Amb a 1.1 and Amb a 2 throughout the molecule [57,87,89], there are regions where the sequences are significantly different, suggesting that both allergens possess a different subset of IgE antibody binding epitopes.

In conclusion, the studies undertaken with short ragweed pollen allergens demonstrate that the Amb a 1 and Amb a 2 family of natural and recombinant proteins play a major role in eliciting an allergic response in susceptible humans. Since the genes coding these individual members of this family of proteins have been cloned and sequenced, the common B- and T-cell human IgE binding epitopes of these allergens can provide rational design of an immunotherapeutic agent with improved efficacy for the treatment of ragweed allergy.

Fungal Spore Allergens

In both the indoor and outdoor environment, fungal spores of *Alternaria alternata, Aspergillus fumigatus* and *Cladosporium herbarum* are the most important source of allergens. The major allergens of these fungi have been characterized. Of these, only the gene encoding a major allergen from *Aspergillus fumigatus*, an 18 kDa protein, has been cloned [90]. The purified 18 kDa protein, Asp f 1, reacted with 85% of IgE from patients with allergic bronchopulmonary aspergillosis (ABPA) or asthma in a solid-phase RIA. On immediate skin testing, four of five patients gave positive intradermal skin tests to Asp f 1 [91]. The expressed fusion protein of Asp f 1 reacted strongly with serum IgE from two ABPA patients on western and dot blots [90]. Using inhibition ELISA, these authors showed that both natural and recombinant Asp f 1 are able to fully inhibit binding of IgE to solid phase recombinant Asp f 1. In skin tests, 5 out of 9 ABPA patients showed a type I skin reaction against recombinant Asp f 1 [90]. Thus, recombinant allergens retain IgE reactivity when compared with natural allergens, and can be used as a tool for the mapping of B-cell epitopes.

CONCLUSIONS

Recombinant allergens offer a number of advantages compared with their natural counterparts. First, the technology permits the production of defined allergens in large quantities, facilitating development of new diagnostic assays that are of far greater specificity than previously possible and providing the potential for international standards [71]. Second, determination of the structure and identification of allergenic epitopes is feasible, providing a new understanding of the molecular basis of IgE interactions. Finally, there are the exciting possibilities offered by modified allergens or peptides as effective therapeutic modalities [92,93].

REFERENCES

1 Roitt I, Brostoff J, Male D. Hypersensitivity-type I. In *Immunology*. London: Gower Medical Publishing, 1987; 19.1–19.18.
2 van Ree R, Driessen MNBM, van Leeuwen WA, *et al*. Variability of crossreactivity of IgE antibodies to group I and V allergens in eight grass pollen species. *Clin Exp Allergy* 1992; **22**: 611–617.
3 Ford SA, Tovey ER, Baldo BA. The spectrum of low molecular weight house dust mite (*Dermatophagoides pteronyssinus*) allergens with emphasis on *Der p* II. *Clin Exp Allergy* 1989; **20**: 27–31.
4 Platts-Mills TAE, Chapman MD. Dust mites: immunology, allergic disease, and environmental control. *J Allergy Clin Immunol* 1987; **80**: 755–775.
5 Chua KY, Stewart GA, Thomas WR *et al*. Sequence analysis of cDNA coding for a major house dust mite allergen, *Der p* I. Homology with cysteine proteases. *J Exp Med* 1988; **167**: 175–182.
6 Chua KY, Doyle CR, Simpson RJ *et al*. Isolation of cDNA coding for the major mite allergen *Der p* II by IgE plaque immunoassay. *Int Arch Allergy Appl Immunol* 1990; **91**: 118–123.
7 Baldo BA, Ford SA, Tovey ER. Toward a definition of the 'complete' spectrum and rank order of importance of the allergens from the house dust mite: *Dermatophagoides pteronyssinus*. *Adv Biosci* 1989; **74**: 13–31.
8 Chapman MD, Platts-Mills TAE. Purification and characterization of the allergen from *Dermatophagoides pteronyssinus*-antigen PI. *J Immunol* 1980; **125**: 587–592.
9 Lind P. Purification and partial characterization of two major allergens from the house dust mite *Dermatophagoides pteronyssinus*. *J Allergy Clin Immunol* 1985; **76**: 753–761.
10 Stewart GA. The isolation and characterization of the allergen Dpt 12, from *Dermatophagoides pteronyssinus* by chromatofocusing. *Int Arch Allergy Appl Immunol* 1982; **69**: 224–230.
11 Heymann PW, Chapman MD, Aalberse RC *et al*. Antigenic and structural analysis of group II allergens (*Der f* II and *Der p* II) from house dust mites (*Dermatophagoides spp*). *J Allergy Clin Immunol* 1989; **83**: 1055–1067.
12 van der Zee JS, van Swieten P, Jansen HM *et al*. Skin tests and histamine release with P_1-depleted *Dermatophagoides pteronyssinus* body extracts and purified P_1. *J Allergy Clin Immunol* 1988; **81**: 884–896.
13 Greene WK, Cyster JG, Chua K *et al*. IgE and IgG binding of peptides expressed from fragments of cDNA encoding the major house dust mites allergen *Der p* I. *J Immunol* 1991; **147**: 3768–3773.
14 Chua KY, Kehal PK, Thomas WR *et al*. High-frequency binding of IgE to the *Der p* allergen expressed in yeast. *J Allergy Clin Immunol* 1992; **89**: 95–102.
15 Chua KY, Dilworth RJ, Thomas WR. Expression of *Dermatophagoides pteronyssinus* allergen, *Der p* II, in *Escherichia coli* and the binding studies with human IgE. *Int Arch Allergy Appl Immunol* 1990; **91**: 124–129.

16 Lynch NR, Thomas WR, Chua Y, *et al. In vivo* biological activity of recombinant Der p II allergen of house-dust mite. *Int Arch Allergy Appl Immunol* 1994; **105**: 70–74.
17 Greene WK, Thomas WR. IgE binding structures of the major house dust mite allergen Der p I. *Mol Immunol* 1992; **29**: 257–262.
18 Stewart GA, Thomas WR, Chua HY *et al.* An allergen and antigenic mapping analysis of a major mite allergen, *Der p* I. *Adv Biosci* 1989; **74**: 297–311.
19 Jeannin P, Didierlaurent A, Gras-Masse H *et al.* Specific histamine release capacity of peptides selected from the modelized *Der p* I protein, a major allergen of *Dermatophagoides pteronyssinus*. *Mol Immunol* 1992; **29**: 739–749.
20 Chua KY, Greene WK, Hehal P *et al.* IgE binding studies with large peptides expressed from *Der p* II cDNA constructs. *Clin Exp Allergy* 1991; **21**: 161–166.
21 Lin K-L, Hsieh K-H, Thomas WR *et al.* Characterization of *Der p* V allergen, cDNA analysis, and IgE-mediated reactivity to the recombinant protein. *J Allergy Clin Immunol* 1994; **94**: 989–996.
22 Sarsfield JK, Boyle AG, Rowell EM *et al.* Pet sensitivities in asthmatic children. *Arch Dis Child* 1976; **51**: 186–189.
23 Thompson RA, Bird AG. How necessary are specific IgE antibody tests in allergy diagnosis? *Lancet* 1983; **1**: 169–172.
24 Leitermann K, Ohmann J. Cat allergen 1: Biochemical, antigenic and allergenic properties. *J Allergy Clin Immunol* 1984; **74**: 147–153.
25 Kleine-Tebbe J, Klkeine-Tebbe A, Jeep S *et al.* Role of the major allergen (*Fel d* I) in patients sensitized to cat allergens. *Int Arch Allergy Appl Immunol* 1993; **100**: 256–262.
26 Dabrowski AJ, Van der Brempt, Soler M *et al.* Cat skin as an important source of *Fel d* I allergen. *J Allergy Clin Immunol* 1990; **86**: 462–465.
27 Anderson MC, Baer H, Ohman JL. A comparative study of the allergens of cat urine, serum, saliva and pelt. *J Allergy Clin Immunol* 1985; **76**: 563–568.
28 Charpin C, Mata P, Charpin D *et al. Fel d* I allergen distribution in cat fur and skin. *J Allergy Clin Immunol* 1991; **88**: 77–82.
29 Chapman MD, Aalberse RC, Brown MJ *et al.* Monoclonal antibodies to the feline allergen *Fel d* I. Single step affinity purification of *Fel d* I, N-terminal sequence analysis and development of a two-site immunoassay to assess *Fel d* I exposure. *J Immunol* 1988; **140**: 812–818.
30 Duffort OA, Carreira J, Nitti G *et al.* Studies on the biochemical structure of the major cat allergen *Felis domesticus* I. *Mol Immunol* 1991; **28**: 301–309.
31 Morgenstern JP, Griffith IJ, Brauer AW *et al.* Amino acid sequence of *Fel d* I, the major allergen of the domestic cat: Protein sequence analysis and cDNA cloning. *Proc Natl Acad Sci USA* 1991; **88**: 9690–9694.
32 Griffith IJ, Craig S, Pollock J *et al.* Expression and genomic structure of the genes encoding FdI, the major allergen from domestic cat. *Gene* 1992; **113**: 263–268.
33 Rogers BL, Morgenstern JP, Garman RD *et al.* Recombinant *Fel d* I: expression, purification, IgE binding and reaction with cat-allergic human T cells. *Mol Immunol* 1993; **30**: 559–568.
34 Bond JF, Brauer AW, Segal DB *et al.* Native and recombinant *Fel d* I as probes into the relationship of allergen structure to human IgE immunoreactivity. *Mol Immunol* 1993; **30**: 1529–1540.
35 Smith PM, Ong EK, Avjioglu A *et al.* Analysis of ryegrass pollen allergens using two-dimensional electrophoresis and immunoblotting. In: Kraft D, Sehon A (eds) *Molecular Biology and Immunology of Allergens*. Boca Raton: CRC Press, 1993; 141–143.
36 Bond JF, Segal DB, Yu X-B *et al.* Human IgE reactivity to purified recombinant and native grass allergens. *J Allergy Clin Immunol* 1993; **91**: 339.

37 Johnson P, Marsh DG. The isolation and characterization of allergens from the pollen of ryegrass (*Lolium perenne*). *Eur Polym J* 1965; **1**: 63–77.
38 Perez M, Ishioka GY, Walker LE *et al*. cDNA cloning and immunological characterization of the ryegrass allergen *Lol p* I. *J Biol Chem* 1990; **265**: 16210–16215.
39 Griffith IJ, Smith PM, Pollock J *et al*. Cloning and sequencing of *Lol p* I, the major allergenic protein of ryegrass pollen. *FEBS Lett* 1991; **279**: 210–215.
40 Singh MB, Hough T, Theerakulpisut P *et al*. Isolation of cDNA encoding a newly identified major allergenic protein of ryegrass pollen: Intracellular targetting to the amyloplast. *Proc Natl Acad Sci USA* 1991; **88**: 1384–1388.
41 Suphioglu C, Singh MB, Taylor P *et al*. Mechanism of grass-pollen-induced asthma. *Lancet* 1992; **339**: 569–572.
42 Silvanovich A, Astwood J, Zhang L *et al*. Nucleotide sequence analysis of three cDNAs coding for *Poa p* IX isoallergens of Kentucky bluegrass pollen. *J Biol Chem* 1991; **266**: 1204–1210.
43 Vrtala S, Sperr WR, Reimitzer I *et al*. cDNA cloning of a major allergen from timothy grass (*Phleum pratense*) pollen; characterization of the recombinant *Phl p* V allergen. *J Immunol* 1993; **151**: 4773–4781.
44 Bufe A, Becker W-M, Schramm G *et al*. Major allergen *Phl p* Va (timothy grass) bears at least two different IgE-reactive epitopes. *J Allergy Clin Immunol* 1994; **94**: 173–181.
45 Matthiesen F, Lowenstein, H. Group V allergens in grass pollens. I. Purification and characterization of group V allergen from *Phleum pratense* pollen, *Phl p* V. *Clin Exp Allergy* 1991; **21**: 297–307.
46 Matthiesen F, Lowenstein H. Group V allergens in grass pollens. II. Investigation of group V allergens in pollens from 10 grasses. *Clin Exp Allergy* 1991; **21**: 309–320.
47 Klysner S, Welinder KG, Lowenstein H *et al*. Group V allergens in grass pollens: IV. Similarities in amino acid compositions and NH_2-terminal sequences of the Group V allergens from *Lolium perenne, Poa pratensis* and *Dactylis glomerata. Clin Exp Allergy* 1992; **22**: 491–497.
48 van Ree R, Driessen MNBM, van Leeuwen WA *et al*. Variability of crossreactivity of IgE antibodies to group I and V allergens in eight grass pollen species. *Clin Exp Allergy* 1992; **22**: 611–617.
49 Avjioglu A, Creaney J, Smith PM *et al*. Cloning and characterization of the major allergen of *Sorghum halepense*, a subtropical grass. In: Kraft D, Sehon A (eds) *Molecular Biology and Immunology of Allergens*. Boca Raton: CRC Press, 1993; 161–164.
50 Laffer S, Valenta R, Vrtala S *et al*. Complementary DNA cloning of the major allergen *Phl p* I from timothy grass (*Phleum pratense*); recombinant *Phl p* I inhibits IgE binding to group I allergens from eight different grass species. *J Allergy Clin Immunol* 1994; **94**: 689–698.
51 Bufe A, Schramm G, Keown MB *et al*. Major allergen *Phl p* Vb in timothy grass is a novel pollen RNase. *FEBS Lett* 1995; **363**: 6–12.
52 Johnson P, Marsh DG. Allergens from common ryegrass pollen (*Lolium perenne*)-I. *Immunochemistry* 1966; **3**: 91–100.
53 Rohac M, Birkner T, Reimitzer I *et al*. The immunological relationship of epitopes on major tree pollen allergens. *Mol Immunol* 1991; **28**: 897–906.
54 Lin Z, Ekramoddoullah AKM, Kisil FT *et al*. Isolation and characterization of *Poa p* I allergens of Kentucky bluegrass pollen with a murine monoclonal anti-*Lol p* I antibody. *Int Arch Allergy Appl Immunol* 1988; **87**: 294–300.
55 Petersen A, Becker W-M, Schlaak M. Characterization of isoforms of the major allergen *Phl p* V by two-dimensional immunoblotting and microsequencing. *Int Arch Allergy Appl Immunol* 1992; **98**: 105–109.

56 Bond JF, Garman RD, Keating KM *et al.* Multiple *Amb a* I allergens demonstrate specific reactivity with IgE and T cells from ragweed-allergic patients. *J Immunol* 1991; **146**: 3380–3385.
57 Griffith IJ, Pollock J, Klapper DG *et al.* Sequence polymorphism of *Amb a* I and *Amb a* II, the major allergens in *Ambrosia artemisifolia* (short ragweed). *Int Arch Allergy Appl Immunol* 1991; **96**: 296–304.
58 Larsen JN, Stroman P, Ipsen H. PCR based cloning and sequencing of isogenes encoding the tree pollen major allergen *Car e* I from *Carpinus betulus*, hornbeam. *Mol Immunol* 1992; **29**: 703–711.
59 Ong EK, Singh MB, Griffith LJ *et al.* Molecular cloning of a group V isoform from rye-grass pollen that demonstrates specific antigenic immunoreactivity. *Gene* 1993; **134**: 235–240.
60 Mehra V, Sweetser D, Young RA. Efficient mapping of protein antigenic determinants. *Proc Natl Acad Sci USA* 1986; **83**: 7013–7017.
61 Zhang L, Olsen E, Kisil FT *et al.* Mapping of antibody binding epitopes of a recombinant *Poa p* IX allergen. *Mol Immunol* 1992; **29**: 1383–1389.
62 Olsen E, Zhang L, Hill RD *et al.* Identification and characterization of the *Poa p* IX group of basic allergens of Kentucky bluegrass pollen. *J Immunol* 1991; **147**: 205–211.
63 Gertzoff ED, Tainer JA, Lerner RA *et al.* The chemistry and mechanism of antibody binding to protein antigens. *Adv Immunol* 1988; **43**: 1.
64 Fedlich PN, Hoeprich PD, Colby CB *et al.* Antibodies that neutralize human β interferon biological activity recognize a linear epitope: Analysis by synthetic peptide mapping. *Proc Natl Acad Sci USA* 1991; **88**: 4040.
65 Savoca R, Schwab C, Bosshard HR *et al.* Epitope mapping employing immobilised synthetic peptides. *J Immunol Methods* 1991; **141**: 245.
66 Appel JR, Pinilla C, Niman H *et al.* Elucidation of discontinuous linear determinant in peptides. *J Immunol* 1990; **144**: 976.
67 van Ree R, van Leeuwen WA, Aalberse RC. Demonstration of human IgE and IgG antibodies against the *Lol p* I C-terminus that crossreact with the C-termini of *Lol p* II and III. *J Allergy Clin Immunol* 1993; **91**: 187.
68 Esch RE, Klapper DG. Cross-reactive and unique grass group I antigenic determinants defined by monoclonal antibodies. *J Allergy Clin Immunol* 1987; **79**: 489–495.
69 Walsh DJ, Matthews JA, Denmeade R *et al.* Cloning of cDNA coding for an allergen of cocksfoot grass (*Dactylis glomerata*) pollen. *Int Arch Allergy Appl Immunol* 1989; **90**: 78–83.
70 Mohapatra SS, Hill R, Astwood J *et al.* Isolation and characterization of a cDNA clone encoding an IgE-binding protein from Kentucky bluegrass (*Poa pratensis*) pollen. *Int Arch Allergy Appl Immunol* 1990; **91**: 362–368.
71 Yang M, Olsen E, Dolovich J *et al.* Immunologic characterization of a recombinant Kentucky bluegrass (*Poa pratensis*) allergenic peptide. *J Allergy Clin Immunol* 1991; **87**: 1096–1104.
72 Valenta R, Vrtala S, Ebner C *et al.* Diagnosis of grass pollen allergy with recombinant timothy grass (*Phleum pratense*) pollen allergens. *Int Arch Allergy Appl Immunol* 1992; **97**: 287–294.
73 Jarolim E, Rumpold H, Endler AT *et al.* IgE and IgG antibodies of patients with allergy to birch pollen as tools to define the allergen profile of *Betula verrucosa*. *Allergy* 1989; **44**: 385–395.
74 Ipsen H, Hansen OC. The NH_2-terminal amino acid sequence of the immunochemically partial identical major allergens of alder (*Alnus glutinosa*) *Aln g* I, birch (*Betula varrucosa*) *Bet v* I, hornbeam (*Carpinus betulus*) *Car e* I, and oak (*Quercus alba*) *Que a* I pollens. *Mol Immunol* 1991; **28**: 1279–1288.

75 Eriksson NE, Wihl JA, Arrendal H *et al.* Tree pollen allergy. III. Cross reactions based on results from skin prick tests and the RAST in hay fever patients: a multi-centre study. *Allergy* 1987; **42**: 205–214.

76 Brieteneder H, Pettenburger K, Bito A *et al.* The gene coding for the major birch allergen, *Bet v* I, is highly homologous to a pea resistance response gene. *EMBO J* 1989; **8**: 1935–1938.

77 Valenta R, Duchene M, Pettenburger K *et al.* Identification of profilin as a novel pollen allergen: IgE autoreactivity in sensitized individuals. *Science* 1991; **253**: 557–560.

78 Seiberler S, Scheiner O, Kraft D *et al.* Characterization of a birch pollen allergen, *Bet v* III, representing a novel class of Ca^{2+} binding proteins; specific expression in mature pollen and dependence of patients' IgE binding on protein-bound Ca^{2+}. *EMBO J* 1994; **13**: 3481–3486.

79 Soutar A, Harker C, Seaton A *et al.* Oilseed rape and seasonal symptoms: epidemiological and environmental studies. *Thorax* 1994; **49**: 352–356.

80 Fell PJ, Soulsby S, Blight MM *et al.* Oilseed rape – a new allergen. *Clin Exp Allergy* 1992; **22**: 501–505.

81 Toriyama K, Okada T, Watanabe M *et al.* A cDNA clone encoding an IgE-binding protein from *Brassica* anther has significant sequence homology to Ca^{2+} binding proteins. *Plant Mol Biol* 1995; **29**: 1157–1165.

82 King TP. Chemical and biological properties of some atopic allergens. *Adv Immunol* 1976; **23**: 77–105.

83 Lowenstein H, Marsh DG. Antigens of *Ambrosia elatior* (short ragweed) pollen III. Crossed radioimmunoelectrophoresis of ragweed-allergic patients' sera with special attention to quantification of IgE responses. *J Immunol* 1983; **130**: 727.

84 Adolphson C, Goodfriend L, Gleich GJ. Reactivity of ragweed allergens with IgE antibodies. *J Allergy Clin Immunol* 1978; **62**: 197–210.

85 King TP, Norman PS, Connell JT. Isolation and characterization of allergens from ragweed pollen. II. *Biochemistry* 1964; **3**: 458–468.

86 Olson JR, Klapper DG. Two major human allergenic sites on ragweed pollen allergen antigen E identified by using monoclonal antibodies. *J Immunol* 1986; **136**: 2109–2115.

87 Rafnar T, Griffith IJ, Kuo MC *et al.* Cloning of *Amb a I* (Antigen E), the major allergen family of short ragweed pollen. *J Biol Chem* 1991; **2**: 1229–1236.

88 Kuo M-C, Zhu X-J, Koury R *et al.* Purification and immunochemical characterization of recombinant and native ragweed allergen *Amb a* II. *Mol Immunol* 1993; **30**: 1077–1087.

89 Rogers BL, Morgenstern JP, Griffith IJ *et al.* Complete sequence of the allergen *Amb a* II: recombinant expression and reactivity with T cells from ragweed allergic patients. *J Immunol* 1991; **147**: 2547–2552.

90 Moser M, Crameri R, Menz G *et al.* Cloning and expression of recombinant *Aspergillus fumigatus* allergen I/a (rAsp*f* I/a) with IgE binding and type I skin test activity. *J Immunol* 1992; **149**: 454–460.

91 Arruda LK, Platts-Mills TAE, Fox JW *et al.* *Aspergillus fumigatus* allergen I, a major IgE-binding protein, is a member of the mitogillin family of cytotoxins. *J Allergy Clin Immunol* 1990; **172**: 1529–1532.

92 Scheiner O. Recombinant allergens: biological, immunological and practical aspects. *Int Arch Allergy Appl Immunol* 1992; **98**: 93–96.

93 Bousquet J, Breitenbach M, Dreborg S *et al.* Diagnosis of allergy and specific immunotherapy using recombinant allergens and epitopes. In: Kraft D, Sehon A (eds) *Molecular Biology and Immunology of Allergens*. Boca Raton: CRC Press, 1993; 311–320.

11 The Use of Peptides for Allergy Immunotherapy

MARK A. EXLEY*, BRUCE L. ROGERS and IRWIN J. GRIFFITH

ImmuLogic Pharmaceutical Corporation, Waltham, Massachusetts, USA.
**Present address: Harvard Medical School, Boston, USA*

INTRODUCTION

The allergic reaction consists of hypersensitivity to non-pathogenic environmental allergens. This allergic reaction can be either chronic or acute and ranges in severity from localized irritation (e.g. mild rhinitis) to systemic anaphylactic shock. Many common allergens are inhaled and initially affect the nasal and bronchial systems. Examples of inhaled allergens are seasonal pollen and non-seasonal household allergens of invertebrates (e.g. mites) or pets. In contrast, bee venom contains an injected allergen that acts systemically. Whatever the nature of the allergen and extent of the hypersensitivity, the common factor of the allergic response is a T cell-dependent production of allergen-specific IgE by B cells [1]. Allergic symptoms represent the cumulative effects of cross-linking this allergen-specific IgE that is bound on the surface of effector cells such as basophils and mast cells (see Figure 11.1). The triggering of effector cells results in degranulation of these cells and bioactive mediator release. We shall concentrate throughout this chapter on the characterization of the T-cell immune response to inhaled allergens, and ways in which this understanding can be translated into effective therapies for allergic disease.

Immunotherapy for the treatment of allergy currently involves hyposensitization by repeated subcutaneous injections of an extract containing the offending allergen [2,3]. This general method has been shown to be efficacious in a number of clinical trials involving atopic patients allergic to ragweed [4], house dust mite [5], domestic cat [6–8] and grasses [9]. Although clinical benefit for some patients has been clearly delineated using this form of immunotherapy, it should be noted that severe side-effects have also been observed. The allergen extracts contain complex mixtures of ill-defined proteins, several of which are capable of binding allergen-specific IgE and triggering the release of histamine from human mast cells and basophils, thus exacerbating symptoms. Further, many atopic patients fail to gain a clinical benefit even after extensive treatment.

The mechanism whereby multiple subcutaneous injections of allergen

Allergic Mechanisms and Immunotherapeutic Strategies. Edited by A.M. Roberts and M.R. Walker.

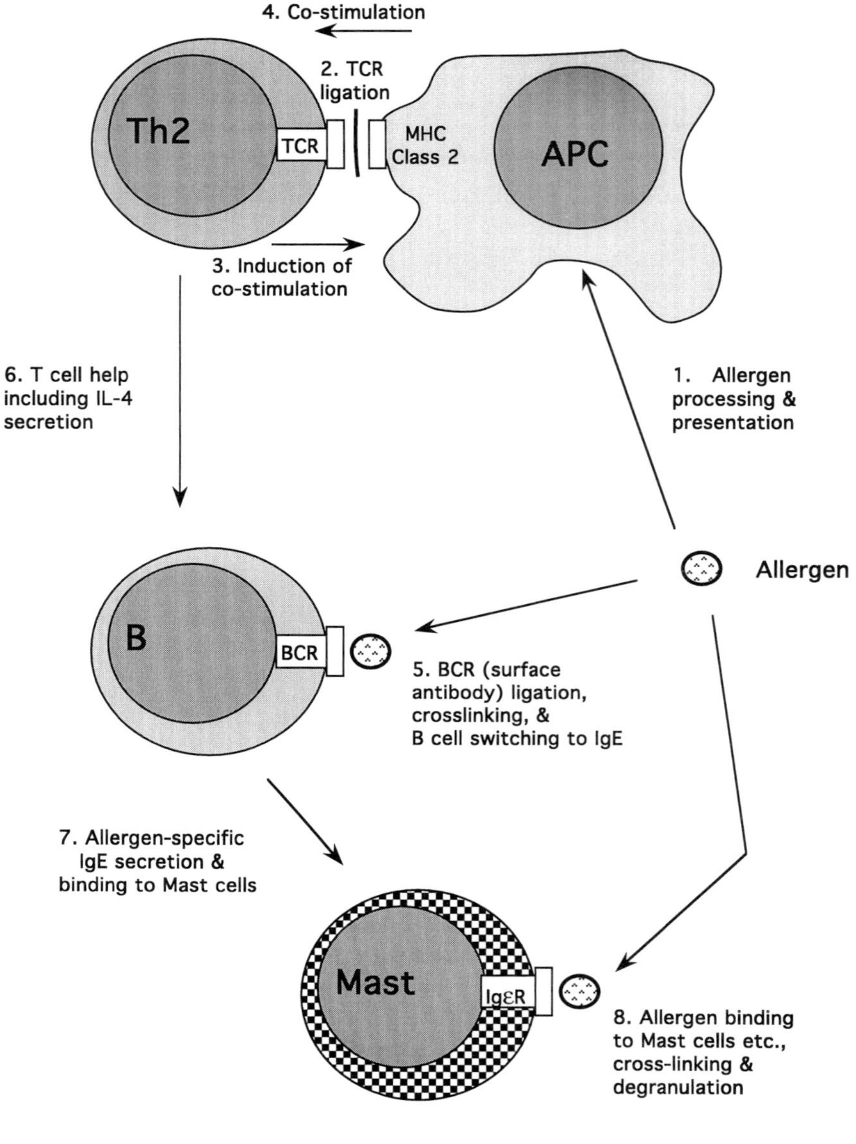

Figure 11.1. Schematic of the pathway leading to allergic reactions. Predominantly IL-4 secreting Th2 cells are activated by allergen peptides presented by APC. B-cell activation results from allergen binding to surface immunoglobulin and T cell help. IL-4 secretion is necessary for B-cell switching to IgE secretion. Allergen-induced cross-linking of IgE bound to the surface of mast cells and basophils leads to subsequent allergic symptoms. Antigen presentation and IL-4 secretion by mast cells and basophils may contribute to the allergic cascade (see text). Eosinophils are also involved in the chronic allergic reaction

extract lead to a diminution of symptoms is unknown. It has been suggested that increased levels of 'blocking IgG antibody' are responsible for the amelioration of the IgE-mediated allergic reaction [10]. However, several studies have been unable to find any significant change in antibody levels that correlate with effective immunotherapy [3,11]. More recently, the function of CD4+ T helper (Th) cells in regulating the allergic response has generated increasing interest. It has now been clearly demonstrated that the secretion of T cell-derived interleukin (IL-4) is required for an IgE response [12,13]. In contrast, the secretion of the lymphokine gamma-interferon (γ-IFN) inhibits an IgE response [13]. The discovery in mice of at least two subtypes of Th cell (Th1 and Th2) with reciprocal generation of γ-IFN and IL-4 [13] has led to a determined effort to define analogous cell types in humans (see Chapter 5). Although the distinction between Th1 and Th2 in humans may not be as unequivocal as in mice, a number of studies with allergen-specific T-cell clones have strongly suggested the existence of CD4+ cells with biased lymphokine secretion [14–17]. Recent evidence that allergen immunotherapy reduces the production of IL-4 during an allergic response *in vitro* is consistent with a role for Th2 cell involvement in allergic responses [18]. Interfering with the Th2 response could reduce allergic symptomology.

A large body of research has also focused on defining the events leading to T-cell activation and subsequent lymphokine secretion. As discussed later, T-cell activation is the result of the T-cell receptor interacting with an antigen fragment (usually peptide) in the context of a major histocompatibility complex (MHC) molecule on the surface of an antigen presenting cell (APC) [19–21]. This has generated a great deal of interest in defining the T-cell epitopes contained within an allergen (T-cell epitope mapping).

It has recently been proposed that a defined T-cell epitope-containing peptide may be used as an effective therapeutic agent for allergic diseases [22–24]. This concept of administering peptides to reduce an ongoing, unwanted, immune response has been examined as a potential therapy for other immune-mediated diseases as well. It has been found that the administration of synthetic peptides can be successfully used to ameliorate symptoms of murine experimental autoimmune encephalomyelitis [25,26], an animal model for multiple sclerosis. The feasibility of using this approach for allergic disease is currently being examined. It has involved a concerted effort to immunochemically characterize and define the primary structure of important allergens, identify the major T-cell epitopes therein and ultimately use such epitope-containing peptides as therapeutic agents.

ALLERGEN CHARACTERIZATION

The purification and biochemical characterization of important allergens commenced almost 30 years ago [27,28]. One of the earliest allergens to be purified and immunochemically defined was Amb a 1 (formerly antigen E)* [29] from short ragweed pollen [27]. This purified protein preparation was subsequently used successfully as an immunotherapy reagent [4]. The definition of Amb a 1 as the major allergen in short ragweed is based on several biological and immunochemical criteria such as the number of allergic patients (atopes) that recognized Amb a 1 as an allergen, the level of IgE binding, the *in vitro* induction of histamine release from basophils and skin test positivity in ragweed-allergic subjects [27,30]. This early body of literature set the stage for the biochemical and immunochemical characterization of important aeroallergens from house dust mites [31–33], cockroaches and other insects [34,35], animal danders [36,37], grasses [38,40], trees [41–43] and weeds [44–46], among others.

The development of antiserum and monoclonal antibodies (mAb) against proteins in crude pollen extracts has also been crucial for allergen purification and characterization. There are now multiple systems where allergens can be purified using immunoaffinity columns. These reagents have also been used in conjunction with human allergic antisera to demonstrate the presence of homologous allergens of related species [47–50] and isoallergens within a given species [51,52]. In particular, mAb have been used to map murine B-cell epitopes and aid in a demarcation of human IgE epitopes within an allergen [53–59].

This work has led to the identification of the major 'target' allergens of many different allergen sources. Target allergens are those recognized by the majority of allergic patients and against which the most IgE is directed. That is, the allergens that are presumed to cause the majority of symptoms in the allergic population. Immunotherapy with T-cell epitope-containing peptides from these allergens is predicted to ameliorate disease symptoms [24].

ALLERGEN SEQUENCES

In order to obtain T-cell epitope maps of the major allergens, it has been necessary to determine their primary amino acid sequence. For small allergens such as Lol p 2 (97 amino acids) and Lol p 3 (97 amino acids) from ryegrass and Amb a 5 (45 amino acids) from short ragweed, it has been possible to determine their sequence by direct amino acid sequence analysis [60–62]. In most cases, however, it has been necessary to clone the gene encoding the allergen of interest using partial amino sequence or monospecific reagents, as described below. The amino acid sequence of the allergen is then predicted from the defined nucleic acid sequence of the cloned gene.

Allergen genes have been cloned using a number of techniques, including

*Allergens are named according to the IUIS approved nomenclature [29].

screening expression libraries with IgE and/or mAb [52,63], screening cDNA and genomic libraries with labelled degenerate oligonucleotide probes or homologous nucleotide sequences (previously cloned isogenes) [64,65] and with the polymerase chain reaction (PCR) [66–74]. With the exception of screening an expression library with antibodies, all of these procedures require some information about the amino acid sequence of the target allergen. The large number of allergen genes that have now been cloned is a tribute to the success of these various techniques [29]. Each of these procedures has strengths and inherent limitations that dictate their use in a given cloning project.

The advent of PCR [75] has arguably had the greatest impact on allergen cloning. This technique has allowed the rapid selection of a large number of separate clones encoding the same allergen, in contrast with other techniques that tend to provide only a few clones for each screening. It should be appreciated that the inherent error rate associated with the thermostable *Taq* polymerase used in this procedure [76] necessitates the analysis of clones from at least two independent amplifications in order to rule out sequence errors introduced during *in vitro* amplification [68]. In spite of this caveat, the application of PCR to cloning allergen genes, as well as the other techniques mentioned above, has rapidly expanded our understanding of allergen complexity.

The cloning of multiple allergen genes showed that major allergens could be encoded by families of genes. For example, Amb a 1 was found to be encoded by a family of four closely related genes [67,68]. These isoallergens, which have now been designated Amb a 1.01–1.04 [29], have 70–90% sequence identity with each other. The biochemically distinct allergen Amb a 2 has also been cloned and found to have 60–70% sequence identity with the Amb a 1 family of gene products [68,69]. Each of the Amb a 1 and Amb a 2 isoallergens has a slightly different predicted molecular weight and pI. In addition, each isoallergen was found to have multiple allelic variants that have approximately 99% sequence identity with the prototype isoallergen sequence [68]. Each of the alleles can have a different predicted pI [77].

Analysis of the genes encoding allergens from multiple sources, including mites [78,79], grass pollen [52,63,64,70,80] and tree pollen [81,82], has shown that the presence of isoforms due to multiple genes or alleles of a single gene is fairly common. This suggests that known allergen complexity within a given pollen source can be due to independent allergens, multiple gene products of a closely related gene family or, possibly, degradation products of each. Each isoallergen and variant has the potential to have unique IgE binding epitopes [82] and, presumably, unique T-cell epitopes. However, homologous allergens from closely related species also have a high degree of cross-reactivity between them. It is this cross-reactivity that provides the opportunity for an effective immunotherapy with isolated allergen gene products or peptide fragments.

Once cloned, the allergen can be expressed by recombinant methods and may be used to assess IgE binding. In some cases, the level of IgE binding by the recombinantly expressed protein cannot be readily distinguished from that of the native allergen (see Chapters 6 and 10). In other cases, the level of IgE binding can depend upon correct folding and/or post-translational modification. For example, mite allergic patients tend to demonstrate low IgE binding to bacterially expressed recombinant (r) Der p 1 [83], but relatively high binding to rDer p 1 expressed in yeast [84]. This shows that IgE binding can depend on allergen tertiary conformation induced by secondary folding and post-translational modifications such as glycosylation.

Theoretically, recombinant allergens can be used for the diagnosis and treatment of allergies. Since the recombinant allergens rBet v 1, rBet v 2 (profilin), rPhl p 1, rPhl p 5 and timothy grass profilin exhibit high levels of IgE binding, it has been suggested that they could be used for the diagnosis of birch and timothy grass allergies, respectively [85,86]. However, this high IgE binding, which makes recombinant molecules attractive as diagnostics, diminishes their potential use in immunotherapy. The IgE binding can lead to the same systemic reactions observed with standard extract immunotherapy.

The deduced amino acid sequence of the cloned allergens can be used to produce an overlapping set of synthetic peptides. These peptides can be used to elucidate the T-cell epitopes in a given allergen, as discussed in more detail below.

T-CELL EPITOPE MAPPING METHODOLOGIES

Determination of the epitopes recognized by the majority of the allergic population is the ultimate goal of T-cell mapping. There are three major methods of T-cell epitope mapping currently exploited to determine this representation. These are: the primary assay, which measures activation of freshly isolated cells; the secondary assay, where an allergen-specific T-cell line is established through one round of *in vitro* antigen-driven expansion; and T-cell clones, which are established through multiple rounds of expansion and selection. Each of these methods has strengths and weaknesses, which are discussed below.

Ideally, the source of lymphocytes for T-cell epitope mapping would be the tissue where the allergen and T cells encounter one another and initiate the allergic immune reaction. This would primarily be the nasal mucosal surfaces, bronchial mucosa, and relevant lymphoid tissue connected via the lymphatic system (draining lymph nodes). Although it is likely that localized T-cell populations are enriched for allergen-reactive cells, it is difficult to obtain large numbers of cells from these sources. Since mucosal and other T cells traffic throughout the body [87], allergen-specific T cells involved in chronic immune responses are represented in the blood. Therefore, for practical reasons, blood remains the primary source of allergen-specific T cells.

Peripheral blood mononuclear leukocytes (PBL) include T lymphocytes, B lymphocytes, and phagocytic APC (monocytes/macrophages). T cells can be stimulated to proliferate in response to allergen proteins in the presence of phagocytes or B cells, both of which constitutively express MHC Class II molecules and can serve as APC. Both B cells and phagocytic APC internalize antigen by receptor-mediated endocytosis and/or fluid phase 'pinocytosis'. The antigen is then proteolytically processed to generate peptide fragments that associate intracellularly with MHC Class II molecules. Peptide:MHC complexes are subsequently expressed at the APC surface and interact with antigen-specific receptors on the T cell. The formation of this triad leads to T cell activation, cytokine release, and proliferation [19].

Cytokine release and/or proliferation are measured after T cells are cultured with the APC and various antigens for several days. Proliferation can be determined by measuring ^{3}H-thymidine uptake into T-cell DNA following stimulation. Several non-isotopic methods are also available commercially that use chromogenic substrates of enzymes expressed by metabolically active or proliferating cells. Cytokine production was originally measured by bioassay of the cell supernatants with factor-dependent cell lines. Currently, ELISAs are available for measurement of most cytokines, and are frequently more specific than bioassays. Other parameters of T-cell activation may also be used in the future.

The nature of the particular T-cell function to be assayed may determine the most appropriate assay to use. Particular T-cell subsets do not necessarily proliferate to the same extent and can have distinct patterns of cytokine release upon stimulation. For example, murine Th2 cells are reported to not proliferate as much as Th1 cells [88]. Further, IFN-γ and IL-4 are differentially produced by murine Th1 and Th2 cells, respectively [13], although IL-2 is produced by both T-cell subsets. Such rigid distinctions are not as readily apparent in humans, even though a Th2-like phenotype is thought to be important in allergy and other antibody-mediated diseases.

COMPARISON OF ALLERGEN REACTIVE PRIMARY, SECONDARY, AND CLONAL T-CELL PROLIFERATION ASSAYS

In primary proliferation assays, PBL isolated from allergic patients are cultured in the presence of antigens for several days and directly assayed for proliferation or cytokine release on approximately day seven. Since APC are present in PBL, additional cells do not need to be added to the culture. These primary proliferation assays involve the least *in vitro* manipulation of any of the T-cell assays discussed here. However, the very low frequency of allergen-specific T cells, and the even smaller number of T cells specific for a given peptide epitope, results in low proliferation indices and poor reproducibility. A primary assay therefore requires large numbers of replicates per assay in order to detect reliably a specific response.

Secondary T-cell assays use T-cell lines enriched for T cells reactive with allergens. These allergen-specific T-cell lines are initiated by stimulation of PBL with the allergen. After several days, antigen-reactive T cells are separated from high density cell debris and unstimulated dying cells. T-cell lines are established by further expansion of the culture with exogenous IL-2 and/or IL-4 for an additional period of up to 20 days after stimulation. At this time the T cells are no longer responsive to lymphokines and cease proliferation (i.e. they are 'rested'). Rested T cells are capable of responding to specific antigen and can be used in secondary allergen- and peptide-driven proliferation assays. However, secondary assays require the presence of exogenous APC. These APC, which can be autologous PBL or EBV-transformed MHC-matched B cells, are treated to prevent proliferation (e.g. γ-irradiated or mitomycin C-treated). After several days of co-culture, T-cell cytokine release and/or proliferation are measured in the same way as in primary assays. The enriched allergen-specific T-cell population allows for greater signal-to-noise ratios (stimulation index, SI) with higher degrees of antigen specificity than found in primary assays. However, assays involving primary cultures and T-cell lines use cells representative of the allergen-specific population. The level of proliferation with primary cultures and secondary T-cell lines is therefore a reflection of responding cell numbers and can be used as an indication of T-cell epitope dominance.

Cloned T cells have been used frequently in T-cell epitope mapping because of the reproducibility of the assays. This is a result of the monoclonal specificity of T-cell clones: rested T-cell clones respond uniformly and synchronously when stimulated with the priming antigen. T-cell clones are also typically unable to respond to other antigens in the cell culture. As a consequence, clones have a large and specific proliferative response (high SI) upon stimulation with antigen. However, T-cell cloning involves considerable *in vitro* manipulation and selection prior to assay. Indeed, there is a significant risk of identifying only a portion of the potential T-cell epitopes since cloning involves multiple rounds of antigenic stimulation usually coupled with limiting dilution. This can lead to selection of clones with the fastest growth characteristics rather than to clones representative of the inherent precursor frequency for a given epitope (assuming that dominance of an epitope is reflected in the number of responding cells). It is therefore more difficult to identify accurately dominant T-cell epitopes with clones than it is with other T-cell assays. Consequently, multiple clones from as many individuals as possible should be used to maximize epitope identification and minimize artefacts attributable to *in vitro* manipulation.

The three main methods of T-cell epitope mapping, primary, secondary, and T-cell clone assays, each have advantages and disadvantages. T-cell epitope mapping aims to determine the set of epitopes most significant in the allergic population. Primary assays involve no prior manipulation, but cannot be relied upon to provide either high success rates or to be more than semi-quantitative in nature. T-cell clones provide homogeneous and reproducible responses to antigenic stimulation, but are the product of considerable *in vitro* manipulation. This manipulation can result in an incomplete epitope map. Further, the relative importance of different epitopes is more difficult to compare with clones than with primary assays or secondary cultures using T-cell lines. Overall, secondary assays with T-cell lines balance high antigen specificity with minimal loss of T-cell receptor repertoire due to *in vitro* manipulation. This allows the relatively rapid analysis of large numbers of patient samples and the identification and ranking of the major T-cell epitopes within the allergic population. Different groups of allergists have concentrated on using each assay; in some cases, data from different methods have been compared (see below).

MAPPING ALLERGEN T-CELL EPITOPES WITH PEPTIDE SETS

T cells respond to minimal peptides, which contain a T-cell epitope, presented in context of a Class II molecule. As discussed previously, these peptides are generated *in vivo* when an APC processes an antigen. *In vitro* assays mimic this by using synthetic peptides. Traditionally, overlapping peptides have been synthesized by conventional chemistry on a modest scale (10–100 μM) and purified by reverse phase HPLC. Although the use of high quality peptides of known sequence and purity represents a considerable advantage in epitope mapping, this approach quickly becomes very expensive as the number of peptides increases. The number of peptides required to map a given allergen is dependent upon the length of the peptides and the amount of their overlap. A minimal peptide length is determined by the MHC Class II molecules, which optimally bind peptides greater than 10 amino acids long [21,89,90]. A maximal peptide length is determined by synthetic capabilities. However, peptides significantly longer than 13–14-mers have an increasing risk of containing more than one T-cell epitope. Increasing or decreasing peptide overlap significantly affects the number of peptides required to map a given allergen. Epitopes may not be detected if there is insufficient peptide overlap. Selection of a synthetic peptide set is therefore a balance between all of these considerations.

Recently, small scale multipeptide synthesis technologies have been able rapidly to produce nanomolar quantities of peptide [91]. However, this method does not control for differences in the efficiency of synthesis for disparate peptide sequences. Further, the peptides are not purified after synthesis [91]. The final crude mixture therefore contains widely variable levels of contaminants, including truncated peptides and peptides with deletions, as well as correctly synthesized material. Accurate dose–response comparisons are difficult without further peptide analysis. The low efficiency of synthesis of longer peptides is also a major limitation. Nevertheless, speed and low cost relative to conventional synthesis have made various forms of this method highly popular.

Recombinant approaches to screening sequences for T-cell reactivity have also recently been developed. One approach couples endonuclease digestion of recombinant plasmids with *in vitro* transcription and translation to create offset peptides [92]. T cells are added to the crude mixture for proliferation assay. A second approach employs microcultures of bacteria synthesizing different fusion proteins containing the peptide set of interest. Several different expression systems have been established. In one such system, protein-A fusion proteins are captured on IgG-coated wells, T cells and APC are then introduced and assayed directly [93]. Overlapping allergen sequences have also been expressed using the glutathione-s-transferase (GST) fusion partner. Purified GST fusion proteins are added directly to cell culture for assay [94].

Another recombinant method is phage display technology [95]. In this approach, usually random oligonucleotides of a desired length are inserted into a phage reporter gene and fusion proteins are expressed on the surface of phage-infected bacteria. Screening identifies individual phage encoding peptides able to stimulate T-cell proliferation. The amino acid sequence of the T-cell epitope is then deduced from the nucleic acid sequence of the phage insert. However, this approach has significant difficulties to overcome for routine application in T-cell epitope mapping. For example, it would be necessary to examine $>20^{10}$ phage to screen all amino acid combinations possible for a 10-mer peptide. It would usually be necessary to use T-cell clones in this procedure so that unlimited numbers of specific cells could be obtained for extensive screening and rescreening. Further, there is no guarantee that the recombinant proteins will be correctly processed by the APC for presentation of a given epitope. Nevertheless, the strong advantages of recombinant and phage display methods may make these approaches very attractive for T-cell mapping in the future.

T-CELL RESPONSES TO ALLERGEN-DERIVED PEPTIDES

The major allergen components of the most prevalent allergen sources have now been subjected to T-cell epitope analysis. From this body of work has come the realization that not all individuals respond to the complete set of epitopes in a given allergen molecule and 'outliers' respond to epitopes not usually seen in a population analysis. It is also apparent that different population pools and assay systems can give only partially overlapping epitope maps. However, certain dominant epitopes are recognized by T cells from the majority of allergic individuals. Where several mapping techniques have been applied, the results are discussed in detail below. Several other allergen T-cell epitope maps (summarized in Table 11.1) [35,96–100] have supported the general conclusions which follow.

Table 11.1. Major allergen epitopes identified by T-cell mapping

Allergen	Method[a]	Peptides[b]	Major epitopes[c]	Reference
Cat major allergen				
Fel d 1	1°	variable	Chain 1: 39–52, 53–66	[97]
	Clones		Chain 2: 9–21*, 22–34, 57–70	
Mite allergens				
Der p 1	Clones	variable	**45–67, 94–104, 117–143**	[103]
Der p 1	1°	MPS, 12 (10)	1–10, **48–57**, 106–116, **120–129**	[104]
Der p 1	1°	recomb. fusions	all fragments, highest within **1–94**	[94]
Der p 2	1° &	variable	**11–50**, 61–86, **78–104**	[105]
	Clones		**11–35***	
Der p 2	1° &	T-bag	**1–15, 20–33, 38–51, 92–105, 116–129**	[106]
	Clones		29–42* **110–129***	
Der p 2	1° &	3 × 15–16	33–47, 58–73, 103–118	[107]
Birch allergen				
Bet v 1	Clones	MPS, 13 (10)	2–22, 77–92, **96–113, 113–124, 145–158**	[96]
	Clones	MPS, 13 (10)	29–50, 61–72, **96–113, 113–124, 145–158**	[98]
Bee venom allergen				
Api m 1	2°	variable	50–69, **83–97**	[99]
	Clones	MPS, 13 (11)	**81–92**, 113–124	[100]
Dipteran haemoglobin				
Chi t	1°	variable/tryptic	all peptides except 102–109	[35]
Grass allergen				
Lol p 1	Clones	20 (10)	**191–210**	[64]
	1°	MPS, 12 (10)	**193–206**	[109]
Lol p 1/Poa p IX	Clones	20 (10)	multiple (15/23 peptides)	[110,111]

[a] Method of T-cell epitope mapping. 1°, primary T-cell cultures; 2°, secondary T-cell lines; clones, T-cell clones.
[b] Method of peptide synthesis and peptide length. MPS, multipin peptide synthesis [91]; T-bag, alternative multi-peptide synthesis procedure [106]; recomb. fusions, recombinant fusion peptides; tryptic, tryptic peptides; variable, variable length; numbers indicate peptide length; numbers in brackets indicate peptide overlap.
[c] The major T-cell epitopes identified in each study. An asterisk (*) indicates epitopes identified with T-cell clones in studies using two methods of T-cell mapping. Epitopes have been aligned to highlight potential common epitopes between different sets of results (**bold**).

Cat Allergen Fel d 1

The major allergen of the domestic cat, Fel d 1, is composed of two disulphide-linked chains. The complete sequence of Fel d 1 chains 1 and 2 [66] allowed the design of overlapping peptides spanning the molecule. Peptides longer than 19 amino acids with overlaps of greater than 9 amino acids were tested in primary and secondary T-cell proliferation assays with a large set of cat-allergic patients. This analysis identified two major epitope contining-peptides in the molecule [101,102].

Mouse strains have been identified that respond to a T-cell epitope contained in amino acids 29–55 of Fel d 1 chain 1 [103]. Significantly, subcutaneous injection of a peptide containing this dominant epitope reduced the response to Fel d 1 chain 1 challenge, even in chain 1-primed mice [103]. This suggests that individual dominant epitopes can down modulate T-cell responses against a whole polypeptide.

Mite Allergens Der p 1 and Der p 2

Several groups have used long-term T-cell lines and T-cell clones from mite-allergic patients to map the T-cell epitopes within the two major mite allergens Der p 1 and Der p 2 [104,105]. The results of these studies are summarized in Table 11.1. Noticeably, different patient groups and different assay systems (particularly clones and secondary assays) produce only partially overlapping epitope identifications. Using multipeptide synthesis technology (12-mer peptides overlapping by 10 residues) and primary T-cell cultures, Stewart *et al.* [105] identified four regions of Der p 1 that contained T-cell epitopes: amino acids 1–10, 48–57, 106–116 and 120–129. In a separate survey using 20-mer peptides overlapping by 10 residues, three T-cell epitope-containing regions were identified with clones: amino acids 45–67, 94–104, and 117–143 [104]. Only one epitope-containing region, amino acids 45–67, was identified in both studies. In a third study, O'Brien *et al.* [94] used GST fusion proteins in primary assays to study T-cell epitopes in Der p 1. The fusion proteins contained between 13 and 113 amino acids of Der p 1 sequence (average Der p 1 fragment size was >50 amino acids). Although T-cell reactivity was detected with every fusion protein tested, the majority of the Der p 1 T-cell reactivity was contained in the first 94 amino acids. This region spans amino acids 45–67, the epitope-containing region identified in the first two surveys. However, the relatively large size of the Der p 1 sequences contained in the fusion proteins makes it impossible to clearly delineate any specific T-cell epitope in this study.

The map differences observed in these three surveys emphasizes the importance of using defined overlapping peptide sets and cells from large numbers of individuals to define accurately the major T-cell epitopes within an allergen. The results also show that analysis with T-cell clones may provide only limited representation of epitopes within the general population and no indication of their relative importance. This demonstrates the importance of using large numbers of clones from many individuals to produce results comparable to the primary and secondary T-cell assays.

Mapping of Der p 2 has identified several regions of human T-cell reactivity (Table 11.1). A combination of results from primary and T-cell clone assays (15–20-mer peptides overlapping by 10 residues) identified T-cell epitopes within amino acids 11–50, 61–86 and 78–104 [106]. The most N-terminal epitope was confirmed and further delineated with T-cell clones [106]. In a separate survey with primary assays (12-mer peptides overlapping by 10 residues, multipeptide 'T-bag' syntheses) van Neerven *et al.* [107] identified several regions containing T-cell epitopes of Der p 2: amino acids 1–15, 20–33, 38–51, 92–105, and 116–129. Only one epitope, contained in amino acids 116–129, was identified with both primary assays and clones. The clones also identified another epitope, contained in amino acids 29–42, that was not seen in the primary assays [107]. Once again, the best representation of T-cell epitopes was obtained from assays of uncloned T-cell populations (Table 11.1). Using primary T-cell assays, Okano *et al.* identified modest T-cell reactivity amongst Japanese allergic subjects to each of three tested regions: >50% responding to amino acids 33–47, less to 58–73, and least to 103–118 [108]. Recently [109], human IgE responses to mite allergens were transiently reconstituted in immunodeficient mice allowing further experimental manipulation of the allergen immune response beyond the constraints of the allergic patient.

Grass Allergen Lol p 1

Initial studies with T-cell clones from three patients showed that a T-cell epitope is contained within amino acids 191–210 (20-mer peptides overlapping by 10 amino acids [64]) of Lol p 1. It was subsequently demonstrated with primary T-cell assays from six patients that the epitope is contained within amino acids 193–206 (12-mer peptides overlapping by 10 amino acids [110]). Subcutaneous injection of the dominant epitope-containing peptides identified *in vitro* also caused the greatest *in vivo* skin reactivity in the patient examined [110].

It can be argued that amino acids 191–210 contain a major T-cell epitope in Lol p 1 since it was identified by clones from three individuals [64] and by primary cultures from five of the six atopes tested [110]. However, this epitope was identified with clones from only two of five atopes examined in a later survey [111]. Further, all patients recognized other epitopes within Lol p 1 [64,110,111]. Indeed, 15 of the 23 20-mer peptides (10 amino acid overlap) examined were found to contain T-cell epitopes [111]. Again it is clear that analysis with a limited number of clones from a few patients will serve to identify the presence of T-cell epitopes, but not to quantitate their dominance.

Therefore, more exhaustive analyses should be done with large numbers of patients in order to identify the number and relative importance of all of the T-cell epitopes in Lol p 1. A feature of the grass antigens is the relatively high homology between the major allergens of a given species and also between the allergens of different grasses [64]. This is reflected at the T-cell level by a high degree of epitope-specific cross-reactivity [17,112]. Therefore, peptide as well as conventional immunotherapy could be expected to provide protection across the large group of clinically relevant grass species and in different locations.

SUMMARY OF ALLERGEN T-CELL MAPPING DATA

T cell epitopes of several major allergens have now been mapped by various combinations of primary, secondary and clonal T-cell assays (summarized in Table 11.1). This body of information has localized regions of the allergens believed to be critical in both initiation and maintenance of the allergic reaction. Several consensus motifs have been identified which provide guides to predict favoured allergen sequences capable of binding with high affinity to Class I and Class II MHC molecules [113–115]. However, these motifs cannot predict whether these peptides are actually produced during processing of the allergen by an APC or are capable of being recognized by the T-cell repertoire in a given individual. Hence, empirical observation of particular allergen T-cell epitopes remains the only approach to identifying such regions. Most importantly, there is not yet any information as to why these allergen sequences provoke T cells that support elevated IgE responses and hypersensitivity in atopes. T-cell dependent B-cell responses involving other immunoglobulin isotypes and conventional immune responses to allergens are common to both atopes and non-atopes. Nonetheless, identification of the major T-cell epitopes within the allergic population provides a therapeutic opportunity against allergic disease. It is now possible directly to test the hypothesis that down-modulation of the allergen-specific T-cell response with peptide immunotherapy will consequently reduce allergic symptoms.

INDUCTION OF T-CELL NON-RESPONSIVENESS

The potential clinical applications of peptide immunotherapy have raised a great deal of interest. Several different approaches have been proposed for this immunotherapy, including enzymatic digestion of allergen into peptides, soluble peptide:MHC complexes, recombinant expression of multiple epitopes in the form of a single molecule (a RECOMBITOPE™ molecule), and free peptide administration. Each of these will be discussed in turn.

The first proposed approach involves the enzymatic digestion of an allergen into peptides [116,117]. This has the theoretical advantage that the peptidic digest will contain many, if not all, of the allergen's T-cell epitopes, allowing down-modulation of the response against the entire molecule. Digestion of the allergen into short fragments can also reduce the number of IgE epitopes, reducing the amount of local and systemic reactions observed during immunotherapy. Treatment with a single peptide derived from a digestion of Api m 1 has been reported to decrease the level of IgE and IgG antibodies in treated individuals with a concomitant decrease in skin test reactivity [116]. Treatment of individuals with an enzymatic digest of an Amb a 1-enriched fraction of short ragweed pollen has also been reported to provide a reduction in symptom-medication scores during the ragweed season [117]. This reduction was comparable to that seen with the Amb a 1-enriched fraction alone. The anti-Amb a 1 IgG titre was increased while the seasonal anamnestic IgE increase was blocked in this small study using 8–10 patients per group [117]. Although this approach is conceptually simple, it is hampered by difficulty in characterization of the digested extract. Not only must the allergen be purified prior to digestion, the peptidic fragments must also be purified away from the contaminating proteolytic enzymes. Further, the peptide fragments must be characterized for completeness of enzymatic digestion, as well as for residual IgE binding by the peptide fragments. Characterization of the digest would be even more difficult if a crude extract or mixture of several allergens were used rather than a single purified protein.

It has recently been proposed that administration of soluble peptide:MHC complexes can down-modulate the response against a protein [118]. This approach has been reported to work effectively in an *in vivo* animal model [118] and an *in vitro* culture with human cells [119]. Such antigen-specific immunotherapy is currently being developed for the treatment of autoimmune diseases including multiple sclerosis, myasthenia gravis and rheumatoid arthritis. It could potentially be applied to the treatment of allergic diseases as well. However, it is perhaps the most labour-intensive of the various methods discussed here. This approach requires the stoichiometric and very stable binding of a defined peptide to a soluble form of a human Class II molecule. This is technically very demanding and presents considerable challenges in pharmaceutical development. Further, the peptide must be presented in context of an individual's own MHC, which may limit the usefulness of this technique due to the high degree of the known Class II polymorphism. The immediate application of this technique may be restricted to situations where there is a single or highly dominant T-cell epitope associated with a single Class II allele (Class II restriction).

The use of RECOMBITOPE™ proteins is another potential approach to maximizing allergen desensitization while minimizing IgE reactivity [120]. A RECOMBITOPE™ molecule is constructed *in vitro* by directly linking DNA sequences that encode T-cell epitopes. Recombinantly expressed RECOMBITOPE™ proteins therefore contain multiple allergen-derived T-cell epitopes. Various configurations of the T-cell epitopes within different RECOMBITOPE™ proteins can be screened to ensure maximal T-cell recognition of each epitope and minimal IgE reactivity.

It was shown that RECOMBITOPE™ proteins containing T-cell epitopes of Fel d 1 can produce strong *in vitro* T-cell responses to the epitopes contained within them [120]. These responses were highly specific and comparable to responses induced by native allergen. Although it has been reported that the synthesis of chimeric peptides can shift the restriction pattern and specificity of T-cell recognition for constituent epitopes [121], no novel T-cell specificities were created in the sequences spanning the junction of different epitopes within the RECOMBITOPE™ protein [120]. All RECOMBITOPE™ proteins showed significant reduction in IgE binding compared to native Fel d 1. However, some RECOMBITOPE™ proteins bound detectable levels of IgE. This indicates that each potential RECOMBITOPE™ protein (with its unique epitope order) must be examined for T-cell reactivity and IgE binding.

The number of potential RECOMBITOPE™ products increases factorially as more T-cell epitopes are incorporated. This is shown clearly by comparing the number of potential RECOMBITOPE™ proteins that can be expressed containing two, three or four T-cell epitopes: two T-cell epitope-containing sequences can be arranged sequentially in only two ways (ab or ba); three T-cell epitope-containing sequences can be arranged in six possible combinations (abc, acb, bac, bca, cab or cba); four T-cell epitope-containing sequences can be arranged in 24 possible combinations. It becomes very difficult to construct and analyse all possible combinations as the number of T-cell epitopes within a RECOMBITOPE™ molecule increases.

Finally, there is the administration of free peptides. These peptides are much easier to characterize in terms of T-cell reactivity, sequence integrity and peptide purity. Peptides can also be selected that do not cause histamine release. These peptides would either not bind IgE or contain only a single monomeric IgE binding site and would therefore not be able to cross-link IgE on the surface of a mast cell or basophil, since IgE cross-linking is essential for histamine release. This lack of histamine release will dramatically reduce the number and severity of systemic reactions and will allow the administration of very large amounts of allergen-specific peptides in a relatively short period of time relative to those associated with standard immunotherapy.

The applicability of peptide immunotherapy is now being addressed in a series of double-blind placebo-controlled clinical trials. Norman *et al.* administered peptides derived from Fel d 1, the major allergen of the domestic cat. Patient symptom scores showed statistical improvement in a dose-related manner after only four injections of peptide [122]. Although 40% of the patients reported mild transient reactions to the first injection, these reactions did not require treatment, disappeared after multiple injections and did not appear to be due to IgE-mediated histamine release. The duration of clinical improvement following peptide immunotherapy is currently under investigation. Further Phase II and III clinical trials of the Fel d 1 derived peptides and also of ragweed Amb a 1 peptides are measuring the effect of peptide immunotherapy on allergic responses including to bronchial allergen challenge.

Peptide immunotherapy was directed against Fel d 1 [122]. Even though IgE is clearly present against other minor allergens in cat pelt, clinical symptom scores showed improvement. This suggests that modulation of the response against the dominant allergens can be efficacious, even though other allergens are also present. Either modulation of the response against the major allergens down-regulates the responses against the minor allergens or the responses against minor allergens are insufficient by themselves to cause the full allergic symptoms.

POTENTIAL MECHANISMS OF T-CELL NON-RESPONSIVENESS

The mechanism(s) by which peptide immunotherapy modulates clinical symptoms of an allergic disease is currently under intense investigation. All available evidence suggests that standard immunotherapy is effective in modulating an ongoing immune response in an allergen-specific fashion. The evidence is consistent with the hypothesis that the effects of immunotherapy are mediated through an action on T cells. It has been proposed that peptide immunotherapy works in a similar fashion [22–24]. There are several potential mechanisms for modulating the T-cell response, including MHC blockade, T-cell deletion, induction of T-cell anergy or tolerization, a redistribution or sequestering of cells, and/or a shift in lymphokines or chemokines [123] secreted by allergen-reactive T cells. Indeed, there is no *a priori* reason why more than one, if not all, of these potential mechanisms may be involved at different stages of standard and peptide-induced immunotherapy. It has also been reported that successful immunotherapy modulates the response of allergen-specific T cells. Immunotherapy appears to affect the relative expression of Th1- and Th2-specific lymphokines *in vivo* and *in vitro* [18,124], as well as decreasing late phase skin test reactivity associated with a decreased number of infiltrating T cells and activated eosinophils [124].

Peptide motifs can be designed that will bind to MHC molecules with relatively high affinity [113–115]. These peptides would bind to MHC molecules upon administration and could block binding of allergen-derived peptides. The blocking peptides would therefore prevent stimulation of allergen-specific T cells. However, it is unlikely that this blockade would have long-term effects since an administered peptide is expected to have a relatively short half-life *in vivo*. This was confirmed experimentally in mice [125], where a high-affinity MHC binding peptide was virtually undetectable in the serum after 10 min. The ability of this peptide to block proliferation against the cognate antigen correlated with the peptide's serum concentration [125]. This suggests that one must identify a method to maintain relatively high serum concentrations of blocking peptides over an extended period of time in order for this therapy to succeed *in vivo*. Further, one would have to select peptides that would effectively bind with very high affinities to multiple MHC molecules without activating allergen-specific T cells. Such a broad blockade could interfere with a patient's ability to mount a normal immune response against many antigens, not just the targeted allergen(s). Therefore, a therapy based on peptide blockade would require the response against an allergen to be linked to a limited set of MHC molecules in order to modulate the allergic disease without immunocompromising the treated individual.

It has been recently reported that large amounts of free peptide or peptide:MHC complexes *in vitro* will lead to clonal deletion of cells through apoptosis [26,119]. Administration of high-dose peptide or protein appears functionally to deplete responsive cells *in vivo* as well. It has not been possible to confirm whether this functional depletion is due to cell death or tolerance since apoptotic cells are rapidly scavenged by macrophages *in vivo*. However, recent work with transgenic mice expressing a single dominant T-cell receptor suggests that cognate peptide administration can lead to T cell non-responsiveness without a direct loss in the number of T cells expressing the transgene [126].

The systemic administration of peptides could affect cells in circulation, in lymphoid organs where immune responses are initiated and amplified and/or in cells in the peripheral sites where allergens are normally encountered (nasal passages and lung bronchi). It may be that the systemic administration of peptide causes an active sequestering or redistribution of allergen-reactive T cells away from the periphery to a more central location. This could have a dampening effect on an allergic reaction by reducing the lymphokine/chemokine secretion associated with T-cell activation at the site of allergen exposure. This mechanism would also necessitate a long-lasting decrease in normal cell circulation patterns. Otherwise, the effects of traditional immunotherapy would be of short duration.

There are several models of T-cell anergy or tolerization where the *in vitro* administration of peptide induces a non-responsiveness in cultured cells without inducing wholesale cell death [127,128]. Such anergy induction affects both proliferation and expression of measured lymphokines. The cells become non-responsive to antigen challenge for some time. The induction of non-responsiveness *in vivo* would lead to a modulation of the on-going T-cell response against an allergen. A shift in available lymphokines upon encounter with an allergen could lead to a shift in the induction and recruitment of new allergen-specific T cells and B cells. Such shifts could also affect the induction of *de novo* shifts in antibody isotypes as well as limiting on-going synthesis of antibodies of specific isotypes. Moreover, a shift from a Th2- to a Th1-like response, either in individual clones or in populations of cells, could lead to a shift in secreted chemokines such as RANTES, and MCP-2, among others [123]. These chemokines can have a profound effect on mast cell, basophil and eosinophil recruitment and activation [123]. Therefore, modulation of the allergen-specific T-cell activation and lymphokine/chemokine secretion pattern can have a profound effect on a number of different and relevant cell types. This mechanism would be consistent with changes observed after immunotherapy [124].

SUMMARY

The epitopes responsible for stimulating allergen-specific T cells of a number of major allergens have been defined (Table 11.1). Murine models and initial clinical results using peptides representing these epitopes suggest that these peptides will provide effective treatments for allergic disease. This may be due to one or more of several effects upon T cells or other players in the allergic cascade. It remains a challenge to understand the mechanisms resulting in the amelioration of disease symptoms following peptide immunotherapy.

ACKNOWLEDGEMENTS

We would like to thank Rich Garman, Geoffrey Sunshine, Tom Briner, Mohammad Luqman, and Barbara Wallner for constructive comments and discussions.

REFERENCES

1 O'Hehir RE, Garman RD, Greenstein JL *et al*. The specificity and regulation of T-cell responsiveness to allergens. *Ann Rev Immunol* 1991; **9**: 67–95.
2 Norman PS. Immunotherapy – state of the art. *N E R Allerg Proc* 1985; **6**: 249–254.
3 Creticos PS. Immunotherapy with allergens. *JAMA* 1992; **268**: 2834–2839.
4 Norman PS, Winkenwerder WL, Lichtenstein LM. Immunotherapy of hay fever with ragweed antigen E: comparisons with whole pollen extract placebos. *J Allergy* 1968; **42**: 93–108.
5 Haugaard L, Dahl R, Jacobsen L. A controlled dose-response study of immunotherapy with standardized, partially purified extract of house dust mite: clinical efficacy and side effects. *J Allergy Clin Immunol* 1993; **91**: 709–722.
6 Sundin B, Lilja G, Graff-Lonnevig V *et al*. Immunotherapy with partially purified and standardized animal dander extracts. I. Clinical results from a double-blind study on patients with animal dander asthma. *J Allergy Clin Immunol* 1986; **77**: 478–487.

7 Hedlin G, Graff-Lonnevig V, Heilborn H *et al.* Immunotherapy with cat- and dog-dander extracts. V. Effects of 3 years of treatment. *J Allergy Clin Immunol* 1991; **87**: 955–964.

8 Alvarez-Cuesta E, Cuesta-Herranz J, Puyana-Ruiz J *et al.* Monoclonal antibody-standardized cat extract immunotherapy: risk–benefit effects from a double-blind placebo study. *J Allergy Clin Immunol* 1994; **93**: 556–566.

9 Varney VA, Gaga M, Frew AJ *et al.* Usefulness of immunotherapy in patients with severe summer hay fever uncontrolled by antiallergic drugs. *Br Med J* 1991; **302**: 265–269.

10 Lichtenstein LM, Norman PS, Winkenwerder WL. A single year of immunotherapy for ragweed hay fever: immunologic and clinical studies. *Ann Intern Med* 1971; **75**: 663–671.

11 Birkner T, Rumpold H, Jarolim E *et al.* Evaluation of immunotherapy-induced changes in specific IgE, IgG and IgG subclasses in birch pollen allergic patients by means of immunoblotting. *Allergy* 1990; **45**: 418–426.

12 Finkelman FD, Katona IM, Urban JF. IL-4 is required to generate and sustain *in vivo* IgE responses. *J Immunol* 1988; **141**: 2335–2341.

13 Mosmann TR, Coffman RL. TH1 and TH2 cells: different patterns of lymphokine secretion lead to different functional properties. *Ann Rev Immunol* 1989; **7**: 145–173.

14 Wierenga EA, Snoek M, de Groot C. Evidence for compartmentalization of functional subsets of CD4+ T lymphocytes in atopic patients. *J Immunol* 1990; **144**: 4651–4656.

15 Parronchi P, Macchia D, Piccinni MP. Allergen- and bacterial antigen-specific T-cell clones established from atopic donors show a different profile of cytokine production. *Proc Natl Acad Sci USA* 1991; **88**: 4538–4542.

16 Del Prete GF, De Carli M, D'Elios MM *et al.* Allergen exposure induces the activation of allergen-specific Th2 cells in the airway mucosa of patients with allergic respiratory disorders. *Eur J Immunol* 1993; **23**: 1445–1449.

17 Baskar S, Parronchi P, Mohapatra S *et al.* Human T cell responses to purified pollen allergens of the grass, *Lolium perenne*. Analysis of relationship between structural homology and T cell recognition. *J Immunol* 1992; **148**: 2378–2383.

18 Secrist H, Chelen CJ, Wen Y *et al.* Allergen immunotherapy decreases interleukin 4 production in CD4+ T cells from allergic individuals. *J Exp Med* 1993; **178**: 2123–2130.

19 Schwartz RH. T-lymphocyte recognition of antigen in association with gene products of the major histocompatibility complex. *Ann Rev Immunol* 1985; **3**: 237–261.

20 Moller G. Antigen requirements for activation of MHC restricted responses. *Immunol Rev* 1987; **98**: 1–187.

21 Brown JH, Jardetzky TS, Gorga JC *et al.* Three-dimensional structure of the human class II histocompatibility antigen HLA-DR1. *Nature* 1993; **364**: 33–39.

22 Chapman MD. Use of nonstimulatory peptides: A new strategy for immunotherapy. *J Allergy Clin Immunol* 1991; **88**: 300–303.

23 Schad VC, Garman RD, Greenstein JL. The potential use of T cell epitopes to alter the immune response. *Semin Immunol* 1991; **3**: 217–224.

24 Gefter ML. A new generation of antigens for immunotherapy. In: Lichtenstein LM, Fauci A (eds) *Current Therapy in Allergy, Immunology, and Rheumatology*. St. Louis: C.V. Mosby, 1992; 376–378.

25 Gaur A, Weirs B, Rothbard J. Amelioration of autoimmune encephalomyelitis by myelin basic protein synthetic peptide-induced anergy. *Science* 1992; **258**: 1491.

26 Critchfield JM, Racke MK, Zuniga-Pflucker JC *et al.* T cell deletion in high antigen dose therapy of autoimmune encephalomyelitis. *Science* 1994; **263**: 1139–1143.

27 King TP, Norman PS, Connell JT. Isolation and characterization of allergens from ragweed pollen. II. *Biochemistry* 1964; **3**: 458–468.
28 King TP, Norman PS, Lichtenstein LM. Isolation and characterization of allergens from ragweed pollen. IV. *Biochemistry* 1967; **6**: 1992–2000.
29 King TP, Hoffman D, Lowenstein H *et al.* Allergen nomenclature. *Int Arch Allergy Appl Immunol* 1994; **105**: 224–233.
30 Adolphson C, Goodfriend L, Gleich GJ. Reactivity of ragweed allergens with IgE antibodies. Analyses by leukocyte histamine release and the radioallergosorbent test and determination of cross-reactivity. *J Allergy Clin Immunol* 1978; **62**: 197–210.
31 Ley V, Saiz JC, Carreira J. Isolation and characterization of the main allergen of *Dermatophagoides farinae* by monoclonal antibodies that recognize IgE related epitopes. *Mol Immunol* 1986; **23**: 1311–1318.
32 Stewart GA. Isolation and characterization of the allergen Dpt 12 from *Dermatophagoides pteronyssinus* by chromatofocusing. *Int Arch Allergy Appl Immunol* 1982; **69**: 224–230.
33 Stewart GA, Butcher A, Lees K *et al.* Immunochemical and enzymatic analyses of extracts of the house dust mite *Dermatophagoides pteronyssinus*. *J Allergy Clin Immunol* 1986; **77**: 14–24.
34 Pollart SM, Mullins DE, Vailes LD *et al.* Identification, quantitation, and purification of cockroach allergens using monoclonal antibodies. *J Allergy Clin Immunol* 1991; **87**: 511–521.
35 Liebers V, Raulf M, Mazur G *et al.* Epitope mapping with peptides of *Chi t* I component III and immunomodulation of the *Chi t* response. *J Allergy Clin Immunol* 1993; **92**: 334–339.
36 Spitzauer S, Rumpold H, Ebner C *et al.* Allergen profiles of dog hair and dander, body fluids and tissues as defined by immunoblotting. *Int Arch Allergy Appl Immunol* 1991; **94**: 346–348.
37 de Groot H, Goei KGH, van Swieten P *et al.* Affinity purification of a major and a minor allergen from dog extract: serologic activity of affinity-purified *Can f* I and of *Can f* I-depleted extract. *J Allergy Clin Immunol* 1991; **87**: 1056–1065.
38 Singh MB, Knox RB. Grass pollen allergens: antigenic relationships detected using monoclonal antibodies and dot blotting immunoassay. *Int Arch Allergy Appl Immunol* 1985; **78**: 300–304.
39 Shen HD, Wang SR, Tang RB *et al.* Identification of allergens and antigens of Bermuda grass (*Cynodon dactylon*) pollen by immunoblot analysis. *Clin Allergy* 1988; **18**: 401–409.
40 Lowenstein H. Isolation and partial characterization of three allergens from timothy pollen. *Allergy* 1978; **33**: 30–41.
41 Vela C, Platas C, Gurbindo C *et al.* Fractionation and biological characterization of *Olea europea* pollen extract. *Int Arch Allergy Appl Immunol* 1982; **68**: 289–294.
42 Belin L. Separation and characterization of birch pollen antigens with special reference to the allergenic components. *Int Arch Allergy* 1972; **42**: 329–342.
43 Yasueda H, Yui Y, Shimuzu T *et al.* Isolation and partial characterization of the major allergen from Japanese cedar (*Cryptomeria japonica*) pollen. *J Allergy Clin Immunol* 1983; **71**: 77–86.
44 de la Hoz F, Polo F, del Prado JM *et al.* Purification of *Art v* I, a relevant allergen of *Artemisia vulgaris* pollen. *Mol Immunol* 1990; **27**: 651–657.
45 Geraci D, Billesbolle KB, Lowenstein H *et al.* Immunochemical characterization of antigens of *Parietaria judaica* pollen. Identification of allergens by means of crossed radio immunoelectrophoresis. *Int Arch Allergy Appl Immunol* 1985; **78**: 421–428.
46 Giulani A, Pini C, Bonini S *et al.* Isolation and purification of a major allergen from *Parietaria officinalis* pollen. *Allergy* 1987; **42**: 434–440.

47 Panzani R, Yashueda H, Shimizu T *et al*. Cross-reactivity between the pollens of *Cupressus sempervirens* (common Cypress) and of *Cryptomeria japonica* (Japanese cedar). *Ann Allergy* 1986; **57**: 26–30.
48 Corbi AL, Cortes C, Bousquet J *et al*. Allergenic cross-reactivity among pollens of *Urticaceae. Int Arch Allergy Appl Immunol* 1985; **77**: 377–383.
49 Standring R, Spackman V, Porter SJ. Distribution of a major allergen of rye grass (*Lolium perenne*) pollen between other grass species. *Int Arch Allergy Appl Immunol* 1987; **83**: 96–103.
50 Brandys J, Grimsoen A, Nilsen BM *et al*. Cross-reactivity between pollen extracts from six *Artemisia* species. *Planta Med* 1993; **59**: 221–228.
51 Olsen E, Zhang L, Hill RD *et al*. Identification and characterization of the *Poa p* IX goup of basic allergens of Kentucky bluegrass pollen. *J Immunol* 1991; **147**: 205–211.
52 Ong EK, Griffith IJ, Knox RB *et al*. Cloning of a cDNA encoding a group-V (group-IX) allergen isoform from rye-grass pollen that demonstrates specific antigenic immunoreactivity. *Gene* 1993; **134**: 235–240.
53 Chapman MD, Heymann PW, Platts-Mills TAE. Epitope mapping of two major inhalant allergens, *Der p* I and *Der f* I, from mites of the genus *Dermatophagoides. J Immunol* 1987; **139**: 1479–1484.
54 Esch RE, Klapper DG. Identification and localization of allergenic determinants on grass Group I antigens using monoclonal antibodies. *J Immunol* 1989; **142**: 179–184.
55 Marc-Series I, Boutin Y, Vrancken ER *et al*. Mapping of *Bet v* I epitopes by using murine monoclonal antibodies. *Int Arch Allergy Appl Immunol* 1990; **92**: 226–232.
56 Lin ZW, Ekramoddoullah AK, Jaggi KS *et al*. Mapping of epitopes on *Poa p* I and *Lol p* I allergens with monoclonal antibodies. *Int Arch Allergy Appl Immunol* 1990; **91**: 217–223.
57 Mourad W, Mecheri S, Peltre G *et al*. Study of the epitope structure of purified *Dac g* I and *Lol p* I, the major allergens of *Dacytylis glomerata* and *Lolium perenne* pollens, using monoclonal antibodies. *J Immunol* 1988; **141**: 3486–3491.
58 Mourad W, Bernier D, Jobin M *et al*. Mapping of *Lol p* I allergenic epitopes by using murine monoclonal antibodies. *Mol Immunol* 1989; **26**: 1051–1057.
59 Han S-W, Chang Z-N, Chang H-H *et al*. Identification and characterization of epitopes on *Cyn d* I, the major allergen of Bermuda grass pollen. *J Allergy Clin Immunol* 1993; **91**: 1035–1041.
60 Ansari AA, Shenbagamurthi P, Marsh DG. Complete amino acid sequence of a *Lolium perenne* (perennial rye grass) pollen allergen, *Lol p* II. *J Biol Chem* 1989; **264**: 11181–11185.
61 Ansari AA, Shenbagamurthi P, Marsh DG. Complete primary structure of a *Lolium perenne* (perennial rye grass) pollen allergen, *Lol p* III: comparison with known *Lol p* I and II sequences. *Biochemistry* 1989; **28**: 8665–8670.
62 Mole LE, Goodfriend L, Lapkoff CB *et al*. The amino acid sequence of ragweed pollen allergen Ra5. *Biochemistry* 1975; **14**: 1216–1220.
63 Singh MB, Hough T, Theerakulpisut P *et al*. Isolation of cDNA encoding a newly identified major allergenic protein of rye-grass pollen: intracellular targeting to the amyloplast. *Proc Natl Acad Sci USA* 1991; **88**: 1384–1388.
64 Perez M, Ishioka GY, Walker LE *et al*. cDNA cloning and immunological characterization of the rye grass allergen *Lol p* I. *J Biol Chem* 1990; **265**: 16210–16215.
65 Griffith IJ, Craig S, Pollock J *et al*. Expression and genomic structure of the genes encoding FdI, the major allergen of the domestic cat. *Gene* 1992; **113**: 263–268.
66 Morgenstern JP, Griffith IJ, Brauer AW *et al*. Determination of the amino acid sequence of *Fel d* I, the major allergen of the domestic cat: protein sequence analysis and cDNA cloning. *Proc Natl Acad Sci USA* 1991; **88**: 9690–9694.
67 Rafnar T, Griffith IJ, Kuo M-c *et al*. Cloning of *Amb a* I (Antigen E), the major

allergen family of short ragweed pollen. *J Biol Chem* 1991; **266**: 1229–1236.
68 Griffith IJ, Pollock J, Klapper DG *et al.* Polymorphism of *Amb a* I and *Amb a* II, the major allergens of *Ambrosia artemisiifolia* (short ragweed). *Int Arch Allergy Appl Immunol* 1991; **96**: 296–304.
69 Rogers BL, Morgenstern JP, Griffith IJ *et al.* Complete sequence of the allergen *Amb a* II: recombinant expression and reactivity with T cells from ragweed allergic patients. *J Immunol* 1991; **147**: 2547–2552.
70 Griffith IJ, Smith PM, Pollock J *et al.* Cloning and sequencing of *Lol p* I, the major allergenic protein of rye-grass pollen. *FEBS Lett* 1991; **279**: 210–215.
71 Breiteneder H, Pettenburger K, Bito A *et al.* The gene coding for the major birch pollen allergen *Bet v* I, is highly homologous to a pea disease resistance response gene. *EMBO J* 1989; **8**: 1935–1938.
72 Larsen JN, Stroman P, Ipsen H. PCR based cloning and sequencing of isogenes encoding the tree pollen major allergen *Car e* I from *Carpinus betulus*, hornbeam. *Mol Immunol* 1992; **29**: 703–711.
73 Breiteneder H, Ferreira F, Reikerstorfer A *et al.* Complementary DNA cloning and expression in *Escherichia coli* of *Aln g* I, the major allergen in pollen of alder (*Alnus glutinosa*). *J Allergy Clin Immunol* 1992; **90**: 909–917.
74 Trudinger M, Chua KY, Thomas WR. cDNA encoding the major mite allergen *Der f* II. *Clin Exp Allergy* 1991; **21**: 33–37.
75 Saiki RK, Scharf S, Faloona S *et al.* Enzymatic amplification of beta-globin genomic sequences and restriction site analysis for diagnosis of sickle cell anemia. *Science* 1985; **230**: 1350–1354.
76 Saiki RK, Gelfand DH, Stoffen S *et al.* Primer-directed enzymatic amplification of DNA with a thermostable DNA polymerase. *Science* 1988; **239**: 487–491.
77 Kuo M-c, Zhu X-j, Koury R *et al.* Purification and immunochemical characterization of recombinant and native ragweed allergen *Amb a* II. *Mol Immunol* 1993; **30**: 1077–1087.
78 Chua KY, Kehal PK, Thomas WR. Sequence polymorphisms of cDNA clones encoding the mite allergen *Der p* I. *Int Arch Allergy Appl Immunol* 1993; **101**: 364–368.
79 Yuuki T, Okumura Y, Ando T *et al.* Cloning and sequencing of cDNAs corresponding to mite major allergen *Der f* II. *Jpn J Allergol* 1990; **6**: 557–561.
80 Silvanovich A, Astwood J, Zhang L *et al.* Nucleotide sequence analysis of three cDNAs coding for *Poa p* IX isoallergens of Kentucky bluegrass pollen. *J Biol Chem* 1991; **266**: 1204–1210.
81 Breiteneder H, Ferreira FD, Hoffmann-Sommergruber K *et al.* Cloning and expression in *E. coli* of four isoforms of *Cor a* I, the major allergen of hazel pollen. *Eur J Allergy Clin Immunol* 1992; **47**: 30 (Abstract).
82 Breiteneder H, Ferreira F, Hoffman-Sommergruber K *et al.* Four recombinant isoforms of *Cor a* I, the major allergen of hazel pollen show different IgE-binding properties. *Eur J Biochem* 1993; **212**: 355–362.
83 Thomas WR, Stewart GA, Simpson RJ *et al.* Cloning and expression of DNA coding for the major house dust mite allergen *Der p* I in *Escherichia coli*. *Int Arch Allergy Appl Immunol* 1988; **85**: 127–129.
84 Chua K-Y, Dilworth RJ, Kehal PK *et al.* Production of recombinant mite allergens. In: Kraft D, Sehon A (eds) *Molecular Biology and Immunology of Allergens*. Ann Arbor: CRC Press, 1993; 135–138.
85 Valenta R, Duchene M, Vrtala S *et al.* Recombinant allergens for immunoblot diagnosis of tree-pollen allergy. *J Allergy Clin Immunol* 1991; **88**: 889–894.
86 Valenta R, Vrtala S, Ebner C *et al.* Diagnosis of grass pollen allergy with recombinant timothy grass (*Phleum pratense*) pollen allergens. *Int Arch Allergy Appl Immunol* 1992; **97**: 287–294.

87 Springer TA. Traffic signals for lymphocyte recirculation and leukocyte emigration: the multistep process. *Cell* 1994; **76**: 301–314.
88 Hunter JCR, Lewis GK. Underestimation of the responder phenotype by conventional T cell proliferative assays. *Clin Biotech* 1990; **2**: 41–46.
89 Srinivasan M, Domanico SZ, Kaumaya PTP *et al*. Peptides of 23 residues or greater are required to stimulate a high affinity class II-restricted T cell response. *Eur J Immunol* 1993; **23**: 1011–1016.
90 Stern LJ, Brown JH, Jardetzky TS *et al*. Crystal structure of the human class II MHC protein HLA-DR1 complexed with an influenza virus peptide. *Nature* 1994; **368**: 215–221.
91 Geysen HM, Rodda SJ, Mason TJ *et al*. Strategies for epitope analysis using peptide synthesis. *J Immunol Methods* 1987; **102**: 259–274.
92 Leary TP, Splitter GA. A method for the rapid identification of T lymphocyte epitopes. *Peptide Res* 1990; **3**: 259–261.
93 Hickling JK, Jones KR, Yuan B *et al*. A method for rapid screening of recombinant proteins for recognition by T lymphocytes. *Eur J Immunol* 1992; **22**: 1983–1987.
94 O'Brien RM, Thomas WR, Tait BD. An immunogenetic analysis of T-cell allergen from the house dust mite, Der p I, with recombinant truncated fragments. *J Allergy Clin Immunol* 1994; **93**: 628–634.
95 Scott JK, Smith GP. Searching for peptide ligands with an epitope library. *Science* 1990; **249**: 386–390.
96 Ebner C, Szepfalusi Z, Ferreira F *et al*. Identification of multiple T cell epitopes on *Bet v* I, the major birch pollen allergen, using specific T cell clones and overlapping peptides. *J Immunol* 1993; **150**: 1047–1054.
97 van Neerven RJJ, van de Pol MM, van Milligen FJ *et al*. Characterization of cat dander-specific T lymphocytes from atopic patients. *J Immunol* 1994; **152**: 4203–4210.
98 Ebner C, Schenk S, Szepfalusi Z *et al*. Multiple T cell specificities for *Bet v* I, the major birch pollen allergen, within single individuals. Studies using specific T cell clones and overlapping peptides. *Eur J Immunol* 1993; **23**: 1523–1527.
99 Dhillon M, Roberts C, Nunn T *et al*. Mapping human T cell epitopes on phospholipase A2: the major bee-venom allergen. *J Allergy Clin Immunol* 1992; **90**: 42–51.
100 Carballido J, Carballido-Perrig N, Kagi M. T cell epitope specificity in human allergic and nonallergic subjects to bee venom phospholipase A2. *J Immunol* 1993; **150**: 3582–3591.
101 Garman RD, Kuo M-c, Counsell CM *et al*. Human T cell reactivity to *Fel d* I, the major allergen of the domestic cat. *J Allergy Clin Immunol* 1992; **89**: 222 (Abstract).
102 Counsell C, Bond J, Ohman J *et al*. Definition of the human T cell epitopes of Fel d 1, the major allergen of the domestic cat. *J Allergy Clin Immunol*. In press.
103 Briner TJ, Kuo M-c, Keating KM *et al*. Peripheral T cell tolerance induced in naive and primed mice by subcutaneous injection of peptides from the major cat allergen, *Fel d* I. *Proc Natl Acad Sci USA* 1993; **90**: 7608–7612.
104 Yssel H, Johnson KE, Schneider PV *et al*. T cell activation-inducing epitopes of the house dust mite allergen *Der p* I. Proliferation and lymphokine production patterns by *Dr p* I-specific CD4+ T cell clones. *J Immunol* 1992; **148**: 738–745.
105 Stewart GA, Armstrong L, Krska K *et al*. Epitope mapping analysis of the major mite allergens using synthetic peptides. In: Sehon AH, Kraft D, Kunkel G (eds) *Epitopes of Atopic Allergens*. Brussels: UCB Institute of Allergy, 1990; 41–47.
106 O'Hehir RE, Verhoef A, Panagiotopoulou E *et al*. Analysis of human T cell responses to the group II allergen of *Dermatophagoides* species: localization of major antigenic sites. *J Allergy Clin Immunol* 1993; **92**: 105–113.

107 van Neerven RJJ, van t'Hof W, Ringrose JH *et al.* T cell epitopes of house dust mite major allergen *Der p* II. *J Immunol* 1993; **151**: 2326–2335.
108 Okano M, Nagano T, Kino K *et al.* Population analysis of cellular responses to synthetic peptides of *Der p* 2, a major allergen molecule of *Dermatophagoides pteronyssinus*, in allergic and non-allergic subjects. *Allergy* 1994; **49**: 436–441.
109 Pestel J, Jeannin P, Delneste Y *et al.* Human IgE in SCID mice reconstituted with peripheral blood mononuclear cells from *Dermatophagoides pteronyssinus*-sensitive patients. *J Immunol* 1994; **153**: 3804–3810.
110 Bungy Poor Fard GA, Latchman Y, Rodda S *et al.* T cell epitopes of the major fraction of rye grass *Lolium perenne* (*Lol p* I) defined using overlapping peptides *in vitro* and *in vivo*. I. Isoallergen clone 1A. *Clin Exp Immunol* 1993; **94**: 111–116.
111 Spiegelberg HL, Beck L, Stevenson DD *et al.* Recognition of T cell epitopes and lymphokine secretion by rye grass allergen *Lolium perenne* I-specific human T cell clones. *J Immunol* 1994; **152**: 4706–4711.
112 Mohaptra S, Yang M, Ansari A *et al.* Molecular basis of cross-reactivity among allergen-specific human T cells: T cell receptor Vα gene usage and epitope structure. *Immunology* 1994; **81**: 15–20.
113 Margalit H, Spouge J, Cornette J *et al.* Prediction of immunodominant helper T-cell antigenic sites from the primary sequence. *J Immunol* 1987; **138**: 2213–2229.
114 Rothbard J, Taylor W. A sequence pattern common to T-cell epitopes. *EMBO J* 1988; **7**: 93–100.
115 Chicz RM, Urban RG, Gorga JC *et al.* Specificity and promiscuity among naturally processed peptides bound to HLA-DR alleles. *J Exp Med* 1993; **178**: 27–47.
116 Litwin A, Pesce AJ, Michael JG. Regulation of the immune response to allergens by immunosuppressive allergenic fragments. 1. Peptic fragments of honey bee venom phospholipase A2. *Int Arch Allergy Appl Immunol* 1988; **87**: 361–366.
117 Litwin A, Pesce AJ, Fischer, T *et al.* Regulation of the human immune response to ragweed pollen by immunotherapy. A controlled trial comparing the effect of immunosuppressive peptic fragments of short ragweed with standard treatment. *Clin Exp Allergy* 1991; **21**: 457–465.
118 Sharma SD, Nag B, Su X-M *et al.* Antigen-specific therapy of experimental allergic encephalomyelitis by soluble class II histocompatibility complex–peptide complexes. *Proc Natl Acad Sci USA* 1991; **88**: 11465–11469.
119 Nicolle MW, Nag B, Sharma SD *et al.* Specific tolerance to an acetylcholine receptor epitope induced *in vitro* in myasthenia gravis CD4+ lymphocytes by soluble major histocompatibility complex class II-peptide complexes. *J Clin Invest* 1994; **93**: 1361–1379.
120 Rogers BL, Bond JF, Craig S *et al.* Potential therapeutic recombitope proteins comprised of T cell epitope containing sequences. *Mol Immunol* 1994; **31**: 955–966.
121 Bhardwaj V, Kumar V, Geysen HM *et al.* Subjugation of dominant immunogenic determinants within a chimeric peptide. *Eur J Immunol* 1992; **22**: 2009–2016.
122 Norman PS, Ohman JL, Long AA *et al.* Early clinical experience with T cell reactive peptides from cat allergen *Fel d* I. *J Allergy Clin Immunol* 1994; **93**: 231 (Abstract).
123 Baggiolini M, Dahinden CA. CC chemokines in allergic inflammation. *Immunol Today* 1994; **15**: 127–133.
124 Varney VA, Hamid QA, Gaga M *et al.* Influence of grass pollen immunotherapy on cellular infiltration and cytokine mRNA expression during allergen-induced late-phase cutaneous responses. *J Clin Invest* 1993; **92**: 644–651.
125 Ishioka GY, Adorini L, Guery J-C *et al.* Failure to demonstrate long-lived MHC saturation both *in vitro* and *in vivo*. Implications for therapeutic potential of MHC-blocking peptides. *J Immunol* 1994; **152**: 4310–4319.

126 Falb D, Briner T, Sunshine G *et al*. Peripheral tolerance in T cell receptor transgenic mice: evidence for T cell anergy. *Proc Nat Acad Sci USA. Eur J Immunol* 1996; **26**: 130–135.
127 Lamb JR, Skidmore BJ, Green N *et al*. Induction of tolerance in influenza virus immune T lymphocyte clones with synthetic peptides of influenza haemagglutinin. *J Exp Med* 1983; **157**: 1434–1442.
128 Higgins JA, Lamb JR, Marsh SGE *et al*. Peptide-induced nonresponsiveness of HLA-DP restricted human T cells reactive with *Dermatophagoides* spp. (house dust mite). *J Allergy Clin Immunol* 1992; **90**: 749–756.

12 Modulation of the Functional Properties of Allergen-specific T Cells by Interferon-α and other Cytokines

ENRICO MAGGI and PAOLA PARRONCHI
Clinical Immunology Department, Institute of Internal Medicine and Immunoallergology, University of Florence, Italy

INTRODUCTION

The protective value of immune responses depends on the pattern of cytokines produced by the T cells involved. Extensive studies on activated T cells have clearly shown that in both mice and humans the production of distinct cytokines is differentially regulated. CD4+ T cells have been distinguished by their cytokine production profile into at least three distinct subsets. Th1 cells produce IL-2, IFN-γ and TNF-β (but not IL-4 and IL-5), whereas Th2 cells secrete IL-4 and IL-5, but not the Th1-type cytokines [1,2]. In addition to cells that fit into the Th1 or Th2 groups, both murine and human CD4+ T-cell clones (TCC) having the capacity to produce both sets of cytokines (Th0) have been reported [3,4]. Since IL-4 is the switching factor for IgE antibody synthesis and IL-5 promotes the differentiation of eosinophils, that are frequently observed in the target organs of allergic patients, Th2 cells may be particularly implicated in the pathogenesis of allergic disorders. The majority of both mouse and human CD8+ T-cell clones exhibit a Th1-like profile of cytokine secretion [5], but human CD8+ T-cell clones with a Th2- or Th0-like profile have also been described, mainly in late phases of HIV infection [6,7]. Besides their profile of cytokine secretion, murine and human Th1 and Th2 clones also differ for several functions. IL-2 is a growth and activating factor for Th1 and Th2 cells, whereas IL-4 and IFN-γ play an opposite regulatory role on proliferation and cytokine synthesis of Th2 and Th1 cells, respectively. Human Th1 and Th2 cells also differ in their helper activity for *in vitro* Ig synthesis by autologous B cells. In the presence of the specific antigen, Th2 clones effectively induce IgM, IgG, IgA and IgE synthesis by autologous B cells. Th1 clones provide help to B cells for IgM, IgG, and IgA, but not IgE, synthesis, but, at high T–B cell ratios, a decline of

Allergic Mechanisms and Immunotherapeutic Strategies. Edited by A.M. Roberts and M.R. Walker.

helper function strictly related to the cytolytic activity of Th1 cells against APC is found [8,9]. This may represent an important mechanism by which Th1 cells down-regulate antibody response *in vivo*; on the other hand, the failure of this regulation by Th2 cells may account, at least in part, for why IgE antibody responses (e.g. to seasonal allergens) are still ongoing a long time after allergen exposure. It has also been clearly shown that cytokines not only determine the functional phenotype of effector lymphocytes, but also represent the main factors affecting their differentiation pathways [7,10,11].

In this chapter we will analyse T helper cell subsets involved in the pathogenesis of allergic disorders as well as the mechanisms regulating Th cell differentiation. In particular, the role of cytokines in determining the development of human T cells into clones showing one or another profile of cytokine secretion will be examined. Finally, we will analyse the activity of IFN-α, not only in modulating Th2 response, but also in promoting the preferential expansion of T cells expressing specific Vβ elements, which may represent a new tool for therapeutic strategies.

Th2 CELLS ARE INVOLVED IN THE PATHOGENESIS OF ALLERGIC DISORDERS

Clear-cut evidence that allergens induce the preferential activation of CD4+ Th2 cells was provided by examining high numbers of *Dermatophagoides pteronyssinus* group 1 (Der p 1), *Lolium perenne* group 1 (Lol p 1) or *Poa pratensis* group 9 (Poa p 9) specific T-cell clones obtained from mite- or grass-sensitive atopic individuals and compared for their pattern of cytokine secretion with purified protein derivative (PPD) or tetanus toxoid (TT) specific T-cell clones derived from the same donors. Virtually all the allergen-specific T-cell clones produced IL-4 (and IL-5) in response to stimulation with phorbol myristate acetate (PMA) plus anti-CD3 antibody, and a proportion of them failed to produce IFN-γ [12]. When assessed with the specific antigen under MHC-restricted conditions, the great majority of allergen-specific T-cell clones behave as Th2-like helper T cells [12]. While most T-cell clones specific for TT produced both IL-4 and IFN-γ (particularly in response to PMA plus anti-CD3 antibody), all T-cell clones specific for PPD produced high amounts of IFN-γ, but most of them did not produce IL-4 and IL-5 [12]. These data suggest that at least *in vitro* allergens preferentially expand CD4+ Th2 cells.

There is a general consensus that Th2 cells and their cytokines are involved in the pathophysiology of IgE-mediated disorders. Higher proportions of IL-4-producing and lower proportions of IFN-γ-producing T-cell clones were obtained from the PB of patients with severe atopic disease than from nonatopic donors [13]. The majority of T-cell clones derived from the conjunctival infiltrates of patients with vernal conjunctivitis were found to express the Th2 cytokine profile [14]. Using an *in situ* hybridization technique, T cells showing mRNA for Th2- but not Th1-type cytokines were found at the site of late-phase reactions in skin biopsies from atopic patients [15] and in mucosal bronchial biopsies or bronchoalveolar lavage from asthmatics [16,17], supporting the view that Th2 cells may selectively accumulate in target organs of atopic patients. To investigate whether the Th2-like cells present in the airway mucosa of patients with allergic respiratory disorders actually reflect a T-cell response to inhaled allergens, biopsy specimens were obtained from the bronchial or nasal mucosa of patients with grass pollen-induced bronchial asthma or rhinitis 48 h after positive bronchial or nasal provocation test with grass pollen extract. High proportions of CD4+ T-cell clones derived from stimulated mucosa were specific for grass allergens and most of them exhibited a clear-cut Th2 profile and induced IgE synthesis in autologous PB B cells [18]. These findings provide convincing evidence that Th2 cells specific for the relevant allergen appear in the mucosa soon after allergen inhalation. These cells, because of their cytokine profile, might well play a triggering role in the initiation of the allergic cascade [18].

Recently, CD30 antigen, a member of the TNF receptor superfamily, has been shown to be a marker associated with the production of Th2-type cytokines [19]. No CD4+CD30+ cells were detected in any of nonatopic donors or atopic patients examined before the grass pollen season, whereas some of the grass-sensitive donors showed small proportions of circulating CD4+CD30+ cells during the period they were suffering from allergic symptoms. Only CD4+CD30+ cells proliferated in response to Lol p 1 and exhibited the ability to produce IL-4 and IL-5, whereas production of both IFN-γ and TNF-β was prevalent in the CD4+CD30– cell fraction [20]. These findings demonstrate that grass allergen-reactive CD30+ T cells inducible to the production of Th2 cytokines can circulate in the peripheral blood of grass-sensitive patients as a consequence of *in vivo* natural exposure to grass pollen allergens.

Further evidence for the role of Th2 cells in the pathogenesis of allergic diseases arises from two recent studies on the effect of specific immunotherapy on the cytokine profile of T cells. Grass pollen immunotherapy did not affect the expression of Th2-pattern cytokines in response to allergen exposure at the level of allergen-induced late-phase cutaneous responses, but expression of mRNA for Th1-type cytokines was enhanced in half of the patients showing clinical improvement [21]. In another study, successful immunotherapy was found to reduce IL-4 production by allergen specific CD4+ T cells to levels observed with T cells from nonallergic subjects, whereas production of IFN-γ was unaffected [22]. Although these reports give contradictory results, they support the concept that the cytokine profiles of allergen-specific memory CD4+ T cells can be manipulated by *in vivo* therapies.

MECHANISMS INVOLVED IN THE REGULATION OF T HELPER DEVELOPMENT

Although in principle Th1 and Th2 cells might arise from distinct precursors, experiments with homogeneous populations of cells from T-cell receptor (TCR) transgenic mice strongly suggest that a single precursor can differentiate into either a Th1 or Th2 phenotype [23]. Reiner and colleagues [24] show that T cells from mice infected with *Leishmania major* express a restricted TCR repertoire in both progressive infection and protective immunity, regardless of histocompatibility haplotypes, further supporting this possibility. According to this model, naive Th precursor (Thp) cells mainly produce IL-2 and progress into early memory Th0 effector cells following a first activation by the specific antigen [10]. These cells would then terminally differentiate into Th1 or Th2 cells upon repeated antigen stimulations [25]. However, the mechanisms responsible for the differentiation of naive Th cells into the Th1 or Th2 phenotype have not yet been completely clarified. Besides the genetic background, attention has been focused on the possible role of types of antigen-presenting cells (APC), nature of antigenic determinants, T-cell repertoire and soluble factors present in the microenvironment at the time of allergen presentation.

GENETIC FACTORS INFLUENCING Th DIFFERENTIATION

The immunogenetic mechanisms underlying heightened IgE responsiveness seen in the atopic diseases can be divided into antigen-specific and non-antigen-specific [26]. The former is strongly influenced by HLA-D-encoded, major histocompatibility complex (MHC) class II genes and involves cognate T cell–B cell interaction. The latter, noncognate regulation of IgE, could involve primarily mast cells, basophils, and possibly other FcRI+ cells, and obviously Th2 cells [26].

Recent evidence for a linkage of overall IgE to markers in chromosome 5q31.1, especially to the IL-4 gene, has been provided [27], suggesting that one or more polymorphisms exist in a coding region or, more probably, a regulatory region of the IL-4 gene. Transcription of IL-4 gene is stringently regulated by multiple promoter elements acting together [27,28]. Other genes map within 5q31.1, including several other candidates which might influence IgE production such as IL-13, IRF1 (whose gene product up-regulates IFN-α) [29,30] and IL-12B (which encodes the β chain of IL-12, a cytokine down-regulating Th2 development) [29,30]. Thus, alterations of molecular mechanisms directly involved in the regulation of IL-4 gene expression, as well as deficient regulatory activity of cytokines responsible for inhibition of Th2-cell development (such as IFN-α and IL-12), or both, may account for the preferential Th2-type response towards environmental allergens in atopic people.

THE APC, ANTIGEN AND T CELL REPERTOIRE TRIAD

Langerhans cells (LC) in the skin, as well as dendritic cells (DC) localized in the respiratory tract, represent the primary contact site between the immune system and allergens coming through the skin or the respiratory mucosa, respectively. These cells transport allergen to regional lymph nodes where allergen presentation to specific CD4+ T cells occurs. Some data suggest that asthmatic patients have higher numbers of intra-epithelial DC than non-asthmatic subjects and that these cells in the presence of allergen molecules can induce T-cell activation and release of IL-4 and IL-5 [31]. However, the role played by professional APC in driving the development of allergen-reactive Th2-like cells remains to be elucidated.

The role of the T-cell repertoire in determining the development of Th1 or Th2-type responses is controversial. In mice infected with *Leishmania major* both Th1 and Th2 cells possessing the same repertoire and recognizing the same peptide have been demonstrated, suggesting that cells with identical T-cell receptor (TCR) can differentiate into either the Th1 or the Th2 phenotype [24]. However, evidence for an important role of specific Vβ-expressing T-cell subsets in the stimulation of IgE production and increased airways responsiveness induced by ragweed allergen has been reported [32]. Thus, it cannot be excluded that the recognition of allergen by the TCR provides a signal or sets of signals that drive the T cells in a certain direction, e.g. to produce IL-4 or alternatively, IFN-γ.

As far as the role of antigen is concerned, recently, large panels of T-cell clones were generated from donors with low or high serum IgE levels specific for two nonapeptides (p92 and p96). Both p92- and p96-specific T-cell clones generated from 'high IgE' donors produced remarkable amounts of IL-4 and low IFN-γ. In contrast, T-cell clones generated from 'low IgE' donors showed a clear-cut difference in their profile of cytokine production: the majority of those specific for p96 produced high amounts of both IL-4 and IFN-γ, whereas most p92-specific T-cell clones showed a Th1-like profile of cytokine production (high IFN-γ and low IL-4).

These data suggest that the nature and/or the intensity of TCR signalling provided by the allergen peptide ligand can influence the cytokine profile of Th cells. However, the above mentioned data clearly indicate that altered regulation of IL-4 production is overwhelming the influence exerted by the allergen peptide ligand. With regard to the possibility that the deregulation of IL-4 production can be due to altered down-regulatory mechanisms, recent experiments suggest a possible role of allergen-specific CD8+ T cells in controlling the Th response against allergens, not only in experimental animals, but also in humans. First, the peptide 92 (see above) expanded higher numbers of CD8+ T cell clones in 'low' than in 'high' IgE producers. In addition, lactalbumin expanded higher numbers of CD8+ T cell clones in nonatopic than in atopic milk-sensitive donors, suggesting that in nonatopic people allergen-specific CD8+ T cells may play an important role (possibly via IFN-γ production) in preventing the differentiation of CD4+ Th cells to the same allergen towards the Th2 pathway. Interestingly, unusual CD8+ T-cell clones showing Th2-like profile of cytokine secretion, ability to provide B-cell help for IgE synthesis, as well as CD30 expression, could be generated from the peripheral blood of patients with AIDS showing high levels of IgE in their serum and hypereosinophilia [34].

MICROENVIRONMENTAL HORMONES

Hormones can also promote the differentiation of Th cells: glucocorticoids enhance Th2 activity, and synergize with IL-4, whereas dehydroepiandrosterone sulphate enhances Th1 activity [35]. Another major prohormone, 25-hydroxy cholecalciferol (25 (OH) vitamin D3) may have a reverse effect on the Th1/Th2 balance [36]. More importantly, calcitriol analogues can rival cyclosporin A in their ability to prolong survival of skin grafts by inhibiting Th1 activity [36]. Finally, progesterone favours the *in vitro* development of human Th cells producing Th2-type cytokines and promotes both IL-4 production and membrane CD30 expression in established human Th1 clones [37]. This may represent one of the mechanisms involved in the Th1/Th2 switch which has been hypothesized to occur at the maternal–fetal interface in order to improve fetal survival and promote successful pregnancy [38].

MICROENVIRONMENTAL CYTOKINES

Attention has recently been focused on the possibility that the type of Th response is dependent upon the factors produced by antigen-presenting cells (APC), or by other cell types during antigen exposure, in determining the development of the specific Th1 or Th2 response.

The factors that regulate the development of human Th1 and Th2 clones have extensively been investigated in our laboratory by using peripheral blood lymphocytes cultured with bacterial antigens and allergens in the presence or in the absence of exogenous cytokines or anti-cytokine antibodies.

Signals Favouring the Th2 Development of T Memory Cells

The effect of cytokines produced by macrophages and/or B cells on the development of Th2 cells seems to be less critical than for Th1 cells. IL-10 has been shown to favour the development of Th2 cells both in mouse and man [23]. IL-1 is a selective co-factor for the growth of some murine Th2 clones [39] and can favour the *in vitro* development of human Th2-like clones [40]. However, in both murine and human systems, IL-4 appears to be the most dominant factor in determining the likelihood for Th2 polarization in cultured cells [29,41–43]. Recently we have looked at both the cytokine profile of CD8+ human T-cell clones and the mechanisms involved in their development. While the majority of CD8+ T-cell clones derived from the peripheral blood of normal individuals showed the same cytokine profile as Th1-type CD4+ T-cell clones, several CD8+ T-cell clones exhibiting a Th0, or even a clear-cut Th2, profile could be derived from peripheral blood of patients with severe atopy, Kaposi's sarcoma skin lesions or unharmed skin of HIV-infected patients [35], and skin lesions of patients with lepromatous leprosy. Furthermore also for CD8+ T cells, IL-4 addition in bulk culture before cloning favours high proportions of CD8+ T cells to shift from the Th1 to the Th0/Th2 like phenotype (Maggi *et al.*, unpublished). Accordingly, IL-4-KO mice fail to generate mature Th2 cells *in vivo* and to produce IgE antibodies [44], suggesting that early IL-4 production by another cell type must be involved.

Possible candidates include a still uncharacterized T-cell subset [45], a double negative (CD4−CD8−) $\alpha\beta$TCR early thymic circulating T-cell subset [46], as well as mast cells and basophils, releasing stored IL-4 in response to FcεR triggering [47,48]. Since helminth antigens or allergens are unable to crosslink these receptors prior to a specific immune response eliciting specific IgG and IgE antibodies, and since mast cell-deficient mice develop normal Th2 responses [49], IL-4 production by mast cells may play a role only in amplifying secondary responses, and not in inducing the Th2 development in primary immune responses. An alternative explanation is that some proteolytic enzymes, which are produced in large quantity by many helminth parasites, trigger mast cells to release IL-4 and other cytokines that induce a Th2 differentiation in the primary response. In this regard, it is of note that some environmental allergens are proteases, and injection of papain in BALB/c mice resulted in a 10–30-fold increase in IL-4 and IL–5 but not IFN-γ or IL-2 in draining lymph nodes [50]. However, the fact that allergens induce Th2-type responses only in selected people suggests that atopic individuals would have genetic dysregulation in the production of IL-4 and/or of cytokines exerting regulatory effects on the development and/or function of Th2 cells.

Signals for the Development of Th1-like Response

The clearest examples of factors affecting the differentiation pathways of both murine and human Th1 cells appear to be cytokines released by APC and/or other cell types at the time of antigen presentation [7,8,51]. Thus, IFN-α, IL-12 and TGF-β produced by macrophages and B cells, particularly in response to intracellular bacteria, have been shown to play an important role in the induction of Th1 expansion in various systems [7,8,29].

In contrast, anti-IL-12 antibody favoured the differentiation of PPD-specific

T cells into Th0 or Th2 instead of Th1 clones [7,29]. IFN-α and IL-12 are produced predominantly by macrophages, cells that have an important role in the presentation of antigen to Th cells. Therefore, it is reasonable to suggest that, given the capacity of viruses and intracellular bacteria to stimulate macrophage production of IFN-α and IL-12 (that induce IFN-γ production by both T cells and NK cells), as well as to activate CD8+ T cells (that produce high amounts of IFN-γ), CD4+ cells may be simultaneously activated by processed antigen plus cytokines that induce them to differentiate towards a Th1 phenotype [7].

Interestingly, allergen-specific T-cell lines, grown in the presence of IFN-α, poly I:C (a synthetic double-stranded RNA contained in different viruses), or influenza virus, contained significantly higher proportions of both CD3+ CD8+ and CD3− CD16+ cells than T-cell lines grown in the presence of allergen alone. More importantly, the removal of either CD8+ or CD16+ cells from PBL populations reduced the capacity of poly I:C to shift the differentiation of allergen-specific T cells from the Th2 to the Th0 or Th1 profile [29]. Taken together, these data suggest that intracellular bacteria and viruses induce specific immune responses of Th1 type at least partly because they either directly stimulate CD8+ T cells and NK cells to produce IFN-γ, or because they induce macrophage production of IFN-α and IL-12 which in turn stimulate NK cell growth and IFN-γ production. However, the production of high concentrations of IFN-γ by NK cells, although important, does not appear to be sufficient for the induction of Th1 responses. Indeed, the addition of anti-IFN-γ antibody to bulk cultures does not prevent or reverse the inhibitory effect of poly I:C on the differentiation of allergen-specific T cells into Th2 clones. Likewise, blocking of IFN-α or IL-12 alone with specific antibodies was ineffective. In contrast, the poly I:C-induced Th0 or Th1 differentiation of allergen-specific T cells could be driven to the Th2 profile by the simultaneous addition of IL-4 plus antibodies reactive with IFN-γ, IFN-α and IL-12 [7,52]. Thus, it is possible that poly I:C interferes with IL-4 production by T cells. It can be concluded, therefore, that viruses and intracellular bacteria induce Th1 responses because the profile of the 'natural' immune response they evoke provides optimal conditions (high concentrations of IFN-γ and absence of IL-4) for the development of Th1 cells.

IFN-α MODIFIES SOME FUNCTIONAL ACTIVITIES OF ALLERGEN-SPECIFIC Th2-LIKE CELLS

It has previously been shown that the great majority of Th1, but only a minority of Th2, CD4+ human T-cell clones exhibited anti-CD3-mediated, lectin-dependent, and MHC-restricted cytotoxic activity [9,53]. We subsequently demonstrated that only a minority of allergen-specific Th0/Th2 clones also showed both lectin-dependent and MHC-restricted cell cytotoxicity [54]. Although a correlation between cytotoxic activity and IFN-γ release by T cells could be observed, IFN-γ itself, as well as other Th1-restricted or related cytokines such as IL-2 and TNF-β, were apparently not responsible for the cytotoxic activity of CD4+ clones. Therefore we asked whether signals able to modulate Th differentiation were also able to regulate the development of cytotoxic activity by CD4+ T cells. Indeed, addition of IL-4 in bulk culture before cloning inhibited not only the differentiation of PPD-specific T cells into Th1-like T-cell lines and clones, but also the development of their cytolytic potential. On the contrary, the addition in bulk culture of IFN-α and IFN-γ favoured the development of Poa p 9-specific T-cell clones showing both Th0/Th1 profile and cytolytic activity [54]. These data suggest that the development of CD4+ T-cell clones with a given profile of cytokine production and the expression of cytolytic activity are similarly regulated.

Besides the effects on the cytokine pattern and cytolytic activity, exogenous IFN-α is able to selectively modulate the epitope specificity of T cells. Indeed, the study of fine specificity of Poa p 9-specific TCC derived in the presence of IFN-α suggests that IFN-α promoted a selective expansion of TCC specific for a single peptide (peptide 26) of the allergen molecule. Although a substantial proportion of both TCC generated in the absence or presence of IFN-α expressed the Vβ2 element, IFN-α favoured the expansion of Vβ2, Vβ17 and Vβ22 positive Poa p 9-specific T cells. The high proportion of Vβ2 positive and p26-specific TCC did not merely reflect the expansion of a single progenitor cell, inasmuch as at least some of them utilized different Jα genes. More importantly, the analysis of some Vβ2 positive Poa p 9-specific clones indicated that none of those generated in the absence of IFN-α recognized the p26 peptide, whereas virtually all TCC generated in the presence of IFN-α responded to this peptide. These data clearly suggest that IFN-α can both shift the cytokine profile of Vβ2 positive T cells and restrict their response to only one peptide.

The ability of IFN-α to promote the preferential expansion of T cells expressing specific Vβ elements was neither limited to a single patient, nor to only one allergen. Moreover, a restricted IFN-α-dependent shift of TCR Vβ repertoire was also observed in Lol p 1-specific T cells from the same patients, suggesting that the modulatory activity of IFN-α on TCR repertoire (and possibly on epitope specificity) of allergen-specific T cells is a more general phenomenon.

At present, the mechanisms by which IFN-α can modulate the epitope specificity of allergen-specific T cells are unclear, but we favour the possibility that IFN-α influences antigen presentation and/or processing by the APC. For example, IFN-α may favour the presentation of particular peptides by modulating the expression of MHC class II determinants on the APC or it may act at the level of antigen processing selectively determining the formation and/or presentation of a given peptide. IFN-γ has been shown to alter the peptidase activity of 20S and 26S proteosomes without affecting the rates of breakdown of proteins or ubiquitinated proteins [55,56]. This suggests that IFN-γ enhances the expression of MHC class I genes which in turn increases the proteosome capacity to cleave small peptides after hydrophobic and basic residues but reduces cleavage after acidic residues. Interestingly, in contrast to the peptides reacting with IFN-α(-) TCC, p26 is extremely hydrophobic in nature and possesses a number of basic residues.

The finding that IFN-α shifts TCR Vβ repertoire and peptide reactivity in parallel to a change in the cytokine secretion profile of allergen-specific T cells suggests a link between recognition of a given peptide and pathway of cytokine production. This does not necessarily imply that Th1 and Th2 cells would have different TCR and recognize different peptides. It was indeed clearly shown that both subsets of CD4+ T cells can use the same receptors, suggesting that the same peptide is able to promote both a Th1- and Th2-type response [57]. Thus, it is possible that, under the influence of IFN-α, different T-cell epitopes are presented by APC, and that these peptides are recognized by TCRs with a different peptide–receptor affinity. Recently, indeed, it has been reported that peptide–ligand affinity may influence the type of cytokine production by T cells by creating an environment of biochemical affinities that triggers activation and development of different T-cell effector functions [24]. Accordingly, in an animal model system of allergic sensitization, it was shown that the development of immediate-type hypersensitivity responses was dependent on the route of sensitization and the stimulation of certain TCR Vβ expressing T cells. In that system, similar to the findings of the present results, different allergens stimulated different TCR Vβ T cells with a differential pattern of T-cell effector functions [58].

Irrespective of the mechanism involved, the results of this study provide a point of departure for new approaches to the development of specific immunotherapy for IgE-mediated diseases. Thus, in principle, a shift from the Th2 response, induced by natural allergen exposure in genetically predisposed individuals, to a Th0/Th1 response could be beneficial for the patient. It remains to be explored whether *in vivo* treatment with IFN-α can achieve a similar shift in the T-cell responses to allergens.

NOVEL STRATEGIES FOR IMMUNOMODULATION OF ALLERGIC DISEASES

The new insights into the pathogenesis of allergic disorders provide novel opportunities for the development of immunomodulatory regimens in allergic diseases. Essentially two new approaches to allergen-specific immunotherapy regimens can be hypothesized: (1) induction of T-cell anergy with allergen-derived peptides [59] and (2) induction of T cell class switch (from Th2 to Th0/Th1). A first possibility is to down-regulate established allergen-specific Th2 responses, i.e. by acting at the level of memory T cells.

Down-regulation of Th2 cells may result from either induction of tolerance, or by selective manipulation of cytokine secretion patterns (reduction of IL-4 production and increase in IFN-γ production). However, a potentially more successful approach should be the up-regulation of allergen-specific Th1 responses, which is directed to prime naive T cells in a way which selects for prevalent Th1 phenotype. Indeed, predominant secretion of Th1-type cytokines in response to allergen will not only result in development and recruitment of different effector responses (IgG, macrophage activation instead of IgE and eosinophil activation), but will also probably inhibit the function of established Th2 responses as a result of cross-regulatory circuits.

Up-regulation of allergen-specific Th1 responses was achieved *in vitro* by using cytokines, such as IFN-γ, IFN-α [54] and IL-12 [29]. It was subsequently demonstrated that the Th1-inducing effect of IL-12 was mainly due to its ability to prime T cells to IFN-γ production [60]. More recently, a strong Th1-inducing effect was also obtained with poly I:C, that appeared to be capable of inducing high production of both IFN-α and IL-12 by macrophages [60]. As we have analysed before, IFN-α was not only found to be able to modulate the cytokine profile of allergen-specific T cells, but also to affect their TCR repertoire. These data suggest that the injection of selected allergen peptides in combination with Th1-inducing cytokines may represent the basis for a novel immunotherapeutic strategy in allergic disorders.

CONCLUDING REMARKS

Studies with both animal and human models provide significant evidence that IL-4 can strongly influence activated CD4+ and CD8+ T cells to differentiate into cells that produce the Th2 set of cytokines. IL-4 also exerts a strong inhibitory effect on the development of cytolytic potential of both types of cells. In humans, at least *in vitro*, IL-1 seems to be also involved in positively regulating the development of Th2-type CD4+ T cells. In contrast, IFN-α and IL-12 (in part via induction of IFN-γ production by both T lymphocytes and NK cells) appear to exert an opposite regulatory effect by favouring the development of CD4+ T cells able to produce the Th1 set of cytokines and to show cytolytic potential. This suggests that a balance between IL-1/IL-4 and IFN-α/IFN-γ/IL-12 at the triad (APC/Ag/Th cell) recognition level might play a critical role in determining the cytokine profile of the specific immune response.

IL-1, IFN-α and IL-12 are produced by macrophages and B cells that act as APC. Thus it is reasonable to suggest that the cytokine profile of the 'natural immunity' evoked by different micro-organisms or soluble antigens plays a critical role in determining the profile of the subsequent specific immune response. In this context, we can speculate that IFN-α production occurs soon after macrophage–antigen first contact, allowing virgin T cells to be activated by the processed antigen, in the presence of a cytokine that induces them to differentiate in a Th1 direction. This may explain why responses against viruses or intracellular bacteria, producing large amounts of IFN-α, usually involve Th1 cells which via their effector activities probably represent highly effective mechanisms in the protection against these infectious agents. In addition, the activity of Th1 cells in mediating killing of APC might down-regulate specific B-cell responses, accounting for the short-lived antibody production frequently observed in successful inflammatory reactions. By contrast, repeated or chronic stimulation by inhaled allergens, that do not evoke strong macrophage activation or high IFN-α production, can allow activation of T cells with Th2-like cytokine secretion profile.

It cannot be excluded that additional IL-4 produced by cells belonging to the mast cell or basophil lineage may further contribute to the maintenance and amplification of an allergen-specific Th2 response. The inability of these cells to kill the APC might explain, at least in part, the chronicity of IgE antibody production present in atopic patients. The finding that IFN-α enables the allergen-specific T cells to kill the APC might be of great interest in view of new approaches to therapy in IgE-mediated diseases. Furthermore, irrespective of the mechanism involved, the results of epitope selection of IFN-α also provide new insights for the development of a novel and specific immunotherapeutic procedure for these patients. The injection of selected allergen peptides in combination with Th1-inducing cytokines or incorporated into adjuvants that select for the Th1 phenotype may represent the basis for a novel immunotherapeutic strategy in allergic disorders.

ACKNOWLEDGEMENTS

This work was supported in part by grants from the Associazione Italiana Ricerca Cancro (AIRC), from the Consiglio Nazionale Ricerche (targeted projects 'Cytokines' and 'ACRO'), from the Istituto Superiore di Sanità (AIDS project) and from the European Community (Biotechnology and FLAIR projects).

REFERENCES

1 Mosmann TR, Cherwinski H, Bond MW, Giedlin MA, Coffman RL. Two types of murine helper T-cell clone. I. Definition according to profiles of lymphokine activities and secreted proteins. *J Immunol* 1986; **136**: 2348–2357.

2 Romagnani S. Human Th1 and Th2: doubt no more. *Immunol Today* 1991; **12**: 256–257.

3 Maggi E, Del Prete GF, Macchia D, Parronchi P, Tiri A, Chretien I, Ricci M, Romagnani S. Profiles of lymphokine activities and helper function for IgE in

human T cell clones. *Eur J Immunol* 1988; **18**: 1045–1051.
4 Mosmann TR, Moore KW. The role of IL-10 in cross-regulation of Th1 and Th2 responses. *Immunoparasitol Today* 1991; **12**: 49–53.
5 Fong TAT, Mosmann TR. Alloreactive murine CD8+ T cell clones secrete Th1 pattern of cytokines. *J Immunol* 1990; **144**: 1744–1752.
6 Salgame P, Abrams JS, Clayberger C, Goldstein H, Convitt J, Modlin RL, Bloom BR. Differing lymphokine profiles and functional subsets of human CD4 and CD8 T cell clones. *Science* 1991; **254**: 279–281.
7 Romagnani S. Induction of Th1 and Th2 response: a key role for the 'natural' immune response? *Immunol Today* 1992; **13**: 379–381.
8 Romagnani S. Lymphokine production by human T cells in disease states. *Ann Rev Immunol* 1994; **12**: 227–257.
9 Del Prete GF, De Carli M, Ricci M, Romagnani S. Helper activity for immunoglobulin synthesis of Th1 and Th2 is limited by their cytolytic capacity. *J Exp Med* 1991; **74**: 809–814.
10 Swain SL. Regulation of the development of distinct subsets of CD4+ T cells. *Immunol Res* 1991; **142**: 14–18.
11 Gajewski TF, Fitch FW. Differential activation of murine Th1 and Th2 clones. *Immunol Res* 1991; **142**: 19–22.
12 Parronchi P, Macchia D, Piccinni M-P, Biswas P, Simonelli C, Maggi E, Ricci M, Ansari AA, Romagnani, S. Allergen- and bacterial antigen-specific T-cell clones established from atopic donors show a different profile of cytokine production. *Proc Natl Acad Sci USA* 1991; **88**: 4538–4542.
13 Romagnani S. Regulation and deregulation of human IgE synthesis. *Immunol Today* 1990; **11**: 316–321.
14 Maggi E, Biswas P, Del Prete G-F, Parronchi P, Macchia D, Simonelli C, Emmi L, De Carli M, Tiri A, Ricci M, Romagnani S. Accumulation of Th2-like helper T cells in the conjunctiva of patients with vernal conjunctivitis. *J Immunol* 1991; **146**: 1169–1174.
15 Kay AB, Ying S, Varney V *et al*. Messenger RNA expression of the cytokine gene cluster, interleukin (IL)-3, IL-4, IL-5, and granulocyte/macrophage colony-stimulating factor, in allergen-induced late-phase cutaneous reactions in atopic subjects. *J Exp Med* 1991; **173**: 775–778.
16 Hamid Q, Azzawi M, Ying S, Moqbel R, Wardlaw AJ, Corrigan CJ, Bradley B, Durham SR, Collins JV, Jeffery PK, Quint DJ, Kay AB. Expression of mRNA for interleukin-5 in mucosal bronchial biopsies from asthma. *J Clin Invest* 1991; **87**: 1541–1546.
17 Robinson DS, Hamid Q, Ying S, Tsicopoulos A, Barkans J, Bentley AM, Corrigan C, Durham SR, Kay AB. Predominant Th2-like bronchoalveolar T-lymphocyte population in atopic asthma. *N Engl J Med* 1992; **326**: 298–304.
18 Del Prete G-F, De Carli M, Maestrelli P, Ricci M, Fabbri L, Romagnani S. Allergen exposure induces the activation of allergen-specific Th2 cells in the airway mucosa of patients with allergic respiratory disorders. *Eur J Immunol* 1993; **23**: 1445–1449.
19 Smith CA, Gruss H-J, Davis T, Anderson D, Farrah T, Baker E, Sutherland GR, Brannan CI, Copeland NG, Jenkins NA, Grabstein KH, Gliniak B, McAlister B, Fanslow W, Alderson M, Falk B, Gimpel S, Gillis S, Din WS, Goodwin RG, Armitage RJ. CD30 antigen, a marker for Hodgkin's lymphoma, is a receptor whose ligand defines an emerging family of cytokines with homology to TNF. *Cell* 1993; **73**: 1349–1360.
20 Del Prete GF, De Carli M, Almerigogna F, Daniel CK, D'Elios MM, Zancuoghi G, Pizzolo G, Romagnani S. Preferential expression of CD30 by human CD4+ T cells

producing Th2-type cytokines. *FASEB J* 1995; **9**: 81–86.
21 Varney VA, Hamid Q, Gaga M, Ying S, Jacobson M, Frew AJ, Kay AB, Durham SR. Influence of grass pollen immunotherapy on cellular infiltration and cytokine mRNA expression during allergen-induced late-phase cutaneous responses. *J Clin Invest* 1993; **92**: 644–651.
22 Secrist H, Chelen CJ, Wen Y, Marshall JD, Umetsu DT. Allergen immunotherapy decreases interleukin 4 production in CD4+ T cells from allergic individuals. *J Exp Med* 1993; **178**: 2123–2130.
23 Hsieh CS, Heimberger AB, Gold JS, O'Garra A, Murphy KH. Differential regulation of T helper phenotype development by interleukin 4 and 10 in an alpha beta T-cell-receptor transgenic system. *Proc Natl Acad Sci USA* 1992; **89**: 6065.
24 Reiner SL, Wang Z-E, Hatam F, Scott P, Locksley RM. Th1 and Th2 cell antigen receptors in experimental Leishmaniasis. *Science* 1993; **259**: 1457–1460.
25 Coffman RL, Chatelain R, Leal LMCC, Varkila K. *Leishmania major* infection in mice: a model system for the study of CD4+ T-cell subset differentiation. *Res Immunol* 1991; **142**: 36–39.
26 Lack G, Renz H, Saloga J, Bradley KL, Loader J, Leung DYM, Larsen G, Gelfand WE. Nebulized but not parenteral IFN-γ decreases IgE production and normalizes airways function in a murine model of allergen sensitization. *J Immunol* 1994; **152**: 2546–2554.
27 Marsh DG, Neely JD, Breazeale DR, Ghosh B, Freidhoff LR, Ehrlich-Kautzky E, Schou C, Krishnaswamy G, Beaty TH. Linkage analysis of IL-4 and other chromosome 5q31.1 markers and total serum immunoglobulin E concentrations. *Science* 1994; **264**: 1152–1156.
28 Murphy KM, Murphy TL, Gold JS, Szabo SJ. Current understanding of IL-4 gene regulation in T cells. *Res Immunol* 1993; **144**: 575–578.
29 Manetti R, Parronchi P, Giudizi M-G, Piccinni M-P, Maggi E, Trinchieri G, Romagnani S. Natural killer cell stimulatory factor (Interleukin 12) induces T helper type 1 (Th1)-specific immune responses and inhibits the development of IL-4-producing Th cells. *J Exp Med* 1993; **177**: 1199–1204.
30 Hsieh C-S, Macatonia SE, Tripp CS, Wolf SF, O'Garra A, Murphy KM. Development of Th1 CD4+ T cells through IL-12 produced by *Listeria*-induced macrophages. *Science* 1993; **260**: 547–549.
31 Schon-Hegrad MA, Oliver J, McMenamin PG, Holt PG. Studies on the density, distribution and surface phenotype of intraepithelial Class II MHC (Ia) antigen-bearing dendritic cells in the conductive airways. *J Exp Med* 1991; **173**: 1345–1356.
32 Renz H, Saloga J, Bradley KL, Loader JE, Greenstein JL, Larsen G, Gelfand EW. Specific Vβ T cell subsets mediate the immediate hypersensitivity response to ragweed allergen. *J Immunol* 1993; **151**: 1907–1917.
33 Daynes RA, Meikle AW, Araneo BA. Locally active steroid hormones may facilitate compartmentalization of immunity by regulating the types of lymphokines produced by helper T cells. *Res Immunol* 1991; **142**: 40–44.
34 Kemeny DM, Diaz-Sanchez D. The role of CD8+ T cells in the regulation of IgE. *Clin Exp Allergy* 1993; **23**: 466–470.
35 Maggi E, Giudizi MG, Biagiotti R, Annunziato F, Manetti R, Piccinni M-P, Parronchi P, Sampognaro S, Giannarini L, Zuccati G, Romagnani S. Th2-like CD8+ T cells showing B cell helper function and reduced cytolytic activity in human immunodeficiency virus type 1 infection. *J Exp Med* 1994; **180**: 489–495.
36 Rook GAW, Hernandez-Pando R, Lightman SL. Hormones, peripherally activated prohormones and regulation of the Th1/Th2 balance. *Immunol Today* 1994; **15**: 301–303.
37 Piccinni M-P, Giudizi M-G, Biagiotti R, Annunziato F, Manetti R, Giannarini L,

Parronchi P, Sampognaro S, Maggi E, Romagnani S. Progesterone favors the development of human T Helper (Th) cells producing Th2-type cytokines and promotes both IL-4 production and membrane CD30 expression in established Th1 clones. *J Immunol* 1995; **155**: 128–133.

38 Wegmann TG, Lin H, Guilberg L, Mosmann TR. Bidirectional cytokine interactions in the maternal-fetal relationship: is successful pregnancy a Th2 phenomenon? *Immunol Today* 1993; **14**: 353–356.

39 Williams ME, Chang TL, Burke SK, Lichtman AH, Abbas AK. Activation of functionally distinct subsets of CD4+ T lymphocytes. *Res Immunol* 1991; **142**: 23–27.

40 Manetti R, Barak V, Piccinni M-P, Sampognaro S, Parronchi P, Maggi E, Dinarello CA, Romagnani S. Interleukin 1 favors the *in vitro* development of type 2 helper (Th2) human T cell clones. *Res Immunol* 1994; **145**: 93–100.

41 Swain SL. IL-4 dictates T-cell differentiation. *Res Immunol* 1993; **144**: 616–620.

42 Maggi E, Parronchi P, Manetti R, Simonelli C, Piccinni M-P, Santoni Rugiu F, De Carli M, Ricci M, Romagnani S. Reciprocal regulatory role of IFN-γ and IL-4 on the *in vitro* development of human Th1 and Th2 clones. *J Immunol* 1992; **148**: 2142–2148.

43 Seder RA, Paul WE, Davis MM, Fazekas de St Groth B. The presence of interleukin 4 during *in vitro* priming determines the lymphocyte-producing potential of CD4+ T cells from T cell receptor transgenic mice. *J Exp Med* 1992; **176**: 1091–1098.

44 Kopf M, Le Gros G, Bachmann M, Lamers MC, Bluthmann H, Kohler G. Disruption of the murine IL-4 gene blocks Th2 cytokine responses. *Nature* 1993; **362**: 245–248.

45 Yashimoto T, Paul WE. CD4^{pos}, NK1.1^{pos} T cells promptly produce interleukin 4 in response to *in vivo* challenge with anti-CD3. *J Exp Med* 1994; **179**: 1285–1295.

46 Zlotnik A, Bean AGD. Production of IL-4 by non-Th2-cell subsets: possible role of CD4-CD8-$\alpha\beta$TCR+ and CD4 subset T cells in T helper subset regulation. *Res Immunol* 1993; **144**: 608–609.

47 Bradding P, Feather IH, Howarth PH, Mueller R, Roberts JA, Britten K, Bews JPA, Hunt TC, Okayama Y, Heusser CH, Bullock GR, Church MK, Holgate ST. Interleukin 4 is localized and released by human mast cells. *J Exp Med* 1992; **176**: 1381–1386.

48 Brunner T, Heusser CH, Dahinden CA. Human peripheral blood basophils primed by interleukin 3 (IL-3) produce IL-4 in response to immunoglobulin E receptor stimulation. *J Exp Med* 1993; **177**: 605–611.

49 Wershil BK, Theodos CM, Galli SJ, Titus RG. Mast cells augment lesion size and persistence during experimental *Leishmania major* infection in the mouse. *J Immunol* 1994; **152**: 4563–4571.

50 Finkelman FD, Urban JF. Cytokines: making the right choice. *Parasitol Today* 1992; **8**: 311–314.

51 McMenamin C, Holt PG. The natural immune response to inhaled soluble protein antigens involves major histocompatibility complex (MHC) Class I-restricted CD8+ T cell-mediated but not MHC Class-II-restricted CD4+ T cell-dependent immune deviation resulting in selective suppression of immunoglobulin E production. *J Exp Med* 1993; **178**: 889–899.

52 Manetti R, Annunziato F, Tomasévic LJ, Giannó V, Parronchi P, Romagnani S, Maggi E. Polyinosinic acid: polycitidylic acid (poly I:C) promotes T helper type 1 (Th1)-specific immune responses by stimulating macrophage production of interferon (IFN)-α and interleukin (IL)-12. *Eur J Immunol* 1995; **25**: 2656–2660.

53 Rotteveel FTM, Kokkelink I, van Lier RAW, Kuenen B, Meager A, Miedema F, Lucas CJ. Clonal analysis of functional distinct human CD4+ T cell subsets. *J Exp Med* 1988; **168**: 1659–1665.

54 Parronchi P, De Carli M, Piccinni MP, Macchia D, Maggi E, Del Prete G-F,

Romagnani S. IL-4 and IFNs exert opposite regulatory effects on the development of cytolytic potential by Th1 or Th2 human T cell clones. *J Immunol* 1992; **149**: 2977–2983.

55 Driscoll J, Brown MG, Monaco JJ. MHC-linked LMP gene products specifically alter peptidase activities of the proteosome. *Nature* 1993; **365**: 262–263.

56 Gaczynska M, Rock KL, Goldberg AL. Gamma-interferon and expression of MHC genes regulate peptide hydrolysis by proteosomes. *Nature* 1993; **365**: 264–266.

57 Howard JC. Restrictions on the use of antigenic peptides by the immune system. *Proc Natl Acad Sci USA* 1993; **90**: 3777–3782.

58 Pfeiffer C, Stein J, Southwood S, Ketelaar H, Sette A, Bottomly K. Peptide ligands can control CD4 T lymphocyte differentiation *in vivo*. *J Exp Med* 1995; **181**: 1569–1574.

59 Yssel H, Fasler S, Lamb J, De Vries J. Induction of non-responsiveness in human allergen-specific type 2 helper cells. *Curr Opin Immunol* 1994; **6**: 847–852.

60 Manetti R, Gerosa F, Giudizi MG, Biagiotti R, Parronchi P, Piccinni MP, Sampognaro S, Maggi E, Romagnani S, Trinchieri G. Interleukin 12 induces stable priming for interferon-γ (IFN-γ) production during differentiation of human T helper (Th) cells and transient IFN-γ production in established Th2 cells clones. *J Exp Med* 1994; **179**: 1273–1283.

Index

Note: Page numbers in *italic* refer to figures and/or tables

Compiled by Caroline Sheard

ASHISH JOSHI

LITIGATING

EVALUATING AND PRESENTING

PARENTAL

AN EFFECTIVE CASE IN COURT

ALIENATION

AMERICANBARASSOCIATION
Family Law Section

Cover design by Kelly Book/ABA Design

Printed in the United States of America.

25 24 5

Library of Congress Cataloging-in-Publication Data

Names: Joshi, Ashish, editor.
Title: Litigating parental alienation : evaluating and presenting an effective case in court / [edited by] Ashish Joshi.
Description: Chicago : American Bar Association, 2021. | Includes bibliographical references and index. | Summary: "How to evaluate and present an effective case in family court"— Provided by publisher.
Identifiers: LCCN 2021009601 (print) | LCCN 2021009602 (ebook) | ISBN 9781641058285 (paperback) | ISBN 9781641058292 (ebook)
Subjects: LCSH: Parent and child (Law)—United States. | Guardians ad litem—United States. | Parental alienation syndrome—United States. | Parental alienation syndrome.
Classification: LCC KF540 .L58 2021 (print) | LCC KF540 (ebook) | DDC 346.7301/7—dc23
LC record available at https://lccn.loc.gov/2021009601
LC ebook record available at https://lccn.loc.gov/2021009602

For Payal, of course

CONTENTS

FOREWORD

Family law judges have hard jobs. One of their most difficult tasks is making custodial determinations, physical and legal. The children's best interests drive those custodial decisions. And best interests are determined by weighing a set of factors the legislature identifies.

The system is often antagonistic. And in many cases, both parents have the same goals—to spend as much time with their children as possible. That means convincing a judge that the child's best interests are better served with one parent, not the other. This can, understandably, get messy.

As the Chief Justice of the Michigan Supreme Court, I oversee the state's court system, including its family courts. In our courts, we presume that it is in a child's best interest to have a strong relationship with both parents. In fact, one of the best interest factors requires these judges to consider the willingness and ability of each of the parties to facilitate and encourage a close and continuing parent-child relationship with the other parent. Courts and the parents who appear before them should all be working to promote positive relationships between children and each of their parents.

But parental alienation poses a serious obstacle to this goal.

Parental alienation is a complex and serious issue that confronts family law judges, practitioners, and court-involved professionals. The key to parental alienation is that it is without justification—not that it is intentional. It is easy to see how unintentional alienation may occur; parents who love their children and zealously want to be their primary caregiver may be inclined to act and speak about the other parent derogatorily to try to influence the children's parenting preference. This is particularly true when the child is old enough to have his or her preference considered by the court in assessing the child's best interests.

But conduct that causes a parent to alienate their child with no objectively reasonable justification cannot be condoned by the courts. Regardless of whether it presents as a diagnosable syndrome in children, our courts can (and should) focus on addressing and curtailing alienating behaviors by parents. Research shows that the consequences of parental alienation can be serious and long-lasting. Early fact-finding and intervention, therefore, is key to halting the alienating behaviors, preventing further harm, and ensuring that children do not grow up carrying views of their parent that are not justified by reality. Doing so not only serves the targeted parent and the children involved, but can also help the alienating parent, who may be engaging in these behaviors unintentionally and without realizing the harm that may be caused.

Given the high-stakes nature of litigating this issue—where custody decisions, the allocation of parenting time, and the future of a healthy parent-child relationship are at stake—it is crucial that attorneys who take on these cases ensure that they are competent and knowledgeable about the law and science of parental alienation. Better-informed practitioners provide stronger advocacy, which allows our courts to make better decisions and produce more just outcomes. When armed with social science, a plan to introduce expert testimony, and an understanding of how other courts have dealt with parental alienation in custodial disputes, family law attorneys are better equipped to inform and aid family court judges with difficult, fact-intensive decisions. Of primary importance is helping to explain, in cases where a child actively rejects one parent, what causes such rejection. Is the rejection driven by justified estrangement, which can look a lot like alienation to the unfamiliar observer, or parental alienation?

Well-informed practitioners can also help the courts craft and implement the appropriate interventions in parental alienation cases, which are key to supporting children's well-being and fostering strong parent-child relationships. Our courts are in a unique position to impact thousands of parent-child relationships. The practitioners who appear before them have a similarly unique responsibility to educate themselves about parental alienation and to familiarize themselves with the tools to competently litigate this delicate and complex area of interpersonal relationships. And that's why resources like this book are so important.

In this book, Ashish Joshi has organized an excellent guide for practitioners that offers a comprehensive overview of the parental alienation phenomenon. He synthesizes the background and science of parental alienation while also taking care to point out the distracting noise and misinformation that makes this topic even more complicated and has the potential to confuse the courts. This book provides practical tips for family law attorneys, from investigating allegations of parental alienation and domestic violence to admitting expert testimony to aid the court in its fact-finding. Still, the main focus is the law, examining the contexts in which this issue comes up, how courts address the subject across the states and worldwide, the role of a guardian ad litem, and the legal interventions available to courts. It is a resource that will make practitioners and court professionals better.

Behaviors that unjustifiably alienate a child from a parent, whether intentional or not, are damaging. They harm children and parents alike. And they make family law judges' work exceptionally difficult to get right. When practitioners know more about the substance of parental alienation, they put themselves in the best position to advocate for their clients and to put the courts in the best position to reach the right results. I am grateful to those—including you, reader—who carry on the important work of advancing the best interests of children and families in promoting, whenever possible, strong relationships between parents and their children.

Bridget Mary McCormack
Michigan Supreme Court Chief Justice

AUTHOR BIO

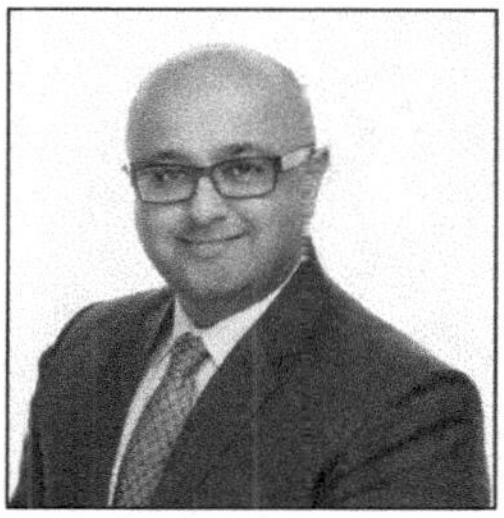

Ashish Joshi is the owner of the law firm, Joshi: Attorneys + Counselors. Mr. Joshi's work focuses on complex family law matters including severe parental alienation, pathological child enmeshment, child abuse, and international child kidnapping. Mr. Joshi has counseled or represented clients in state and federal courts across the United States and internationally, including in India, United Kingdom, Canada, Luxembourg, Hong Kong, British Virgin Islands, Japan, and China. Mr. Joshi has been admitted to the Bar of the Supreme Court of the United States, State Bars of New York, Michigan, District of Columbia, and Gujarat, India.

Mr. Joshi has published a number of articles and co-authored books on parental alienation and child abuse. He serves as a senior editor for *Litigation*, the journal of the American Bar Association's Section of Litigation, on the Advisory Board for *Champion*, the journal published by the National Association of Criminal Defense Lawyers, and on the board of directors of the Parental Alienation Study Group.

INTRODUCTION

I am a trial lawyer. Like other trial lawyers, I am the ultimate generalist. While my practice overwhelmingly focuses on litigating and trying complex cases involving parental alienation in American family courts and internationally, I, ultimately, am a generalist. I have no formal education or training in medicine, psychology, social work or other related disciplines. But as Ed Zschau, the polymath professor at Princeton, once said, I learn the most the fastest when I don't know what I'm doing. In order to present a case involving parental alienation, I first had to educate myself on the concept of alienation, the empirical science supporting the theory, the Five-Factor Model that's used to diagnose parental alienation, the effective legal and mental health interventions. That was the easy part. Then came the hard part: Educating the judges and persuading them to intervene in cases involving parental alienation.

Judges too are generalists, almost all of them. Like trial lawyers, judges have to be able to solve legal problems that can touch on almost anything. And that is why judges do not depend upon their own knowledge of everything, but on how to assess and evaluate the arguments of the lawyers. It's the lawyers who have to understand. It's the lawyers who have to marshall the evidence that's needed to persuade and empower a judge to do the right thing. A good trial lawyer can teach anything. She will break it into parts. She will explain it so a judge (or a jury) could understand it. And she will do it in a manner that speaks to common sense, devoid of dogma or ideology. This book is meant for the lawyers—lawyers who have to educate themselves about parental alienation, break it down into parts, master the topic, and then explain it to judges. So, when judges say, to quote Dickens, "Barkis is willing," the lawyers are able to respond, "We'll help."

I owe debt and gratitude to the experts who have helped me understand the theory of parental alienation and have been unfailingly generous with their time and knowledge to answer my questions. First and foremost, I acknowledge my mentor and former law partner, Demosthenes Lorandos, Ph.D., J.D., who got me interested in this area of practice and encouraged me in my efforts. To him I owe an immense debt of gratitude and I thank him for all that he has done. I also wish to acknowledge the work and support of William Bernet, M.D., Richard Warshak, Ph.D., Amy J. L. Baker, Ph.D., Steven G. Miller, M.D., and Linda Gottlieb LMFT, LCSW-R. I am a dwarf standing on the shoulders of these and other giants who have significantly contributed to the field of parental alienation. Of course, any errors or omissions in this book are mine alone and should not be attributed to these scholars or experts.

A few words about the legal cases that I have cited and referred to in this book. Family law is the domain of state law and jurisdictions vary in their approach towards parental alienation. A New York family court's orientation towards parental alienation may differ, at times, from that of California's. Even within a state, a court in the urban area that has significantly more experience in handling cases involving mental health issues may take a different approach than a rural court, which may not have had similar opportunities. A domestic relations judge in Chicago, for instance, may be more familiar with the theory of parental alienation and the effective interventions that are required to remediate it than a judge who presides over a domestic relations docket in a rural Illinois county. The cases cited in this book are not cited for their precedential, binding value— in fact, there may be none since very few cases involving parental alienation have been adjudicated by state supreme courts. So why cite them? For two reasons.

First, it is important for a lawyer representing a targeted parent (a parent who is the target of the alienating parent's behaviors) to understand that regardless of the jurisdiction, the underlying behaviors of an alienating parent and the symptoms of an alienated child remain the same. Whether one is a family court practitioner in Alaska or Arizona, when confronted with cases involving parental alienation, one will find a similar set of behaviors, facts, and circumstances. It is important to note that some cases do not actually use the term "parental alienation" or derivations thereof. But they are still useful and illustrative of the tactics employed by alienating parents. While the diagnosis of parental alienation is limited to children who meet the criteria of the Five-Factor Model, many high-conflict cases have evidence of alienating behaviors that may have mild to severe effect on the children. The judicial opinions written by trial and appellate courts of such cases can be instructive as they may illustrate how judges, lawyers, parties, and other court-appointed or court-involved professionals manage, navigate, confront, and put an end to these alienating behaviors. I have found it helpful to read the judicial decisions from various courts around the country (and internationally). It is always interesting to me to see how a lawyer presented the case in one particular jurisdiction, what theories together with evidence were presented to the court, how the presiding judge reacted to it, what, if any, was the legal intervention, and finally, in case of an appeal, whether the decision was sustained at an appellate level.

Second, while a judicial opinion from a foreign jurisdiction may not have precedential value, it may still end up having significant educational value and might empower a judge in another jurisdiction. As the Supreme Court Justice Stephen G. Breyer explained in his book, *The Court and the World*, there's something to be said about learning from foreign sources: "[I]f someone with a job roughly like my own, facing a legal problem roughly like the one confronting me, interpreting a document that resembles the one I look to, has written a legal opinion about a similar matter, why not read what that judge has said? I might learn from it, whether or not I end up agreeing with it." Breyer, S., *The Court and the World*, 240 (Knopf, 2015). When a lawyer before a Michigan family court is trying to persuade the court to order a specialized program on reunifying the alienated child with the targeted parent, it may be helpful to show to the court what a Maryland judge did when faced with a similar situation. The wheel doesn't need to be invented every time. Perhaps the Michigan judge may agree with the Maryland judge's decision or reasoning; perhaps not. But a lawyer can certainly try and use the similarities between the two cases to put forward a persuasive argument to empower a judge who otherwise might not feel inclined to blaze a new trail in ordering effective mental health interventions to remediate alienation.

A review of judicial decisions from the courts around the country demonstrate that parental alienation is widely acknowledged and used as a concept by courts and practitioners. But there is push back. Some opponents of the concept of parental alienation are detractors who will stoop to any level and will turn a blind eye to emerging research, empirical studies, and judicial decisions that are increasingly in support of the concept of parental alienation. For them, there is no such thing as parental alienation and despite significant evidence to the contrary, it doesn't exist. Some are concerned about the weaponization of the theory of parental alienation and how it is misused against abused women as a legal strategy to win custody disputes. Others cherry pick the research findings or conflate different phenomena. Together these opponents of the concept of parental alienation create smokescreens and confuse the field by conflating theories, draw sweeping contradictory conclusions about the parental alienation theory, present strawman arguments, and put forward ideologies masquerading as science. The result is confusion, misinformation, fallacies, myths, and *woozles*—unsupported and misleading claims that are widely disseminated and often repeated. Hopefully, this book will help the practitioners to separate the wheat from the chaff.

As this book will demonstrate, there is no doubt that parental alienation exists and that American courts have acknowledged the concept. At the same time, it should be acknowledged that the theory of parental alienation is, on occasions, misused. There are cases where the concept of alienation has been used to counter evidence of abusive behaviors and justified rejection of an abusive parent by the child victim. However, this is true of any theory or phenomenon. In the area of domestic violence, courts have seen and called out false or orchestrated allegations of "abuse." We don't discredit the concept of domestic violence or intimate partner violence due to some rogue actors misusing or abusing the theory to suit their nefarious agenda. To do so would be to throw the baby out with the bathwater. The same could be said of the concept of parental alienation. In fact, it is ironic that the current struggle to legitimize the concept of parental alienation and to give it a place that it deserves in social science research is reminiscent of the struggle, decades ago, made by the advocates against domestic violence and child abuse.

Litigating cases involving parental alienation is tough. It is gut wrenching to see a parent use their child as a pawn and weapon to hurt the other parent. Having a practice that is devoted to litigating these cases, day in and day out, in courts around the country and internationally could easily result in burnout. I am fortunate to have support of a team of professionals without whom my work (and the writing of this book) would not have been possible. I am thankful to my colleague and associate, Andrew Bossory and research assistants, Laura Tobon, Dana VanKleeck, and Elle Murphree.

I acknowledge and am grateful for the help, encouragement, patience, and camaraderie of my wife, Payal and the support of our two children, Arya and Arjun. Finally, I am thankful for the unconditional love and support of my parents, Kishori and Shailesh, who have always inspired me to give any endeavor my best.

Ashish Joshi
Ann Arbor, November 30, 2020

CHAPTER 1

Parental Alienation: An Introduction

A divorce aspires for a healthy closure of a marriage. Where the couple has had children together, a post-divorce parent-child relationship continues to exist and necessitates that the parents, despite their divorce, continue to co-parent the child. At the healthiest end of this spectrum, a child has positive relationships with both parents and desires time with each of his or her parents. The majority of post-divorce children fit into this category. At the other end of this spectrum is an unhealthy, toxic, and often pathological situation wherein a child rejects a parent. Where the rejection is unequivocal, strident, without guilt or ambivalence, absolute and without justification, we encounter the phenomenon known as "parental alienation."

More often than not, the first signs of the corrosive legacy of parental alienation are contact refusal or visitation interference. "The children refuse to see their mother!" Or in another case, "they refuse to leave their mother's house and get in the car when the father shows up for his parenting time." In yet another case: "I am 16 years old and no judge is going to tell me whether or not I want to see my father." Such scenarios confound and frustrate the judges, lawyers, guardians *ad litem*, child representatives, child custody evaluators, parenting coordinators, child therapists, mediators, and last but not the least, rejected parents who are caught up in the intricate web of family court litigation dynamic. Court professionals often report being stymied by children's such refusals to cooperate and abide by the court-ordered parenting time schedules.[1]

1. Warshak, R. (2015). Parental alienation: Overview, management, intervention, and practice tips, *Journal of the American Academy of Matrimonial Lawyers*, 28, 181–182.

For frustrated litigants—fathers, mothers, grandparents—who are caught up in the tentacles of the alienation monster and attempt to seek redress from the family court system, the words of the actor Alec Baldwin ring true: "to be pulled into the American family law system in most states is like being tied to the back of a pickup truck and dragged down a gravel road late at night. No one can hear your cries and complaints, and it is not over until they say it is over."[2]

Parental Alienation: Old Wine in a New Bottle

Parental alienation is not a new phenomenon; the mental condition has been described in the legal cases since the early 19th century and in the scientific literature since the 1940s.[3] The concept of parental alienation has been acknowledged and addressed by English-speaking courts for the last two hundred years. Family law judges, attorneys, guardians *ad litem*, and mental health professionals routinely deal with cases involving parental alienation, even though they may not be aware of the condition or be familiar with the term, its origin, or its implications. Which begets the question: *What is parental alienation?*

Scientists and mental health experts have defined the condition known as parental alienation in several different ways. One of the most widely accepted definitions explains it as a "mental condition in which a child—usually one whose parents are engaged in a high-conflict separation or divorce—allies himself or herself strongly with an alienating parent and rejects a relationship with the 'target' parent without legitimate justification."[4]

When we peel the layers of this definition, three key features of the phenomenon come to light. First, parental alienation can be conceptualized as a mental condition present in the *child*, i.e., the child has a distorted or false belief that the rejected or disfavored parent is "evil," "dangerous," or somehow unworthy of love or affection. Second, the child's rejection of the alienated or target parent is *without legitimate justification*. And this is an important distinction: If there is a documented history of the rejected parent being abusive or severely neglectful, the child's rejection of that parent could be legitimate, and, if so, it would not be a case of parental alienation. Third, it is important to note that the rejected parent is not expected to be a "perfect" parent and may even have contributed to the child's dislike or hatred of him or her. More often

2. Baldwin, A. (2008). *A Promise to Ourselves*, St. Martin's, 3.

3. *See, e.g.*, "*Westmeath v. Westmeath*: The Wars Between the Westmeaths, 1812–1857," in Stone, L. (1993). *Broken Lives: Separation and Divorce in England, 1660–1857*, 284; Levy, D. M. (1943). *Maternal Overprotection*, Columbia University Press, 153.

4. Lorandos, D., Bernet, W., & Sauber, R. (2013). Overview of parental alienation. In Lorandos, D., Bernet, W., & Sauber, R. (Eds.), *Parental Alienation: The Handbook for Mental Health and Legal Professionals*, Charles C. Thomas, 5.

than not, a rejected parent reacts to the alienation dynamic in frustration, even anger. But such *reaction* to the sabotaging and breakdown of the parent-child relationship should not be confused with its *causation* and the essential feature of parental alienation remains that the child's rejection of the alienated parent is far out of proportion to anything that parent has done.[5]

Aside from the experts, family courts too have defined the phenomenon of parental alienation and the courts' definitions encapsulate the key features of the condition as defined by the mental health professionals.

Perhaps the most succinct but comprehensive summary of North American case law on parental alienation (PA) is to be found in the book, *Parental Alienation—The Handbook for Mental Health and Legal Professionals* (2013). In his chapter summarizing North American law on PA "distilled from 3,000 PA cases in the United States and Canada," attorney-psychologist Demosthenes Lorandos wrote:

> The purpose for building this chapter was twofold: *First,* to give the reader representative examples of parental alienation (PA) cases from the United States and Canada . . . .
>
> *Second,* to provide brief but accurate descriptions of many alienation cases across a twenty-five-year period to illustrate that PA deniers do not seem to know the data . . . . Like global warming deniers and creationists, the PA deniers thrive in a post-fact/Fox News world.[6]

Distilling thousands of U.S. and Canadian courts' decisions, Dr. Lorandos wrote about scores of cases over a twenty-five-year period where the North American courts not only acknowledged parental alienation but decisively intervened to provide appropriate mental health and legal interventions.[7] Having updated his research and findings, Dr. Lorandos published his 2020 chapter, "Parental Alienation in U.S. Courts, 1985 to 2018," in the book *Parental Alienation—Science and Law.*[8] He found thousands of cases all over the United States where the term "parental alienation" or "alienation" or a variant thereof was discussed. On restricting the query to focus on cases where an independent evaluating expert testified on the subject of parental alienation (whether or not the expert found parental alienation), or where the court found on any basis that there was parental alienation (whether or not there was expert testi-

5. Bernet, W. (2020). Introduction to parental alienation. In Lorandos, D., & Bernet, W. (Eds.), *Parental Alienation: Science and Law,* Charles C. Thomas, 1–2.

6. Lorandos, D. (2013). Parental alienation and North American law. In Lorandos, D., Bernet, W., & Sauber, R. (Eds.), *Parental Alienation: The Handbook for Mental Health and Legal Professionals,* Charles C. Thomas, 348.

7. Lorandos, D., Bernet, W., & Sauber, R.. (2013). Overview of parental alienation. In Lorandos, D., Bernet, W., & Sauber, R. (Eds.), *Parental Alienation: The Handbook for Mental Health and Legal Professionals,* Charles C. Thomas, 5.

8. Lorandos, D., & Bernet, W. (Eds.) (2020). *Parental Alienation: Science and Law,* Charles C. Thomas.

mony), Dr. Lorandos and his team identified 1,181 cases where the construct of parental alienation was determined to be material, probative, relevant, admissible, and discussed.[9] For a practitioner who is skeptical of American family courts' acceptance of the phenomenon of parental alienation, the entire list of the 1,181 cases, which feature recognition of parental alienation by both trial courts and appellate courts, is found in the appendix of the book, *Parental Alienation—Science and Law.*

In an attempt to simplify the issues, eschew esoteric terminology, and perhaps inject common sense in dealing with the practical matters at hand, family court judges have acknowledged that "[p]arental alienation is the flipside of a concept long used by the . . . courts to decide disputed custody matters; i.e., the 'willingness to foster a relationship between the child and [the opposite] parent.'"[10] In analyzing this bedrock concept of American custody law, courts have generally focused on "interference" by one parent in the other parent's relationship with the children in a manner inconsistent with their best interests.[11] In parental alienation cases, conduct by a parent is transformed, usually through expert testimony, from "interference" to more intentional, egregious, and far more damaging "alienation" behavior.[12]

While the detractors continue to manufacture controversy over the phenomenon of parental alienation—especially regarding the Parental Alienation Syndrome (PAS)[13]—American courts have unhesitatingly defined the condition and intervene where they have found evidence of alienating behaviors. For instance, in *Meadows v. Meadows,* the Michigan Court of Appeals defined parental alienation as "[t]he process of one parent trying to undermine and destroy to varying degrees the relationship that the child has with the other parent."[14] It is important to note that the *Meadows* court focused more on the "process"—the alienating behaviors through which the alienating parent attempts to "undermine and destroy" the relationship that the child has with the target parent.

On the other hand, in *McClain v. McClain,* the Tennessee Court of Appeals, in defining parental alienation, has focused on the mental condition of the child and has defined the phenomenon as "primarily a description of the psychological condition of [a] child."[15] Acknowledging the essential feature of parental alienation that the mental health professionals agree on, the *McClain*

9. Lorandos, D. (2020). Parental alienation in U.S. courts, 1985 to 2018. In Lorandos, D., & Bernet, W. (Eds.), *Parental Alienation: Science and Law,* Charles C. Thomas, 370–371.

10. J.F. v. D.F., 61 Misc.3d 1226(A), 2018 N.Y. Slip Op. 51829(U)), 2018 WL 6530810, at *3, n. 4. (citing Matter of Sweeney v. Daub-Stearns, 2018 NY App.Div.Lexis 7923 (3d Dept 2018)).

11. Musachio v. Musachio, 137 AD3d 881 (2d Dept 2016).

12. J.F. v. D.F., *supra.*

13. *See, e.g.,* Gillespie v. Gillespie, No. 1849, 2016 WL 1622890, at *12 (Frienman, J. concurring).

14. Meadows v. Meadows/Henderson, 2010 WL 3814352 (Mich.App.) (Unpublished).

15. McClain v. McClain, 539 S.W.3d 170, 182 (2017).

court further opined: "The essential feature of parental alienation is that a child . . . allies himself or herself strongly with one parent (the preferred parent) and rejects a relationship with the other parent (the alienated parent) without legitimate justification."[16]

As a New York trial judge concluded: "[T]here is no doubt that parental alienation exists."[17] In this 2018 decision, the New York court analyzed the concept of parental alienation and offered a *legal* definition of the phenomenon. Wrestling with the somewhat amorphous concept of "unjustified behavior" of an alienating parent, the judge struggled for a "more demanding definition of parental alienation to more explicitly describe the concept of what constitutes 'unjustified behavior.'"[18] Borrowing a chapter from the elements of the tort of Intentional Infliction of Emotional Distress, the New York court defined the condition to require that "(1) the alleged alienating conduct, without any other legitimate justification, be directed by the favored parent, (2) with the intention of damaging the reputation of the other parent in the children's eyes or which disregards a substantial possibility of causing such, (3) which proximately causes a diminished interest of the children in spending time with the non-favored parent and, (4) in fact, results in the children refusing to spend time with the targeted parent either in person, or via other forms of communication."[19]

In spite of the variations in how the family courts have defined parental alienation, they all seem to agree that that there are certain *behaviors*, which, when manifested by an alienating parent, result in damaging a child's relationship with the other parent. These behaviors need not be intentional; they could be reckless or even inadvertent but still end up causing significant damage to a parent-child relationship. On occasions, family court judges have even witnessed a parent engaging in alienating behaviors in front of their eyes. As a long serving domestic relations judge from Cook County, Illinois,[20] recalled:

> One day in court, a mother was seeking an increase in child support from her former husband. The father testified that his income had declined dramatically. After the case was over, I was riding down the elevator with the mother and the parties' teenage daughter. They did not notice I was there or did not recognize me out of my black robe. The mother was sharing details of the case with the daughter, as I would not let the daughter come into the courtroom. The mother was telling her what a liar and manip-

---

16. *Id.*
17. J.F., *supra*, *8.
18. *Id.*
19. *Id.*
20. Michele Lowrance is a former domestic relations judge in Cook County, Illinois. She has written and presented extensively on the topic of parental alienation and judicial interventions.

ulator her father was, fully expecting the daughter to agree. I doubted this child would ever be able to hear her father's side of the story. Even if the father was lying, I wondered why the mother could not share her frustration with her sister, her neighbor, or even the cashier at the corner store; anyone but the child. I was saddened because I knew that sharing this information with the daughter might forever affect the way the girl viewed her father and ultimately how she viewed men in general. Would they all be liars and manipulators to her? The daughter had no way to defend her trust in her father against this onslaught; she would certainly question it and probably cease to rely on it. Could the mother be sure the daughter would heal from believing her father is manipulative, uncaring, and a liar? I don't believe the mother considered the long-term effects. If she had, would she have intentionally hurt her daughter?[21]

Mental health professionals and experts have used different terms to describe these behaviors.[22] For example, Dr. Stanley Clawar, a sociologist, and Brynne Rivlin, a social worker, used the terms "programming," "brainwashing,"[23] and "indoctrination" when describing the behaviors that cause parental alienation.[24] The authors explained that these behaviors

> hinder the relationship of the child with the other parent due to jealousy, or draw the child closer to the communicating parent due to loneliness or a desire to obtain an ally. These techniques may also be employed to control or distort information the child provides to a lawyer, judge, conciliator, relatives, friends, or others, as in abuse cases.[25]

Dr. Richard Warshak, a clinical professor of psychiatry, has used the term "pathological alienation" that results from such alienating behaviors:

> a disturbance in which children, usually in the context of sharing a parent's negative attitudes, suffer unreasonable aversion to a person or per-

21. Lowrance, M. (2013). A judge's perspective on parental alienation. In Lorandos, D., Bernet, W., & Sauber, R. (Eds.), *Parental Alienation: The Handbook for Mental Health and Legal Professionals*, Charles C. Thomas, 507.

22. See the discussion in Lorandos, D., Bernet, W., & Sauber, R., (2013). Overview of parental alienation. In Lorandos, D., Bernet, W., & Sauber, R. (Eds.), *Parental Alienation: The Handbook for Mental Health and Legal Professionals*, Charles C. Thomas, 8.

23. Jennifer H. v. Paul F., 800 N.Y.S.2d 348, 2004 WL 3131979, at *10 (Suffolk Co., N.Y. Fam. Ct. June 9, 2004).

24. Clawar, S., & Rivlin, B. (1991). *Children Held Hostage: Dealing with Programmed and Brainwashed Children*, American Bar Association Section of Family Law. Also *see* Clawar, S., & Rivlin, B. (2013). *Children Held Hostage: Identifying Brainwashed Children, Presenting a Case, and Crafting Solutions*, Second Edition, ABA.

25. *Id.* at 15.

sons with whom they formerly enjoyed normal relations or with whom they would normally develop affectionate relations.[26]

At times, judges have used terms other than "parental alienation" to criticize the very behaviors underlying the condition but have chosen to call it by another name. For instance, in *Martin v. Martin*, the Nebraska Supreme Court found a custodial parent to have used "passive aggressive techniques" in undercutting the non-custodial parent's relationship with the children.[27] While the words "parental alienation" were not used by the Nebraska court, its detailed discussion of the custodial parent's alienating behaviors and strategies leave little room for doubt that the court was addressing the phenomenon of parental alienation. In the end, the consensus amongst the courts, experts, and mental health professionals appears to be that the phenomenon of parental alienation involves "a child's reluctance or refusal to have a relationship with a parent without a good reason."[28]

As to *how* parental alienation takes place, Dr. Amy J. L. Baker and her colleagues' research describing the Five Factor Model of parental alienation, which is discussed in detail in Chapter 4 of this book, "Presenting a Case of Parental Alienation in Court," is widely used and accepted by mental health professionals.[29] As one of the five factors that need to be carefully evaluated before making a diagnosis of parental alienation, Dr. Baker describes seventeen alienating strategies that are most prevalent in the alienation process. They include badmouthing, limiting contact, confiding in the child, asking the child to spy on the target parent, referring to the target parent by first name, withholding important information from the target parent, and undermining the authority of the target parent. Not all strategies have to be present for alienation to occur. One could have a case of parental alienation, even severe parental alienation, with less than half of the seventeen strategies put into play.

In terms of the severity of the symptoms or behaviors that are manifested in the child, parental alienation can be termed as mild, moderate, or severe.[30] Mild parental alienation "means that the child resists contact with the target parent but enjoys the relationship with that parent once parenting time is underway."[31] Moderate parental alienation "means that the child strongly

26. Warshak, R. (2006). Social science and parental alienation: Examining the disputes and the evidence. In Gardner, R. A., Sauber, S. R., & Lorandos, D. (Eds.), *The International Handbook of Parental Alienation Syndrome: Conceptual, Clinical and Legal Considerations*, Charles C. Thomas, 361.

27. Martin v. Martin, 294 Neb. 106 (2016).

28. Bernet, W., Wamboldt, M., & Narrow, W. (2016). Child affected by parental relationship distress. *Journal of the American Academy of Child & Adolescent Psychiatry*, 55(7), 575.

29. Baker, A., & Fine, P. (2013). Educating divorcing parents: Taking them beyond the high road. In Baker, A., & Sauber, S. (Eds.), *Working with Alienated Children and Families: A Clinical Guidebook*, Routledge Press.

30. Lorandos, D., Bernet, W., & Sauber, R. (2013), *supra*, 23.

31. *Id.*

resists contact and is persistently oppositional during parenting time with the target parent."[32] Severe parental alienation "means that the child persistently and adamantly refuses contact and may hide or run away to avoid being with the target parent."[33]

Regardless of the varying definitions of parental alienation, or even the nomenclature (as discussed *supra*, the phenomenon has been referred to by other names), the consensus amongst the mental health and legal professionals was aptly put forward by the New York Supreme Court as "there is no doubt that parental alienation exists."[34]

Alienation versus Estrangement

Not all cases where a child rejects a parent or refuses to see a parent after separation or divorce are cases of parental alienation. While the common denominator in both parental alienation and parental estrangement is the child's refusal to have a relationship with one of his or her parents, the distinguishing feature of parental alienation is that the child's rejection of the target parent is *without legitimate justification*. If, for example, a rejected parent has a documented history of family violence, abuse or neglect, the child's rejection of that parent could be justified.[35] Most mental health professionals call this legitimate rejection of a parent by a child "estrangement" or "realistic estrangement."

Courts too have distinguished alienation from estrangement. For example, here's how the Tennessee Court of Appeals, in *McClain v. McClain*, differentiated alienation from estrangement:

> Alienation and estrangement . . . are not interchangeable or synonymous concepts. The difference between estrangement and alienation resides in the presence vs absence of a reasonable objective basis for a child's severe and persistent rejection and denigration of a parent. Rejection and denigration of a parent with a reasonable objective basis is estrangement; rejection and denigration without such basis is parental alienation.[36]

It is important to note that the *McClain* court, in its attempt to distinguish alienation from estrangement, was careful to point out that not only does there have to be a legitimate justification for a child's rejection of a parent, such justification has to be considered from an "objective" basis. Family law practitioners should keep this distinction in mind and not let unfounded or undocumented

---

32. *Id.*

33. *Id.*

34. J.F. v. D.F., *supra*.

35. Kelly, J., & Johnston, J. (2001). The alienated child: A reformulation of parental alienation syndrome, *Fam. Ct. Rev.*, 39, 249, 253.

36. McClain v. McClain, *supra*, at 182.

allegations of "abusive" behavior on the part of rejected parent provide an easy justification for a child's rejection of a parent.

In addition, while estrangement may also result in a child rejecting a parent and may necessitate court and therapeutic intervention, it does not necessarily negate the existence of parental alienation. The existence of the former does not necessarily mean an absence of the latter. At times, despite a pattern of abuse or neglect demonstrated by a rejected parent, there may *also* exist evidence of alienating behaviors. These cases are known as "hybrid" cases. And it is possible that what was once a hybrid case may turn into an alienation case with the passage of time coupled with the improved behavior from one parent and no change from the other.

Consider a recent case out of Michigan courts. In *Martin v. Martin*, the Michigan Court of Appeals affirmed the trial court's finding that the father, who in the past was found to have been "controlling," changed his behavior while the mother, despite the change in the father's behavior, continued to interfere with and obstruct the children's relationship with their father:

> Since at least 2010, [Mother] has denigrated her now ex-husband . . . to their three children. [Father] was not blameless, and the trial court found in 2012 that he was controlling and misused corporal punishment in times of anger. During a four-year period during which [Mother] effectively prevented any parenting time, [Father] engaged in extensive counseling and showed marked improvement. Even so, [Mother] continued to obstruct her children's counseling and parent-child reunification efforts, adding to the strain on [Father's] relationship with his children . . . We discern no error in the circuit court's conclusion that awarding [Father] sole custody and preserving that parent-child relationship was in the child's best interest.[37]

In evaluating a case for presence of alienation or estrangement, it is also important to look for the objective evidence supporting the reason for rejection. If abusive or neglectful behavior is alleged of a parent, it is important to look for independent evidence corroborating such behavior. It is important to look at the relationship as it existed *prior* to the divorce and/or separation. If the father is being accused of having an anger problem, was this complaint made by the child (*not* the spouse) prior to the separation or divorce? If the mother is being accused of neglect, did this problem manifest prior to the divorce or separation? Were there any findings made by the child protective services or by an independent factfinder such as a jury or a judge in an ancillary proceeding that corroborated the allegations of such abusive behavior? Are there eyewitnesses who have witnessed the alleged abusive behavior of the accused parent? *Why*

37. Martin v. Martin, Michigan Court of Appeals No. 349261 (January 28, 2020).

is it important to thoroughly investigate the allegations of abusive behavior that arguably led to the rejection of the parent by the child? It is important to do so for several reasons.

First, it is important because in a forensic setting—such as a courtroom—a factfinder is asked to determine a more objective "truth" than what practicing clinicians and therapists are asked to evaluate behind closed doors. Second, it is dangerous to simply assume the abuse allegations to be true. The argument of some special interest groups—for example, "the fact that there is no evidence doesn't mean it didn't happen"—has no place in a courtroom, especially an American courtroom, where an accused has a presumption of innocence. Allegations of physical, sexual, or other kinds of abusive behavior can have life-changing ramifications for the accused, his or her reputation, career, and, more importantly, his or her access to the children. Third, it is a common alienating strategy for the alienating parent to falsely accuse or orchestrate the false allegations against the target parent. Such repeated false allegations of "domestic violence" or "abuse" that lead to investigations by protective services or the police have been seen by courts as an "abusive use of conflict," which is an alienating strategy.[38] Fourth, young children, adolescents, and even adults can be coached or manipulated into making false allegations of "abuse"—a fact supported both by legal and scientific literature.[39] Fifth, alienators attempt to triangulate, misuse, and often abuse the court process, child protective services' investigations, and law enforcement resources to further solidify parental alienation by denigrating the parent who has been falsely accused of abuse in the eyes of the child (and the world at large) and deprive the accused parent access to the children.[40]

When confronted with solid evidence of their alienating behaviors—behaviors that have been shown to severely harm a parent-child relationship—alienators often resort to making unfounded claims in an attempt to obfuscate the issues. One claim, made often, argues that the theory of parental alienation is nothing but a gambit that has been manufactured to protect abusive men from being held accountable for their actions. Sometimes this strawman argument is taken to preposterous levels. For example, one of the well-known detractors of parental alienation wrote a letter to the *Diagnostic and Statistical Manual*, Fifth Edition (DSM-5) Task Force alleging that advocates of parental alienation

---

38. *See* Delekta v. Delekta, 2019 WL 2711294 (Mich. Court of Appeals) (Unpublished); In the Matter of the Marriage of Reichert v. Reichert-Randazzo, 2 Wash.App.2d 1063 (2018) (Unpublished).

39. Sternjohn v. John, 2019 WL 3000751 (Court of Appeals of Minnesota) (Unpublished); Ahern, E. et. al. (2011). Young children's emerging ability to make false statements, *Developmental Psychol.* 47(1), 61–66; Ceci, S., Crotteau-Huffman, M., Smith, E., Loftus, E. et. al. (1994). Repeatedly thinking about non-events: Source misattribution among preschoolers, *Consciousness and Cognition*, 3, 388; Chrobak, Q. et. al. (2008). Inventing stories: Forcing witnesses to fabricate entire fictitious events leads to freely reported false memories, *Psychonomic Bull. & Rev.*, 15, 1190–1195.

40. Sternjohn v. John, *supra.*

include "father's rights' groups who don't like to be interfered with when they are sexually abusing their children."[41] The detractor subsequently withdrew his outrageous statement, saying, "I apologize for suggesting that all fathers who accuse mothers of [Parental Alienation Syndrome] are sexually abusing their children. That was clearly an overstatement that I retract . . . . I do not deny that parental alienation occurs and that a lot of people are hurt when there is an alienator."[42]

Abuse, regardless of gender, race, or sexual orientation, should never be condoned. When proven, such behavior has to be confronted with swift, decisive, and effective action. However, in a forensic setting, it is important to thoroughly investigate the *allegations* of abuse. "Determining when a child's negative feelings about one parent are rational or irrational is more often than not quite challenging. In some respects, the process is similar to differentiating a non-bizarre delusion from a persistent, justified worry."[43] A child who has been alienated typically "has a false belief that the rejected parent has been abusive or neglectful. Children with false beliefs about events that never actually occurred may develop false memories . . . memories of non-events."[44] In evaluating a case for the presence of alienation and/or estrangement, the court appointed evaluators and/or experts must investigate whether the reasons given for contact refusal are true, accurate and/or justified. Fortunately, there is good research that shows how to do it.[45]

A thorough and robust investigation into allegations of abuse is necessary not only to rule out the possibility of estrangement but also to check for presence of any alienating behaviors. Domestic violence is about control and domination. A perpetrator of domestic violence is likely to continue his or her "violent" pattern by controlling the children also. Research has demonstrated that "abusive ex-partners are likely to attempt to alienate the children from the other parent's affection (by asserting blame for the dissolution of the family and telling negative stories), sabotaging family plans (by continuing criticism or competitive bribes), and undermine parental authority (by explicitly instructing the children not to listen or obey).[46] A parent who has been found to be abusive or controlling and domineering is more likely to continue his or

41. Bernet, W. (2013). Parental alienation, DSM-5, and ICD-11. In Lorandos, D., Bernet, W., & Sauber, R. (Eds.), *Parental Alienation: The Handbook for Mental Health and Legal Professionals*, Charles C. Thomas, 494.

42. *Id.*

43. *Supra* 10, citing Ceci, S., Crotteau-Huffman, M., Smith, E., Loftus, E. et. al. (1994). Repeatedly thinking about non-events: Source misattribution among preschoolers, *Consciousness and Cognition*, 3, 388–407.

44. *Supra* 28 at 577.

45. *See, e.g.*, Bernet, W., & Freeman, B. (2013). The psychological assessment of contact refusal In Lorandos, D., Bernet, W., & Sauber, R. (Eds.), *Parental Alienation: The Handbook for Mental Health and Legal Professionals*, Charles C. Thomas, 47–73; Drozd, L., & Olesen, N. (2004). Is it abuse, alienation, and/or estrangement? A decision tree. *J Child Custody* 1, 65–106.

46. Jaffe, P., Johnston, J., Crooks, C., & Bala, N. (2008). Custody disputes involving allegations of domestic violence: Toward a differential approach to parenting plans. *Family Court Review*, 46(3), 500–523.

her harassing and controlling pattern by manipulating the children to turn against the victim parent.[47]

Another differentiating aspect between estrangement and alienation is the level or magnitude of rejection of a parent by the child. An alienated child is polarized in his or her views of the rejected parent: The child views the world in black and white. The target parent is often characterized as "horrible"; the preferred parent is praised as "perfect." The level of polarization in severe alienation cases is pathological. While non-alienated children recover quickly from whatever caused their resentment, alienated children "never," "ever" want to see the target parent. Though it sounds counter-intuitive, research shows that an alienated (and non-abused) child may be *more* negative toward the rejected parent than a child who was actually abused:

> It is remarkable that abused children frequently remain attached to their abusive parents, whom they might perceive as charming and charismatic. . . . a maltreated child may have ambivalent feelings toward the abusive parent; however, the alienated child almost always has highly negative attitudes toward a non-abusive parent.[48]

Parental Alienation versus "Parental Alienation Syndrome"

Courts often get dragged down the rabbit hole of being asked to adjudicate whether the "Parental Alienation Syndrome" has sufficient scientific validity and reliability, or general acceptability amongst the scientific community, to be admissible as expert evidence. A parent who is accused of engaging in alienating *behaviors* may attempt to obfuscate the issues by presenting expert opinion that "Parental Alienation Syndrome" has no scientific underpinning and, therefore, the court must disregard any and all evidence of parental alienation. This is a red herring and family law practitioners who represent the alienated parents in court must rise to the challenge to reframe the issue for the court. The focus of the factfinder must not be on the "syndrome," it be must be on the alienating *behaviors*. But first, it is important to understand this so-called controversy.

The term "Parental Alienation Syndrome" was formulated by the child psychiatrist Richard Gardner. As Dr. Gardner—certified in psychiatry and child psychiatry by the American Board of Psychiatry and Neurology—explained:

> the parental alienation syndrome is a disorder that arises primarily in the context of child-custody disputes. . . . It results from the combination of

47. Warshak, R. (2010). Family bridges: Using insights from social science to reconnect parents and alienated children. *Family Court Review*, 48, 48–60.
48. *Supra* 28 at 577.

a programming (brainwashing) parent's indoctrinations and the child's own contributions to the vilification of the target parent.[49]

Dr. Gardner's formulation of Parental Alienation Syndrome was lauded by some and criticized by others. The criticism that was levied at Dr. Gardner mainly consisted of "*ad hominems* and shoddy scholarship" that found him pilloried.[50] However, since Dr. Gardner's formulation of the Parental Alienation Syndrome in the mid-1980s, several mental health professionals and researchers, working *independently* of Dr. Gardner, have studied the behaviors that are considered as alienating behaviors and reached a consensus that parental alienation is real and it constitutes "child abuse."[51] The Clawar / Rivlin findings that were published by the American Bar Association in their book titled *Children Held Hostage*, Dr. Richard Warshak's description of a pattern of coercive control and domination by a parent, Leona Kopetski's research, Barry Bricklin's work, and Johnston / Kelly's paper referring to parental alienation as "an insidious form of emotional abuse of children that can be inflicted by divorced parents," *all* ultimately culminated into a proposal that parental alienation be included in DSM-5.[52]

The difference between the term *parental alienation* and "Parental Alienation Syndrome" is that Dr. Gardner's definition focuses solely on the *child's* behavior after he or she has been successfully alienated from the targeted parent; whereas the term *parental alienation* "focuses on the behavior and actions of the aligned parent, rejected parent, and the child."[53] The fact that there may be some controversy surrounding the former does not negate the robust science underlying the latter. As the Connecticut Superior Court acknowledged in *Mastrangelo v. Mastrangelo*, the "strategies" of alienation are "scientifically present and reliable, and thus pass the . . . *Daubert* test."[54] They also pass the *Frye* test.[55] In an informal poll of members of the Association of Family and Conciliation Courts (AFCC) conducted in 2010, 98 percent of the 300 respondents agreed with the question: "Do you think that some children are manipulated by one parent to irrationally and unjustifiably reject the other parent?"[56] While the term "Parental Alienation Syndrome" may continue to generate irrelevant controversy, there is no disagreement amongst the courts or mental health pro-

---

49. Lorandos, D. (2013). Parental alienation. In Morewitz, S., & Goldstein, M. (Eds.), *Handbook of Forensic Sociology and Psychology*, Springer, 323.

50. Ibid.

51. *Id.* at 324.

52. *See* Bernet, W. (2008). Parental alienation disorder and DSM-5, ***Am.*** *J. Fam. Therapy*, 36, 349, 366; Bernet, W. (2010). *Parental Alienation, DSM-5, and ICD-11*, Charles C. Thomas.

53. Mastrangelo v. Mastrangelo, 55 Conn. L. Rptr. 245 (2012) (Unreported).

54. *Id.*

55. H.L.J. v. R.G.J., Jr. No. 2014 MDA 2019 (Superior Court of Pennsylvania, July 28, 2020).

56. Baker, A., Jaffee, P., Bernet, W., & Johnston, J. (2011). Brief report on parental alienation survey. *The Association of Family and Conciliation Courts eNEWS*, 30(2).

fessionals on the phenomenon of parental alienation and the toxic *behaviors* manifested by the alienating parent, which cause significant harm to the targeted parent's relationship with the child.

Family courts have increasingly refused to get drawn into the meaningless controversy surrounding the "Parental Alienation Syndrome" and instead focused their attention on an alienating parent's behaviors. For instance, in *Martin v. Martin*, the Michigan Court of Appeals, refusing to take the bait on adjudicating the controversy over the "syndrome," instead held:

> [Mother] . . . essentially contends that 'parental alienation' is junk science. While there may be a dispute in the scientific community about whether there is diagnosable, pathological condition called parental alienation syndrome . . . there is no reasonable dispute that high-conflict custody disputes frequently involve acts by one parent designed to obstruct or sabotage the opposing parent's relationship with the child.[57]

Parental Alienation and DSM-5

Another argument lobbed against parental alienation is that it is not included in the American "bible" of mental disorders—the DSM-5. Therefore, the argument goes, it must not be good science. This is another red herring. Prior to the publication of DSM-5, "there was a proposal to include parental alienation disorder as a new diagnosis."[58] The members of the DSM-5 Task Force "never said that they doubted the reality or the importance of parental alienation."[59] "However, they concluded that parental alienation did not meet the standard definition of a mental disorder, that is, 'the requirement that a disorder exists as an internal condition residing within an individual.'"[60] Accordingly, the DSM-5 Task Force "said that parental alienation should be considered an example of a relational problem because it involves a disturbance in the child's relationship with one or both parents."[61]

In 2016, two of the authors who contributed to DSM-5, along with Dr. William Bernet of Vanderbilt University School of Medicine, published a paper in the peer-reviewed *Journal of the American Academy of Child & Adolescent Psychiatry*.[62] The authors pointed out that "one of the new terms introduced in the DSM-5 was 'child affected by parental relationship distress' (CAPRD)."[63] The

57. Martin v. Martin, Michigan Court of Appeals No. 349261 (January 28, 2020), FN 2.
58. Bernet, W., Wamboldt, M., & Narrow, W. (2016), *supra*, at 575.
59. *Ibid.*
60. *Ibid.*
61. *Ibid.*
62. *Id.* at 571–579.
63. *Id.* at 571.

authors elaborated that their purpose of publishing the article was "to explain how clinicians and researchers can use the new terminology of CAPRD."[64] They pointed out that "since two of the authors of [the] article" wrote the chapter on "Other Conditions" in the DSM-5, their article was consistent with the structure, content, and intentions of the DSM-5.[65] The authors proposed that the CAPRD category should be used by clinicians "when the focus of clinical attention is the negative effects of parental relationship distress on a child in the family, including effects on the child's mental or medical disorders."[66] The term "parental relationship distress," authors pointed out, includes behaviors such as "persistent disparagement of one or both parents by the other parent."[67] Typically, as a result of such behaviors, "a child affected by parental relationship distress displays impaired functioning in behavioral, cognitive, affective, and/or physical domains. Examples of behavioral problems include oppositionality and the child's reluctance or refusal to have a relationship with a parent without a good reason (parental alienation)."[68] Examples of "cognitive problems" may include the child "adopting the false belief that the rejected parent is evil or dangerous (parental alienation)."[69] The authors clarified that "children who experience parental alienation almost always fulfill the definition of CAPRD."[70]

The concept of parental alienation is covered by DSM-5 under three specific diagnoses: (1) Child affected by parental relationship distress (V61.29), (2) Parent-child relational problem (V61.20), and (3) Child psychological abuse (995.51).[71]

The psychological damage associated with parental alienation has been well researched and documented.[72] Heeding the clarion call of anguished parents and frustrated mental health professionals, courts around the country have intervened in cases involving parental alienation and taken remedial

64. *Id.* at 572.
65. *Ibid.*
66. *Ibid.*
67. *Ibid.*
68. *Ibid.*
69. *Ibid.*
70. *Id.* at 575.
71. *See* American Psychiatric Association. (2013). *Diagnostic and statistical manual of mental disorders* (5th ed.) (DSM-5), Author, 715–716, 719.
72. Wallerstein, J., & Blakeslee, S. (1989). Second chances: Men, women, and children a decade after divorce, Ticknor & Fields; also *see* Baker, A. (2005). The long-term effects of parental alienation on adult children: A qualitative research study. *American Journal of Family Therapy*, 33, 289–302.

action.[73] Week after week, family courts around the country issue judicial opinions that acknowledge the phenomenon of parental alienation. In the three decades since Dr. Gardner first published his formulation of a Parental Alienation Syndrome, American courts have seen a significant increase in parental alienation cases. It is imperative that professionals, both from legal and mental health professions, understand the solid research in the area of parental alienation. Given the body of scientific research and legal literature in support of parental alienation, diligent professionals can easily and effectively refute the skeptics who claim that the phenomenon doesn't exist or cannot be accepted by courts because of the underlying insufficient data.

73. Matter of Marriage of Reichert, No. 48783-7-II, 2018 WL 1393794, at *7 (Wash Ct App, March 20, 2018); *In re* HM, No. G057128, 2019 WL 3522043, at *26 (Cal Ct App, August 2, 2019); Hiller v. Hiller, 919 NW2d 548, 558 (SD, 2018); SternJohn v. John, No. A18-1838, 2019 WL 3000751, at *5 (Minn Ct App, July 1, 2019); Delekta v. Delekta, No. 345006, 2019 WL 2711294, at *3 (Mich Ct App, June 27, 2019); Geary v. Geary, 27 NE3d 877, 895 (Ohio Ct App, 2015); McClain v. McClain, 539 SW3d 170, 223 (Tenn Ct App, 2017); Rodman v. Friedman, 33 AD3d 400, 401; 826 NYS2d 1, 2 (2006); Bergin v. Bergin, No. HAN-19-77, 2019 WL 3788326, at *3 (Me, August 13, 2019).

CHAPTER 2

Admissibility of Expert Testimony on Parental Alienation

It is undeniable that family law courts in the United States accept the phenomenon of parental alienation. As far back as 1804, parental alienation was asserted in the courts of England.[1] Over the next two hundred years, courts across the world acknowledged parental alienation and attempted to provide appropriate interventions. It is no different in the United States.[2] A survey of parental alienation cases in the United States from 1985 through 2018 examined the question "Have the courts in the United States found the construct of parental alienation material in high-conflict child custody cases?" and the resounding answer was yes![3]

While parental alienation as a phenomenon is widely accepted by both mental health and legal professionals, the admissibility of the construct—expert evidence in support of parental alienation—is at times challenged in the courtroom. Detractors of parental alienation (and attorneys representing

1. King v. De Manneville, 5 East 221, 102 Eng. Rep. 1054 (K.B. 1804). *See also*: Shelley v. Westbrook, 37 Eng. Rep. 850 (Ch. 1817); Earl of Westmeath v. Countess of Westmeath. 162 Eng. Rep. 992 (1826); *In re* Barry, 42 F. 113 (S.D.N.Y. 1844); *In re* Burrus, 136 U.S. 586 (1890).

2. Bernet, W. (2020). Introduction to parental alienation. In Lorandos, D. & Bernet, W. (Eds.), *Parental Alienation: Science and Law*, Charles C. Thomas; Clawar, S., & Rivlin, B. (2013). *Children Held Hostage: Identifying Brainwashed Children, Presenting a Case, and Crafting Solutions*, Second Edition, ABA; Gardner, R. A. et al. (Eds.) (2006). *The International Handbook of Parental Alienation Syndrome*, Charles C. Thomas, 158, 169, 433–437; American Professional Society on the Abuse of Children. (2017). *Practice Guidelines: The Investigation and Determination of Suspected Psychological Maltreatment of Children and Adolescents*, APSAC, https://www.apsac.org/9235fgnl8.

3. Lorandos, D. (2020). Special issue: Parental alienation in U.S. courts, 1985 to 2018. *Fam. Ct. Rev.*, 58, 322, 326.

parents who are alleged to have engaged in parental alienation) all too often make misleading arguments that parental alienation does not exist, is not scientific, and has no place in the family law courtroom. However, a close look at the empirical research and studies in support of the theory of parental alienation and the current admissibility standards in American courtrooms provides a solid framework to support the admissibility of the construct of parental alienation. Let us examine the criteria for the admissibility of expert testimony, how parental alienation meets these criteria, and how to present expert evidence regarding parental alienation to the court.

The admission of expert evidence, including evidence concerning parental alienation, is governed by state and federal evidence rules and admissibility standards are further clarified and expanded through common law—that is, judicial decisions. Generally speaking, expert evidence must be relevant, probative, and material if it is to be admissible.[4] Additionally, all relevant evidence is generally admitted[5] unless: "[I]ts probative value is substantially outweighed by a danger of . . . unfair prejudice, confusing the issues, misleading the jury, undue delay, wasting time, or needlessly presenting cumulative evidence."[6] For instance, a court may strike an expert report as cumulative if the report offers the same evidence as previously admitted evidence. Evidence is relevant if it "has 'any tendency to make the existence of any fact that is of consequence to the determination of the action more probable or less probable than it would be without the evidence.'"[7] Materiality looks to the relation between the supporting evidence and the issues in the case.[8] A trial court must first make a preliminary determination of materiality when assessing the admissibility of the evidence.[9] In family courts, "a trial judge is vested with broad discretion to determine the materiality and relevance of proposed evidence."[10] Finally, evidence is probative if it "tends to prove or disprove a point in issue."[11]

The requirement that preliminary questions concerning the admissibility of evidence shall be determined by the court is born from the Federal Rule

4. F.R.E. Rule 401 Pub. L. 93-595, §1, Jan. 2, 1975, 88 Stat. 1931; Apr. 26, 2011, eff. Dec. 1, 2011.

5. The Daubert trilogy is: Daubert v. Merrell Dow Pharmaceuticals, Inc, 509 US 579; 113 S Ct 2786 (1993); Joiner v. General Elec Co, 78 F3d 524, 529 (CA 11, 1996), reversed as: General Electric Co. v. Joiner, 522 US 136; 118 S Ct 512 (1997); Kumho Tire Company, Ltd. v. Carmichael, 526 U.S. 137; 119 S.Ct. 1167 (1999).

6. *See*: Daubert v. Merrell Dow Pharmaceuticals, Inc, 509 US 579; 113 S Ct 2786 at 2795; n. 9, (1993) "In a case involving scientific evidence, evidentiary reliability will be based upon scientific validity." Emphasis in original. And *see*: Kumho Tire Company, Ltd. v. Carmichael, 526 U.S. 137; 119 S.Ct. 1167 at 1174: Expert testimony must demonstrate a valid connection to the pertinent facts as a precondition to admissibility.

7. Daubert v. Merrell Dow Pharm., Inc., 509 U.S. 579, 587, 113 S. Ct. 2786, 2794, 125 L. Ed. 2d 469 (1993) (Quoting Fed. R. Evid. 401).

8. Brown, K. S. et. al. (Eds.) (2006). *McCormick on Evidence*, 6th Edition, Thomson/West, 306–307.

9. Vandivier v. State, 822 N.E.2d 1047, 1052 (Ind. Ct. App. 2005). See, also, Miller, 770 N.E.2d at 772; State v. Fodor, 179 Ariz. 442, 880 P.2d 662, 674 (1994) (citing Franzi v. Superior Court, 139 Ariz. 556, 679 P.2d 1043, 1049 (1984)).

10. *In re* Shane Chayann Orion S., 79 A.D.3d 430, 912 N.Y.S.2d 46 (2010).

11. Garner, B. A., & Black, H. C. (2004). *Black's Law Dictionary*, 8th Edition, Thomson/West.

of Evidence 104(a) (and the equivalent state rule thereto). This rule allows the court to hold an evidentiary hearing to make a preliminary determination that an expert is properly qualified, and that the expert's underlying reasoning or methodology is scientifically valid and can be applied to the facts of the case.[12] Federal Rule of Evidence 104 (c) provides in part that hearings on preliminary matters, such as *Daubert* hearings, may be conducted when the interests of justice require. In the exercise of its gatekeeping function, as enunciated and clarified by the *Daubert* trilogy, a trial court must undertake a preliminary determination of whether the methodology of the expert's proposed testimony is scientifically reliable. A *Daubert* hearing is the appropriate way to challenge an expert whose methodology is questionable.[13] In answering these gatekeeping questions, the courts must evaluate the experts, their opinions, and the foundations for those opinions on a case-by-case basis.[14] In conducting these hearings, the trial judge may rely on another expert's evaluation of underlying data.[15] However, the final determination—the gatekeeping role—belongs to the judge, *not* the expert. The court's reliance on experts must neither abandon nor override its role as a gatekeeper.[16,17]

Admissibility Standards

Currently in the United States, there is no uniform system of admitting evidence. Most states model their evidence rules on the Federal Rules of Evidence; however, each state differs in how it applies its admissibility standards. (See

---

12. *See, e.g.,* Smelser v. Norfolk Southern Ry. Co., 105 F.3d 299, 302-303, 46 Fed. R. Evid. Serv. (LCP) 468, 1997 FED App 33P (6th Cir. 1997); cert denied, 118 S.Ct. 67, 139 L. Ed.2d 29 (US 1997). When applying Daubert, the trial court resolves preliminary questions on admissibility of expert testimony under FRE 104(a), and must determine whether expert testimony reflects scientific knowledge and whether findings are based on scientific knowledge and derived by the scientific method. In Smelser, the trial court did not apply Daubert factors in admitting the testimony of a biomedical engineer and the verdict for a plaintiff in FELA suit was reversed. See, also: Watkins v. Schriver, 52 F.3d 769 (8th Cir 1995); Eagleston v. Guido, 41 F.3d 865 (2nd Cir. 1994), cert denied, 116 S.Ct 53 (1996).

13. *See, e.g.,* United States v. Vitek, 144 F.3d 476 (7th Cir. 1998). The trial court held a lengthy and exhaustive Daubert hearing.

14. *See, e.g.,* Soden v. Freightliner Corp., 714 F-2d 498, 502- 505 (5th Cir. 1983) Fed R. Evid. 703 requires courts to examine reliability of expert's sources on a case-by-case basis.

15. *See, e.g., In re* Japanese Elec., Prod. Antitrust Litig., 723 F.2d 238, 285 (3d Cir 1983), rev'd on other grounds sub nom. Matsushita Elec. Indus. Co. v. Zenith Radio Corp., 473 U.S. 574 (1986). Proper inquiry is not what the court deems reliable but what experts in relevant discipline deem it to be.

16. Daubert v. Merrell Dow Pharmaceuticals, Inc., 509 U.S. 579, 113 S. Ct. 2786, 2793-2799, 125 L. Ed. 2d 469, 485 (1993); *In re* Paoli R.R. Yard PCB Litigation v. Southeastern Pa. Trans., 35 F.3d 717, 742 (3d Cir. 1994). Daubert clearly holds that Fed. R. Evid: 703 requires an independent gatekeeping role.

17. *See, e.g.,* Head v. Lithonia Corp. Inc., 981 F.2d 941. 944 (10th Cir. 1989). It is reversible error when a trial court fails to make a preliminary determination that data underlying an expert's opinion is of kind reasonably relied on by experts in field. And *see*: University of Rhode Island v. A.W. Chesterton Co., 2 F.3d 1200,1217-1218 (1st Cir. 1993); *In re* Agent Orange Prod. Liab. Lit., 611 F. Supp. 1223,1246 (E.D.N.Y. 1985), aff'd, 818 F.2d 187 (2d Cir. 1987), cert. denied, 487 U.S. 1234 (1988); Advent Sys. Ltd. v. Unisys Corp., 925 F.2d 670, 682 (3d Cir. 1991); Wilder Enters., Inc. v. Allied Artists Pictures Corp., 632 F.2d 1135,1144 (4th Cir. 1980).

Appendix D for a chart of admissibility of expert evidence standards in different states.) In the post-*Daubert* era, while most states apply the *Daubert* model of gatekeeping, a handful continue to apply the old *Frye* model and some, still yet, apply a hybrid of both tests or their own admissibility standards.[18]

State Admissibility Standards

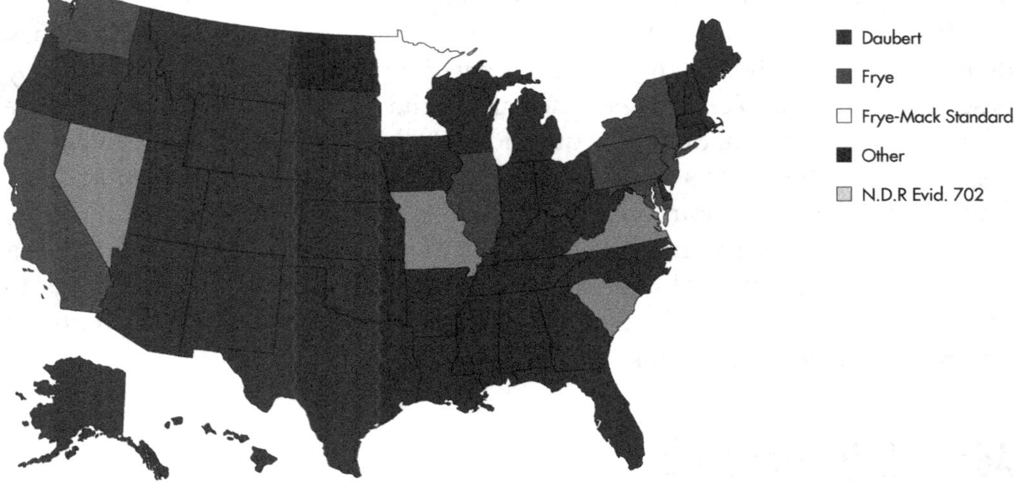

Nonetheless, the two main threshold tests to determine admissibility of expert evidence are the *Daubert* test and its predecessor the *Frye* test. The *Frye* test is a threshold evidentiary admissibility standard for novel scientific ideas.[19] Under *Frye*, "expert testimony based on scientific principles or procedures is admissible but only after a principle or procedure has 'gained general acceptance' in its specific field."[20] The new or novel scientific procedure "need not be 'unanimously endorsed' by the scientific community but must be 'generally accepted as reliable.'"[21] In a *Frye* hearing "the burden is on the proponent to 'show the generally accepted reliability of such procedure in the relevant scientific community through judicial opinions, scientific or legal writings, or expert opinion other than that of the proffered expert.'"[22] A *Frye* type hearing is generally held prior to the trial to give the "defendant the opportunity to establish admissibility of expert testimony on the theory."[23]

18. For instance, Connecticut applies a Porter test, while California applies both Frye and Kelly standards.

19. *See* Zafran v. Zafran, 740 N.Y.S.2d 596 (2002).

20. People v. Fortin, 706 N.Y.S.2d 611 (2000) (quoting People v. Wesley, 83 N.Y.2d 417 (1994)).

21. Zafran v. Zafran, 740 N.Y.S.2d 596 (2002) (quoting People v. Middleton, 54 N.Y.2d 42 (1981)).

22. *Id.* (quoting Cameron v. Knapp, 520 N.Y.S.d 917 (Sup.Ct., N.Y. County, 1987).

23. *See, e.g., Id.*

The *Daubert* test is an evidentiary threshold test based on Rule 702 of the Federal Rules of Evidence which is used in federal courts and has also been adopted in most state courts.[24] The *Daubert* court ruled that "a federal trial court has the responsibility to determine, pursuant Rule 702, whether the proffered evidence will 'assist the trier of fact.'"[25] The *Daubert* court decided on a two-part test. At the outset of the hearing, the trial judge must determine, "pursuant to Rule 104(a), whether the expert is proposing to testify to (1) scientific knowledge that (2) will assist the trier of fact to understand or determine a fact in issue."[26] This requires an assessment of whether the methodology underlying the testimony is "scientifically valid and of whether that reasoning or methodology properly can be applied to the facts in issue."[27] The *Daubert* court held that: "Many factors will bear on the inquiry, and we do not presume to set out a definitive checklist or test."[28] The key questions the *Daubert* court proffered to determine scientific validity are: "(1) Whether it can be, and has been, tested; (2) whether the theory or technique has been subjected to peer review and publications; (3) the known of potential rate of error, including the existence and maintenance of standards controlling the technique's operation; and (4) whether the technique is generally accepted in the relevant scientific community."[29] In a *Daubert* hearing a trial judge should determine "whether sufficient indicia of legitimacy exists to support the conclusion that evidence derived from the principle may be considered by a fact finder at trial."[30] This is important because applying a *Daubert* test instead of *Frye* gives the court the ability to reject evidence that may have been generally accepted but not scientifically valid—what many term "junk science."

Expert evidence that supports parental alienation is based in the social sciences.[31] Parental alienation can be observed by mental health practitioners and forensic scientists during therapy, custody evaluations, supervised parenting, etc. In order to allow testimony regarding these observations and subsequent testing used by the practitioner, the court must determine reliability of measurement tools used to categorize parental alienation. Therefore, courts must be well versed in the way social scientists determine reliability of measurement tools. Generally, social scientists determine reliability of measurement

---

24. Mastrangelo v. Mastrangelo, 2012 WL 6901161 *3.
25. *Id.* (quoting FRE 702).
26. Daubert v. Merrell Dow Pharm., Inc., 509 U.S. 579, 592–93, 113 S. Ct. 2786, 2796, 125 L. Ed. 2d 469 (1993).
27. *Id.*
28. *Id.*
29. *Id.* at 4.
30. *Id.*
31. Baker, A. J. L. (2013). Parental alienation and the Daubert standards. In Lorandos, D., Bernet, W., & Sauber, R. (Eds.), *Parental Alienation: The Handbook for Mental Health and Legal Professionals*, Charles C. Thomas, 326.

tools by: "(1) interrater/interobserver reliability, (2) test-retest reliability, (3) parallel-forms reliability, and (4) internal consistency reliability."[32]

The first of the reliability standards, *interrater reliability,* is important because it demonstrates consistency in the results of the measurement tool. For instance, if a group of researchers observed the same scenario, it would be expected that the testing scores would be similar for that observation. Interrater reliability is statistically measured. Discussing how interrater reliability works, Dr. Baker states: "Interrater reliability is typically considered adequate if it is .80 or better. So, for example, if two custody evaluators review ten case files and agree on nine of them regarding the presence or absence of PAS in the child then interrater reliability, if expressed as the percentage of agreement, would be 90 percent. As a kappa, the figure would depend on the nature of the scoring and the types of agreement and disagreement. A kappa statistic is usually lower than the percentage of agreement. For example, even with 90 percent agreement, the kappa could be considerably lower depending upon the pattern of responses."[33] Interrater reliability is a crucial component of a measurement tool. When a measurement tool demonstrates low levels of interrater reliability, it is indicative that the procedure frequently leads to mistaken findings.

The second way social scientists determine reliability of measurement tools is by *test-retest reliability.* This type of reliability refers to testing a subject and then retesting the subject at a later date to determine the similarity in the subject's test answers. It would be expected that the subject would have similar answers despite the span of time in between testing sessions. However, this is only true if there have not been any changes in the test subject between the testing sessions. For instance, if the test subject was a child who suffered from alienation, and if interventions were introduced after the first testing session, it would be expected that the second testing session would result in different answers. Dr. Baker notes that it is not appropriate to apply the test/retest reliability standard when a change of circumstances has happened. Additionally, she notes that it would not be appropriate to test a "child once when brought by the favored parent and once when brought by the rejected parent. If the child is brought to one session by the alienating/favored parent and to the second session by the rejected/targeted parent, the child's responses might vary widely from one testing session to another. This does not necessarily indicate lack of reliability of the measure. Rather it reflects that alienated children behave differently depending upon which parent is observing them."[34]

Parallel-forms reliability is similar to test/retest reliability in that it compares the test answers among two separate questionnaires. However, parallel-forms

32. *Id.*
33. *Id.*
34. *Id.*

reliability is set up in a way that it provides the test taker with two separate forms that have similar questions and then compares the answers of the parallel forms—which the test taker takes at the same time. It is only appropriate to use this type of reliability method if the inventory has the same question types. For instance, "[i]f there is a thirty-item personality test with ten items about depression and ten items about anxiety and ten items about cognitive styles, parallel-forms reliability would not be appropriate."[35]

The last type of reliability standard used by social scientists is *internal consistency*. Internal consistency reliability is a measure of how well a test addresses different constructs and delivers reliable scores. The scores are generally measured by the correlation between the different constructs. A practitioner who provides summary scores must determine that there is internal consistency between the individual items on the test. "A statistic known as a Cronbach's alpha can be calculated to determine whether there is sufficient internal consistency of the items to allow for the creation of a summary score. An alpha of .80 or above is considered adequate internal consistency for the creation of a summary score. An option when conducting a Cronbach's alpha is to examine what the alpha would be if each item were removed. This allows the researcher to determine whether a particular item is actually reducing the internal consistency and should be removed. One bad item can lower the alpha, and it is allowable to create a summary score omitting one item if the analysis suggests that this is warranted."[36]

Now let's turn to the concept of validity. In addition to the expert's measurement tools being reliable, they must also be valid. For a measurement tool to be "valid," it must measure what it intends to measure. For instance, "a depression scale is supposed to measure depression . . . an anxiety scale is supposed to measure anxiety . . . a measure of a child's unwarranted rejection of a parent is supposed to measure a child's unwarranted rejection of a parent."[37] There are six types of validity: (1) face validity, (2) content validity, (3) predictive validity, (4) concurrent validity, (5) convergent validity, and (6) discriminate validity.[38] Both face validity and content validity are the less stringent of the six types of validity. Face validity refers to a subjective assessment of whether the measurement procedure used in a study appears to be a valid measure of a given construct. For instance, if a measurement tool sought to measure school performance, a question that asks, "How many AP classes have you taken?" would appear to have face validity because the question appears to be related to school performance. However, taking AP classes is not in itself indicative of

35. *Id.*
36. *Id.*, 329.
37. *Id.*, 330.
38. Lorandos, D., & Campbell, T. (2005). *Benchbook in the Behavioral Sciences–Psychiatry–Psychology–Social Work*, Carolina Academic Press, 373.

school performance, so while the measurement tool may have face validity, it may not in and of itself be valid. Likewise, content validity is a nonstatistical measure that ensures that the content on a measurement tool is related to the subject being tested. For example, "if a researcher constructed a measure of the child's alienation, a review of Gardner's eight behavioral manifestations would be a good starting place to determine whether the items on the measure cover all eight."[39]

The next four types of validity are more stringent and provide a stronger basis to determine validity of measurement tools. For instance, predictive validity tells you how well a certain measure can predict future behavior. Predictive measurement tools are "also useful for developing interventions and for evaluating treatment outcomes because factors selected are measures of the extent to which goals are met."[40] A depression scale has predictive validity because it can be used to predict future behaviors of people who test for depression. Concurrent validity is used to test new measurement tools. A new measurement tool will be used concurrently with an older measurement tool that has already been determined to be valid. If the scores from the new measurement tool are statistically similar to the scores of the older valid measurement tool, it can be said that the new measurement tool is concurrently valid.[41] "Concordance of .80 or higher is considered an indication of concurrent validity. Of course, there are not always existing reliable and valid measures of the construct of interest, which would rule out this form of validity."[42] Convergent validity is shown when tests having the similar constructs are highly correlated. To test convergent validity, a practitioner would (1) "correlate the scores between two assessment tools or tools' sub-domains that are considered to measure the same construct" and (2) use the "multitrait-multimethod matrix approach,"[43] which "organizes convergent and discriminant validity evidence for comparison of how a measure relates to other measures."[44] An example of convergent and discriminate validity is found when "a measure of PA strategies [are] associated with some type of Axis II personality disorder but not

39. Baker, A. J. L. (2013), *supra*. *See also*: Gardner, R. A. (1998). *The Parental Alienation Syndrome: A Guide for Mental Health and Legal Professionals*, Creative Therapeutics.

40. Johnston, J. R., & Sullivan, M. J. (2020). Parental alienation: In search of common ground for a more differentiated theory, *Fam. Ct. Rev.*, 58, 270, 282.

41. Baker, A. J. L., (2013), *supra*.

42. *Id.* at 331.

43. Chin, C. L., & Yao, G. (2014). Convergent validity. In Michalos, A. C. (Ed.), *Encyclopedia of Quality of Life and Well-Being Research*, Springer.

44. Campbell, D. T., & Fiske, D. W. (1959). Convergent and discriminant validation by the multitrait-multimethod matrix. *Psychological Bulletin*, 56, 81–105.

necessarily an Axis I disorder. Thus, a measure of PA strategies could be convergently and discriminately validated with measures of Axis I and Axis II diagnoses.'[45]

While seemingly complex, it is essential that the family law attorney who endeavors to present expert evidence on parental alienation understand the concepts of reliability and validity and their applicability to the theory of parental alienation. Understanding these reliability standards will provide the framework for challenging an opposing expert or detractors of parental alienation and assist the family court in making the right decision. By having a sound understanding of the fundamentals of social sciences and how they apply to admissibility of expert testimony, the attorney, through argument and expert testimony, can educate and assist the court to admit expert evidence in support of parental alienation. The more informed the court is during the hearing, the better the chances of getting in reliable testimony regarding parental alienation. While some judges are well versed on parental alienation, methodology, and reliability of test measurements, other judges are not. It is the attorney's responsibility to educate and inform the court regarding measurements used to test parental alienation.

Admissibility of Parental Alienation Evidence under the *Frye* Test

Admissibility under the *Frye* test is based on the general acceptance of the theory being proffered. The *Frye* test is still used in a handful of states: Alabama, California, Florida, Illinois, Maryland, New York, Pennsylvania, Utah, and Washington. The *Frye* test has its roots in the 1923 case *Frye v. United States.* The case, which disputed the admissibility of a polygraph test report, held that the admission of expert testimony must be based on scientific methods that are sufficiently established and accepted. The *Frye* court held that "Just when a scientific principle or discovery crosses the line between the experimental and demonstrable stages is difficult to define. Somewhere in this twilight zone the evidential force of the principle must be recognized, and while the courts will go a long way in admitting experimental testimony deduced from a well-recognized scientific principle or discovery, the thing from which the deduction is made must be sufficiently established to have gained general acceptance in the particular field in which it belongs."[46] *Frye* is most commonly recognized as the general acceptance theory and essentially puts the gatekeeping role into the hands of the scientific community.

45. *Id.*
46. Frye v. United States, 293 F. 1013, 1014 (D.C. Cir. 1923).

For the states that do use the *Frye* test, the attorney must notice a *Frye* hearing in order to establish the admissibility of parental alienation.[47] Keep in mind that the admissibility standard under *Frye* is that the theory or construct is generally accepted, so an expert should testify "as to the scientific theory" and submit "peer-reviewed journals . . . to establish whether the scientific community has generally accepted parental alienation syndrome."[48] For instance, to establish admissibility of parental alienation, an attorney "submitted 136 peer-reviewed articles regarding parental alienation syndrome and the testimony of four experts."[49] During a *Frye* hearing, an expert may testify as to their familiarity of parental alienation and their opinion as to whether parental alienation is generally accepted in the scientific community. Importantly, under *Frye*, "the particular scientific approach need not be unanimously endorsed by the scientific community, but rather, it must be generally accepted as reliable."[50] Consequently, the party offering the proof has the burden to "show the generally accepted reliability of the procedure in the relevant scientific community through judicial opinions, scientific or legal writings, or expert opinion other than the proffered expert."[51]

Expert evidence of parental alienation is supported by the *Frye* standard. Recently, a Pennsylvania appellate court affirmed a trial court's ruling—admitting expert testimony on parental alienation and the appropriate mental health intervention required to remedy the child's indoctrination and brainwashing—using the *Frye* test.[52] "To date, more than 1,000 books, book chapters, and articles have been published in mental health or legal professional journals on the subject of parental alienation."[53] Here's how one family court in Florida, in the case *Kilgore v. Boyd*,[54] ruled:

> If I do have to apply a *Frye* test [Dr. Gardner] has passed the *Frye* test. And I find that parental alienation syndrome has passed the *Frye* test in my courtroom, which is a Circuit Court Courtroom in the Family Law division, based on the evidence and the argument before me. The evidence and the argument before me, the testimony and the CV of Dr. Gardner, together with an excerpt of his writings. There was also proffered an

47. 127 Am. Jur. Proof of Facts 3d 237 (Originally published in 2012). *See also*: Zafran v. Zafran, 191 Misc. 2d 60, 740 N.Y.S.2d 596 (Sup 2002).

48. *Id.* See, for example, *In re* Marriage of Bates, 212 Ill. 2d 489, 289 Ill. Dec. 218, 819 N.E.2d 714 (2004).

49. *Id.*

50. 127 Am. Jur. Proof of Facts 3d 237 (Originally published in 2012). *See* Zafran v. Zafran, 191 Misc. 2d 60, 740 N.Y.S.2d 596 (Sup 2002).

51. 127 Am. Jur. Proof of Facts 3d 237 (Originally published in 2012).

52. H.L.J. v. R.G.J., Jr., Superior Court of Pennsylvania (No. 2014 MDA 2019), filed July 28, 2020.

53. Harman, J. et al. (2018). Parental alienating behaviors are family violence, *Psychological Bulletin*, 144(12), 1275–1299, 1278.

54. Kilgore v. Boyd, Circuit Court of the 13th Judicial Circuit of the State of Florida, Hillsborough County, Family Law Division. Case no. 94-7573, Div. D.

article from the Florida Bar Journal which, quite frankly, I read when it came out and at the time I read it I placed some credibility in it. I'm also impressed by the fact that Dr. Gardner is cited in the footnote in at least one of the cases, I believe it's *Schultz vs. Schultz*.[55]

The theory of parental alienation is generally accepted in the scientific community. There is a "very high consensus" amongst the mental health community of professionals that "mothers, fathers, children, young adults, and counselors have been able to describe the explicit behaviors that may be perpetrated by one parent and have the capacity to distance, damage, or destroy a child's relationship with the other parent."[56] In addition, there is also "consensus as to what outcomes are associated with different levels of severity of parental alienation in children. This consensus is found across many different studies using different methods and samples. Therefore, there has been noteworthy professional agreement about the types of alienating behaviors that A[lienating] P[arents] use, and research has demonstrated reliable identification of clusters of symptoms in children who have been alienated."[57]

Despite the availability of peer-reviewed and other research and consensus on the topic, some legal commentators continue to express skepticism regarding the admissibility of expert testimony of parental alienation.[58] For instance, *People v. Fortin* was the first appellate case in New York to make Parental Alienation the subject of a *Frye* hearing. In order to determine the admissibility of the expert testimony on parental alienation the court in *Fortin* held that it must consider whether the expert's opinion is "based on a theory or technique generally accepted in the scientific community, the need of the jurors for specialized information, and the relevance of the expert's opinion to the issue in the case."[59]

The *Fortin* court first focused on whether parental alienation is generally accepted in the scientific community. The proponent of the expert testimony must "lay a proper foundation establishing that the processes and methods employed by the expert in formulating his or her opinions adhere to accepted standards of reliability within the field."[60] There are two ways to establish that reliability: either where "the general acceptance would be so notorious that the court could take judicial notice" or where "acceptance could be established by reference to legal writings and opinions."[61] In this case, the court heard

---

55. *Id.*

56. Harman, J. et al. (2018), *supra*, 1278.

57. *Id.*

58. § 73:16. Specific expert testimony—Psychological processes—Parental alienation syndrome, 4 Criminal Procedure in New York § 73:16 (2d).

59. People v. Fortin, 706 N.Y.S.2d 611, 613 (2000).

60. *Id.* at 614.

61. *Id.*

testimony at the *Frye* hearing on PAS from Dr. Gardner, the leading expert on the theory.[62] The court found that based on the testimony, "the defendant has not established general acceptance of Parental Alienation Syndrome within the professional community which would provide a foundation for its admission at trial."[63,64] But it is noteworthy that the *Fortin* case focused on "Parental Alienation Syndrome," not the phenomenon or theory of parental alienation. Generally speaking, while New York courts have expressed skepticism over the scientific validity of "Parental Alienation Syndrome," "there is no doubt that parental alienation exists."[65]

In *People v. Sullivan*, the defendant's expert witness' testimony on parental alienation was excluded.[66] The expert witness in this case, Dr. Rand, testified that "on over 20 occasions he had testified on parental alienation syndrome; that parental alienation syndrome is accepted in the psychological scientific community [and] that there are more than 100 professional articles on the topic."[67] Even though the trial judge did not order a *Frye* hearing, the judge ruled that "the testimony was not scientific enough to satisfy the Kelly-Frye rule."[68] The Court of Appeals affirmed finding the testimony was correctly excluded under section 801 of the Federal Rules of Evidence, not because of the *Frye* rule.[69] Under Section 801 an expert's testimony must be limited "to a subject that is sufficiently beyond common experience that the opinion of an expert would assist the trier of fact."[70] The appellate court found that "the concept that a parent would encourage a child to lie in a divorce case is commonly understood."[71]

In the case *In re Marriage of Bates*, the wife moved to bar the expert testimony of Dr. Gardner regarding Parental Alienation Syndrome.[72] The court ordered a *Frye* hearing to test the admissibility of the testimony on PA.[73] The husband, as the proponent of the expert testimony, had the burden of proving its general acceptance and "proffered three expert witnesses and 136 articles from peer-reviewed publications as exhibits."[74] All three expert witnesses testified

---

62. *Id.*
63. *Id.*
64. Interestingly, the court cites to another New York case debating the admissibility of DNA evidence, saying that "it is not for a court to take pioneering risks on promising new scientific techniques, because premature admission both prejudices litigants and short-circuits debate necessary to determination of the accuracy of a technique." *Id.* (quoting People v. Wesley, 83 N.Y.2d 417, 437 (1994).
65. J.F. v. D.F., 61 Misc.3d 1226(A), 2018 N.Y. Slip. Op. 51829(U).
66. *See* People v. Sullivan, 2003 WL 1785921 (2003).
67. *Id.* at 12.
68. *Id.* at 13.
69. *Id.*
70. *Id.*
71. *Id.*
72. *See In re* Marriage of Bates, 212 Ill.2d 489, (2004).
73. *Id.* at 499.
74. *Id.* at 500.

that PA was generally accepted and cited many peer-reviewed publications.[75] Dr. Barden testified that PA is "a useful and clear description of a set of symptoms or clusters, commonly seen in child custody proceedings."[76] Dr. Gardner also testified that PA arises "primarily, if not exclusively, in the context of child custody disputes."[77] This testimony helped to establish the general acceptance and relevance of the expert testimony and the court found that "the principle of Parental Alienation Syndrome is sufficiently established to have gained general acceptance in the particular field."[78]

In a 2014 New Jersey child custody case, the trial court introduced a custody expert who testified regarding parental alienation.[79] The Superior Court found that the trial court erred by not subjecting the PAS testimony to a *Frye* hearing. The court noted that at the time of the trial "PAS was not a recognized syndrome in the DSM-IV" and that "the Supreme Court and this court have not yet determined that PAS is a scientifically reliable or generally accepted theory."[80] The court stated that the "admission of novel scientific material like PAS must meet the test established in *Frye*, that is, that the opinions are 'generally accepted within the relevant scientific community.'"[81] In this case neither the "scientific reliability nor general acceptance of PAS was established."[82] The court did not issue an opinion on whether "evidence of PAS may ever be properly admitted."[83] While PAS was not held as a generally accepted theory in New Jersey in 2014, Florida had already held that PAS is generally accepted in the scientific community as discussed above in the *Kilgore* case.

Admissibility of Parental Alienation under the *Daubert* Test

With the landmark case *Daubert v. Merrell Dow Pharmaceuticals* in 1993, the role of gatekeeper was essentially transferred from the scientific community to the judge. In the *Daubert* case, the Supreme Court held that the Federal Rules of Evidence superseded *Frye* as the standard for admissibility of expert evidence in federal courts.[84] In *Daubert*, the Court agreed on the following guidelines for admitting scientific expert testimony:

---

75. *Id.* at 500–501.
76. *Id.* at 500.
77. *Id.*
78. *Id.* at 501.
79. *See* M.A. v. A.I., 2014 WL 7010813 *2.
80. *Id.* at *5.
81. *Id.*
82. *Id.*
83. *Id.*
84. Daubert v. Merrell Dow Pharm., Inc., 509 U.S. 579, 587, 113 S. Ct. 2786, 2793, 125 L. Ed. 2d 469 (1993). (Stating they contend that the Frye test was superseded by the adoption of the Federal Rules of Evidence. We agree.)

> (1) the judge is the gatekeeper, ensuring that scientific expert testimony truly proceeds from scientific knowledge. (2) The trial judge must ensure that the expert's testimony is "relevant to the task at hand" and that it rests "on a reliable foundation." (3) The judge must find it more likely than not that the expert's methods are reliable and reliably applied to the facts at hand. That is, the knowledge is gained through the scientific method, defined as (a) the process of formulating hypotheses and then conducting empirical experiments to prove or falsify the hypotheses, (b) being subject to peer review and publication, (c) having a known or potential error rate and the existence and maintenance of standards and controls concerning its operation, and (d) having theory and technique that is generally accepted by the relevant scientific community.[85]

While the *Daubert* test holds the expert to higher scrutiny, a problem has become apparent. The legal community is ill prepared for analyzing and interpreting scientific evidence.

> Research has demonstrated that legal education does not improve either methodological or statistical reasoning abilities. Comprehensive research demonstrates that our courts are not prepared to evaluate science and some commentators have stridently argued that lawyers and judges are simply science illiterates.[86]

Nonetheless, the *Daubert* decision was critical because it determined that expert testimony must not only be generally accepted—as the *Frye* Court held—but also that expert testimony must be derived from the scientific method. As described above, to be deemed scientific, a method must be based on empirical and measurable evidence. "In brief, the scientific method involves researchers proposing hypotheses and designing studies to test these hypotheses using reliable and valid measures. Findings are subject to peer review

---

85. *Id.*

86. Lorandos, D. (2017). Expert evidence post Daubert: The good, the bad, and the ugly, *Litigation* (Spring). *See also*: Lehman, D. R., Lempert, R. O., & Nisbett, R. E. (1988).The effects of graduate training on reasoning: Formal discipline and thinking about everyday life events, *American Psychologist*, 43, 431, 443: Judges are not seen to be more skilled in the evaluation of science than lay people. In fact, Lehman and colleagues demonstrated that legal education does not improve either methodological or statistical reasoning abilities. *See also*: Kovera, M. B., & McAuliff, B. D. (2000). The effects of peer review and evidence quality on judge evaluations of psychological science: Are judges effective gatekeepers? *Journal of Applied Psychology*, 85, 574–586, 583: "the scientific training judges receive is insufficient to help them recognize flawed psychological research." *See also*: Gatowski, S. I. et al. (2001). Asking the gatekeepers: A national survey of judges on judging expert evidence in a post-Daubert world, *Law and Human Behavior*, 24, 433, 452: This October 2001 study with a survey frame of "9,715 state trial court judges from all 50 states and the District of Columbia" concluded that "although judges surveyed reported that they found Daubert criteria useful for determining the admissibility of proffered expert evidence, the extent to which judges understand and can properly apply the criteria when assessing the validity and reliability of proffered scientific evidence was questionable at best."

and when found worthy are published in peer-reviewed journals."[87] In order for the Court to qualify an expert and determine if the proposed testimony is appropriate under *Daubert,* the court must determine whether the proposed expert will be helpful to the trier of fact. The inquiry ends if a determination is made that the expert or the subject matter are not helpful.

After helpfulness is determined, the court must then determine if the proposed expert is qualified to offer the proffered testimony. Following their decision in Daubert, the Supreme Court passed on a Third Circuit ruling in *DeLuca v. Merrell Dow Pharmaceuticals, Inc.*[88] In *DeLuca* the Third Circuit reasoned that: "Rule 703 is satisfied once there is a showing that an expert's testimony is based on the type of data a reasonable expert in the field would use in rendering an opinion on the subject at issue."[89] Experts are permitted wide latitude in their opinions and are not required to base their pronouncements on first-hand knowledge; the *Daubert* Court required that "the expert's opinion must have a reliable basis in the knowledge and experience of his discipline."[90] In this analysis, courts are required to excuse proposed experts who do not have a grasp of the "knowledge and experience of [their] discipline."[91] Highlighting that the "focus . . . . must be solely on principles and methodology,"[92] the Court's analysis cites *United States v. Smith*[93] and informs that "error rate" in the predictions and techniques espoused in the opinions of the experts must be considered.[94]

Further, in the case *Kumho Tire Co. v. Carmichael,* the Court expanded on *Daubert* by holding that

> an expert, whether basing testimony upon professional studies or personal experience, employs in the courtroom the same level of intellectual rigor that characterizes the practice of an expert in the relevant field. Nor do we deny that, as stated in *Daubert,* the particular questions that it mentioned will often be appropriate for use in determining the reliability of challenged expert testimony. Rather, we conclude that the trial judge must have considerable leeway in deciding in a particular case how to go about determining whether particular expert testimony is reliable. That is to say, a trial court should consider the specific factors identified

87. Baker, A. J. L. (2013). Parental alienation and the Daubert standards. In Lorandos, D., Bernet, W., & Sauber, R. (Eds.), *Parental Alienation: The Handbook for Mental Health and Legal Professionals,* Charles C. Thomas.

88. DeLuca v. Merrell Dow Pharmaceuticals, Inc., 911 F 2d 941, (3rd Cir. 1990) aff'd without op. 6 F 3d 778 (3rd Cir. 1993) cert denied, 114 S Ct 691 (1994).

89. *Id.* at 953 (emphasis added).

90. 113 S Ct at 2796.

91. *Id.*

92. 509 U S 579, 113 S Ct at 2797.

93. United States v. Smith, 869 F2d 348, 353-354 (CA7 1989).

94. *Id.* 509 U S 579, S Ct at 2797; 125 L Ed 2d at 483.

> in *Daubert* where they are reasonable measures of the reliability of expert testimony.[95]

The *Kumho* court held that the courts must have considerable leeway in deciding whether the proposed testimony and the proposed expert is reliable.

> Rule 702 does not distinguish between "scientific" knowledge and "technical" or "other specialized" knowledge but makes clear that any such knowledge might become the subject of expert testimony. It is the Rule's word "knowledge," not the words (like "scientific") that modify that word, that establishes a standard of evidentiary reliability."[96]

This imposes a duty on the court to determine the validity of the expert's qualifications and the reliability of the proposed testimony.[97] The *Kumho* court holds experts to demonstrate a valid connection to the pertinent facts as a precondition to admissibility.[98]

The *Joiner* case furthered this discussion by adding that "experts must have a more rigorous connection between underlying data and conclusions than merely their own ('ipse dixit') say so."[99] In any case, *Joiner* instructs that

> conclusions and methodology are not entirely distinct from one another. Trained experts commonly extrapolate from existing data. But nothing in either *Daubert* or the Federal Rules of Evidence requires a district court to admit opinion evidence that is connected to existing data only by the ipse dixit of the expert. A court may conclude that there is simply too great an analytical gap between the data and the opinion proffered.[100]

Justice Breyer, concurring, stated that

> [t]his requirement will sometimes ask judges to make subtle and sophisticated determinations about scientific methodology and its relation to the conclusions an expert witness seeks to offer—particularly when a case arises in an area where the science itself is tentative or uncertain, or where testimony about general risk levels in human beings or animals is offered to prove individual causation. Yet . . . judges are not scientists and

---

95. Kumho Tire Co. v. Carmichael, 526 U.S. 137, 152, 119 S. Ct. 1167, 1176, 143 L. Ed. 2d 238 (1999).
96. *Id.*
97. *Id.* at 1176–1177.
98. *Id.* at 1176.
99. Joiner, 118 S.Ct. at 519.
100. Gen. Elec. Co. v. Joiner, 522 U.S. 136, 146, 118 S. Ct. 512, 519, 139 L. Ed. 2d 508 (1997). *See also*: Turpin v. Merrell Dow Pharmaceuticals, Inc., 959 F.2d 1349, 1360 (C.A.6), cert. denied, 506 U.S. 826, 113 S.Ct. 84, 121 L.Ed.2d 47 (1992).

> do not have the scientific training that can facilitate the making of such decisions.[101]

Justice Breyer explained that the lack of scientific training does not excuse the court from "exercising the 'gatekeeper' duties that the Federal Rules of Evidence impose."[102] The court must determine whether

> particular expert testimony is reliable and "will assist the trier of fact," Fed. Rule Evid. 702, or whether the "probative value" of testimony is substantially outweighed by risks of prejudice, confusion or waste of time, Fed. Rule Evid. 403. To the contrary, when law and science intersect, those duties often must be exercised with special care.[103]

If the court does determine that the proposed expert is qualified, the court must determine that the proffered testimony is reliable. The *Daubert* court grounded its admissibility analysis in the principles and methodology of science, notes:

> that scientists typically distinguish between 'validity' (does the principle support what it purports to show?) and 'reliability' (does application of the principle produce consistent results?) . . . our reference here is to evidentiary reliability–that is, trustworthiness . . . . In a case involving scientific evidence, evidentiary reliability will be based upon scientific validity.[104]

For testimony relating to parental alienation, the Four-Factor Model (the precursor of the Five-Factor Model) as a determinative test for the presence of parental alienation is considered reliable and valid.[105] This model of parental alienation was developed as a framework to "ensure that information about all parties is factored into custody assessments."[106] The Four-Factor model of PA differentiates alienated children from estranged children by showing whether there was "(1) a prior positive relationship between the child and the now rejected parent; (2) absence of maltreatment by the rejected parent; (3) use of alienating behaviors by the favored parent; and (4) presence of behavioral manifestations of alienation in the child."[107] The only difference between the Four-Factor model and the Five-Factor model that is currently being applied by mental health professionals is the addition of the factor requiring that the

---

101. *Id. See also*: Brief for Trial Lawyers for Public Justice as Amicus Curiae 15; Brief for New England Journal of Medicine et al. as Amici Curiae 2 ("Judges . . . are generally not trained scientists").

102. Gen. Elec. Co. v. Joiner, 522 U.S. 136, 147–48, 118 S. Ct. 512, 520, 139 L. Ed. 2d 508 (1997).

103. *Id.*

104. Daubert, 509 U S 579, 113 S Ct at 2795 n. 9 (emphasis in original).

105. Baker, A. J. L. (2018). Reliability and validity of the four-factor model of parental alienation. *Journal of Family Therapy*, 0:1–2. doi: 10.1111/1467-6427.12255.

106. *Id.*

107. *Id.*

child has demonstrated a rejection of a parent or is strongly resisting contact with the rejected parent—*sine qua non* for a case involving parental alienation.

The Five-Factor model of parental alienation is critical for the admission of expert evidence because it negates the assumptions made by parental alienation detractors regarding the construct of parental alienation. For instance, a common challenge to the validity of parental alienation evidence is that alienation presupposes that a rejection of the target parent is without legitimate cause. However, the model ensures that a determination of alienation is only made when there is no evidence of prior abuse and there is evidence of a prior positive relationship—thus lending to the reliability of the model.[108] An important consideration arising out of the model is "a highly counterintuitive feature of PA, that is, most abused children continue to seek a relationship with their abusive parent, while alienated children (who were never abused) strongly reject a relationship with the targeted parent."[109]

Detractors of parental alienation may also incite several misleading arguments in an attempt to undermine the reliability and validity of parental alienation. For example,

> An argument against the admissibility of parental alienation theory may take the form of condemning the person who coined the term, Dr. Gardner, for self-publishing one of his books, for supposedly not accurately portraying his credentials and several patently false allegations . . . pointing out that it is not mentioned by name in the Diagnostic and Statistical Manual of the American Psychiatric Association, or . . . that the science behind parental alienation theory is not sound.[110]

These arguments do not help further the discussion of a phenomenon that is obviously injurious to families—and for those courts that may not be as well informed—these arguments can confuse and conflate the issues surrounding the phenomenon of parental alienation. In addition to detractors confusing the issues surrounding parental alienation, the general public also has a repertoire of false beliefs about parental alienation. These false beliefs can "lead therapists and lawyers to give bad advice to their clients, evaluators to give inadequate recommendations to courts, and judges to reach injudicious decisions. The increasing recognition of the phenomenon of children's pathological alienation from parents brings with it a proliferation of mistaken assumptions

108. *Id.*

109. Baker, A. J. L. (2020). Parental alienation and empirical research. In Lorandos, D., & Bernet, W. (Eds.), *Parental Alienation: Science and Law*, Charles C. Thomas.

110. *Id.*

about the problem's roots and remedies. These assumptions fail to hold up in the light of research, case law, or experience."[111]

The Five-Factor model of parental alienation goes a long way to quash these arguments. The model requires that a prior positive relationship between the child and the target parent must have existed. A prior positive relationship negates the argument that is often proclaimed that there has never been a bond between the target parent and the child. Additionally, the existence of a prior positive relationship screens for parents who were "habitually absent, uninvolved, and uncaring from claiming that they are victims of parental alienation."[112] The model's third factor, absence of abuse and/or neglect, screens for parents who "have engaged in behaviors that warrant a child's rejection."[113] The fourth factor applies the seventeen strategies of parental alienation, which must be observed.[114] Notably, the "Baker Strategy Questionnaire" has been shown to be both reliable and valid.[115] The final factor describes the child's presentation of the eight behaviors commonly displayed in children suffering from parental alienation.[116] "There is both clinical and research support that alienated children behave quite differently than children who are realistically estranged from a parent."[117]

It would be helpful to the proponent of the expert evidence on the theory of parental alienation to take a methodical, step-by-step approach in qualifying an expert. Dr. Demosthenes Lorandos and Dr. Terence Campbell have offered such an analysis.[118] The authors explain that the first determination to be made is helpfulness—will the proposed expert testimony assist the trier of fact. Next, the court must determine whether to qualify the witness as an expert. Last, the court must determine, through a three-part analysis, that the proffered evidence is reliable and valid.[119]

---

111. Warshak, R. A. (2015). Ten parental alienation fallacies that compromise decisions in court and in therapy, *Prof'l Psychol.: Research & Practice*, 46, 235.

112. *Id.*

113. *Id.*

114. Baker, A. J. L., & Ben-Ami, N. (2011). To turn a child against a parent is to turn a child against himself. *Journal of Divorce and Remarriage*, 54(2), 203–219.

115. Baker, A. J. L., (2020), *supra*.

116. *Id.*

117. *Id.*

118. Lorandos, D., & Campbell, T. (2005). *Benchbook in the Behavioral Sciences–Psychiatry–Psychology–Social Work*, Carolina Academic Press, 45–46.

119. *Id.*

Lorandos & Campbell Decisional Template for Expert Testimony

FIRST Make A Determination of Helpfulness:

"If scientific, technical, or other specialized knowledge will assist the trier of fact to understand the evidence or to determine a fact in issue..."

Require an Offer of Proof or a Rule 26 (a)(2) statement

Conduct a Rule 104 analysis of relevancy considering materiality and probative value

Conduct a Rule 403 analysis of probative value vs. countervailing reasons for exclusion

If "NO" move on to other witnesses →

If "YES" continue ↓

SECOND Make A Determination of Expert Qualifications:

". . . a witness qualified as an expert by knowledge, skill, experience,training, or education, may testify thereto in the form of an opinion orotherwise. . . "

Require an Offer of Proof or a voir dire analysis of the proposed expert's knowledge, skill, experience, training, or education

If "NO" move on to other witnesses →

If "YES" rule that the witness qualifies as an expert and continue ↓

THIRD Make A Determination of Reliability – In Three Parts:

". . . if (1) the testimony is based upon sufficient facts or data. . ."

This is a Qualitative Analysis

Require an Offer of Proof or conduct a Daubert hearing and determine the identity and quantum of the facts and/or data the proposed expert has relied upon

If "NO" ask:

"Can the factual basis or the data upon which the expert's proposed testimony is based be significantly improved?"

If "NO" move on to other witnesses →

If "YES" determine amount of time allowable before re-assessment if any and continue ↓

If "YES" or once a sufficiency determination of the basis of the proposed testimony has been made, continue ↓

". . . (2) the testimony is the product of reliable principles and methods."

This is a Qualitative Analysis

Require an Offer of Proof or conduct a Daubert hearing and determine the validity and reliability of the principles and methodology the proposed expert has utilized

If "NO" move on to other witnesses →

If "YES" continue ↓

" . . . and (3) the witness has applied the principles and methods reliably to the facts of the case."

This is a "Fit" Analysis

Require an Offer of Proof or conduct a Daubert hearing and determine the "fit" of the proposed expert's conclusions to the reliability criteria and the facts of the case.

If "NO" move on to other witnesses →

If "YES" rule that proposed testimony is ADMISSIBLE

In the recent Maine case *Bergin v. Bergin,* the Supreme Judicial Court of Maine affirmed the trial court's inclusion of expert testimony regarding parental alienation. The *Bergin* court held that

> Maine Rule of Evidence 702 provides that an expert may testify in the form of an opinion if her specialized knowledge "will help the trier of fact to understand the evidence or to determine a fact in issue." To be admissible, expert testimony must (1) "meet a threshold level of reliability," (2) be "relevant pursuant to M.R. Evid. 401," and (3) "assist the trier of fact in understanding the evidence or determining a fact in issue."[120]

The *Bergin* court reasonably concluded that all three requirements were met.

> The expert testified extensively as to her work in the field of parental alienation, her education, her publications, the general acceptance of the field, her previous work as an expert in judicial proceedings, and the methods that she applied in this specific case. The evidentiary hearing included substantial discussions of the mother's role in preventing the father from having contact with the children, making the expert's testimony relevant, and the testimony aided the court by providing "a counterintuitive explanation as to the dynamics . . . present in [the] situation."[121]

120. Bergin v. Bergin, 2019 ME 133, ¶¶ 9-10, 214 A.3d 1071, 1074 (Quoting Tolliver, 2008 ME 83, ¶ 29, 948 A.2d 1223 (quotation marks omitted).)

121. *Id.*

In particular, the court found that the mother's persistent and unrelenting efforts to prevent the children from having a healthy relationship with their father outweighed other factors regarding the children's best interests. The record supports the court's finding that, despite a previously "strong relationship" with the father, the children were left without a meaningful relationship with their father as a result of the mother's interference, frequent moves, and refusal to allow and support regular contact between the children and the father. The court's thorough and thoughtful findings regarding the best interests of the children reflect an appropriate application of the legislatively established policy encouraging children's connections with both parents.[122]

Connecticut first adopted the gatekeeping rationale of the *Daubert* test in *State v. Porter*.[123] In this case the Superior Court of Connecticut held a "Porter" hearing to determine the admissibility of expert testimony on Parental Alienation Syndrome using the *Daubert* test. Dr. Baker testified as to her "15 articles on the topic of parental alienation, the strategies, syndromes and their interrelationships."[124] Dr. Garber also testified as to the distinction between Parental Alienation and Parental Alienation Syndrome and how the "syndrome focuses solely on the behavior and actions of the child or children, as contrasted to the concept of parental alienation, which, instead, focuses on the behavior and actions of the aligned parent, rejected parent *and* the child or children."[125] Based on the testimonies at the Porter hearing, the court found "a general acceptance of the concept of 'strategies' of alienation employed by an aligned parent against a rejected parent toward their child or children." Because the testimonies showed reliability and acceptance, the court ruled that parental alienation, *not* PAS, passed the *Daubert* test.[126]

In the Texas case, *Matter of Marriage of Koenig*, the Mother argued that the Father failed to preserve error of admitting expert witness testimony regarding Parental Alienation. The Court found that for purpose of its review, Father preserved error and found the trial court properly admitted expert testimony regarding parental alienation. The Court found:

> If scientific, technical, or other specialized knowledge will assist the trier of fact to understand the evidence or to determine a fact in issue, a witness qualified as an expert by knowledge, skill, experience, training or education may testify thereto in the form of an opinion or otherwise.[127]

---

122. *Id.*
123. M.A. v. A.I., 2014 WL 7010813 *2.
124. *Id.* at 5.
125. *Id.* at 9.
126. *Id.*
127. Cooper Tire & Rubber Co. v. Mendez, 204 S.W.3d 797, 800 (Tex. 2006) (quoting Tex. R. Evid. 702); *see also* Daubert v. Merrell Dow Pharm., Inc., 509 U.S. 579, 588–89 (1993).

The court also found that "there is no rigid formula to determine whether a particular witness is qualified to testify as an expert . . . there must be a fit between the subject matter and the expert's familiarity with that subject matter."[128] Dr. Alvarez's testimony revealed that the Father was

> engaged in parental alienation and such actions had negatively affected the children's relationship with their mother. Dr. Alvarez also testified that Charles was an obstacle to co-parenting the children. As examples of the alienation, Dr. Alvarez testified the children would call Kimberly by her first name; they were concerned with adult issues; and the oldest child made statements indicating he was aligned with Charles in promoting Charles's agenda and felt responsible for Charles's emotions. Additionally, Dr. Alvarez testified that Charles's parents engaged in a pattern of alienation, including saying derogatory things about Kimberly to the children, and did not consider Kimberly to be the children's mother. Dr. Alvarez observed varying degrees of anxiety in each of the children during her visits, which she attributed to Charles's behavior. Dr. Alvarez testified that she did not observe an intention on Kimberly's part to ruin the relationship between the children and Charles. Dr. Alvarez opined that Charles should have supervised visitation until he completed counseling related to parental alienation.[129]

Again, in the Delaware parental alienation case *J.H. v. J.D.*, the court found that the expert's testimony and report regarding parental alienation were admissible based on *Daubert*. The court explained:

> In assessing the reliability of the proffered expert testimony, the Court examines "(1) whether a theory or technique has been tested; (2) whether it has been subjected to peer review and publication; (3) whether a technique had a high known or potential rate of error and whether there are standards controlling its operation; and (4) whether the theory or technique enjoys general acceptance within a relevant scientific community." These Daubert factors "are not a definitive checklist or test," as the Court's inquiry must be tied to the facts of the particular case.[130]

The testimony offered by the expert witness regarding parental alienation was admitted. The court noted that

> Dr. R____ frequently offers expert testimony in this Court regarding issues related to custody and visitation. This Court has noted that

---

128. Mega Child Care, Inc. v. Tex. Dept. of Protective and Regulatory Servs., 29 S.W.3d 303, 310 (Tex. App.–Houston [14th Dist.] 2000, no pet.) Broders v. Heise, 924 S.W.2d 148, 153 (Tex. 1996).

129. In the Matter of the Marriage of Koenig, 2017 WL 2704081, Not Reported in S.W.3d (2017).

130. J.H. v. J.D., 2017 WL 4403331, Not Reported in A.3d (2017).

> "Dr. R____ is a clinical psychologist with extensive training in family therapy," and that "[a] significant proportion of his practice consists of performing custody evaluations." Besides qualifying as an expert, Dr. R____ offered relevant evidence based upon reliable methods that assisted the Court in determining D____'s best interests.[131]

Arkansas courts have dealt with the admissibility of parental alienation as early as 1997, where the court relied on expert testimony to determine the alienation ongoing in the case. In *Turner v. Benson* the court found

> [w]hether one parent is alienating a child from the other is an important factor to be considered in change of custody cases, for, just as the chancellor noted below, a caring relationship with both parents is essential to a healthy upbringing. The testimony of several witnesses left the chancellor with the clear impression that Ben was happy during visitation with appellee, but was uncomfortable in expressing his enjoyment when he returned to appellant.[132]

Then, in 2000, in *Chambers v. Chambers*, an Arkansas court determined that a change of circumstances had occurred because of the ongoing parental alienation justifying an enforcement order for visitation.[133] In the 2006 Arkansas case, *Linder v. Johnson*, the court held that

> [T]his case . . . turns on the credibility of the witnesses and whether the trial court erred in relying on Dr. DeYoub's conclusions instead of Dr. Thomas's. We hold that the trial court did not err in relying on Dr. DeYoub's conclusions. . . . Although Dr. DeYoub met with the parties for a briefer period than Dr. Thomas did, the statements to Dr. DeYoub made by the children and Jennifer support his conclusion that Jennifer deliberately and successfully alienated her children from Deron. Based on those statements, Dr. DeYoub concluded that this case was "an egregious" case of parental alienation.[134]

In Colorado in 2007, relying on the testimony offered by an expert witness in the case, the court admitted evidence showing that in an "extensive, longitudinal study in Colorado, parental alienation has been found to occur in twenty percent of cases involving custody and parenting time."[135] Also, in Connecticut,

131. *Id.* at 8.
132. Turner v. Benson, 59 Ark.App. 108, 953 S.W.2d 596, 598-99 (Ark.App. 1997) (emphasis added).
133. Chambers v. Chambers, 2000 WL 795278 at *1 (Ark.App. 2000).
134. Linder v. Johnson, 2006 WL 3425021 at *5 (Ark.App. 2006) (emphasis added).
135. *In re* Marriage of Hatton, 160 P.3d 326, 334 (Colo.App. 2007) (citing Kopetski, Leona M., Identifying Cases of Parent Alienation Syndrome-Part I, 27 Colo. Law. 65, 68 (Feb.1998)) (emphasis added).

Eric Frazer, a court-appointed psychologist, conducted an evaluation of the child and testified at trial. The court qualified Frazer as an expert in the field of forensic psychology, custody evaluations and parental alienation. Frazer met with the child once, outside the presence of the mother or father. Frazer defined parental alienation "as a circumstance where one parent portrays the other parent in a negative light, and the child takes note of such portrayal. The child has less or no contact with the alienated parent based on the perception put forth by the other parent."[136]

Again, in Connecticut in 2007, the court found parental alienation evidence admissible when it held that

> Dr. Black's testimony and his reports are clear that it is his opinion that a "state of alienation" exists as between the boys and the Defendant . . . Dr. Black testified that . . . (1) The child exhibits antagonism toward the alienated parent; 2) Specific and few events are present that could be used as a basis for the antagonism, all of which cannot reasonably justify the antagonism; 3) When a child is asked why he/she feels negatively toward the alienated parent, the response is generalized, i.e., "He's mean"; 4) The child is very aligned with the alienating parent; and 5) The child doesn't want to be with the alienated parent . . . [T]he Court finds Dr. Black's findings [and] conclusions . . . trustworthy.[137]

Next, in the troubling 2003 case of *In re Marriage of McCord,* when the mother challenged the expert's opinion that the mother had severely alienated the child against the father, the court stated:

> We have not passed upon the issue of whether parental-alienation syndrome is a reliable theory. We find it unnecessary to do so now. Rather, we look at the evidence introduced and draw our own conclusion. Because this is a de novo review, we look only at the evidence we deem admissible. We consider the opinions of all the experts as we do the other testimony. We give opinion testimony the weight we consider it deserves after considering, among other things, the expert's education, experience, familiarity with the case, reasons given for the opinion, and interest, if any, in the case. We find no reason to reverse on this ground.[138]

The court found troubling a report of a licensed independent social worker who was requested by a child abuse investigator to do an evaluation. The court noted that the social worker concluded there were "many indicators of the

136. *In re* Jaime S., 120 Conn.App. 712, 727, 994 A.2d 233 (2010).
137. Krukiel v. Krukiel, 2007 WL 241257 at *6 (Conn.Super.,2007) (emphasis added).
138. *In re* Marriage of McCord, 674 N.W.2d 685 (Table), 2003 WL 23219961 at *5 (Iowa App. 2003) (emphasis added).

sexual-allegations-in-divorce syndrome and the parental-alienation syndrome present and recommended a change in custody."[139] The court then noted that another licensed independent social worker who was ordered to counsel the child had "grave concerns about the repeated and unsubstantiated allegations made by the child and her mother and noted the family situation fits the criteria for the most severe form of parental-alienation syndrome."[140] The court noted the licensed independent social worker recommended custody be changed as soon as possible and that therapy continue for the child and contact with her mother and grandmother be monitored and supervised.[141]

Again, in the 2010 Kentucky case *L.S. v. B.S.*,[142] the court admitted expert evidence relating to parental alienation when the parents of the case entered into an agreed order pursuant to which a licensed psychiatrist was appointed to undertake counseling and such treatment of the children as she saw "fit and appropriate." The order stated:

> [t]he court requests recommendation of how best to establish and maintain an ongoing relationship with the children, with each of the parents herein and with specific recommendations for how parenting by each of the parents could be improved to implement and enhance the well-being of the children, minimize any actual or possible parental alienation and properly incorporate the significant others of each of the parents into a comprehensive treatment and parenting plan.[143]

When the psychiatrist filed the report with the court, it stated that the psychiatrist was "gravely concerned about the apparent parental alienation created by the mother, which she stated had a negative impact on the children and interfered with the father's ability to maintain a healthy relationship with his children." When the mother argued that the trial court improperly relied on the theory of Parental Alienation Syndrome (PAS) to alter the visitation terms, the court held that

> [w]e have carefully reviewed the family court's order, and find no reliance on a "theory" of parental alienation syndrome. The trial court found that the mother "demonstrates no real understanding that it is important and desirable that both children feel free to love and enjoy their father as well as their mother." This conclusion was based on the evidence offered at trial, not on an abstract theory of parental alienation syndrome.[144]

---

139. *Id.*
140. *Id.*
141. *Id.*
142. L.S. v. B.S., 2010 WL 4366367 at *1, 3, 6 (Ky.App. 2010).
143. *Id.*
144. *Id.*

In the 2009 Louisiana case *Palazzolo v. Mire*, the court-appointed psychologist/custody evaluator was qualified as an expert in the field of clinical psychology. According to the psychologist, "Ms. Mire engaged in some alienation tactics in the beginning, but that was not the primary reason why the child currently desired not to see Ms. Palazzolo." Another doctor was then qualified as an expert in clinical psychology and was appointed by the court to conduct a second custody evaluation on Ms. Palazzolo's behalf. The second custody evaluator conducted her evaluation over a three-month period. According to the second custody evaluator, "a more accurate description of what Dr. Jordan [another qualified expert] found to be a lack of maternal bonding was a significant disruption in the maternal bonding or evidence of severe parental alienation."[145]

> Dr. Lockman, who was qualified as an expert in the area of development psychology and child development, testified [as to] possible causes of disruption of the attachment [being] a parent leaving, having a psychotic problem, changing dramatically, being absent, or being the subject of parental alienation.[146]

Crucially, the testimony offered that

> Parental alienation . . . has been recognized as a psychological condition that can be harmful to a child's long term emotional development. Moreover, "the conduct of one parent in denigrating the other parent and undermining the child's relationship with that parent, an adult with whom the child has had a very important relationship, is a form of emotional abuse."[147]

Michigan courts have taken a similar stance on the admissibility of parental alienation evidence. As early as 1996, Michigan courts have admitted evidence concerning parental alienation. For instance, in *Bielaska v. Orley*,

> Dr. Campbell testified that the children were subjected to suggestibility. He testified that there is evidence of "parental alienation syndrome" where the children are being alienated from their father to the extent that they don't even recognize that he is their father, and that that foretells very serious consequences for these children unless it is corrected.[148]

However, in 1999, in the case *Krieger v. Krieger*,

> Dr. Richard Gardner testified for the defense that he prepared a report and concluded that defendant was not engaging in parental alienation,

145. Palazzolo v. Mire, 10 So.3d 748, 761, (La.App. 4 Cir. 2009) (emphasis added).
146. *Id.* at 764–765.
147. *Id.* at 774 (emphasis added) (citing Bala, N., Fidler, B.-J., Goldberg, D., & Houston, C. (2007). Alienated children and parental separation: Legal responses in Canada's family courts, *Queen's L.J.*, 33, 79, 88).
148. Bielaska v. Orley, 1996 WL 33324080 at *23 (Mich.App.) (emphasis added).

> that defendant should be awarded custody of the four children, and that the problems between the children and plaintiff were a result of plaintiff's own neglect and abuse, and plaintiff's being schizophrenic, paranoid, delusional and psychotic.[149]

Then, in the 2000 case *In re Spencley*, the court upheld the admissibility of evidence relating to parental alienation when the appellate court held that

> we believe that petitioner properly responds that the family court's factual findings are amply supported by the record and that the term "parental alienation syndrome" is merely a way of describing appellant's actions as they related to the circumstances of this case. At trial, one of the psychologists who had worked with the family, described appellant's behavior as "parental alienation syndrome" simply as a way of describing her behavior. In other words, there was evidence that appellant was, during the course of the divorce, attempting to alienate the children from their father . . . Although appellant disputes the legitimacy of this theory, we agree with petitioner that the psychologist's use of this theory at trial was merely a way to explain appellant's behavior to deprive the children of their emotional well-being. In fact, there was a great deal of evidence that appellant was manipulating the children to alienate them from their father.[150]

Then, in 2005, in *Ostermann v. Ostermann*,[151] the court qualified an expert who discussed the parental alienation in the case and found that the "Defendant engaged in parental alienation as well, albeit to a lesser degree."[152] The expert, who also "pointed out plaintiff's parental alienation, found no evidence of significant mental problems in either party."[153] Moreover, in the 2009 case *Lopez-Negrete v. Lopez-Negrete*,

> Dr. Hobbs also testified regarding her psychological evaluation of defendant. According to Dr. Hobbs, defendant had problems with anger and "her distaste for her husband negates his being in a sense." She further stated that defendant was "so consumed with her negativity and her anger at her husband that the air he breathes is toxic." Dr. Hobbs also stated that defendant's anger toward plaintiff could lead to a situation called parental alienation, in which a child will not acknowledge a single positive thing about the other parent.[154]

---

149. Krieger v. Krieger, 1999 WL 33453292 at *2 (Mich.App.) (emphasis added).
150. *In re* Spencley, 2000 WL 33519710 at *4 (Mich.App.) (emphasis added).
151. Ostermann v. Ostermann, 2005 WL 2323410 at *2 (Mich.App.) (emphasis added).
152. *Id.*
153. Ostermann v. Ostermann, 2005 WL 2323410 at *2 (Mich.App.) (emphasis added).
154. Lopez-Negrete v. Lopez-Negrete, 2009 WL 1506668 at *15 (Mich.App.) (emphasis added).

Also, in the 2010 *Meadows v. Meadows/Henderson* case,

> [P]sychologist John D. Ulrich, Ph.D., testified that he concluded that defendant had engaged in a pattern of parental alienation . . . Ulrich described parental alienation as "[t]he process of one parent trying to undermine and destroy to varying degrees the relationship that the child has with the other parent." . . . This finding is also not against the great weight of the evidence.[155]

On January 28, 2020, the Michigan Court of Appeals issued a published opinion in a case involving parental alienation wherein it affirmed a trial court's award of sole physical and legal custody to a target parent along with a temporary no-contact order that restrained the alienating parent from having any unsupervised contact with the child. In *Martin v. Martin*, the Court, similar to several other courts around the country, refused to get drawn into the meaningless controversy surrounding the "Parental Alienation Syndrome" and instead focused its attention on the alienating parent's *behaviors*:

> [Mother] . . . essentially contends that "parental alienation" is junk science. While there may be a dispute in the scientific community about whether there is diagnosable, pathological condition called parental alienation syndrome . . . there is no reasonable dispute that high-conflict custody disputes frequently involve acts by one parent designed to obstruct or sabotage the opposing parent's relationship with the child.[156]

Notably, in the 2010 Missouri case, *Noland Vance v. Vance*, Dr. Aram, a clinical psychologist interviewed the Father, the Mother, and the two children. The doctor also reviewed available records, including medical records; performed various diagnostic testing; and interviewed other individuals identified by the parties. Dr. Aram's written evaluation was admitted in evidence at the hearing. Dr. Aram found no credible evidence, however, that Father had physically abused the children. Although Mother and the children made such allegations, Dr. Aram noted that the children mentioned the same litany of facts as Mother and used phraseology similar to hers. Dr. Aram also observed that Mother overstated or exaggerated facts to support her version of events that purportedly occurred. Dr. Aram opined that Mother's allegations of child abuse were mistaken, but sincere. As a consequence of Mother's mistaken belief that abuse had occurred, she sincerely believed Father posed a danger to the children. Dr. Aram opined that Mother would do everything in her power to keep the children from Father "with a near religious zeal." By doing so, Dr. Aram opined that Mother was emotionally abusing the children by alienating their

155. Meadows v. Meadows/Henderson, 2010 WL 3814352 at *3 (MichApp) (emphasis added).
156. Martin v. Martin, Michigan Court of Appeals No. 349261 (January 28, 2020), FN 2.

affections for Father. Moreover, Mother's alienating behavior was constant and consistent. While Mother claimed to encourage the children to be loving and respectful toward Father, Mother admitted that she never said anything positive about Father to the children. Similarly, neither Elle nor James had anything positive to say about Father, except that James did say that he wished his Father would "change." Dr. Aram concluded that Mother's constant negativity towards Father, by berating him in front of the children and inciting their fear of him, had caused the children to suffer severe trauma. Relying upon literature in the field, Dr. Aram explained that there were ten indicators of parental alienation. All ten indicators were present in this case. Dr. Aram described this situation as the worst case of parental alienation he had ever seen. As a mandatory reporter of child abuse, Dr. Aram believed he was required to report this form of emotional abuse to the court. Dr. Aram diagnosed Mother as having an adjustment disorder not otherwise specified (NOS) that resulted in the alienation of the children from their father in a high-conflict marriage and divorce.[157]

Finally, in another notable 2010 case, this time in New Mexico, *Kimbrell v. Kimbrell*, the court appointed a "Rule 11-706 expert," Dr. Zieman, who submitted a final report in which he concluded that "Husband and Wife's disagreements were intractable and that joint custody was no longer feasible or in the best interests of the children."[158] The record reflects that Dr. Zieman evaluated the family and submitted extensive reports about the emotional and mental health of the children. The district court's custody determination was based, in part, on Dr. Zieman's recommendations. The GAL observed that Husband and Wife's inability to co-parent and Husband's inability to place the children's well-being and relationships with one another above his own desire to alienate Wife necessitated an award of sole custody. Dr. Zieman reached the same conclusion but was far more explicit in condemning both Husband and Wife's conduct. In Dr. Zieman's view, Husband and Wife were not concerned with the best interests of their children but were primarily focused on defeating one another and winning control over financial resources. Accordingly, Dr. Zieman concluded that sole legal custody was not only prudent but necessary. This arrangement, Dr. Zieman found, would most effectively limit the amount of interaction between Husband and Wife which would in turn protect the children from being further ensnared in Husband and Wife's ongoing and intractable feud. This evidence plainly supports the district court's conclusion that the circumstances since the initial custody determination had changed materially and that joint custody was no longer in the children's best interests.[159]

---

157. Noland-Vance v. Vance, 321 S.W.3d 398 (Mo.App. 2010) (emphasis added).
158. Kimbrell v. Kimbrell, 2010 WL 4060974 at *1, 3, 5 (N.M.App.) (emphasis added).
159. *Id.*

The Road Ahead

American family courts have a long history of struggle with the construct of parental alienation. However, the above litany of cases demonstrates that the phenomenon of parental alienation is not only firmly entrenched in our courts, but also the theory is also admissible through expert evidence. Parental alienation is admissible under the reliability and validity standards of *Daubert* and the general acceptance standard of *Frye*. A look at cases involving parental alienation shows how debilitating to the family unit it is and how it requires significant court intervention to remediate its affects. To establish the necessity of court intervention, expert testimony proving parental alienation and on appropriate specialized reunification programs is essential.

In order to get the court to provide the appropriate intervention, the practitioner must be able to provide the right tools to the factfinder. A good expert would be a licensed mental health professional who is knowledgeable about the peer-reviewed and other professional literature on parental alienation, who can discuss the empirical studies conducted on parental alienation, who can educate the court on the issues of reliability and validity of the research supporting the theory of parental alienation research, who can discuss both the qualitative and quantitative research on the topic, the application of appropriate measurement tools, and finally, how the available research and data informs the facts of the particular case. Additionally, the expert should be able to demonstrate the general acceptance of parental alienation in the scientific community. The expert should be prepared to discuss not only the devastating symptoms and behaviors seen in children affected by parental alienation, but also discuss the risk of inaction, importance of appropriate court intervention and proper treatment programs. If the facts of the case so necessitate, the expert should be able to show how parental alienation can cause the child to make "complaints about the parent with no specific recollection as to events causing the complaint. Such complaints will include physical, emotional, or sexual abuse with little or no substantiation."[160] The expert should discuss how each treatment option can either remediate or intensify the most common parental alienation symptoms on the child—some of which include distress, anxiety, panic, anger, and withdrawal.[161]

The practitioner should always keep in mind that the expert testimony that is to be proffered must meet the rigorous standards set forth in the tests discussed in this chapter. To be admissible, the testimony must be relevant, probative, and material. In the end, it is the responsibility of the attorney to draw out

160. *Id.*

161. 127 Am. Jur. Proof of Facts 3d 237 (Originally published in 2012). *See also*: *In re* Marriage of Bates, 212 Ill. 2d 489, 289 Ill. Dec. 218, 819 N.E.2d 714 (2004).

for the factfinder the appropriate tools and highest quality research and data to use in determining the reliability and validity of the expert's testimony. And there's plenty available. The bibliography in Dr. Amy J. L. Baker's chapter in the recent book, *Parental Alienation: Science and Law* (2020), alone attests to the fact that the results of the parental alienation research have been subjected to peer-review and have been published in peer-reviewed journals.

It is critical to understand what level of training the judge has had, how many parental alienation cases she/he has presided over, how he/she has ruled on these cases, and what evidence he/she has admitted and under what circumstances. Understanding this basic information will go a long way in determining how to get the message across. Additionally, it is critical to find an expert who can help the legal team understand the science so that the legal team is in a good position to inform and educate the court and to effectively cross-examine an opposing expert should the other side bring one to challenge the theory of parental alienation.

The identification, analysis, and intervention of parental alienation have come a long way since 1804, when the theory was first discussed in the courts of England. To misconstrue alienation as nonexistent or as an abuser's ruse helps no one and ultimately puts children at risk. As the *Bergin* court found in Maine, proper expert evidence can indeed assist the trier of fact to understand this phenomenon and its counterintuitive nature:

> The expert testified extensively as to her work in the field of parental alienation, her education, her publications, the general acceptance of the field, her previous work as an expert in judicial proceedings, and the methods that she applied in this specific case. The hearing included substantial discussions of [Mother's] role in preventing [Father] from having contact with the children, making the expert's testimony relevant, and the testimony aided the court by providing "a counterintuitive explanation as to the dynamics . . . present in [the] situation.[162]

162. Bergin, *supra* at 116.

CHAPTER 3

Interventions in Parental Alienation Cases

Parental alienation has been described in legal cases since the early 19th century and in scientific literature since the 1940s.[1] One of the most widely accepted definitions of parental alienation is a "mental condition in which a child—usually one whose parents are engaged in a high-conflict separation or divorce—allies himself or herself strongly with an alienating parent and rejects a relationship with the 'target' parent without legitimate justification."[2] When examining parental alienation, three salient features of the phenomenon come to the light. First, parental alienation is a psychological condition present in the child. For instance, a child may present with a distorted or false belief that the rejected or disfavored parent is "evil," "dangerous," or somehow unworthy of love or affection. Second, the child's rejection of the alienated or target parent is without legitimate justification. This is critical. If there is a documented history of the rejected parent being abusive or severely neglectful, the child's rejection of that parent could be legitimate and, if so, it would not be a case of parental alienation. Third, the rejected parent is not expected to be a "perfect" parent and may even have contributed to the child's dislike or hatred of him or her. Often, a rejected parent reacts to the alienation dynamic in frustration,

1. *See, e.g.*, Westmeath v. Westmeath: The wars between the Westmeaths, 1812–1857, in Stone, L. (1993). *Broken Lives: Separation and Divorce in England, 1660–1857*, Oxford Press, 284; Levy, D. M. (1943). *Maternal Overprotection*, Columbia University, 153.

2. Lorandos, D., Bernet, W., & Sauber, R. (2013). Overview of parental alienation. In Lorandos, D., Bernet, W., & Sauber, R. (Eds.), *Parental Alienation: The Handbook for Mental Health and Legal Professionals*, Charles C. Thomas, 5.

even anger. This can be a normal response to continued rejection by a child. This reaction to the sabotaging and breakdown of the parent-child relationship should not be confused with its causation. The essential feature of parental alienation remains that the child's rejection of the alienated parent is *far out of proportion* to anything that parent has done.[3]

When addressing parental alienation, family courts have generally focused on *behaviors* manifested by an alienating parent and the signs of alienation in the affected child. For instance, in *Meadows v. Meadows*, the Michigan Court of Appeals acknowledged parental alienation by focusing on the behaviors of an alienating parent: "[t]he process of one parent trying to undermine and destroy to varying degrees the relationship that the child has with the other parent."[4] Of course, the signs or symptoms of alienation present in the child are important as well, as the Tennessee Court of Appeals, in *McClain v. McClain*, found by focusing on the mental condition of the child: "The essential feature of parental alienation is that a child . . . allies himself or herself strongly with one parent (the preferred parent) and rejects a relationship with the other parent (the alienated parent) without legitimate justification."[5]

Interventions in cases of parental alienation have two primary goals. First, to correct the distortions and false perception that the alienated child harbors of the targeted or rejected parent. And, second, to reunify the alienated child with the targeted or rejected parent with a long-term aspirational goal of the child having a healthy relationship with both the parents. A child subjected to alienating behaviors has been exposed to a form of psychological or emotional abuse—regardless of the different terms used to describe these behaviors.[6] For example, Dr. Stanley Clawar, a sociologist, and Brynne Rivlin, a social worker, used the terms "programming," "brainwashing," and "indoctrination" when describing the behaviors that cause parental alienation.[7] These behaviors, the authors explain, are pathological and severely damage the relationship of the child with the other parent due to the alienating parent's jealousy, or attempting to draw the child closer due to loneliness or a desire to obtain an ally. As time progresses and the child continues to be subjected to brainwashing and programming, these techniques are also employed to control or distort information the child provides to a lawyer, judge, conciliator, relatives, friends, or third parties.[8] In a similar vein, Dr. Richard Warshak, a clinical professor of psychiatry, has written about "pathological alienation" that results from

---

3. Bernet, W. (2020). Introduction to parental alienation. In Lorandos, D., & Bernet, W. (Eds.), *Parental Alienation: Science and Law*, Charles C. Thomas, 1–2.

4. Meadows v. Meadows/Henderson, 2010 WL 3814352 (Mich. App.) (Unpublished).

5. McClain v. McClain, 539 S.W.3d 170, 182 (2017).

6. Lorandos, D., Bernet, W., & Sauber, S. R., *supra*, at 8.

7. Clawar, S., & Rivlin, B. (2013). *Children held hostage: Dealing with programmed and brainwashed children*, American Bar Association Section of Family Law.

8. *Id.* at 15.

similar alienating behaviors: [a] disturbance in which children, usually in the context of sharing a parent's negative attitudes, suffer unreasonable aversion to a person or persons with whom they formerly enjoyed normal relations or with whom they would normally develop affectionate relations.[9]

Courts have found that such brainwashing, programming, and alienating behaviors are "a form of emotional abuse that should not be tolerated."[10] A child subjected to such alienating behaviors needs urgent intervention.

Courts Intervene to Check the Emotional Abuse of Parental Alienation

Professional literature—including peer-reviewed scientific papers—and legal opinions from the family courts around the country make one thing clear: Parents (including third parties or allies of the alienating parent, such as a grandparent, aunt, uncle, sister, etc.) who manifest alienating behaviors perpetrate emotional abuse on their children. Alienating parents are abusive parents. The *Diagnostic and Statistical Manual of Mental Disorders,* Fifth Edition (DSM-5), describes child psychological abuse as "nonaccidental verbal or symbolic acts by a child's parent or caregiver that result, or have reasonable potential to result, in significant psychological harm to the child."[11] A parent's manifestation of alienating behaviors has a potential to result in and often does result in psychological harm to the child. Indeed, in the context of parental alienation, professional literature "identifies two core elements of child abuse: parental alienation as a significant form of harm to children that is attributable to human action. As a form of individual child abuse, parental alienation calls for a child protection response."[12]

Alienating parents attempt to distort their child's worldview by using tactics designed to manipulate the child and disparage the other parent or portray him or her in a false light. As Dr. Jennifer Harman, one of the leading experts in the area of parental alienation, writes together with her colleagues:

> Parental alienation refers to a child's reluctance or refusal to have a relationship with a parent . . . for illogical, untrue, or exaggerated reasons . . . While alienating behaviors will not always lead to severe parental alienation,

9. Warshak, R. (2006). Social science and parental alienation: Examining the disputes and the evidence. In Gardner, R. A., Sauber, S. R., & Lorandos, D. (Eds.), *The International Handbook of Parental Alienation Syndrome: Conceptual, Clinical and Legal Considerations*, Charles C. Thomas, 361.

10. McClain v. McClain, *supra*, at 200.

11. American Psychiatric Association. (2013). *Diagnostic and Statistical Manual of Mental Disorders* (5th ed.) (DSM-5), Author, 719.

12. Kruk, E. (2018). Parental alienation as a form of emotional child abuse: Current state of knowledge and future directions for research. *Family Science Review*, 22(4), 141–164 (page 141, emphasis added).

> which is the complete rejection and refusal of contact with the [targeted parent], they still impact the child and other parental figure in many negative ways, even in the mildest of circumstances.[13]

For the child subjected to parental alienating behaviors, it causes a significant mental disturbance and distortions, based on a false belief that the alienated parent is a dangerous and unworthy parent. The long-term consequences of this emotional abuse are immense. For instance, research shows that adults who were emotionally abused as children have a higher prevalence of intrapersonal problems, emotional problems, social competency problems, learning problems, behavioral problems, and physical health problems.[14]

Emotional abuse against children is prohibited for good reason. In *Stern-John v. John*, a Minnesota court defined child endangerment as "an 'unusually imprecise' concept[15] that encompasses danger to emotional health or development, such as risk of harm flowing from emotional abuse, including parental alienation."[16] American courts are not alone in condemning such emotional abuse of children. For instance, an Ontario court described a parent's act in alienating a child as irresponsible "and demonstrates that parent's inability to act in the best interests of their children." The Ontario court likened this alienating behavior to encouraging the child to not take care of its physical health:

> It is the responsibility of good parents to manage their children's health and safety issues without necessarily the consent or joy of their children. A healthy relationship with both parents is a health and safety issue that good parents ensure takes place.[17]

Because parental alienation is so harmful to children, it is critical to intervene in these cases and such intervention has to be swift, sufficient, and strong. Checking the ongoing emotional abuse and remedying the ill effects of alienation is critical to the child's healthy development. However, resolving family law cases involving alienation can be tricky at best. The longer the alienation has occurred, the more entrenched families become with their roles of alienator, target parent, and manipulated child. In instances where false allegations of abuse are made, the alienator and the manipulated child may release

---

13. Harman, J., Kruk, E., & Hines, D. (2018). Parental alienating behaviors: An unacknowledged form of family violence, *Psychological Bulletin*, 144(12), 1275–1276.

14. Hart, S. N., Brassard, M. R., Baker, A. J. L., & Chiel, Z. A. (2017). Psychological maltreatment of children. In Kilka, J. B., & Conte, J. R. (Eds.), *APSAC Handbook on Child Maltreatment*, Fourth Edition, Sage, 145–162 (pages 150–152).

15. SternJohn v. John, No. A18-1838, 2019 WL 3000751, at *4 (Minn. Ct. App. July 1, 2019). *See also*: Goldman, 748 N.W.2d at 285 (quotation omitted).

16. *Id. See also*: Amarreh, 918 N.W.2d at 232, Minn. Stat. § 518.18(d)(iv).

17. McAlister v. Jenkins, 2008 CarswellOnt 4266, paragraph 36.

a blitzkrieg of accusations in the hopes of forever severing the bond between the target parent and children. A Michigan court, *Harner v. Harner*, found that

> [there] was evidence of numerous, ever-growing, increasingly-egregious, and highly-suspect claims of abuse by the children that were unsubstantiated and called into question by several witnesses, giving rise to a reasonable conclusion that no abuse occurred, along with a reasonable inference that the claims were attributable to conduct, coaching, and communications by defendant, which can be properly characterized as acts fostering parental alienation.[18]

Partly because of this type of entrenchment, family therapy often is ineffective, with a more coordinated and specialized effort required of the court and experts trained to recognize and treat issues surrounding parental alienation. Parties who are in the midst of high-conflict litigation need advocates who can help the court recognize the alienating behaviors so the court can assist the family with remediation.

> The solution to post separation parenting disputes is a family justice system that mandates early intervention by judges and clinicians based on established and accepted legal principles and social science. The real issue which needs to be addressed is the conflict between the parents that prevents the children from enjoying a meaningful relationship with each of their parents postseparation.[19]

In any instance, "exposing the children to unregulated emotional turmoil, verbal denigration of the other parent, withholding access of parenting time, and a hostile atmosphere can instill fear and anxiety in a child who has very little resilience."[20] Helping the court understand what kind of intervention is needed and how to enforce it is critical to alleviating the alienation.

Recognizing Available Interventions

Courts have options when confronted with parental alienation. Before the court can determine the appropriate intervention, it must be presented with evidence supporting the severity of alienation. The severity of alienation can be measured on a spectrum: mild, moderate, or severe.

---

18. Harner v. Harner, No. 338746, 2018 WL 521863, at *4 (Mich. Ct. App. Jan. 23, 2018).

19. Fidler, B., & Bala, N. (2010). Children resisting postseparation contact with a parent: Concepts, controversies, and conundrums, *Fam. Ct. Rev.*, 48, 10.

20. Darnall, D. C. (2013). Mild cases of parental alienation. In Lorandos, D., Bernet, W., & Sauber, R. (Eds.), *Parental Alienation: The Handbook for Mental Health and Legal Professionals*, Charles C. Thomas.

> The level of severity of the [parent child contact problem] will depend on duration, frequency, and intensity of child and parent behaviors, the child's age, maturity, and vulnerability, and the other factors in the circle diagram. Indices of the type and severity may be found in the child's behavior, the parent's behavior, or the outcome of resistance or rejection.[21]

Understanding the severity of the parental alienation is important because the intervention is different depending on the severity. Courts have ordered a variety of therapies, treatment programs, no contact orders, and changes in custody in attempt to alleviate and remedy parental alienation. Throughout the years, both legal and mental health professionals have surveyed and evaluated what remedial options work best for alienation and under which circumstances. When early intervention is possible and the alienation is mild, family therapy may be successful. Mild parental alienation refers to "situations in which the child objects to and criticizes the target parent but yet enjoys the presence of the target parent once time passes or the location is no longer in close proximity to the alienating parent."[22]

In fact, early identification of potential alienation cases is one way the court system can help to resolve the phenomenon of parental alienation. At its early stages, there is a lot a court can do to curb its growth. For instance, the court can craft parenting plan orders, rigorously enforce court orders, and provide parents with education and resources with an eye towards addressing any alienation issues. Research suggests that

> [f]ormalizing the parents' consent to treatment in a court order is often prudent, because as previously noted, it is difficult to know in advance which cases may become severe, and usually, the longer the alienation lasts, the worse it gets and more difficult it becomes to remedy, even if there is reconciliation many years later.[23]

The best resolution of mild and moderate alienation cases is to catch them in early stages, often through judicial exhortation, encouragement of counseling, and enforcement of a settlement. This, however, requires an early identification of high conflict cases and cases involving alienating behaviors, coupled with proactive case management at the pre-resolution, resolution, and enforcement stages.[24]

---

21. Fidler, B., & Bala, N. (2020). Concepts, controversies and conundrums of "alienation": Lessons learned in a decade and reflections on challenges ahead, *Fam. Ct. Rev.*, 58, 576, 580.

22. Darnall, D. C. (2013). Mild cases of parental alienation. In Lorandos, D., Bernet, W., & Sauber, R. (Eds.), *Parental Alienation: The Handbook for Mental Health and Legal Professionals*, Charles C. Thomas.

23. Fidler, B., & Bala, N. (2020). Concepts, controversies and conundrums of "alienation": Lessons learned in a decade and reflections on challenges ahead, *Fam. Ct. Rev.*, 58, 576, 580.

24. *Id. See also* (Martinson, 2010).

In reality, however, parties come to court already entrenched in the thick of an embittered alienation struggle. Once the alienation passes this threshold and is entrenched, more aggressive intervention measures are warranted. At this point, traditional therapies almost never work.[25] Research suggests the more severe the alienation, the "more interventionist solutions" must be engaged "if long lasting and meaningful change (second order), not only surface or superficial change (first order), is to come about."[26] This is because behavioral changes can often "precipitate a shift in attitudes and emotions."[27] As exasperating as it is for everyone involved, it is critical to remain vigilant and challenge the alienating behavior at every turn. This requires intensive therapy and enforcement measures. The court interventions must first address the safety, permanence, and well-being of the alienated child. In a child abuse and neglect construct, this is often accomplished by providing mental health psychoeducational services to the family and through a temporary or permanent separation of children from an unsafe or risky environment. Court ordered services "should be considered safety strategies because they are intended not only to remediate the harm due to past [child abuse and neglect] but also to lower the risk of future [child abuse and neglect]."[28] These interventions are "only as good as the level of family participation."[29] Because "many parents . . . dispute the contention that they are abusive or neglectful,"[30] successful intervention requires "specific efforts to overcome barriers to participation."[31] When a court orders specific intervention, the alienating parent's insight into his or her behaviors and compliance with the treatment must be evaluated because better insight is "associated with . . . lowered assessed clinical risk of maltreatment."[32] The critical factor involved is "the impact that condition has on parenting abilities."[33] Parents who are repeat offenders and are simply unable to refrain from "a repeated pattern" of "interfering with or directly undermining the child's important relationships" are upsetting the "child's basic psychological needs."[34] Such behavior has been identified as "exploiting/corrupting" psychological maltreatment and is associated with encouraging a child to "develop

25. *Id.*

26. *Id. See also* (Watzlawick, Weakland, & Fisch, 1974).

27. *Id.*

28. Berliner et al. (2015). Report of the APSAC task force on evidence-based service planning guidelines for child welfare, *Child Maltreatment*, 20(1), 6–16 (at 7).

29. *Id.* at 9, 14.

30. *Id.* at 9.

31. *Id.* at 14.

32. Montgomery, S. A., & Street, D. F. (2011). Visitation arrangements for impaired parents, *Child and Adolescent Psychiatric Clinics of North America*, 20(3), 295–503 (at 500–501).

33. *Id.* at 495.

34. American Professional Society on the Abuse of Children. (2017). *Practice Guidelines: The Investigation and Determination of Suspected Psychological Maltreatment of Children and Adolescents*, APSAC, https://www.apsac.org/9235fgnl8, 4.

inappropriate behaviors and attitudes."[35] In the end, whatever intervention is used, it must be aimed at contact and reunification with the rejected parent. "The collective weight of the literature, despite limitations such as small sample sizes and lack of random assignment to treatment conditions, suggests that contact with the rejected parent is essential to healing a damaged parent-child relationship . . . Sending a child for what they are calling 'reconciliation therapy' for an hour a week is never going to work if the child is then returned to the programmer for the other 167 hours in that week."[36]

Early Intervention and Prevention

Custody cases need individualized approaches. From a case management perspective, when a case enters the judicial system, it is important to assess the risk factors for parental alienation. This is because

> the inception of alienation may be very subtle; it may begin with a disapproving frown at the mention of the other parent's name, refusal to acquiesce to the child's request for additional time, refusal to give the child private time for phone calls, or irrational criticism about the target parent's parenting skills.[37]

In fact, "[t]hese divorce and parental conflict-related alignments, which may not be unjustified initially, may, if not remedied early on, develop into alienation where the child's reaction becomes disproportionate to the reality of their experience with the rejected parent."[38] To properly assess for parental alienation, a court has a variety of assessment tools at its disposal. For example, a comprehensive evaluation focusing on issues related to parental alienation, estrangement, enmeshment, and child alignment may be helpful.

> A comprehensive evaluation must take into account different assessment techniques including interviews, standardized instruments, parenting and personality assessments, collateral sources, observations of parent-child interaction, review of documents, family histories, and so on, as well as new instruments that are being developed for PA screening.[39]

---

35. *Id.*

36. Warshak, R. A. (2020). Risks and realities of working with alienated children, *Fam. Ct. Rev.*, 58, 432, 438.

37. Darnall, D. C. (2013). Mild cases of parental alienation. In Lorandos, D., Bernet, W., & Sauber, R. (Eds.), *Parental Alienation: The Handbook for Mental Health and Legal Professionals*, Charles C. Thomas.

38. Fidler, B., & Bala, N. (2010). Children resisting postseparation contact with a parent: Concepts, controversies, and conundrums, *Fam. Ct. Rev.*, 48, 10.

39. Worenklein, A. (2013). Moderate cases of parental alienation. In Lorandos, D., Bernet, W., & Sauber, R. (Eds.), *Parental Alienation: The Handbook for Mental Health and Legal Professionals*, Charles C. Thomas.

However, this usually requires stringent case management on the part of the court, and greater advocacy on behalf of the targeted or rejected parent. It is critical for the attorney representing the targeted or rejected parent to not fall prey to the common fallacies and pitfalls that compromise and undermine the outcomes in litigating cases of parental alienation.[40] "Identifying the early signs of alienation is a precursor to preventing moderate to severe alienating behavior from occurring."[41] On the one hand, the court could preemptively create parenting orders with the back thought of preventing alienation issues. It would follow then that the court would strictly enforce its orders. Early enforcement of all court orders sends the implicit but clear message to both parties—and the children—that orders are meant to be followed. Court orders that are flouted with impunity or not adhered to are meaningless and not worth the paper they are printed on.

Equally important is the urgency for courts to keep the child's best interests above the child's wishes, which may sometimes conflict. What a minor child wants may not be what's in the child's best interests—especially in a case where the child has been manipulated, brainwashed, programmed, and alienated by a parent to reject the other parent. A North Dakota court reversed a modification that relied on the child's wishes instead of the child's best interests: "the court may not rely solely on the child's wishes in visitation enforcement and modification actions, but the child's wishes and evidence of parental alienation are factors that may be considered in the best interest of the child analysis."[42] Similarly, a Michigan Court of Appeals recently affirmed a trial court's disregard of the testimony of two alienated children when the court found that the children, having being manipulated and alienated, were unable to express a reasonable preference.[43]

Providing guidance on what is helpful in alienation cases, a Louisiana court, in *Palazzolo v. Mire*[44] stated:

> [W]hat helps is early prevention of alienation, a good assessment of the multiple factors that contribute to alienation within the child and family, clear court orders that affirm parental rights and restore an appropriate access plan (one that the child can tolerate); ongoing case management, and family-focused therapy (not just parent-child reunification). What

40. *See* Chapter 9, *infra*.

41. Darnall, D. C. (2013). Mild cases of parental alienation. In Lorandos, D., Bernet, W., & Sauber, R. (Eds.), *Parental Alienation: The Handbook for Mental Health and Legal Professionals*, Charles C. Thomas.

42. Votava v. Votava, 2015 ND 171, ¶ 15, 865 N.W.2d 821, 825. *See also* Lind v. Lind, 2014 ND 70, ¶ 14, 844 N.W.2d 907; Loll v. Loll, 1997 ND 51, ¶¶ 15–16, 561 N.W.2d 625; *see also* Milligan v. Milligan, 149 So.3d 623, 628 (Ala.Civ.App.2014) (holding that under the circumstances the trial court abused its discretion when it allowed teenage children to determine whether they would visit their father).

43. Brown v. Pentoney, No. 349532 LCNo. 12-108147-DM (Mich. Court of Appeals, May 7, 2020).

44. Palazzolo v. Mire, 10 So.3d 748 (2009).

> hurts is to do nothing, long delays where the child has no contact with the rejected parent, draconian punishments and threats, "parentectomies" (severing the child's relationship with the aligned parent abruptly), ongoing litigation in the adversarial legal system, and total disregard for the child's ongoing distress or the teenager's need to have some choice in those more difficult cases that are resistant to resolution.[45]

Early intervention no doubt is helpful. On the other hand, an ounce of prevention is worth the pound of cure. Parents could be required to obtain education on the harmful effects of alienation on the child and on the family.

> Sometimes alienating parents will get defensive if they are made to feel they are to blame for their behavior, but parents engaged in mild alienation are typically receptive to education once the behavior is pointed out to them in a supportive and gentle manner.[46]

It may be helpful to offer divorce and custody litigants an opportunity to attend education classes upon filing for divorce or custody. When discussing education programs available for parents, some experts have noted that

> these programs provide information about the effects of separation on children, and tend to emphasize the importance of parental communication and co-operation, while recognizing the need to protect children from parental conflict, violence, and abuse. Most of these programs, however, offer only a few hours of didactic education, and have value only if parental conflict is relatively low and parents are able to focus on the interests of their children.[47]

The alienating strategies deployed by some parents are crippling weapons that are used without thinking of the harmful effects such strategies or behaviors can have on the child. Proper education would promote the idea of putting the child first, enabling a healthier post-separation family dynamic. When the severity of alienation is mild, parents are more likely to be able to change their behavior with education.[48]

---

45. *Id.* (quoting from Johnston, J. R. (2005). Children of divorce who reject a parent and refuse visitation: Recent research and social policy implications for the alienated child, *Fam. L.Q.*, 38, 757, 774–775).

46. Darnall, D. C. (2013). Mild cases of parental alienation. In Lorandos, D., Bernet, W., & Sauber, R. (Eds.), *Parental Alienation: The Handbook for Mental Health and Legal Professionals*, Charles C. Thomas.

47. Fidler, B., & Bala, N. (2020). Concepts, controversies and conundrums of "alienation": Lessons learned in a decade and reflections on challenges ahead, *Fam. Ct. Rev.*, 58, 576, 580.

48. Darnall, D. C. (2013). Mild cases of parental alienation. In Lorandos, D., Bernet, W., & Sauber, R. (Eds.), *Parental Alienation: The Handbook for Mental Health and Legal Professionals*, Charles C. Thomas.

Traditional Therapy Does Not Work in Resolving Parental Alienation

Targeted parents who have been victims of alienation when subjected to traditional therapy sessions together with their alienated children feel trapped. It is tantamount to living one's life in a surreal manner reminiscent of *Groundhog Day*. Alienated children never run out of excuses for not wanting to see or have a relationship with the targeted parent. More often than not, these excuses have no connection with reality and are a result of the alienating parent's brainwashing, programming, and manipulation of the child. The therapist, working in the classic clinical mode, attempts to validate the child's feelings, emotions, and perceptions, and this usually leads to the child being further entrenched in the distortions. It is like a never-ending rollercoaster ride that targeted parents are desperate to get off. Severely alienated children often lack critical thinking skills thanks to the ongoing manipulation of the alienating parent.[49] The relationship between the alienating parent and the alienated child has been likened to a cult leader and his followers.[50] When a child has been this severely alienated, the child's ability to mislead legal and mental health professionals increases.[51] At this degree of alienation, traditional therapy is often ineffective. This is troubling because family law practitioners and courts often advocate counseling or "therapy" to litigants. It is also usually a judge's first tool of choice in trying to resolve a conflict: Kids do not want to see the mom or dad? Go work it out in therapy!

In the 2010 Ohio case *Rooney v. Rooney*,[52] it was found that the mother had engaged in parental alienation. The expert

> rated Mother's degree of parental alienation as somewhere between mild and moderate. The doctor discussed parental alienation and the negative effects it has on the child's relationship with the parent being alienated as well as the child's future relationships with others. [The expert] noted research has shown traditional therapy does not work in parental alienation cases, and the only solution in the instant matter was a change of custody. In his opinion, a change of custody of the children would be less harmful to them than the continued alienation.[53]

Even children who are moderately alienated are almost always involved in a "significant campaign of denigration, particularly at transition times." Their

49. Reay, K. M. (2015). Family reflections: A promising therapeutic program designed to treat severely alienated children and their family system, *American Journal of Family Therapy*, 43, 197–207 (at 205).

50. *Id.*

51. *Id.*

52. Rooney v. Rooney, 2010-Ohio-2439, ¶ 8.

53. *Id.*

malevolence towards the target parent is not as pervasive as a severely alienated child, though.

In alienation cases, research demonstrates that traditional therapy, while children remain under the care of their favored parent, is unlikely to repair the strained parent-child relationship and in fact, may make things worse.[54] Why? One reason why phobia-reduction techniques fail to overcome children's refusal to spend time with a parent is that most of these children, except preschoolers, do not really fear their rejected parent. If they act "frightened" of the parent, often this is a ruse to avoid contact and a result of the loyalty-bind that the children are trapped in. The lack of genuine fear is evident in the children's uninhibited denigration, expressions of hatred, and disrespect toward the rejected parent, as opposed to the obsequious or withdrawn behavior typical of children's interactions with a feared adult.[55]

Counterintuitive it may seem, but often an alienated child's anger towards the rejected parent masquerades as "fear." "Alienated children hold on to their anger and use the anger to rationalize and perpetuate the hatred. If a child's anger appears to be out of proportion to the offense and the healing never happens, one has to ask who or what is preventing the healing from occurring."[56] Traditional therapy can magnify and solidify the animosity and hatred that the alienated child feels towards the target parent. Another noteworthy roadblock to therapy with an alienating parent is the "bias that therapists have, which is believing that our clients are always truthful."[57] Instead of helping, this bias reinforces the alienating parent's ability to manipulate the situation. It is critical, when court ordering treatment, that the judge is aware of any biases between the therapist and the alienator. As former judge, Hon. Michele Lowrance, who spent a long time adjudicating contentious matrimonial cases in one of the busiest family courts in the country, found:

> I have seen traditional therapists allow the child to determine how long it will be (if ever) before they agree to see the target parent. Because the child is aligned with the alienating parent, they are emotionally required to keep rejecting contact with the target parent. Remember, alienated chil-

54. Warshak, R. A. (2015). Ten parental alienation fallacies that compromise decisions in court and in therapy, Prof'l Psychol.: Research & Practice, 46, 235. *Id.* at 243 (citing Weir, K., & Sturge, C. (2006). Clinical advice to courts on children's contact with their parents following parental separation, *Child and Adolescent Mental Health*, 11, 40; Fidler, B., & Bala, N. (2010). Children resisting postseparation contact with a parent: Concepts, controversies, and conundrums, *Fam. Ct. Rev.*, 48, 10; Garber, B. (2013). Cognitive-behavioral methods in high-conflict divorce: Systematic desensitization adapted to parent-child reunification interventions, *Family Court Review*, 53, 96; and others).

55. *Id.* at 243.

56. *Id.*

57. Darnall, D. C. (2013). Mild cases of parental alienation. In Lorandos, D., Bernet, W., & Sauber, R. (Eds.), *Parental Alienation: The Handbook for Mental Health and Legal Professionals*, Charles C. Thomas.

dren are often told that if they are nice to the target parent, it could be used "against" them in court.[58]

Reunification, Not Therapy

Reunification, "reunification therapy," or "reunification counseling," is a relatively new term that is gaining traction in the family courts. It is important to understand that reunification is *not* therapy. In his recent book, *Parent-Child Reunification,* Dr. Stanley S. Clawar writes:

> Reunification is a special type of intervention that is not, per se, psychotherapy (clinical); it is not family therapy, nor is it any other type of the presently practiced (forensic) therapeutic interventions. This is important to know because many therapists who come from different schools of thoughts and methodologies are applying their particular brand of therapy to this social and legal dilemma—usually without much success.[59]

There is confusion amongst legal practitioners and, at times, even mental health professionals between traditional psychotherapy and court-ordered reunification. The latter refers to a forensic setting in which the process and the professional providing the services are accountable to the court. Eminent forensic psychologist, Dr. S. Richard Sauber, has offered a detailed comparison chart, comparing traditional therapy with reunification.[60] Some primary distinctions between the two are presented below:

Issue	Psychotherapy	Reunification
1. Whose client is patient/ litigant?	Mental health practitioner	Court retains the jurisdiction and maintains accountability
2. Applicable privilege	Therapist-patient privilege	Informed consent and court order for full disclosure and non-confidentiality to ensure accountability
3. Who pays?	Patient or family member or insurance	Predetermined by a court order; insurance coverage unlikely

58. Lowrance, M. (2013). A judge's perspective on parental alienation. In Lorandos, D., Bernet, W., & Sauber, R. (Eds.), *Parental Alienation: The Handbook for Mental Health and Legal Professionals,* Charles C. Thomas, 503.

59. Clawar, S. (2020). *Parent-Child Reunification–A Guide to Legal and Forensic Strategies,* ABA, 2.

60. Sauber, S. R. (2013). Reunification planning and therapy. In Lorandos, D., Bernet, W., & Sauber, R. (Eds.), *Parental Alienation: The Handbook for Mental Health and Legal Professionals,* Charles C. Thomas.

Issue	Psychotherapy	Reunification
4. Goals	Goals are mutually determined between the therapist and the patient	Court defines the objective of reunification
5. Process variables	Addressing specific symptoms or behaviors	Overcoming visitation refusal, fears, or phobias of reconciliation with target parent and correction or reframing of foundation for the rejection
6. Selection of the therapist/professional	Self-referral	Through court process
7. Attitude of the therapist/ professional	Supportive, empathetic	Direct, neutral, objective, detached, goal-driven without distraction or deviation
8. Degree of alliance	A helping relationship; allies or advocacy, rarely confrontational or adversarial	A helping relationship based upon judicial findings of facts, detailed documentation, external pressure for compliance together with consequences for non-compliance
9. Role of historical truth	Patient report with minimum external scrutiny	Litigant information supplemented with and verified by collateral sources. Often, findings of court after a trial or an evidentiary hearing
10. Criteria for success	Patient satisfaction	Ability for alienated child and target parent to be able to interact and maintain a consistent visitation schedule; reestablish a strong emotional bond and attachment with one another

The aim of reunification is to repair or rehabilitate a "fragmentation of the family unit."[61] The goals of reunification can move beyond the initial reunification and can include

> facilitating global healthy child adjustment and coping mechanisms. This includes correcting the child's distorted and polarized views and

61. *Id.*

> replacing them with more realistic views of each parent, improving the child's healthy relationships with both parents, addressing divorce-related stress, boundaries and age-appropriate autonomy and restoring adequate parenting, co-parenting and parent-child roles.[62]

This is usually accomplished by starting with an initial obligatory visit between the parent and the child, then progressing to a fun, shared activity; and eventually reliving the time-sharing as if it were in the "'good old days' of a genuine, mutually expressed, loving, and caring relationship."[63]

In the 2019 Oregon case *Al-Ani v. Wafeek,*[64] the court described this case as "the worst case of parental alienation of my legal career." Initially, the court found the mother to be the primary parent and awarded her custody. But, because mother had severely alienated the child from the father, even to the point of "brainwashing," the court required that both parties, along with the child, participate in reunification therapy, designed to rebuild father's relationship with the child. The court deferred a determination of parenting time until after the completion of the reunification therapy. In the end, and pointedly because of mother's noncompliance, the court awarded custody to the father, with limited parenting time to the mother. In some cases of severe alienation, therapy may have to be suspended and the courts may have to think about other "elective interventions that provide transformative experiences that help children relinquish negative attitudes while saving face."[65]

If counseling or therapy—of whatever kind—is not helping and appears to aggravate the situation, the therapist may feel ethically bound to inform the court that treatment should be discontinued.[66] This was the case in a 2019 Florida case, *Foreman v. James,*[67] where the court expressed "exasperation with the reunification efforts and announced his intention to order the parties to participate in the Family Bridges program. . . . The trial judge expressed how the child's alienation from the Father was causing long-term emotional damage to the child."[68] In cases involving alienation, the child must be reunified with the target parent. To increase the success of reunification, it is critical that the court issue orders that explicitly state "it is in the best interest of the alienated child to be reunified and resume contact with the previously target parent."[69]

---

62. Fidler, B., & Bala, N. (2010). Children resisting postseparation contact with a parent: Concepts, controversies, and conundrums, *Fam. Ct. Rev.*, 48, 10.

63. Sauber, S. R. (2013). Reunification planning and therapy. In Lorandos, D., Bernet, W., & Sauber, R. (Eds.), *Parental Alienation: The Handbook for Mental Health and Legal Professionals*, Charles C. Thomas.

64. Al-Ani v. Wafeek, 300 Or.App. 710, 712 (2019).

65. Warshak, R., *supra* at 243, 245.

66. *Id.* at 244.

67. Foreman v. James, 2019 WL 4854380 (Fla. Ct. App., 2019).

68. *Id.* at 1.

69. Worenklein, A. (2013). Moderate cases of parental alienation. In Lorandos, D., Bernet, W., & Sauber, R. (Eds.), *Parental Alienation: The Handbook for Mental Health and Legal Professionals*, Charles C. Thomas.

Additionally, in some mild to moderate cases of parental alienation, it may be just as important to involve the alienating parent with the reunification process if the alienating parent has demonstrated an understanding of the harm such behaviors cause and is genuinely open to psychoeducational counseling. In some instances, isolating the alienating parent has shown to "exacerbate the intensity of the dynamics, leading to a greater degree of anxiety and a resulting increase in alienation."[70] Again, the methodology and effectiveness of the reunification is linked to the severity of the alienation.

In addition, it is crucial that the reunification therapist provide detailed progress to the court, so a conjoined effort can be made between the legal and mental health systems to 1) effectively remediate the alienation and 2) control the alienating parent's ability to manipulate or sabotage the process. In cases where reunification was unsuccessful, it is typically due to the alienating parent's interference with the reunification process. For instance, in *D.B. v. M.B.V.*,[71] an Indiana court conducted hearings wherein an expert testified that he had worked with the family for several years. The expert had conducted a custody evaluation and reunification therapy. In the expert's opinion, reunification between the father and his children was undermined by the mother's "systematic alienation of the children from their father."[72] The expert testified that his observations of the children's aggression toward the father in that the children would "bait, taunt, and insult" the father. The expert finally "expressed concerns that unsupervised parenting time would subject the father to the risk of false accusations of abuse and possible arrests."[73] Ultimately, a reunification plan will be dependent on a comprehensive family evaluation and a finding of whether the case is of mild, moderate, or severe alienation. Each case will require an independent analysis to come up with a proper reunification strategy.

Specialized Intensive Treatment Programs: The SWAT Teams to Combat Severe Parental Alienation

One effective solution when confronting severe cases of alienation is to order the family to partake in an intensive treatment program, such as Family Bridges or Turning Points for Families. These types of programs require restricting contact or temporarily ceasing contact between the alienating parent and the child while the target parent and child are reunited and educated through

70. *Id.*
71. D.B. v. M.B.V., 913 N.E.2d 1271, 1273 (Ind.App. 2009).
72. *Id.*
73. *Id.*

a program designed to restructure the alienated child's concept of the target parent. Contrary to what some may believe, research shows us that "[o]nce children are removed from the favored parent, and any other extended family members involved in the alienation dynamics, they begin to feel emotionally safe and steadfastly reconnect with the rejected parent."[74] This is true even if initial transient stress is present.[75] Experts have witnessed the magnitude of alienated children's resilience and the speed with which they recover their submerged ability to reconnect with the rejected parent once a court orders them to be placed with the rejected parent and suspend contact with the favored parent for a temporary period.[76] In order for intensive treatment programs such as Family Bridges to work, "intervention for parental alienation needs to be court-mandated . . . with court sanctions for non-compliance."[77] This is because many alienating parents "have come to believe during prolonged litigation that noncompliance with court orders . . . brings no negative consequences."[78] Additionally, it sends the implicit message to the alienated child that the law and authority need not be respected.[79] Moreover, intensive treatment programs protect the child from the alienator's psychological abuse. "If the court determines that the favored parent's behavior constitutes psychological abuse of the children or creates an extremely unhealthy environment, a no-contact order protects children from further mistreatment."[80] Even when the court determines alienation exists, but does not rise to the level of abuse, a no-contact order for the duration of the treatment is essential because the child will require protection from the "constant cues, communications, attitudes, and influence that undermine the children's relationship with the other parent."[81]

---

74. Reay, K. M. (2015). Family reflections: A promising therapeutic program designed to treat severely alienated children and their family system, *American Journal of Family Therapy*, 43, 197–207 (at 205).

75. Templer, K., Matthewson, M., Haines, J., & Cox, G. (2017). Recommendations for best practice in response to parental alienation: Findings from a systematic review, *Journal of Family Therapy*, 39(1), 103–122 (at 118). Citing to: Dunne, J., & Hedrick, M. (1994). The parental alienation syndrome: An analysis of sixteen selected cases, *Journal of Divorce and Remarriage*, 21, 21–38; Gardner, R. A. (2001). Should courts order PAS children to visit/reside with the alienated parent? A follow up study, *American Journal of Forensic Psychology*, 19, 61–106.

76. Warshak, R. (2013). Severe cases of parental alienation. In Lorandos, D., Bernet, W., & Sauber, R. (Eds.), *Parental Alienation: The Handbook for Mental Health and Legal Professionals*, Charles C. Thomas.

77. Templer, K., Matthewson, M., Haines, J., & Cox, G. (2017). Recommendations for best practice in response to parental alienation: Findings from a systematic review, *Journal of Family Therapy*, 39(1), 103–122 (at 115).

78. Kelly, J. B. (2010). Commentary on "Family Bridges: Using insights from social science to reconnect parents and alienated children" (Warshak, 2010), *Family Court Review*, 48(1), 81–90 (at 85).

79. *Id.*

80. Warshak, R. A. (June 12–13, 2014). Parental alienation: What it is; How to manage it. In The University of Texas School of Law AAML, Texas Chapter (Ed.), *Innovations—Breaking Boundaries in Custody Litigation*, Author, 27.

81. *Id.*

It is a documented fact that alienated children suffer from severe behavioral, emotional, and cognitive impairments.[82] Specialized reunification programs (which are radically different from "therapy") are designed to repair the damaged relationship between alienated parents and the children. They often require a temporary no-contact period between the favored parent and the children, together with the parent's compliance with some conditions before the resumption of regular contact. Resumption of contact is dependent on the favored parent's willingness and demonstrated ability to modify his or her alienating behaviors—behaviors that would no doubt sabotage the gains made during the reunification program in an absence of a no-contact order. Also, "optimal timing" to resume regular contact would depend on a number of factors,

> such as the favored parent's ability to modify behaviors that create difficulties for the children, the children's vulnerability to feeling pressured to realign with a parent, the duration of the alienation or estrangement prior to the Workshop, and the favored parent's past conduct and compliance with court orders.[83]

In cases of severe parental alienation, experienced and knowledgeable clinicians recommend "a period of 3–6 months before regular contacts resume" between a formerly favored parent and the child "to allow a child to consolidate gains and work through the numerous issues that arise in living with the rejected parent free from the influence of the favored parent."[84] While the regular (unsupervised) contact is held off for a limited period, therapeutically monitored contacts between a formerly favored parent and child may occur sooner.[85] It is critical to understand why family courts order the temporary no-contact periods between the favored parent who has been found to have engaged in alienating behaviors and the child. When contact resumes, it usually occurs first during sessions with a professional who can monitor its impact upon the child who is going through (or has just been through) a reunification program. Such precautions are necessary because research demonstrates that it is *very* hard for alienating parents to change their behaviors. If contact is restored prematurely or without proper safeguards, the children become "re-alienated," reverting to their old behaviors and back to rejecting the target parent.[86] The pathology of parental alienation is so severe that some alienators chose to go for months "without seeing [their] children or working towards

82. Warshak, R. (2013). Severe cases of parental alienation. In Lorandos, D., Bernet, W., & Sauber, R. (Eds.), *Parental Alienation: The Handbook for Mental Health and Legal Professionals*, Charles C. Thomas, 5.
83. Warshak, R. (2010), *supra*, at FN 95.
84. *Id.*
85. *Id.*
86. *Id.* at 69.

meeting conditions for renewal of contact."[87] Some refuse to cooperate with court orders and want "no contact with [the] children because [they] take their [the children's] reconciliation with [the target parent] as a personal rejection."[88] Some "chose to cut off all contact with [the child] and said that when the boy turns 18 he could choose to renew contact."[89]

Separating Children from an Alienating Parent Is Not Traumatic

In court, it is often argued that because an alienated child is so aligned—so "close" or so "bonded"—with the alienating parent, abrupt removal from the alienating parent's care will be "traumatic" for the child. This is nonsense and, at best, pure speculation. More often than not, such argument is intended to chill an otherwise incendiary judicial response to parental alienation and stop the psychological abuse being perpetrated on the alienated child.

Research demonstrates that alienation *abates* when children are required to spend time with the parent they claim to hate or fear.[90] Despite this, lawyers, guardians ad litem, children's attorneys, and other court-involved professionals predict dire consequences to children if the court fails to endorse their strong and strident preferences to avoid a parent. Usually such predictions "are vulnerable to reliability challenges because the experts cite undocumented anecdotes, irrelevant research, and discredited interpretations of attachment theory."[91] A court, when presented with such "sky is falling" predictions, should remember the following three salient facts: (1) no peer-reviewed study has documented harm to severely alienated children from the reversal of custody; (2) no study has reported that adults, who as children complied with expectations to repair a damaged relationship with a parent, later regretted having been obliged to do so; and (3) studies of adults who were allowed to disown a parent find that they regretted that decision and reported long-term problems with guilt and depression that they attributed to having been allowed to reject one of their parents.[92] Professionals who attempt to persuade courts to not separate children from an alienating parent (or oppose a temporary no-contact order between the alienating parent and the children) generally cite attachment theory to support their predictions of "trauma" or psychological damage to children. Such arguments are flawed, misleading, and "rooted in research with children who

87. *Id.*

88. *Id.*

89. *Id.*

90. Warshak, R. A. (2015). Ten parental alienation fallacies that compromise decisions in court and in therapy, *Prof'l Psychol.: Research & Practice*, 46, 235–249.

91. *Id.*

92. *Id.*, citing Baker, A. L. J. (2005). The long-term effects of parental alienation on adult children: A qualitative research study, *American Journal of Family Therapy*, 33, 289–302.

experienced prolonged institutional care as a result of being orphaned or separated from their families for other—often severely traumatic—reasons."[93] A consensus of leading authorities on attachment and divorce shows that this theory does not support generalizing the negative outcomes of traumatized children who lose *both* parents to a case involving parental alienation, where children leave one parent's home to spend time with their other parent, under a court order.[94]

Attorneys for targeted parents should challenge these professionals who argue against the no-contact orders to unpack their evocative jargon if they attempt to dissuade a court from intervening in an alienation case by using terms like "trauma" and "attachment."[95] When these professionals predict that the child will be "traumatized," what they usually mean is that the child will be "unsettled."[96] Such pessimistic predictions not only lack empirical support but are blissfully ignorant of (or perhaps, willfully blind to) the well-documented benefits of removing a child from an alienating parent whose behavior is considered psychologically abusive.[97] Sure, removing a child from a drug-infested household would no doubt cause anxiety to the child and the whole experience may be unsettling. But would a court or protective services workers hesitate to remove a child from a home when confronted with strong evidence of drug abuse or other dangerous behaviors manifested by a parent? Science tells us—and courts have agreed—that parental alienation is psychological or emotional abuse. Research has demonstrated that the harms associated with psychological abuse or maltreatment are equal and sometimes more than other forms of abuse, including physical and sexual abuse.[98] Effective interventions—including separating the child from an alienating parent and temporarily suspending contact between the two—provide experiences that help uncover the positive bond between the child and the targeted parent. "These experiences can help [the children] to create a new narrative about their lives, one that is more cohesive, more hopeful, and allows them to begin to see themselves in a new place."[99] In *Martin*, the Michigan Court of Appeals acknowledged how alienation behaviors are alarming and psychologically abusive: "[T]hese are not minor disputes over contempt and parenting time. These are matters that could have a significant effect on the child's life, including on her long-term mental and emotional

93. *Id.*, citing Ludolph, P. S., & Dale, M. D. (2012). Attachment in child custody: An additive factor, not a determinative one, *Family Law Quarterly*, 46, 1–40.

94. *Id.*

95. *Id.*

96. *Id.*, citing Zervopoulos, J. A. (2013). *How to Examine Mental Health Experts*, American Bar Association.

97. Clawar, S., & Rivlin, B., *supra.*

98. Spinazzola, J. et al. (2014). Unseen wounds: The contribution of psychological maltreatment to child and adolescent mental health and risk outcomes, *Psychol. Trauma: Theory Res. Prac. & Pol'y*, 6(S1), at S18.

99. *Id.*, citing Norton, C. L. (2011). Reinventing the wheel: From talk therapy to innovative interventions. In Norton, C. L. (Ed.), *Innovative Interventions in Child and Adolescent Mental Health*, Routledge, 2.

health: having to maintain the perception of hatred and contempt toward her father—which she may or may not share with her mother—will undoubtedly affect her mental and emotional health as well as her long-term relationship with her father."[100] Given the significant damage to children who remain alienated from a parent, removing the child from an alienating parent's custody and entering a temporary no-contact order between the two is ultimately "far less harsh or extreme than a decision that consigns a child to lose a parent and extended family under the toxic influence of the other parent who failed to recognize and support the child's need for two parents."[101]

Modification of the Custodial Environment

In cases involving severe alienation, courts have modified custody if it is the best interest of the alienated child.[102] A review of cases from trial and appellate courts around the country demonstrates that family courts have not shied away from changing custody when presented with evidence of parental alienation.[103] Considering both the short- and long-term consequences alienation has on the child, it is not surprising that the courts have changed custody. The risks associated with a change of custody are minimal and the risk of allowing the child to continue to be in the care and custody of an alienating parent are severe. It is not acceptable to err on the side of complacency when a child is being emotionally abused. Research suggests that

> a significant concern in addition to the child not having a relationship with the rejected parent and often the entire extended family, is the alienating parents' intrusive and overprotective parenting and the exploitation, indoctrination, induction of fear and hatred and, in some cases, paranoia, in children. Important distinctions need to be made between the strength and quality of an attachment; a strong bond does not necessary mean it is healthy.[104]

100. Martin v. Martin (Michigan), *supra*, at 9.

101. Warshak, R. (2015), *supra*, at 244.

102. *See*, generally, Lorandos, D. (2020). Parental alienation in U.S. courts, 1985 to 2018. In Lorandos, D., & Bernet, W. (Eds.), *Parental Alienation: Science and Law*, Charles C. Thomas, 365–385.

103. Lorandos, D. (2013). Parental alienation and North American law. In Lorandos, D., Bernet, W., & Sauber, R. (Eds.), *Parental Alienation: The Handbook for Mental Health and Legal Professionals*, Charles C. Thomas, 348–424.

104. Fidler, B., & Bala, N. (2010). Children resisting postseparation contact with a parent: Concepts, controversies, and conundrums, *Fam. Ct. Rev.*, 48, 10.

Research also shows that "environmental changes may be very effective in helping children overcome unreasonable negative attitudes."[105] In fact, the benefits of changing custody in cases of severe alienation show an improvement of "90 percent of 400 cases in which an increase in the child's contact with the target parent was court ordered."[106]

For a court to grant a change in custody, a party usually must show either proper cause or a substantial change in circumstances requiring such modification. Evidence of parental alienation satisfies the threshold and provides proper cause and a substantial change of circumstances. For instance, as held by a Minnesota court, "A majority of courts, including Minnesota courts, agree that a sustained course of conduct by one parent designed to diminish a child's relationship with the other parent is unacceptable and may be grounds for denying or modifying custody."[107] Parental alienation "can justify a post-dissolution request for a modification of a time-sharing designation in a final judgment."[108] For instance, in the 2005 Florida case, *Wade v. Hirschman*, the court found evidence of parental alienation amongst other factors and concluded that the evidence satisfied the threshold of "substantial and material changes in circumstances justifying modification of child custody."[109]

Additionally, an Illinois court awarded a father sole custody based on a showing that "mother engaged in pattern of parental alienation, made repeated allegations of sexual abuse against father, none of which were substantiated, and made numerous disparaging comments about father in front of child and others."[110] Another Illinois court modified custody based on evidence of substantial parental alienation:

> In making its ruling, the trial court found by clear and convincing evidence that there had been a change in circumstances and that modification was necessary to serve the best interest of the child. The trial court found evidence of substantial parental alienation, which would require

105. Lorandos, D., Bernet, W., & Sauber, R. (2013). Overview of parental alienation. In Lorandos, D., Bernet, W., & Sauber, R. (Eds.), *Parental Alienation: The Handbook for Mental Health and Legal Professionals*, Charles C. Thomas.

106. *Id.*

107. Amarreh v. Amarreh, 918 N.W.2d 228, 231–32 (Minn. Ct. App. 2018) Lemcke v. Lemcke, 623 N.W.2d 916, 919 (Minn. App. 2001), review denied (Minn. June 19, 2001); *see also*, Nies v. Nies, 407 N.W.2d 484, 487 (Minn. App. 1987) (noting district court's finding that "consistent interference with visitation endangered the children's emotional health and development"); Chafin v. Rude, 391 N.W.2d 882, 886 (Minn. App. 1986) (affirming modification of custody based on expert's opinion that mother's inability or unwillingness to support healthy relationship between son and his father posed real and serious danger to son's healthy development).

108. Korkmaz v. Korkmaz, 200 So. 3d 263, 265 (Fla. Dist. Ct. App. 2016). *See also*, McKinnon v. Staats, 899 So.2d 357, 361 (Fla. 1st DCA 2005).

109. Wade v. Hirschman, 903 So. 2d 928 (Fla. 2005) (abrogating, Perez v. Perez, 767 So. 2d 513, Gibbs v. Gibbs, 686 So. 2d 639, Metcalfe v. Metcalfe, 655 So. 2d 1251, Johnson v. Adair, 884 So.2d 1169, Leng-Gross v. Gross, 898 So.2d 241. West's F.S.A. § 61.13(3)(a-j, m)).

110. Hanson v. Spolnik, 685 N.E.2d 71 (Ind. Ct. App. 1997). I.C. 31–1–11.5–22(d) (1995 Supp.).

> that [child] spend an extended period of time with [Father] with less interference from [Mother].[111]

Below are some additional examples of cases wherein courts have intervened and modified custody or granted other appropriate relief to remedy parental alienation.

Case Examples

Wylie v. Wylie[112]

In this 2019 Louisiana case, the court considered evidence introduced in the case and testimony from several witnesses, including court-appointed mental health experts and experts specializing in parental alienation. The court opined that the alienation of the child from her father would continue unless a change is made. The PA expert testified that if alienation continues or is intentional, then the child should be relocated to Florida with her father. The court accepted this expert's recommendation and found that the mother had acted to intentionally alienate the child from her father and either failed or refused to recognize the pattern of alienation and lacked the ability to self-correct or rehabilitate that well-settled pattern of behavior.

Dean v. Valinho[113]

In 2011, in a case involving years of severe alienation by the mother, a Connecticut court was left with the decision to

> remove custody of the child from the mother and risk permanently destroying the child's relationship with his father, or, leave the child with his mother and hope that family psychotherapy will take hold and reverse a decade of harm to this child that mental health professionals to date have had no success in stemming.

After mother's expert recommended leaving the child with the alienating mother and severing the relationship with the father completely, the court stated that it would "not entertain an order severing the child's relationship with his father as part of a cease fire" as this would tantamount to leaving the child with an abusive parent and having "no antidote to the mother's continued undermining of any remaining positive feelings toward his father." The court ultimately found that the present custody orders were not in the best interest of the minor child and awarded the father sole legal custody.

---

111. *In re* Marriage of Divelbiss, 308 Ill. App. 3d 198, 206, 719 N.E.2d 375, 380 (1999).
112. Wylie v. Wylie, 52,800 (La. App. 2 Cir. 5/22/19), 273 So. 3d 1256, 1264.
113. Dean v. Valinho, 2011 WL 8204118 (Conn. Super. Ct., 2011).

In re Marriage of Moore[114]

In this 2018 Illinois case, the court's expert found that the child "suffered from a severe case of parental alienation syndrome." The expert explained "that parental alienation syndrome occurred when a child [is] aligned with one parent who confronts or questions the safety or love of another parent by making the other parent appear 'evil or unsafe.'" The expert stated that the child displayed signs of all the parental alienation criteria. He further explained: "[the child] was alienated from his mother. At one time he had a very loving relationship with her, and that all changed after he had these numerous visits with his father and the unsupervised time." Because this case of parental alienation was so severe, the expert recommended that the child have no contact with the father until interventions were made. The expert stated that parental alienation was emotional abuse because it put "a ton of pressure on kids." The expert opined that the children's contact with the father should be limited to avoid further psychological damage. As a result, the trial court suspended the father's visitation.

Martin v. Martin[115]

In this early 2020 Michigan case, the court awarded father sole custody and mother supervised visitation after a long and contentious struggle with alienation by mother. The child's therapist testified that he had "never seen such a lack of engagement in 25 years of counseling with a child." The therapist believed the children (in addition to the minor child who was the focus of the court decision, there were two other children who were not within the jurisdiction and the reach of the court any longer) suffered from post-traumatic stress disorder from mom's continued campaign against the father. The therapist stated, "I feel like they've been provided inaccurate information by mom that has resulted in them having a very intense level of fear, anxiety, and anger at their dad that is not warranted." The therapist had observed mom being "openly hostile towards [father] in front of the children and said things that simply weren't accurate." The therapist testified that the father, on the other hand, had been appropriate, tried to engage the children in activities, and had reacted appropriately even when the children were "angry and in his face and yelling and screaming." Ultimately, the therapist rated this case of parental alienation as a nine and asserted that the child should have no contact with her mother; the maternal side of his family; or her community, which included dance, church, and school.

The court found that

---

114. *In re* Marriage of Moore, 2018 IL App (3d) 170279-U.
115. Martin v. Martin, 2020 WL 448325 (Mich. App. Ct., 2020).

> [i]t has been shown that [mother's] stubborn hatred of [father] and her undermining of the agreed custodial relationship has been significant and ongoing, and that it has grown to involve surreptitious communications with [the child] to enlist the child as a co-conspirator in that effort. These are not minor disputes over contempt and parenting time. These are matters that could have a significant effect on the child's life, including on her long-term mental and emotional health: having to maintain the perception of hatred and contempt toward her father—which she may or may not share with her mother—will undoubtedly affect her mental and emotional health as well as her long-term relationship with her father.

Sneed v. Sneed[116]

In this 2018 North Carolina case, the Court temporarily suspended the alienating mother's visitation so the father and child could attend Family Bridges. On appeal, the Court stated that the trial court "had ample evidence before him to justify a conclusion that [Mother] had purposefully engaged in a course of conduct designed to alienate the child[ren]'s affections for [their] father, and that these actions were detrimental to the child[ren]'s welfare."[117] Moreover, the court did not permanently deny Mother the right of reasonable visitation; rather, the court specifically found and concluded that "Defendant/Mother is a fit and proper person to exercise visitation with the minor children, however, it is in the minor children's best interests and welfare that Defendant/Mother's visitation with the minor children be suspended pending completion of the Family Bridges program[.]" The court's order thus complied with the requirements of N.C. Gen. Stat. § 50-13.5(i). In its finding, the court stated it has wide discretion to fashion an order which will best serve the interests of the child; thus, "[t]he decision of the trial court regarding custody will not be upset on appeal absent a clear showing of abuse of discretion, provided that the decision is based on proper findings of fact supported by competent evidence."[118]

Begins v. Begins[119]

This 1998 Vermont case was remanded after the trial court found that

> father did not "deserve to win custody," yet reasoned that he had "effectively done so" as a result of his own misconduct, and thus concluded that it had no other choice but to award custody to father. . . . We categorically reject such reasoning. "[A] parent who willfully alienates a child

---

116. Sneed v. Sneed, 820 S.E.2d 536 (2018).
117. Woncik v. Woncik, 82 N.C. App. 244, 247, 346 S.E.2d 277, 281 (1986).
118. *Id.* at 279.
119. Begins v. Begins, 168 Vt. 298, 302, 721 A.2d 469 (Vt. 1998).

from the other parent may not be awarded custody based on that alienation." Although obviously well intended, the court's decision effectively condoned a parent's willful alienation of a child from the other parent. Its ruling sent the unacceptable message that others might, with impunity, engage in similar misconduct. Left undisturbed, the court's decision would nullify the principle that the best interests of the child are furthered though a healthy and loving relationship with both parents.[120]

Walton v. Walton[121]

Brenda used the allegations of physical abuse, not just in support of her position in court, but also as a justification for her clearly concentrated effort to alienate her sons against Philip. Among the ways in which she interfered with Philip's relationship with the boys were her repeated refusals to allow Philip his turn in court-ordered parenting rotations. In addition, Brenda purchased and permitted the boys to install key-locks on their bedroom doors in order that the boys could avoid meals and other contact with Philip during those times he was in charge . . . [C]ourt-appointed custody evaluator, psychologist Dr. Wayne Graves . . . observed: "[M]other's psychological status is so dysfunctional that I do not see any remediation possible within any short term time frame as within several years of intense psychological assistance. I do not expect change to occur there so that she could become by some rehabilitation primary parental responsibility."[122]

Horning v. Wolff[123]

Based on MMPI results [the child] Daisy shows indications of Parental Alienation Syndrome. Apparently, [the mother] Gidget would not facilitate any relationship between Daisy and her father absent the court's intervention. . . . Dr. Milsaps-Linger, who conducted a parental alienation evaluation for the trial court, stated in her report that appellant's responses to the Minnesota Multiphasic Personality Inventory–2 test "resulted in a profile the indicated significant mental health issues" and that appellant had a "tendency toward hypochondriasis." She further opined that appellant's general profile suggested a "mixed affective disturbance" and that appellant's "current level of day-to-day coping and self-sufficiency appears uneven and disorganized." In short, from our review of the trial

120. *Id.*
121. Walton v. Walton, 2007 WL 2405329 at *2 (Ohio App. 6 Dist.).
122. *Id.*
123. Horning v. Wolff, 2006 WL 3505864 at *4 (Ohio App. 5 Dist. 2006).

court's November 4, 2005 Judgment Entry, it is apparent that the trial court considered all of the best interest factors set forth in R.C. 3109.04(F) . . . [T]he trial court . . . clearly found that, based on consideration of all of the factors, it was in Daisy's best interest for custody to be granted to [the father].[124]

MM v. AM[125]

By Order dated February 24, 2009, after a hearing which included the testimony of the court-appointed therapist, Dr. Jennifer Campbell, plaintiff was awarded temporary custody of the parties' daughters, 'V' and 'I' (Bivona, J., J.S.C.). Justice Bivona based the change in custody "upon a finding of defendant having engaged in a continuous pattern of aggressive parental alienation." By Order dated May 8, 2009, Justice Bivona referred the issue of permanent sole and legal custody of 'I', 'V' and 'C' to trial. Subsequently, the plaintiff withdrew his application for permanent custody of 'C'.[126]

G. (M.) v. G. (D.)[127]

Whatever the cause, it is clear that their daughter has become alienated from her father. The convictions of the Plaintiff are firm. The frustration of the Defendant is evident. The alienation of their daughter from her father is profound. The cause of that alienation is in dispute. . . . Dr. Aubé came to the conclusion that there had been parental alienation . . . the parties and their daughter be referred to a clinical counselor experienced in psychoanalytic child therapy so that the recommendation of that counselor can guide the parties and their daughter back to a healthier relationship between mother and daughter and father and daughter. . . . In the interim, I see no useful purpose in continuing the supervised access, as it has resulted in absolutely no communication or relationship between father and daughter. In fact, I find that these visits have harmed the relationship between father and daughter. Access will be removed until the new counselor is in the position to recommend that it be resumed and, if resumed,

124. *Id.*
125. MM v. AM, 32 Misc.3d 1205(A) at *2, 932 N.Y.S.2d 761 (Table) (N.Y.Sup. 2011).
126. *Id.*
127. G. (M.) v. G. (D.), 2009 CarswellBC 1629, 2009 BCSC 809, [2009]; B.C.W.L.D. 5440, [2009] B.C.W.L.D. 5444, [2009] B.C.W.L.D. 5460, [2009]; B.C.W.L.D. 5467, [2009] B.C.W.L.D. 5487, [2009] W.D.F.L. 3530, [2009]; W.D.F.L. 3442, [2009] W.D.F.L. 3462, [2009] W.D.F.L. 3401, [2009] W.D.F.L.3411 (British Columbia Supreme Court 2009) [¶¶ 3, 53, 60, 63].

the nature of access, including telephone access and personal access with or without supervision.[128]

Conclusion

Courts in the United States have made significant advances in remediation of parental alienation. It can no longer be argued that the court system does not recognize parental alienation or its symptoms. There is growing case law on its admissibility as well as strategies on how to deal with it once parental alienation is recognized. It is not a one-stop shop. Where mild cases of parental alienation can be managed by therapy and early court interventions, severe cases require strong measures, including, but not limited to, custody reversal. The safety of the child exposed to parental alienation requires such vigilance. There must be a coordinated effort from the court and mental health experts to devise an appropriate plan to meet the best interests of the child. Additionally, parental alienation cases require advocates who are familiar with the literature and who can help their clients achieve effective outcomes—for instance, knowing when therapy will and will not help address the alienating issues. Sometimes this means educating the client on alienation and how the client's reactions to the alienation can either harm or progress their case.

And while there has been movement towards addressing alienation as it occurs, our justice system still has a long way to go. One important aspect is ensuring the court is offered all information regarding the parental alienation dynamic. As a family law practitioner, one of the most critical aspects of the case is helping the court understand the science underlying parental alienation, presenting evidence of a parent's alienating behaviors together with signs of alienation in the child, and then offering a solution. It is essential for courts to prioritize risk assessment to ensure "that the safety of parents and their children is not endangered by the court."[129] This can be accomplished by providing "unambiguous, detailed court orders for the interventions and for there to be court monitoring of implementation of orders, and any modifications to parenting plans and interventions."[130]

---

128. *Id.*

129. Fidler, B., & Bala, N. (2020). Concepts, controversies and conundrums of "alienation": Lessons learned in a decade and reflections on challenges ahead, *Fam. Ct. Rev.*, 58, 576, 589.

130. *Id.*

CHAPTER 4

Presenting a Case of Parental Alienation in Court

Family court judges routinely make findings, both of law and fact. Judges make findings of fact that ultimately support their decisions of child custody, parenting time, visitation, restraining orders, and mental health interventions. Parental alienation is a significant factor that has the potential to dramatically change a court's decision on child custody and parenting time orders. Indeed, in cases of severe parental alienation, the primary focus of the court should be on protecting the child from ongoing psychological abuse, not reunification with the rejected or targeted parent. Courts have also viewed presence of parental alienation as proper cause or a change of circumstances necessitating an evidentiary hearing that could lead to change of custody and other remedial intervention. Some courts have opined that presence of parental alienation and evidence of alienating behaviors manifested by a parent could trump all other factors that a court typically considers in awarding custody to a parent.

In order to make a finding of parental alienation, a court must have *evidence*—not allegations, speculations, or assumptions—that one parent has manifested alienating behaviors, and, as a result of those behaviors, the child exhibits signs or symptoms that are commonly found in alienated children, including, but not limited to, rejection of the targeted parent. It is not necessary that the child should completely reject the targeted parent. In mild to moderate cases of parental alienation, a child often continues to have contact with the targeted parent, but the overall relationship suffers and the child refuses to engage with the parent and overall considers the parent unworthy of love or affection. It is also not necessary that a case of parental alienation be viewed in binary terms. That is, it is not necessary that the alienating parent bears one hundred percent responsibility for the child's rejection of the targeted parent. The targeted parent could have demonstrated behaviors (or reactions to the child's rejection of the parent) that could be considered sub-optimal parenting or worse and could have contributed to the family dynamics. And in presenting a case of parental alienation, the lawyer for the targeted parent needs to consider all of these issues, marshal the necessary evidence, organize it, and present it in a manner that not only helps a court understand the phenomenon of parental alienation and its severity, but also empowers a judge to order an appropriate legal and mental health remedial intervention.

Expert Testimony: One Tool in the Litigator's Toolbox

In most cases, an attorney for a targeted parent presents expert testimony in court to lay out a case of parental alienation. An expert typically testifies as to what is meant by parental alienation, why and how it is harmful to children, and more importantly, what the court can and should do about it. When making a decision on whether to use an expert to present a case of parental alienation, there are several considerations to keep in mind. First, know your judge. Ask yourself if the judge in your case is generally receptive to hearing expert testimony. While cases involving parental alienation generally involve expert testimony, it is not a requirement. A trier of fact can make a finding of parental alienation by finding presence of alienating behaviors together with a child's unjustified rejection of a parent due to those behaviors. In fact, an Ontario Court of Appeals recently held that a trial court doesn't need an expert report to make a finding of alienation as a primary causal factor in family dysfunction.[1] Second, it is important to figure out whether the parent can afford the services of an expert. While a court can (and often does) award attorney fees and costs upon making a finding of parental alienation, it is the target parent who initially bears the burden of proving the existence of parental alienation. Depending on the case, its litigation history, and availability of proofs, retaining an expert to conduct a forensic record review could be an expensive proposition. Third, determine whether a local professional, often court-appointed, such as a guardian ad litem, a friend of the court investigator, or a custody evaluator, has already made the determination that parental alienation is present. If so, an outside expert paid by one side may not be necessary.

If it is determined that an outside, privately retained expert is necessary, the next step then to consider is whether such expert should function

1. *See* A.M. v. C.H., 2019 ONCA 764 (Ontario Court of Appeals).

as a "general," education-only expert or as a "specific," education-and-case-specific expert. The former would not be privy to the facts of the case and would not offer an opinion as to whether parental alienation is present in that particular case. Such an expert would typically describe the phenomenon of parental alienation, the peer-reviewed scientific literature in support of the condition, the Five-Factor Model for determining whether parental alienation is present, typical behaviors of an alienating parent, typical symptoms of an alienated child, short-term and long-term sequalae of parental alienation, and, last but not least, why the court should intervene in cases involving parental alienation—and intervene early rather than late. Such general expert can also answer hypothetical questions from attorneys and/or court, which can help link the educational testimony to the facts of the case. For example, after having an expert explain what is meant by a "Borrowed Scenario," where one finds a rehearsed quality to a child's litanies, together with phraseology that is not commonly used by the child, an attorney can ask a hypothetical question to the expert: *Dr. Smith, if the court were to find evidence of the presence of "Borrowed Scenarios" in this case, would such evidence be consistent with symptoms typically manifested by an alienated child?*

In contrast, a case-specific expert would be familiar with the underlying facts of a given case, having conducted a detailed review of the pertinent records of the case, and would proffer an opinion as to whether parental alienation exists in that case, and if so, what evidence supports such a finding. Of course, the case-specific expert would also offer educational or instructional testimony as to the phenomenon of parental alienation and other related topics that a general expert would testify to. But with this kind of an expert, the attorney need not ask hypothetical questions. Rather, the attorney can direct the examination toward specific facts or issues present in the case, which leads the expert to opine on the existence of parental alienation. For instance, the expert can testify about the examples of alienating behaviors manifested by a favored or alienating parent in the case, together with evidence of signs of alienation demonstrated by the child.

As is often the case, there are pros and cons associated with each kind of expert. Offering general expert testimony has three primary advantages. First, the expert is protected from the accusation of being a "hired gun," i.e., bias. The expert will not be seen as tailoring the descriptions of alienating behaviors and symptoms to the facts of the case since the expert will not be aware of the facts of the case. Some courts may see this apparent weakness of not knowing the facts of the case as strength, and this can protect the expert against a claim of bias. Second, if the attorney is skilled at weaving hypothetical questions appropriately tied to the facts of the case, the court may readily recognize the behaviors and symptoms being described by the expert despite the expert not knowing the facts of the case. This can contribute to the credibility of the expert's testimony and the weight accorded to it by the court. Third, the fees for the general expert witness should cost significantly less compared to a special expert (who has to spend a large amount of time reviewing records and learning the facts of the case), and the report, if one is being produced, should be available quickly.

The primary disadvantage of such an expert is that the expert does not know the facts of the case and his or her testimony may come off as irrelevant or unhelpful. Further, if the attorney in charge of direct examination is not skilled or experienced in framing the hypothetical questions during the direct examination, the testimony may get mired in evidentiary objections and fail to "connect the dots" for the court. Worse, there is a risk that the opposing counsel or a court that is skeptical of the presence of parental alienation in a particular case may ask hypothetical questions of their own, which could result in the general expert responding in a manner that undermines the case. In short, one could end up winning the battle but losing the war: having the court afford credibility and weight to the expert but discounting the testimony nonetheless because it did not fit the facts of the case.

Similarly, there are pros and cons to using a specific expert witness. The primary advantage of a specific expert is that the expert will be familiar with the facts of the case: the particular behaviors of the alienating parent and the case-specific symptoms of the alienated children. This allows the expert to testify not only what alienation is, as described by professional literature, but why it is present in a particular case at hand, providing particular case-specific examples for the trier of fact. This makes the expert's testimony powerful and compelling. The other advantage of having a specific expert testify is that the witness, having conducted a detailed review of the case records, is less likely to concede critical facts or issues during the cross examination. Of course, this is true only if the attorney proffering the expert testimony was diligent enough to provide all relevant (good and bad) information to the expert and not just cherry-picked information that supports a particular narrative. If relevant negative information was suppressed, any ethical professional will concede that such information could change her position on whether alienation is, in fact, present. Another factor to consider when hiring a specific expert witness is the background and credentials of the person. It may be important to hire someone who is a licensed mental health professional simply to mitigate the criticism that reviewing a case file containing mental health records constitutes "clinical work" and therefore requires a licensed clinician. This is not necessarily true, and a case file review is not necessarily clinical work, but some courts may be persuaded by this argument, so, all else being equal, having a clinician do the work may be easier. This is especially true in jurisdictions in which such an expert would be allowed to make recommendations about proper treatment or interventions. Opposing counsel or the court may object to a non-clinician doing so.

Best Interest Factors—Totality of Circumstances

Expert testimony is a tool, but it is not the only tool in a litigator's toolbox to persuade a court that parental alienation exists in a particular case. Courts routinely make a finding of the presence of parental alienation by relying on evidence that includes more than just an expert opinion. For instance, in *Rodman v. Friedman*, a New York appellate court affirmed a trial court's finding of parental alienation and held:

> [The trial judge] found plaintiff mother had alienated the child from defendant father . . . The court based its finding that the mother had alienated the child from the father not simply on the forensic report, but also on its in camera interview with the child, another forensic report, and numerous documents, interviews and court appearances.[2]

While expert testimony can no doubt be very compelling (and empowering) for a court to reach a conclusion on whether parental alienation is present in a particular case, courts, more often than not, look to the totality of the evidence. As an Ohio court held in *Geary v. Geary*:

> The testimony of [Expert] alone did not establish parental alienation. The trial court specifically noted it was making a finding of parental alienation based on the "totality of the evidence," including the testimony of appellant and appellee . . . The trial court placed particular emphasis on the testimony of appellant with her conflicting statements and her admission that she lied under oath.[3]

When confronted with an argument that a targeted parent had not presented expert testimony to support an argument that the child had suffered serious harm due to the alienating behaviors manifested by a favored parent, a Tennessee appellate court opined:

> Respectfully, "[the] trial judge, as the trier of fact finder, is not required to check his or her common sense at the door when considering evidence . . . Expert testimony is only necessary "when the subject matter requires that the court and jury have the aid of knowledge or experience not held by ordinary witnesses . . . and where common knowledge furnishes no criteria for judgment or where proof depends upon observation and analysis outside the common experience of jurors . . . When faced with undisputed evidence that the child suffers what might be described by a laymen as a "panic attack" . . . the trial court correctly found that the child's emotional needs were not being met by Mother even if the absence of expert proof

2. Rodman v. Friedman, 33 A.D.3d 400, 400-401 (2006) (N.Y. Slip. Op. 07264).
3. Geary v. Geary, 27 N.E.3d 877 (2015) (Court of Appeals of Ohio).

to that effect. In her continued campaign to make Father and Stepmother unhappy or uncomfortable, Mother largely ignored the impact that her outbursts were having on her child.[4]

The Alaskan Supreme Court has affirmed a trial court's finding of parental alienation in absence of expert testimony where "the record presents a mound of evidence from which the [c]ourt can fairly easily draw conclusions about the relationship that are characteristic of the parental alienation dynamic."[5]

There is no dispute that parental alienation (or even "attempts at parental alienation") are not in a child's best interests, and evidence of such may form the basis for a change of custody.[6] Courts have found that

> [t]he great weight of authority holds that conduct by one parent that tends to alienate the child's affections from the other parent is so inimical to the child's welfare as to be grounds for a denial of custody to, or a change of custody from, the parent guilty of such conduct.[7]

And, as the Supreme Court of North Dakota held,

> A material change in circumstances may be present when one parent attempts to alienate a child's affection for the other parent, or when the child's parents are openly hostile towards each other and the child is negatively affected by that hostility.[8]

Finally, as a Michigan court[9] lamented:

> I feel very strongly that alienating a child against a father or a mother and consistently attempting to do that and denying that it's occurring; and consistently . . . saying the parent sexually abused the child, when it didn't occur; saying the parent neglected or abused the child, and calling CPS when it didn't occur; taking the child to the hospital and saying there's injuries when you shouldn't; taking the child to into another state in an attempt to keep the child from the parent, I believe [all] this goes to a parent's moral fitness. And that's very concerning to me.

4. Fiala v. Fiala, unpublished Tenn. Ct. App. 2019, 2018 WL 4523206.

5. Joy B. v. Everett B., 2019 WL 5656351, unreported case in Alaskan Supreme Court (No. S-17129) (November 1, 2019). Also see Eisenlohr v. Eisenlohr, 135 Conn.App. 337, 348 (2012).

6. Sundstorm v. Sundstorm, 177 Vt. 577, 580 (2004); Stone v. Pellegrini-Stone, 2014 IL App (3d) 130977-U.

7. Renaud v. Renaud, 168 Vt. 306, 309, 721 A.2d 463, 466 (1998). Also see *In re* Gorcyca, 500 Mich. 588, 597 n 4; 902 N.W.2d 828 (2017); McClain v. McClain, 539 S.W.3d 170, 189 (2017); Hibbard v. Hibbard, 139 Conn. App. 10, 25; 55 A.3d 301 (Conn. App. Ct. 2012).

8. Hankey v. Hankey, 861 N.W.2d 479, 482 (2015).

9. Poag-Emery v. Emery, 2014 WL 1618359 (Mich. Ct. App).

The Five-Factor Model

Proving parental alienation in court usually involves explication of the Five-Factor Model and presentation of evidence through the prism of the model. The Five-Factor Model is based on the work of Amy J. L. Baker, Ph.D., and her colleagues.[10] According to the parental alienation theory, when a court or a professional is asked to determine the presence of (or rule out) parental alienation, such determination cannot be made without considering the actions, behaviors, and attitudes of all the relevant players, to wit: the child, the rejected parent, and the favored parent. One way to make this determination is to consider the five factors proposed by Dr. Baker and her colleagues: (1) the child actively avoids, resists, or refuses a relationship with a parent; (2) presence of a prior positive relationship between the child and the now rejected parent; (3) absence of abuse or neglect or seriously deficient parenting on the part of the now rejected parent; (4) use of multiple alienating behaviors by the favored parent; and (5) exhibition of many or all of the eight behavioral manifestations of alienation by the child. When all five factors are present, one can determine that the child is alienated.

The Five-Factor Model is not a speculative, academic theory; the model has been empirically supported in a study of sixty-eight mental health professionals who rated sixteen variations of a vignette.[11] As Dr. Baker explains,

> [a]ll ratings of the vignette with Factors 2–5 present indicated that alienation was the most likely cause of a child's rejection of the other parent. When only one or no factor was present, there was an agreement that it was not a case of alienation.[12]

The Model offers family law practitioners and judges a framework to ensure that information about all relevant parties is factored into making an assessment or a finding. More importantly, the Model can be used to differentiate alienated from estranged children.[13] Let's consider each factor and how it fits in presenting a case of parental alienation in court.

---

10. Baker, A. J. L., Bone, M., & Ludmer, B. (2014). *High Conflict Custody Battle Survival Guide 101*, New Harbinger.

11. Baker, A. J. L. (2020). Parental alienation and empirical research. In Lorandos, D., & Bernet, W. (Eds.), *Parental Alienation: Science and Law*, Charles C. Thomas, 207–253.

12. Baker, A., (2020), *supra*, at 209 (citing Baker, A. (2018). Reliability and validity of the four-factor model of parental alienation, *Journal of Family Therapy*, 42(1).)

13. Baker, A. (2018). Reliability and validity of the four-factor model of parental alienation, *Journal of Family Therapy*, 42(1).

Factor One: Child Resists a Relationship with a Parent

The threshold consideration in determining whether parental alienation exists is that the child is refusing, resisting, or avoiding having a positive relationship with a parent. This might involve complete rejection and contact refusal on part of the child, but it doesn't necessarily have to. Parental alienation may exist in cases where a child agrees to contact but resists or refuses attempts on the part of the parent for communication, affection, and interaction. In such situations, the child goes on visitation or parenting time to see the targeted parent and is physically present but is emotionally absent and not involved or engaged with the parent. For example, the child may go on visitation but spends the entire time in his or her room ignoring the targeted parent, refusing to eat meals together, refusing to do any activities, and refusing to engage with the parent. At times, the child might even insist on going on visitation, only to act as a spy for the favored parent and snoop for information belonging to the targeted parent that could be used (or abused) by the favored parent. It is not necessary that for a case to be determined as a case of parental alienation, there must be a complete and absolute contact refusal by a child.

Further, there is a false belief or a misconception that the Parental Alienation theory claims that all rejected children are victims of alienation. The theory of parental alienation posits that the children who are aligned with one parent and reject the other parent *may* be alienated (where the child rejects a parent without legitimate justification and as a result of undue influence of the favored parent) or estranged (where the child rejects a parent for justifiable reason, such as serious abuse or neglect) or a combination of both (a "hybrid" case, including features of both alienation and estrangement). But just because a child resists contact with or rejects a parent doesn't mean that a court can *assume* that the child is alienated. The child's resistance or rejection is simply a factor to be considered when evaluating a case using the Five-Factor Model.

Factor Two: Prior Positive Relationship with the Rejected Parent

It is important to consider the prior, "baseline," relationship between the now rejected parent and the child. Was this relationship once healthy? Was the parent who is now rejected and found unworthy of love and affection once an active participant in the children's lives? Did the parent help coach or otherwise participate in the children's sporting or extracurricular activities? Did s/he attend the children's medical appointments? Did s/he attend the parent-teacher conferences? Did the parent go on regular vacations with the children? Did they enjoy their time together during the vacations, such as swimming, snowmobiling, hunting, sporting events, travel, etc.? Did the parent help the children with homework? Participate in the bedtime routines? Was the parent an involved parent in the children's regular and routine lives? These are some of the important questions that need to be answered when evaluating Factor Two of the Model.

The fundamental premise of the phenomenon of parental alienation is that the child's resistance to or rejection of a parent is disproportionate or without justification and that the favored parent has manifested behaviors that have enabled or helped turn the child against the other parent, with whom the child once had a healthy and loving relationship. Thus, it is essential to determine that a normative relationship must have once existed and that the parent who is now being rejected once had a positive, loving bond with the child. A prior positive relationship also provides evidence that the parent who is now rejected once had the ability or capacity to provide adequate caretaking of the child and to provide guidance, love, and affection. As Dr. Richard Gardner wrote in describing the Parental Alienation Syndrome, "I am referring here only to those who have been good, dedicated parents."[14]

In *Noland-Vance v. Vance*, a Missouri trial judge juxtaposed a child's close and positive relationship with the targeted parent with his attitude towards the parent upon alienation:

> Of primary importance to this Court was . . . voice mail recordings from [Father's] cell phone made by the oldest son, James. James called [Father] at the beginning of the separation of the parties when all the children were at their grandparents' house . . . James called [Father's] phone eight (8) times over three days and left messages on his voice mail. This is evidence of James' close relationship with his father. He asked his father repeatedly to come to . . . pick him up. . . . He expressed his love for his father during each call. He was not fearful of [Father] . . . James clearly wanted to be with his father and the Court considered this evidence as very credible. In his words and actions James did not act as though he had been subjected to extensive abuse as described by [Mother] . . . James' attitude toward his father has changed and been influenced by the conduct of [Mother].[15]

Further, when we consider a child's (or the favored parent's) "justification" for the child's resistance to or rejection of the rejected parent, we should be careful in not holding the rejected parent to an unrealistic standard. It is not required that the rejected parent should have been an ideal or perfect parent. In fact, the rejected parent, like all parents, will almost always be imperfect and may be far from being an "ideal" parent. In fact, in cases involving allegations of parental alienation, we will almost always find episodic evidence of sub-optimal or even poor parenting. The relevant question is not whether the

14. Gardner, R. (1998). *The Parental Alienation Syndrome*, Second Edition, Creative Therapeutics, 209.
15. Noland-Vance v. Vance, 321 S.W.2d 398, 413 (Mo. App. 2010).

rejected parent is "perfect." Rather, the relevant question is "whether this parent has engaged in normative parenting, which encompasses a wide spectrum of parenting styles and behaviors."[16] Many professionals and courts make the mistake of putting the targeted parent on trial in an attempt to justify the child's rejection of that parent and in doing so, they try to establish that the flaws of that parent (which more often than not are normative and found in an overwhelming number of parents all over) are the cause of the child's rejection. In cases of parental alienation, it would be a serious error to do so.

First, in most instances, the supposed flaws or shortcomings of the rejected parent emerge after the child has already rejected the parent. And "from a purely logical point of view, B cannot cause A if B followed A."[17] Second, it is highly likely that the favored parent, being human, is equally as flawed as the targeted parent. Nevertheless, the child, far from rejecting the favored parent, idealizes the parent in a polarized manner. In the child's mind, the rejected parent can do nothing good; the favored parent is "perfect" and has no flaws. This exposes the fallacy that an alienated child is reacting to the parents in a reality-based manner. Third, the supposed flaws of the rejected parent probably pre-existed the rejection and did not bother the child prior to the divorce or separation. For instance, a parent who has an ingrained habit of being too neat ("neat freak") doesn't suddenly change his or her behavior after the divorce or separation. If this "flaw" did not interfere in the parent-child relationship up until divorce, it is not plausible that it would result in the child rejecting the parent and suddenly finding him or her unworthy of affection after the divorce. Therefore, a child's justification in resisting or rejecting a parent should be carefully and critically evaluated. Overall, Factor Two requires that when evaluating a case for parental alienation, a trier of fact must ascertain whether the child had a previously existing positive relationship with the now rejected parent.

Factor Three: Lack of Abuse by Rejected Parent

It bears repeating that it is important to remember that just because a child rejects a parent does not mean that the child is alienated. Just because a child is rejecting a parent does not mean that the parent did something to "deserve it." A highly counterintuitive feature of parental alienation is that most abused children continue to seek a relationship with their abusive parent, while alienated children (who were never abused) strongly reject a relationship with a targeted parent. It is rare and aberrant for a child to actually reject a parent, especially in such a strident and absolute manner as occurs in parental alienation cases.

16. Baker, A. (2020), *supra*, at 210.
17. Baker, A. (2020), *supra*, at 211.

"Even children who have been beaten, molested, and abandoned by a parent generally do not behave in a callous and extreme manner when dealing with an abusive parent."[18] Research in the field of child maltreatment shows at least six sources of evidence for the phenomenon that scientists refer to as "bonded to the abuser"—that despite the abuse and neglect experienced at the hand of a parent, most children *want to maintain a relationship with the abuser*.[19] Children are hard-wired to form and maintain attachment relationships with caregiving adults, even abusive caregivers. Even in cases of actual abuse or maltreatment, what is affected is the *quality* of the attachment, not whether there is an attachment. Family law professionals should understand just how uncommon it is for the children to reject a parent, even a truly abusive parent (who is likely to be much more aberrant in his or her parenting than the rejected parent in an alienation case). Clinicians and mental health experts have found that physically abused children *want to* maintain relationships with abusive caregivers.[20] That's what's so counterintuitive about parental alienation cases—to be confronted with children who, alleging "abuse" by a rejected parent, have unequivocally rejected the parent without any ambivalence.

That being said, Factor Three of the Five-Factor Model does require a trier of fact to determine that the now rejected parent did not engage in abuse, neglect, or seriously deficient parenting of the kind and severity that could reasonably be expected to cause a child to reject a parent. In other words, this factor requires an evaluator to determine whether a child's rejection of the target parent is far out of proportion to anything that parent has done to justify the rejection. When considering allegations of abuse, neglect, or maltreatment made against a rejected parent, it is important to bear in mind that the definition of child maltreatment varies from state to state as a result of the federal child abuse law, the Child Abuse Prevention and Treatment Act.[21] It is also important to determine whether independent or formal child abuse investigations have concluded that the rejected parent had in fact engaged in any form of abusive action constituting child maltreatment. This is important for several reasons.[22]

First, if the rejected parent has abused or neglected the child, the case cannot be considered a pure alienation case (regardless of the behaviors of the favored parent and child). The case could be hybrid (if there is evidence of alienating behaviors on the part of the favored parent) or it might be a case of

18. Baker, A. (2020), *supra*, at 211.

19. Baker, A., & Schneiderman, M. (2015). *Bonded to the Abuser: How Victims Make Sense of Childhood Abuse*, Rowman and Littlefield.

20. Baker, A. et al. (2019). The Assessment of Attitudes and Behaviors about Physically Abused Children: A Survey of Mental Health Professionals, Journal of Child and Family Studies, published online 11 September 2019.

21. Child Abuse Prevention and Treatment Act (CAPTA) of 1974, 42 U.S.C. §§ 5101-5116i (2019).

22. Baker, A. (2020), *supra*, at 212–215.

realistic estrangement, but it cannot, by definition, be a pure case of parental alienation. Second, the treatment intervention that is appropriate in an alienation case is not appropriate in a case involving abuse or neglect. In the latter case, the reunification treatment should be designed for abusive parents, not alienated parents. As Dr. Amy J. L. Baker explains,

> abuse-specific treatment models, such as Alternatives for Families: A Cognitive Behavioral Therapy (AF-CBT), are designed to decrease the reliance on punitive parenting styles of an abusive parent and increase the use of non-punitive behavior management strategies on the part of the parent, while simultaneously helping the child process the trauma from the abuse.[23]

In contrast, an alienation-specific treatment intervention is designed to provide the child with opportunities to correct the distorted thoughts and feelings about the rejected parent and to provide experiential opportunities for the alienated parent to function once again as a safe, loving, and available attachment figure for the child.[24] It is critical for the health and well-being of children (and the parent(s)) that they receive the right treatment. Third, it is important to thoroughly investigate whether the now rejected parent actually engaged in abusive behavior because in alienation cases such allegations are likely to continue to be made by the favored parent and/or the children and it is necessary to fully investigate this issue in order to resolve it one way or the other. If not, allegations of abuse or maltreatment will continue in the litigation and the process and, if repeated often enough, pose a risk of becoming a truth in the mind of the child (as well as in the perceptions and beliefs of the legal and mental health professionals) even if abuse never actually happened. As a Washington family court held in *Reichert v. Reichert-Randazzo,* false allegations that lead to child protective services and/or police investigations constitute an "abusive use of conflict" on the part of the alienating parent and "are detrimental to [a child] because they deprive him of a normal childhood, normal sibling relationships, and a normal relationship with [the targeted parent]."[25]

---

23. Baker, A. (2020), *supra,* at 213 (citing Kolko, D., & Swenson, C. (2002). *Assessing and Treating Physically Abused Children and their Families: A Cognitive Behavioral Approach*).

24. *See, e.g.,* Gottlieb, L. (2013). The application of structural family systems therapy to the treatment of parental alienation syndrome. In Baker, A., & Sauber, R. (Eds.), *Working with Alienated Children and Families: A Clinical Guidebook,* 209; Warshak, R., & Otis, M. (2010). Helping alienated children with Family Bridges: Practice, research and the pursuit of "humbition," *Fam. Ct. Rev.,* 48, 91; Warshak, R. (2019). Reclaiming parent-child relationships: Outcomes of Family Bridges with alienated children, *Journal of Divorce & Remarriage,* 60(8), 645–667.

25. In the Matter of the Marriage of Reichert v. Reichert-Randazzo, 2 Wash.App.2d 1063 (2018) (Unpublished); also see Delekta v. Delekta, 2019 WL 2711294 (Mich. Court of Appeals) (Unpublished).

Factor Four: The Alienating Behaviors by the Preferred Parent

In order for a child to be considered alienated, s/he must have been exposed or subjected to parental alienation behaviors by the favored parent (and/or third parties). Again, it is important to note that it is not sufficient to assume or infer that the behaviors have occurred. Rather, these behaviors must have been observed through actions, attitudes, written statements (including email, text messages, social media posts, voicemails, etc.), behaviors, etc.[26] As a practice pointer, lawyers representing the target parents should try not to get bogged down on the unwarranted debate or litigation over the scientific support underlying "PAS" or the "syndrome." Rather, the focus should be on the *behaviors*—the alienating behaviors that are so harmful the child and the child's relationship with the target parent. As a Louisiana court held:

> Although parental alienation has not been recognized as a true psychological syndrome, it has been recognized as a psychological condition that can be harmful to a child's long-term emotional development. Moreover, "the conduct of one parent in denigrating the other parent and undermining the child's relationship with that parent, an adult with whom the child has had a very important relationship, is a form of emotional abuse."[27]

Professional literature demonstrates that a child who is exposed or subjected to these behaviors develops thoughts and feelings about the rejected parent that are due to the influence of the other /favored parent (instead of a child's direct experience of the rejected parent).[28] Several research studies have established the reliability and validity of these alienating behaviors. For example, Baker and Chambers presented the Baker Strategy Questionnaire (BSQ) as a brief assessment of adult recall of parental use of alienating behaviors.[29] The measure was found to be both reliable and valid. The internal consistency (also called inter-item consistency) was above .90.[30] As Dr. Baker explained,

> [i]n over half a dozen subsequent studies, the BSQ has been used with over 2500 research participants from an array of locations, ages, experiences, and sampling strategies. In each study the BSQ was found to have

26. Baker, A. (2018), *supra*, at 4.
27. Palazzolo v. Mire, 10 So.3d 748 (La.Ct.App. 2009).
28. Baker, A. (2018), *supra*, at 4, citing Baker, A. J. L., & Ben-Ami, N. (2011). To turn a child against a parent is to turn a child against himself. *Journal of Divorce and Remarriage*, 54(2), 203–219; Baker, A., & Brassard, M. (2013). Adolescents caught in parental loyalty conflicts, *Journal of Divorce and Remarriage*, 54, 393–413; Baker, A., & Chambers, J. (2011). Adult recall of childhood exposure to parental conflict: Unpacking the black box of parental alienation, *Journal of Divorce and Remarriage*, 52(1), 55–76.
29. Baker, A. (2018), *supra*, at 5, citing Baker, A., & Chambers, J. (2011), *supra*.
30. Practitioners who wish to know what role internal consistency and other statistical measures play in evaluating reliability and validity of research studies—a critical ingredient of a Daubert hearing—should read: Lorandos, D., & Campbell, T. (2005). *Benchbook in the Behavioral Sciences–Psychiatry–Psychology–Social Work*, Carolina Academic Press.

extremely high internal consistency scores as well as being associated with the relevant reliable and valid measures of outcomes that theory suggests would be associated with exposure to alienating behaviors such as depression, low self-esteem, anxiety and difficulties trusting others.[31]

These harmful behaviors have been found by family courts to constitute "emotional abuse" (which mandatory reporters of child abus,e are obligated to report),[32] and can lead to a child's alienation and unjustified rejection of the targeted parent. There is no single definitive list of alienating behaviors. However, there is a great deal of consensus in the field that the behaviors or tactics outlined below constitute alienating behaviors.[33]

1. Badmouthing or Denigrating the Other Parent.

> The alienating parent speaks ill of the other parent to the children and within the children's hearing in a steady stream of negative messaging that is not balanced by anything positive [or] emphasizes the negative aspects of the other parent's personality and choices [or] vilifies the other parent in the children's community.[34]

This tactic creates a belief in the children that the target parent is unsafe or dangerous, unloving, and undeserving or unworthy of love or affection. A New York court summed it up well when it held, "an excellent indicator of a parent's concern for the emotional well being of a child is . . . their treatment of the other parent in the presence of the children and the image they portray of the other parent to the children."[35] In *Weaver v. Weaver*, the Vermont Supreme Court affirmed the trial court's order restricting a mother's access to her child's records and forbidding her from having contact with the child's school personnel and medical providers upon finding that she engaged in a "campaign of parental alienation" by communicating with "virtually everyone who had a

31. Baker, A. (2018), *supra*, at 5.

32. Noland-Vance v. Vance, 321 S.W.2d 398, 405 (Mo. App. 2010) ("Dr. Aram described this situation as the worst case of parental alienation he had ever seen. As a mandatory reporter of child abuse, Dr. Aram believed he was required to report this form of emotional abuse to the court."). Also see Fiala v. Fiala, unpublished Tenn. Ct. App. 2019, 2018 WL 4523206 ("The term emotional abuse . . . means 'to injure (a person) physically or mentally' . . . To be abusive, to be 'characterized by wrongful or improper use,' or to be 'habitually cruel, malicious, or violent[.]' . . . Here, Mother's behavior towards Father . . . can be described as nothing short of abusive. . . . We cannot conclude that Mother's action in directly exposing the child to the abuse directed at. . . . Father does not also constitute a form of emotional abuse . . . these interactions have a profound negative effect on the child.").

33. Baker, A. (2020), *supra*.

34. Descriptions of all parental alienation strategies are quoted from Baker, A. J. L., & Fine, P.R. (2014). *Surviving parental alienation: A journey of hope and healing*, Rowman and Littlefield, 8–10.

35. D.D. v. A.D., 63 N.Y.S.3d 304, 2017 N.Y. Slip Op. 50807(U).

substantial relationship with father or [child] . . . to disparage father and undermine his relationship with [child]."[36] The Court found that these contacts "were all part of mother's persistent and unremitting effort to alienate [child] from father."[37] Similarly, in *McNutt v. Yates*, an Arkansas appellate court affirmed the trial court's modification of custody where a mother engaged in a campaign of false information and denigration, accusing the father of sexual deviance, burglary, and killing the children's dog and made disparaging remarks about the father in front of the children, in public, and to people at the children's school.[38] In *In re Anya*, an Illinois appellate court affirmed the trial court's grant of custody to a father where the mother had engaged in various alienating behaviors, disparaged the father by freely and openly speaking negatively about him directly to the child and in front of her (including calling the father a "child molester" and saying "die, die, die" in the father's direction when the child was present), "oblivious to the impact that her words . . . were having on [child]."[39] The child's "reaction to this extreme negativity was clearly expressed in her body language when she would hang her head or actually crawl under a chair or table when [mother] [was] discussing [father]."[40] Further, in *Hanson v. Spolnik*, an Indiana court granted the father sole custody where a mother, in an attempt to destroy the relationship between the child and the father, made false allegations of sexual abuse and called the father names in front of the child, including "Satan."[41] In *McClain v. McClain*, a severe case of parental alienation, a Tennessee court documented a father's duplicitous behavior wherein he sent some text messages in an apparent show of support of the child's time with the mother, but then sent other messages that undermined the child's relationship with the mother by telling the child that the mother was "mentally ill," that the child had "a right to be ugly to [mother]," and "[child] will never like her. Nobody likes her. It is impossible."[42] Repeated, unfounded allegations of abuse made by one parent can be grounds for granting custody to the other parent. An alienating parent's campaign of denigration in an attempt to portray the target parent as "dangerous" or "abusive" can take a serious toll on the child's mental health and his or her relationship with

36. Weaver v. Weaver, 2019 WL 1504095 (Vermont).
37. *Id.*
38. McNutt v. Yates, 2013 Ark. 427; 430 S.W.3d 91 (Ark. 2013).
39. *In re* Anya J.K., unreported, 2013 IL App (2d) 121194-U; 2013 WL 1932716 (Ill App. Ct. 2013).
40. *Id.*
41. Hanson v. Spolnik, 685 N.E.2d 71 (Ind.Ct.App. 1997). Also see Arms v. Arms, 803 N.E.2d 1201 (Ind. Ct.App. 2004); Albright v. Bogue, 736 N.E.2d 782 (Ind.Ct.App. 2000); Maddux v. Maddux, 40 N.E.3d 971 (Ind. Ct.App. 2015); S.D. v. B.D., 962 N.E.2d 702 (Ind.Ct.App. 2012).
42. McClain v. McClain, 539 S.W.3d 170, 195 (Tenn. Ct. App. 2017).

the target parent. As an Illinois court found in a case where the mother made unfounded accusations of abuse against the father, the children were "negatively impacted" and were "exposed to a constant mantra that [father] does bad things to them."[43]

2. Limiting Contact. "The alienating parent interferes with the amount of face-to-face time the children spend with the other parent such as coming early for pick-ups and late for drop-offs [or] does not produce the children for the other parent's parenting time [or] shows up during the other parent's parenting time and monopolizes the children's attention."[44] This tactic thwarts, reduces or limits the target parent's opportunities to enjoy his or her time with the children, to create loving memories, and to counter the badmouthing message by demonstrating to the children that the parent is involved, safe, loving, and deserving of love and affection. As an Illinois appellate court opined in *In re Marriage of Debra N. and Michael S.*, it is appropriate to modify custody arrangement and transfer custody to the non-custodial parent where "the custodial parent has made attempts to thwart the noncustodial parent's efforts to visit and maintain a close relationship with the child.[45] In the same vein, a Mississippi appellate affirmed a trial court's finding that limiting contact and "interference with visitation" constituted "a material change in circumstances given sufficient severity."[46] "Indeed, 'a non-custodial parent's right to visitation has been described as a right more precious than any property right.'"[47] One example of such behavior could be "intentionally setting up activities during the summer for [child] that would substantially interfere with [targeted parent's] visitation time."[48] Another example of such tactic would be, as a New York court found, a parent "regularly show[ing] up at random locations where [other parent] was with the subject children and demand immediate parenting time."[49]
3. Interfering with Communication.

> The alienating parent makes it difficult for the children and targeted parent to speak on the phone (or communicate by other means) during periods of separation [or] blocks e-mails and text

---

43. Stone v. Pellegrini-Stone, 2014 IL App (3d) 130977-U ("Mommy wants me to say daddy does bad things to me, but he doesn't and I love daddy.")

44. *Supra* 34.

45. *In re* Marriage of Debra N. and Michael S., 2013 ILApp (1st) 122145. Also see Eisenlohr v. Eisenlohr, 135 Conn.App. 337 (2012).

46. Ellis v. Ellis, 952 So.2d 982 (Miss. Ct. App. 2006).

47. *Id.*, citing Mord v. Peters, 571 So.2d 981, 983 (Miss. 1990) quoting Biamby v. Biamby, 114 A.D.2d 830, 494 N.Y.S.2d 741, 742 (1985).

48. *Id.*

49. D.D. v. A.D., 63 N.Y.S.3d 304, 2017 N.Y. Slip Op. 50807(U).

> messages [or] does not share cell phone numbers [or] does not answer calls [or] does not deliver gifts and letters.

This tactic makes it difficult for the targeted parent and the children to stay in touch and share each other's lives in a meaningful way. In *Sundstorm v. Sundstorm*, a Vermont court found "crystal clear" evidence of this alienating behavior where a mother "had intentionally and repeatedly sabotaged father's ability to have telephone contact with the children"[50]:

> The court found that . . . mother had continued to interfere with father's telephone contact with the children. The court explained that when father tried to call the children every day, as permitted by the divorce decree, one of several things happened: there was a busy signal; the phone would go unanswered; mother would answer and say the children were unavailable; the call would be automatically forwarded to a business; or mother would answer and tell father that until he paid her all the money she felt she was due, he would never get to talk to the children. The court found that when the father had spoken to the children, he heard mother on many occasions in the background telling the children what to say. Mother also stated to father, when he asked her when a good time to call would be, "There is no good time to call. Stop calling us and move on with your life."[51]

Similarly, an Indiana court found the mother to have engaged in interfering with the father's parenting time when the mother called police to perform "wellness checks" on father and child during the father's parenting time.[52] Orchestrating interference in communication or contact between the child and the targeted parent is the key part of this alienating tactic. It could be done through omission (e.g., not making the child available for a visitation or a phone call) or done through commission (e.g., repeatedly contacting the child during the other parent's visitation, calling the police or protective services for wellness checks, asking a neighbor to check on the children, parking the car outside or near the targeted parent's house, or visiting a neighbor of the targeted parent while the children are with the targeted parent). Some courts have insisted on requiring the custodial parent to post a bond to discourage interference with the other parent's visitation rights.[53]

---

50. *Supra* 34.
51. Sundstorm v. Sundstorm, 177 Vt. 577, 579-580 (2004).
52. *In re* Paternity of N.W., 35 N.E.3d 674 (Ind.Ct.App. 2015).
53. Shindell v. Shindell, 322 P.3d 1270 (WY. 2014).

4. Interfering with Symbolic Communication.

   > The alienating parent makes it difficult for the children to think about, talk about, or look at pictures of the other parent during periods of separation [or] eliminates photographs [or] does not discuss the other parent (unless badmouthing) [or] discourages the children from thinking about the targeted parent.

   This tactic instills a tribal mentality into the children, undercuts the children's attachment and feelings of closeness with the targeted parent. The children come to believe that it's simply not "acceptable" to show affection or even speak of the other parent while they are with the alienating parent.
5. Withholding Love and Approval from the Children. "In order to keep their attention directed toward themselves, the alienating parent becomes emotionally cold and distant when the children show positive feelings and thoughts towards the targeted parent."[54] This tactic creates anxiety in the children about losing the love and affection of the alienating parent while at the same time increasing the children's need for the alienating parent's approval. In *Fiala v. Fiala*, a Tennessee court found "overwhelming" evidence of a mother engaging in

   > a pattern of hostile behavior toward Father while the child was present. Mother's inappropriate behavior includes: (1) telling the child that Father did not love him; (2) accusing Father of kidnapping the child even though the child was returned to Mother on time; (3) telling the child that Father "brainwash[ed]" the child; (4) calling Stepmother "whore," "bitch," and other names in the child's presence and encouraging the child to have nothing to do with Stepmother, including even hugging her; and (5) refusing to allow the child to participate in activities because Stepmother was present.[55]

   The Court found that the child was "profoundly affected by the hostility" and "Mother's outrageous behavior."[56]
6. Telling the Children that the Targeted Parent Does Not Love Them.

   > The alienating parent encourages the children to falsely believe that the targeted parent has done things that are hurtful and selfish because that parent does not really care about or value them [or] conflates the end of the marriage with the end of the targeted parent's love of the children.[57]

---

54. *Supra* 34.
55. Fiala v. Fiala, unpublished Tenn. Ct. App. 2019, 2018 WL 4523206.
56. Fiala v. Fiala, unpublished Tenn. Ct. App. 2019, 2018 WL 4523206.
57. *Supra* 34

This tactic creates a false belief in the children by "brainwashing them" into believing that they are unwanted or rejected by the targeted parent, which in turn generates anger towards that parent.[58] A New York court case[59] provides an example of such behavior:

> Husband told the children that "mommy is filing for divorce and throwing me out, she does not love us anymore . . . In another telling choice made by Husband, he got a permanent tattoo on his arm of a dead 'family tree' being stabbed by Wife's favorite flower and surrounded by tombstones. He then made the poor choice of showing it to his daughter while implying that it was a depiction of how Mommy destroyed their family."

7. Allowing or Forcing the Children to Choose between Parents. "By offering desirable alternatives to visitation and/or psychologically pressuring the children to forgo parenting time with the targeted parent, the alienating parent creates situations in which the children will feel compelled to reject the targeted parent."[60] This tactic creates or heightens a need in the children to justify their choice, which focuses them on the negative qualities in the targeted parent. It also creates conflict between the children and the targeted parent, who becomes hurt and angry at the children's "choice." The more the children reject the targeted parent and justify their rejection by focusing on the supposed "flaws" of the parent, the more frustrated and hurt the targeted parent is. This toxic dynamic often leads to sub-optimal parenting or poor judgment on the part of the targeted parent, which then is used as an excuse to justify the children's rejection.
   Courts have also found that over-empowering a child to allow him or her to choose whether or not to spend time with a parent is an alienating behavior. For instance, an Indiana court[61] found:

   > Sadly, this child believes that he has the ability to make a choice as to whether or not to spend time with Father. [Child] believes that he is in charge. The Court believes this to be a result of mother's destructive behavior and influence. Mother disparages Father in presence of [Child]. Mother allows [Child] to choose when he will see his Father. Mother makes it incredibly difficult for Father to be involved in the minor child's life.

---

58. Barnard v. Barnard, 1997 WL 379617 (Oh.Ct.App.) ("the father . . . has embarked upon a campaign to discredit the mother in the eyes of the children, brainwashing them to believe the mother is a liar and does not love them and that she steals their clothes").
59. D.D. v. A.D., 63 N.Y.S.3d 304, 2017 N.Y. Slip Op. 50807(U).
60. *Supra* 34.
61. *In re* Paternity of N.W., 35 N.E.3d 674 (Ind.Ct.App. 2015).

8. Creating the Impression that the Other Parent is Dangerous. "The alienating parent does and says things, such as planting false memories of harm or misinterpreting events to falsely create this impression, that suggest or imply that the other parent has or will cause harm to the children."[62] This tactic is designed to create fear and sow doubt in the minds of the children about the targeted parent's capacity or ability to love them and keep them safe. For instance, as an Arkansas court found a mother to be engaging in parental alienation by telling the children or third parties, without any proof, that the targeted parent had "killed the children's puppy," or burglarized the home.[63] Or where a Missouri court determined that the mother had a mistaken belief that the father posed a danger to the children, did everything in her power to keep the children from the father "with a near religious zeal," and by doing so was "emotionally abusing the children by alienating their affections for Father."[64] In *Hibbard v. Hibbard*, a Connecticut court held a mother in contempt of the visitation orders when she unilaterally suspended her daughter's visits with the father on unsubstantiated allegations of abuse.[65] In *Stone v. Pellegrini-Stone*,[66] an Illinois court listed "a pattern of manipulative behavior" engaged in by a mother to alienate the children from their father:

> The court concluded that [mother] engaged in a pattern of manipulative behavior in order to destroy her children's relationship with their father by becoming overly emotional at visitation exchanges, making disparaging remarks about [father] in the children's presence, encouraging the children to say bad things about [father], alienating the children from [father], and making false allegations of physical and sexual abuse against him . . . [mother] filed six police reports and petitions for orders of protection against [father], claiming both physical and sexual abuse. All of those allegations were investigated by the police and DCFS and determined to be unfounded. In contrast to [mother's] manipulative, harmful and alienating behavior, the trial court determined that [father] has tried to and would continue to facilitate a positive relationship between the children and [mother].

9. Confiding in the Children. "The alienating parent shares personal information with the children about the targeted parent that induces

---

62. *Supra* 34.
63. McNutt v. Yates, 2013 Ark. 427; 430 S.W.3d 91 (Ark. 2013).
64. Noland-Vance v. Vance, 321 S.W.2d 398, 405 (Mo. App. 2010). Also see Eisenlohr v. Eisenlohr, 135 Conn.App. 337 (2012).
65. Hibbard v. Hibbard, 139 Conn. App. 10; 55 A.3d 301 (Conn. App. Ct. 2012).
66. Stone v. Pellegrini-Stone, 2014 IL App (3d) 130977-U.

the children to feel anger or shame about that parent and protective of the parent who is engaging in this behavior."[67] This tactic creates psychological distance between the children and the targeted parent due to the propaganda of misinformation planted by the alienating parent. It also creates a loyalty bind and a tribal mentality—"us versus him/her"—in the children. A commonly used tactic is inappropriate "sharing" of information regarding court or litigation with the children, such as alleged non-payment of child support or maintenance. As one court found:

> The court found that . . . mother would place the children on the phone and tell father that he needed to get a job and pay mother. Father presented two tapes of the children making the following statements to him. "Hi Dad, leave us alone. Pay your child support. Get a job, OK?" . . . The court found it beyond doubt that the mother told the children to make these statements to father, and explained that it was "entirely inappropriate for a parent to place a child in the middle of the parenting dispute over child support or maintenance."[68]

Often, there is evidence of pathological enmeshment—lack of proper boundary between a parent and the child—in addition to the alienation dynamic. The alienating parent has difficulty in separating himself from the child and thinks of himself and the child as a "team." In one case of parental alienation, a Michigan court found an alienating parent freely discussing her extramarital and post-divorce affairs with her teenage children. After an evidentiary hearing on parental alienation, the trial judge found:

> These boundary issues extended to [the mother's] discussion with the children of her pre- and post-divorce extramarital affairs. [She] testified that she . . . had discussed these matters with the children as a way of "taking that away from him." When asked about it on cross-examination, [the mother] admitted these disclosures, but denied that it denigrated [the father] to be talking with the children about her search for a "strong man." . . . [S]he wanted [the children] to know "why I built relationships with other men while still married to [the father]" and that their son correctly reported to the counselor that "she was looking for

67. *Supra* 34.
68. Sundstorm v. Sundstorm, 177 Vt. 577, 580 (2004).

love." [The father] testified that he had never discussed such matters with the children.[69]

10. Forcing the Children to Reject the Targeted Parent. "The alienating parent creates situations in which the children will personally inform the targeted parent that he or she has been excluded from important events in their lives."[70] This tactic pressurizes the children to focus on the negative qualities of the targeted parent in order to justify their rejection of that parent. At the same time, it incites hurt and anger in the targeted parent and has the potential to create a vicious and toxic cycle of the targeted parent reacting to the rejection and showing frustration and anger, which then is used as an excuse to justify the rejection.
11. Asking the Children to Spy on the Targeted Parent. "By such requests as asking the children to look through the targeted parent's mail, cell phone call log, or desk drawer, the alienating parent encourages or induces the children to betray the targeted parent's trust."[71] This tactic creates a sense of guilt in the children for betraying the targeted parent's trust, which is then turned into a desire to avoid the parent and a need to justify the rejection by focusing on the negative qualities of that parent.
12. Asking the Children to Keep Secrets from the Targeted Parent.

    > By involving the children's self-interest (e.g., don't tell your father we are going to take a vacation next year because he will try to stop us), the alienating parent encourages the children to withhold important information from the targeted parent despite that parent's having a right or need to have access to that information.

    This tactic, similar to the one above, creates a sense of guilt in the children, which is then turned into a desire to avoid the parent whom they betrayed and a need to justify such betrayal by focusing on the negative qualities of that parent.
13. Referring to the Targeted Parent by First Name When Speaking to the Children and/or Encouraging the Children to Do the Same. "For example, 'Frank [not Dad] is on the phone' or 'You just need to tell Jane [not Mom] that you are not going there this weekend."[72] This tactic sends a message to the children that the targeted parent is not an authority figure and undermines his or her role as a parent. For instance, a Missouri court was troubled to find that "[t]he two youngest children . . . referred to [Father] as 'Brent,' which was disturbing given their young ages."[73]

---

69. Boterenbrood v. Boterenbrood, Ottawa County Circuit Court Case No: 11-71079-DM (Michigan), pg. 11.
70. *Supra* 34.
71. *Supra* 34.
72. *Supra* 34.
73. Noland-Vance v. Vance, 321 S.W.2d 398, 412-413 (Mo. App. 2010).

Similarly, in a Massachusetts case, a trial judge was extremely troubled to learn that the mother had allowed and encouraged the children to call their father by his first name and call their step-father "Papa":

> Mother is hereby restrained from permitting the children to refer to their Father, in her presence, by any other name than "Dad" or "Father." The Court remains extremely troubled by the Mother's inappropriate allowances of the children calling their father by his first name, and referring to and calling their step-father "Papa" (which means father in German). Mother is further restrained from permitting the children to continue to call their step-father "Papa" or "Dad." Mother's instructions to the children shall be to refer to their step-father [by his first name]. Mother's failure to adhere specifically to the terms contained in this Paragraph shall invoke an immediate review by this Court of the custodial or parenting orders then in place.[74]

14. Referring to a Stepparent as "Mom/Dad" and Encouraging the Children to Do the Same. "'This is your new daddy,' or 'Mommy and I' (when the father is speaking of himself and his new wife)." This tactic replaces the targeted parent with a stepparent and conveys to the children that the alienating parent's new partner is the real parent and should matter to the children. It also creates an impression in the children's community—teachers, coaches, parents of their friends—that the replaced "parent" is the real parent and thereby generates feelings of hurt and anger in the targeted parent. As a New York court[75] found:

> The testimony established that . . . elements of parental alienation, instigated by actions of the mother, arose in the child's relationship with the father. More particularly, the mother allowed the child to believe that the fiancé was her actual father, allowed the child to refer to the deceased fiancé as "dad" and to the father by his first name, allowed the child to wear clothes memorializing the fiancé during visits with the father, and encouraged discussion in her household about the father's presumed participation in an alleged conspiracy to "ruin" the family.

15. Withholding Medical, Social, Academic Information from the Targeted Parent and Keeping That Parent's Contact Information Off Relevant Forms. "The alienating parent does not share team lists, class lists, rosters, schedules, homework assignments, and the like with the targeted

74. Wardell v. Wardell, Docket No. MII7D1619 (Middlesex Division Probate and Family Court), Further Temporary Orders, dated August 12, 2020.

75. Russell v. Russell, 173 A.D.3d 1607 (2019). Also see Williams v. Ramsey, 101 Ark. App. 61 (2007).

parent and does not put the parent's name and number on enrollment and contact forms."[76] This tactic robs the targeted parent of opportunities to parent the children while creating a false impression that s/he does not care enough to participate in the important events in the children's lives.[77] As one trial judge in Vermont found: "mother had filed a form with the children's school that listed her boyfriend as the children's stepfather, which meant that father was not permitted to obtain information about the children."[78] In another instance, an Arkansas court[79] gave custody to the father when it found the mother to have engaged in parental alienation: "The record is replete with [mother's] attempt to alienated [father] from his son—for example, her refusal to keep [father] apprised of medical information, especially in light of [son's] serious medical conditions."

16. Changing the Children's Names to Remove the Association with the Targeted Parent. "The alienating parent (if the mother) uses her maiden name or her new spouse / boyfriend's last name as the children's last name, or (if the father) creates a new nickname or uses only his portion of the hyphenated last name."[80] This tactic attempts to erase the connection between the targeted parent and the children. In *Mullins v. Mullins*, an Illinois court found that a mother's "overall conduct constituted a 'scheme' to destroy the father-child relationship," which included her behavior to remove the father's name from the children's school records and instead use her maiden name:

    > a change of surname of a child of divorced parents may contribute to estrangement of the child from his father. . . . A change of name imposed upon a child could represent to him a rejection by his father; or evidence that his father is deserving of rejection or contempt; or a statement by his mother and stepfather that his true identity is a shame and embarrassment to them and others. Such consequences could be enormously harmful to the child.[81]

17. Undermining Authority of the Targeted Parent / Inducing Dependency on Him-/Herself. "The alienating parent does and says things that encourage the children to believe that he or she is the only authority figure and that the rules, regulations, and values of the targeted parent are not valid or important."[82] This tactic undermines the targeted

---

76. *Supra* 34, at p.90.
77. Barnard v. Barnard, 1997 WL 379617 (Oh.Ct.App.) ("father attempted to remove the mother from 'the loop' as far as school activities were concerned").
78. Sundstorm v. Sundstorm, 177 Vt. 577, 580 (2004).
79. Sharp v. Keeler, 99 Ark. App. 42 (2007).
80. *Supra* 34.
81. Mullins v. Mullins, 142 Ill. App.3d 57; 490 N.E.2d 1375, 1388 (Ill. App. Ct. 1986).
82. *Supra* 34.

parent in the eyes of the children, incites conflict between the children and the targeted parent, and over-emphasizes the importance and control of the alienating parent in the children's lives.

Factor Five: Children Exhibit Alienation Behaviors

The final factor, Factor Five, focuses on a child exhibiting some or all of the eight behaviors or signs that research has determined to differentiate alienated children from non-alienated ones. Similar to the Factor Four behaviors or tactics, Factor Five behaviors are well established by clinical and research support. For instance, there is both clinical and research support that alienated children behave very differently than children who are realistically estranged from a parent due to the parent's neglect or abusive behavior. In their reformulation paper, Kelly and Johnston state that, "For the most part our observations of the behaviors and emotional responses of alienated children are similar to those reported by others."[83] Dr. Baker and other researchers' empirical observations found that only alienated children claimed to have no positive memories of the rejected parent, failed to identify a single positive aspect of that parent, expressed no interest in reparation of the relationship, and failed to see any flaws in the non-rejected parent.[84] In addition, psychiatrist William Bernet and his colleagues, while developing the Parental Acceptance-Rejection Questionnaire (PARQ), similarly found no expression of ambivalence or mixed feelings in alienated children. These children viewed one parent as all "good" and other as all "bad," something that was not observed even in children who had actually been neglected, abused, or abandoned by a parent.[85] In contrast (and to underscore the highly counterintuitive nature of the parental alienation phenomenon), truly abused and neglected children who had been removed from home have consistently been found to miss their abusive parent, want to be reunited with that parent, blame themselves for the abuse, and minimize the negative impact of the abuse.[86] The behaviors outlined next are unique and specific to alienated children are typically not exhibited by a child even toward an abusive parent.[87]

83. Kelly, J., & Johnston, J. (2001). The alienated child: A reformulation of parental alienation syndrome, *Family Court Review*, 39, 249–266; *see also* Gardner, R. (1998). *The Parental Alienation Syndrome: A Guide for Mental Health and Legal Professionals*, Creative Therapeutics.

84. Baker, A., Burkhard, B., & Kelly, J. (2012). Differentiating alienated from not alienated children: A pilot study, *Journal of Divorce and Remarriage*, 53(3), 178–193.

85. Bernet, W., Gregory, N., Reay, K., & Rohner, R. (2017). An objective measure of splitting in parental alienation: The Parental Acceptance-Rejection Questionnaire, *Journal of Forensic Science*, August, 776–783.

86. Baker, A., Creegan, A., Quinones, A., & Rozelle, L. (2016). Foster children's views of their birth parents: A review of the literature, *Children and Youth Services Review*, 67. 177–183.

87. Baker, A. (2020), *supra*, at 227.

1. Campaign of Denigration.

   > The child behaves in a rude, arrogant, disrespectful, and entitled manner toward the targeted parent. The child has no qualms about denigrating that parent to others in the community. The child has difficulty recalling or acknowledging any positive memories of the targeted parent.[88]

   Alienated children typically present a laundry list of "flaws" that a targeted parent suffers from. Without prompting, or, at times, after minimal prompting by an authority figure such as a lawyer, judge, mental health professional, or child protective services investigator, the child's rehearsed performance will be turned on and provide a command performance.
2. Weak, Frivolous, or Absurd Reasons for Rejecting the Targeted Parent. Alienated children provide irrational and often ridiculous justification for rejecting a parent.

   > The child will offer reasons such as the floors being scratched or not liking the hairstyle or clothes of the targeted parent. The child will sometimes refuse to even offer a reason, claiming to have done so too many times before when that it is not the case.

   In *McClain v. McClain*, a Tennessee court found that the alienated children's preference for the favored parent was not "reasonable . . . in light of the 'vitriolic' statements . . . made against Mother without a reasonable basis in fact."[89] In another case, *Duke v. Duke*, the court found that the children rejected the mother and "criticiz[ed] her behaviors, no matter what she does, e.g., whether she laughs, cries, or tries to help them":[90]

   > [Father] and the children began to assert that [Mother] was sick, that she was dangerous, and that she was nice to the children for the sake of court proceedings. None of these beliefs or accusations had a factual basis. As a result, the children became hostile and upset toward [Mother]. They criticized her for virtually everything that she did. They criticized [her] over trivial matters. They criticized her for being a stay-at-home mother and not seeking employment outside the home, even though that had been her role throughout their entire lives.

88. Examples of all manifestations of symptoms of parental alienation in the children are quoted from Baker, A. J. L., & Fine, P. R. (2014). *Surviving Parental Alienation: A Journey of Hope and Healing*, Rowman and Littlefield, 12.

89. McClain v. McClain, 539 S.W.3d 170, 207 (Tenn. Ct. App. 2017).

90. Duke v. Duke, 2014 WL 4966902 (Tenn.Ct.App. 2014).

3. Lack of Ambivalence toward His/Her Parents. All human relationships, including the parent-child relationship, are ambivalent and contain mixed feelings. This is not the case in a situation involving an alienated child. Here,

   > [t]he child claims to worship the alienating parent beyond what is appropriate, necessary, or realistic, while claiming to despise the targeted parent. Both responses are unrealistic and show an inability to see each parent as a mix of good and bad qualities.

   In *Noland-Vance v. Vance*, a Missouri court found striking evidence of this behavior from severely alienated children:

   > The glowing way in which the children perceive their mother, and the way in which they uncritically describe her as being the perfect parent stands in stark contrast to their descriptions of their father. The three oldest girls were exceptionally derogatory towards their father. When asked by the [GAL] to tell one redeeming quality of [Father], they could not give an answer. The three oldest girls denied anything positive in their relationship with [Father] to an unnatural extreme. The three youngest children were very articulate to the point of sounding rehearsed in their testimony. They seemed like "little adults." The two youngest children . . . referred to [Father] as "Brent," which was disturbing given their young ages. The three youngest children did their best to mimic the extreme hatred toward their father as shown by the three oldest children. The children's negative view of their father is out of all proportion to reality.[91]

4. Independent Thinker Phenomenon.

   > The child strenuously insists that the alienating parent played no role in his/her rejection of the targeted parent despite the alienating parent's obvious influence.[92]

5. Lack of Guilt Regarding Poor Treatment of the Targeted Parent. "While behaving in a rude and callous manner, the child fails to manifest awareness of or caring about the pain being inflicted on the targeted parent."[93] The child displays a complete absence of gratitude for anything that the parent has done, such as love, affection, giving gifts, or financial assistance.

---

91. Noland-Vance v. Vance, 321 S.W.2d 398, 412-413 (Mo. App. 2010). *See also*: Costley v. Benjamin, 2005 WL 1950114 (Tn.Ct.App. 2005).

92. *Supra* 87.

93. *Supra* 87.

6. Reflexive Support for the Alienating Parent in All Parental Conflicts. "The child sides with the alienating parent, no matter how absurd, illogical, or inconsistent that parent's position is."[94]
7. Presence of Borrowed Scenarios. "The child uses words, phrases, and concepts that are not understood, cannot be defined, and are readily attributable to the ideas and beliefs of the alienating parent."[95] One often hears the child use phraseology that is not commonly used by the child (e.g., "My dad / mom is a narcissist." "S/he does not validate my feelings."). In *Noland-Vance v. Vance*, a Missouri court found that the children had been seriously affected and influenced by mother's negative statements about the father and, as a result, mentioned "the same litany of facts as Mother and used phraseology similar to hers."[96]
8. Spread of Animosity to Friends and Family of the Targeted Parent. "The child cuts off and/or denigrates formerly beloved friends, neighbors, and family based on their association with the targeted parent."[97] Cousins, uncles, aunts, grandparents—all of whom may have had a loving relationship with the child—are viewed as being "in the other camp" and untrustworthy.

Programming / Brainwashing Techniques Used by Alienating Parents

In addition to the Five-Factor Model, professionals also consider other tactics or strategies employed by alienating parents. For example, Stanley Clawar and Brynne Rivlin, in their book *Children Held Hostage*[98], discuss eleven brainwashing techniques that alienating parents use to influence their children to reject a "good enough" targeted parent. After an intensive review of 1,000 cases of family counseling / therapy, mediation, reconciliation, and forensic evaluation, it was apparent to the researchers that there are often negative dimensions to the communications that parents have with their children about the other parent. Such covert and overt communication between a parent and the child surrounding the other parent may contain techniques for undermining the targeted parent in the eyes of the child, undermining the relationship of the child with the other parent, or controlling or distorting the information the child provides to a lawyer, judge, a custody evaluator, or other court professional. These techniques could

---

94. *Supra* 87.
95. *Supra* 87.
96. Noland-Vance v. Vance, 321 S.W.2d 398, 405 (Mo. App. 2010).
97. *Supra* 87.
98. Clawar, S., & Rivlin, B. (2013). *Children Held Hostage*, Second Edition, American Bar Association, 31–63.

be used consciously, intentionally, and deliberately, or unwittingly, by an alienating parent. Regardless, it is important to understand the power these techniques have on inculcating, modifying, and solidifying belief systems and attitudes in the children who are exposed to such techniques. Once they are solidified, the alienated child internalizes the beliefs and attitudes, causing others, including professionals, to view the child as having an independent, even principled belief. An alienating parent can employ these techniques for an extended period of time, often without detection, causing a significant impact on the children and polarizing their relationships with the alienating parent and targeted parent.

1. Denial of Existence Technique.

   > One of the basic techniques parents use to assault the character of the other parent is to deny or not acknowledge the social existence of the other parent. The manner of denial can vary greatly. One common technique is simply never to talk about the other parent. By excluding any discussion of the other parent or ignoring the topic when raised by the child, the brainwashing parent can send a subtle message to the child that the other parent is not significant. He or she does not exist in our conversation, and therefore, he or she does not, in social terms, exist.[99]

   Another technique employed by an alienating parent is to employ body language or non-verbal signs that communicates to the child that the targeted parent is unworthy or insignificant. Children who have been exposed to the regular use of such technique will frequently mirror this behavior. Examples of this technique include an alienating parent destroying family photo albums; blatantly ignoring the other parent at social events, games, weddings, or religious ceremonies; denying or refusing to acknowledge that the children have had (or should have) positive experiences with the targeted parent; and creating or encouraging a fiction that the targeted parent never really was "into" parenting and was never interested in the children's activities, community, or events.
2. The "Who, Me?" Technique. "A subtle but powerful technique is to make indirect attacks on the other parent. When questioned about such attacks, the brainwashing parent will say, 'Who, me?'"[100] The alienating parent will then remonstrate that s/he meant no such thing and that the listener or child was certainly misinterpreting what was said. The typical pattern followed by the alienators is to attack the character, lifestyle, career choice, extended family, past, present, or future of the

99. Descriptions of brainwashing techniques are quoted from Clawar, S., & Rivlin, B., *supra*, 31–63.
100. *Supra* 99.

targeted parent. For instance, making statements such as "Lawyers are very corrupt and are getting worse and worse reputations with the public today," where the targeted parent is an attorney.

3. Middle-Man Technique: "By speaking to the child about issues that should be first discussed with the other parent, the programmer/brainwasher can compromise and/or damage the child's relationship with or image of the target parent."[101] This can happen by an alienating parent asking questions to the child such as, "Do you think you would like to have more time with Mom?" This places the child in the middle and pressures him or her to make a choice in front of the inquiring parent. In doing so, it can have an effect of closing down communications because the child gets the message that the alienating parent does not want to hear, ever, that the child could enjoy his or her time with the targeted parent.
4. Circumstantial Technique:

   > By manipulating, changing, rearranging, and commenting on time, the programming parent tries to gain dominance in the eyes of the children. "Your mother's always late for delivery and pickup. I wonder if she would be late for her own funeral." The other parent told her children, "He's always early for pickup, but late for delivery." These parents are attacking character by discussing punctuality.

   This behavior signifies to the children that the other parent lacks importance. If the targeted parent does not show up for an event, the alienating parent can say, "Well, it's just like it's always been—everything comes before the kids." A farmer father who has to attend a meeting of the Farm Bureau in Washington, DC, is portrayed to his children by the alienating mother as someone who missed a school event so he could attend another "farm bureau drunk fest."
5. "I Don't Know What's Wrong with Him" Technique: "Many parents have developed a technique whereby they create and/or exaggerate differences between themselves and the other parent in front of the children."[102] The alienating parent will use a phrase or present an idea or employ snickers or facial grimaces—anything that he or she consciously or unconsciously knows will "push the buttons" of or incite the other parent. The instigating parent is often so skilled at this technique that when the targeted parent reacts, usually with frustration or anger, the instigating parent will profess that his or her motives are sincere or noble and that the other parent is "crazy," "bananas," "paranoid,"

101. *Supra* 99.
102. *Supra* 99.

"unstable," or "in need of therapy." Children who are exposed to this technique may mirror the dysfunctional communication style observed by them with their siblings or friends.

6. Ally Technique:

   Attempting to get the children to side with one parent against the other occurs both in and outside of marriage. At the time of divorce or custody conflict, however, the attempt to ally the children is stronger. It can happen that the children will create an ally relationship with their mother or father against the target parent. An example would be asking the children direct questions such as, "Don't you think your mother is wrong to try to get all the money she can from us?"

   Children who are exposed to this technique are forced to choose between their parents and denounce one over the other. The counter-intuitive nature of parental alienation poses a risk; to an untrained or unsophisticated eye, the children allied with the alienating parent may appear to be "close" and very attached. However, it may be due to the result of them being subjected to constant, regular, and devious brainwashing and programming.

7. Morality Technique:

   Programming behaviors often include moral judgments against the target parent concerning his/her values, lifestyle, choice of friends, successes or failures in life (career, financial, relational), or residential choice. These criticisms are intended to elevate one's own position in comparison with the target parent, who becomes diminished by this good/bad dichotomy.

   Children exposed to such techniques are no longer able to accept both parents as equally worthy or good. The child's perception of the targeted parent changes from its original, more positive view, to conform to the alienating parent's distorted and negative opinion. Over a period of time, the child's view of the targeted parent becomes so ingrained that the alienating parent, who instilled the beliefs, no longer has to promote the desired perceptions on a regular basis. Such beliefs have been given life within the child's own mind.

8. Threat of Withdrawal-of-Love Technique:

   This is a coercive, powerful, and almost universally successful technique utilized by parents who programme. Here, the children come to fear rejection or loss of love from a parent if they express love or a desire to be with the other parent. It becomes implicitly or

> explicitly understood that to be loved and accepted, the child must become a cohort and also turn against the other parent.

For instance, while the child is at the targeted parent's home, the alienating parent remains in constant contact with the child through telephone calls, emails, or texts, hoping to confirm that the child is not enjoying himself or herself, is not being cared for appropriately, or desperately longs for the alienating parent. Any negative report made by the child regarding the targeted parent is "rewarded" with love, affection, understanding, and sympathy, showered by the alienating parent. The ultimate result is that the alienating parent now has an ally who "understands" his or her plight. In essence, the children are taught by words and behaviors, "Now you know what I went through."

9. "I'm the Only One Who Really Loves You" Technique: "The intent is to create the belief that the target parent or those who are associated with that parent are not sincere in their love and caring for the child. Genuine love, interest, and involvement, by contrast, exist only in the heart of the programmer."[103] An often-used technique by alienating parents is to over-inform children or share inappropriate information with them on adult matters. For instance, "If only your father would pay what he owes us in child support, I wouldn't have to worry about putting food on the table." The message conveyed to the child is that the targeted parent is attempting to hurt "us," the alienating parent and the child, who are portrayed as if they were one entity. In some instances, parents form a close bond with their children, becoming intensely enmeshed. Although this may satisfy a parent's social-emotional need, it is pathological and has severe negative ramifications for the children.
10. "You're an Endangered Species" Technique:

> One method of instilling distrust, fear, lack of love, or the belief that a parent is unable to care properly for the child is accomplished through a procedure of judgmental, opinionated, and negative commentary and/or physical inspection and interrogation once the child arrives "home" again.

Being exposed to this technique over a period of time, the child comes to believe that anything associated with the targeted parent is unsafe, dangerous, or wrong and perceives at being risk when in contact with the parent. Minor injuries such as bumps, scratches, or bruises obtained accidentally or through normal play or sport are checked for severity and intent. The child is taken for a medical examination or a report is made to the child protective services. The child is repeatedly questioned and pressured to spend less time with the other parent.

---

103. *Supra* 99.

11. Rewriting Reality Technique:

> Through rewriting reality, the brainwasher attempts to convince a child to doubt his or her ability to perceive reality. A child may observe a scenario unfold from beginning to end, but as the brainwashing parent repeatedly goes over the scenario and resists the child's interpretation, the original and 'true' reality is ultimately filtered out and rewritten script is eventually adopted.

Soon, the "new reality" is accepted and the alienated child takes on the role of the Director and becomes the tribal hero, the warrior who is aligned with the alienating parent and feels compelled to protect the parent from the perceived dangerousness of the targeted parent. The alienating parent rarely needs to be involved anymore because the rewritten reality now lives within the child.

Single Factor Model versus Multi-Factor Models

Generally speaking, there are two theories or models that have evolved over time that attempt to explain how or why parental alienation occurs: a single factor model and multi-factor model. The single factor model asserts a primary causal relationship between the alienating behaviors of the favored or preferred parent and an alienated child. In other words, the model asserts that the favored parent's alienating behaviors caused parental alienation. Some professionals believe that this model leads to a false dichotomy and is an overly simplistic view of the phenomenon of parental alienation.[104] In response, some professionals have advocated for a multi-factor model to assess a situation where a child is resisting or refusing contact with a parent. Here, the alienating behavior by the preferred parent is viewed as an important but not the only (nor necessarily the dominant) factor accounting for children's resistance or refusal of contact with a parent.[105] Other factors, such as the child's relationships with siblings, rejected parent's reaction, divorce conflict and litigation, extended families, lack of functional coparenting, etc., all play part in the multi-factor model.

From a practice standpoint, litigating a case of parental alienation using multi-factor models is too complex, too vague, too costly, and inefficient. "Compared to the single factor model, they are more difficult to explain, and they may appear less useful to the court or legal professionals."[106] Using such a model may generate not just confusion but also lead to ineffective legal and mental

104. *See, e.g.*, Johnston, J., & Sullivan, M. (2020). Parental alienation: In search of common ground for a more differentiated theory, *Family Court Review*, 58(2), 270.

105. *Id.* at 279.

106. *Id.* at 282.

health interventions. Progress towards goals and outcomes in treatment are difficult to evaluate when we have myriad factors—not just alienating behaviors manifested by a favored parent—that allegedly contribute to the problem. In reviewing hundreds of cases where a court found parental alienation to exist, I did not come across a single case that focused on a multi-factor model for fact-finding or to provide remedial measures to combat alienation. In cases where there is significant and strong evidence of parental alienating behaviors by a favored parent, together with a lack of abuse or neglect by the rejected parent, it is effective and efficient to present the case in court using the single factor model.

Conclusion

To sum up, parental alienation is not a new phenomenon; the mental condition has been described in the legal cases since the early 19th century and in the scientific literature since the 1940s.[107] Detractors who oppose the theory of parental alienation more often than not attempt to engage in needless debates and litigation over the "controversy" of "PAS" or the "syndrome." As shown in this chapter, this is a strawman argument. Courts around the country are increasingly refusing to get bogged down by meaningless controversy surrounding the "Parental Alienation Syndrome" and instead focus attention on the alienating parent's *behaviors*. At the end of the day, a court cannot control, contain, or modify esoteric, nebulous, speculative theories. What it can control, contain, and hopefully, modify are behaviors manifested by a parent—behaviors that are unquestionably harmful to the child's mental health and his or her relationship with the other parent. As the Michigan Court of Appeals recently held:

> [Mother] . . . essentially contends that "parental alienation" is junk science. While there may be a dispute in the scientific community about whether there is diagnosable, pathological condition called parental alienation syndrome . . . there is no reasonable dispute that high-conflict custody disputes frequently involve acts by one parent designed to obstruct or sabotage the opposing parent's relationship with the child.[108]

107. *See, e.g.*, Westmeath v. Westmeath: The wars between the Westmeaths, 1812–1857, in Stone, L. (1993). *Broken Lives: Separation and Divorce in England, 1660–1857*, Oxford Press, 284; Levy, D. M. (1943). *Maternal Overprotection*, Columbia University, 153.

108. Martin v. Martin, Michigan Court of Appeals No. 349261 (January 28, 2020), FN 2.

CHAPTER 5

The Role of Guardian ad Litem and Child Representative

Consider this vignette: There is an ongoing contentious divorce litigation with the parties fighting for custody. The child has aligned herself with her father ("favored parent") and is resisting and refusing to spend any time with her mother ("target parent"). Despite a significant history of maternal love and care the child claims that the mother has "abandoned us" and, despite no evidence to support it, alleges that her mother has a "drinking problem." Court-ordered parenting time and visitation orders are routinely and consistently violated. Exchanges turn into nightmarish scenarios as the child refuses to go with the target parent. Police and child protective services investigators are summoned to investigate reports of "abuse." The frustrated target parent keeps demanding court intervention without success. The court, also frustrated, appoints a guardian ad litem (GAL) or child's representative to help resolve the situation. Upon arrival on the scene, the GAL tries to make sense of the ongoing mayhem. Given the child's refusal to go to court-ordered parenting time, the GAL recommends a "cooling off" period and recommends that the target parent not compel the child to go on visitation for a limited time. The GAL selects a therapist to provide "family therapy" or "reunification therapy" to help reunify the mother with the child.

In therapy, the child tells tales of "abusive" behavior: Mom abandoned "us," is mean, yells "for hours," and "drinks." The therapist validates the child's perceptions, emotions, and behavior and uncritically accepts every statement that the child makes, regardless of the mountain of evidence to the contrary. The mother, who participates in some joint sessions, is advised not to challenge the daughter's version of events and is asked to shove aside all the "evidence" she has put together showing a healthy, loving, and close relationship with her daughter prior to the filing of divorce. Instead, the mother is advised to show "empathy." The child's behaviors of acting-out and her fear and rejection of the mother gets worse. Months go by without any parenting time. Lawyers spend time on phone conferences and file motions that don't result in any change in the status quo. Soon, legal fees and costs spiral out of control. The time comes when the target parent is either supremely frustrated, out of money, or both. Something must give.

Unfortunately, this scenario is not uncommon and plagues family courts around the country. Time after time, courts look to the GALs or children's representatives to help resolve these issues in the best interests of the children. The hope, if not the goal, is to move towards a collaborative model where divorcing parties treat each other with dignity and mutual respect, where child clients are treated like adult clients and have a voice in the process of decision-making.[1] In contentious cases, some courts are increasingly appointing attorneys for children—mainly to protect them, give them a "voice" in the proceedings, and promote their best interests, but also with a hope that a neutral quasi-judicial professional may help the parties reach a resolution.

Parental alienation, however, changes everything.[2] The underlying pathology of parental alienation and its effect on the alienated children compels us to take a skeptical look at the child-centered model, forcing each case—with its unique set of facts and circumstances—to be viewed through a critical lens. While the child-centered model might be suitable for non-alienation high-conflict cases, it would be disastrous to use such a model in parental alienation cases because, in alienation cases, unlike estrangement, the child's rejection of the target parent is based on a false or unreasonable belief that is *significantly disproportionate* to the child's actual experience.[3] To give "voice" to an alienated child and give weight to such child's custodial preference would be detrimental to the child's best interests.

It's understandable why a family law judge, when faced with the complex allegations of contact refusal, interference with visitation, and parental alienation, would appoint a GAL. The court, understandably, wants another pair of eyes and ears to analyze the situation and recommend what's in the best interests of the child. However, what many courts fail to realize is that parental

1. *See* Elrod, L. D. (2007). Client-direct lawyers for children: It is the "right" thing to do, *Pace L. Rev.*, 27, 869, 905.

2. Rosen, J. (2013). The child's attorney and the alienated child: Approaches to resolving the ethical dilemma of diminished capacity, *Family Court Review*, 51(2), 330.

3. Rosen, *supra*, 331; *see also* Harner v. Harner, 2018 WL 521863, (Mich., January 23, 2018) (". . . there were reasons to believe that the children's claims of neglect and abuse were not founded on actual experiences . . . [and] suggested coaching by [the mother]").

alienation is not only a specialized area, but it is also highly counterintuitive and generally misunderstood. Further, there is a lack of training[4] and dearth of easily accessible resources for the various third parties involved with the children who are victims of alienation.[5] Errors of commission and/or omission are easy to make through inadvertence, misinformation, and lack of diligence or competence or experience. And such errors may not only constitute violations of professional codes of ethics but can have significant and, at times, irreversible, impact on the result of the case. Nevertheless, despite the risks involved, little effort is made in ensuring that the GAL or the child's representative has the requisite knowledge, skill, and/or experience in dealing with cases involving parental alienation.[6]

GALs and Child Representatives: Experts by Default?

Family court judges generally appoint a GAL to conduct an investigation and make recommendations as to custody and/or parenting time that are in the best interests of the child.[7] Despite the regularity with which GALs are appointed by family courts around the country, no consensus exists on standards applicable to these professionals, their duties, form of advocacy, or their allegiance. As one law-review article stated, the role of the GAL is very broad and a professional often wears more hats than one:

> The guardian ad litem has been defined as any and all of the following: a court-appointed investigator who makes recommendations to the court about who should have custody; a lawyer who represents a child; an advocate for the "best interest" of the children; and a facilitator/mediator. The GAL is sometimes called the "eyes and ears of the court." In some states, GALs are allowed to provide facts and opinions to the court without taking the witness stand or being subject to cross-examination. Consequently, everything they are asked to report to the court about their conversations

---

4. The National Court Appointed Special Advocate Association (NCASAA) trains and provides volunteer guardians ad litem for use by courts nationwide. However, the organization's focus is not on private child custody litigation where the majority of parental alienation cases originate, but rather on training professionals to represent children who have experienced abuse or neglect, including those targeted for sex trafficking, affected by the opioid crisis, and preparing to age out of the foster care system.

5. Ludmer, B. (2018). Understanding ethical issues in a parental alienation case, *PASG Newsletter*, 4(3), 9.

6. *See* Haralambie, A., & Glaser, D. (1995). Practical and theoretical problems with the AAML Standards for Representing "Impaired" Children, *Journal of the American Academy of Matrimonial Lawyers*, 13, 57, 75. ("One of the major benefits of requiring that children's attorneys be specially trained [*e.g.* A.A.M.L. Standard 1.2] is that attorneys will have particular competence to fulfill advocacy roles which are somewhat different than those ordinarily performed by attorneys for adult clients.")

7. *See, e.g.*, Michigan statute MCL 722.27; Wilburn v. Wilburn, 169 Ohio App.3d 415 (2006); Ex Parte J.G. (*In re*: J.G. v. B.G.), 281 So.3d 371 (Alabama 2019; Dissenting Opinion).

> with children and parents is hearsay. GALs serve "a quasi-judicial role . . . cloaked in judicial immunity."[8]

In addition to being vague and ambiguous, a GAL's role is also controversial:

> The GAL essentially serves as an expert witness without any expert qualifications and without having to be a witness. First of all, a GAL cannot be qualified as an "expert" because there is no such thing as a lay or attorney "expert" in custody cases. And unlike child custody evaluators, who are frequently psychologists, GALs are not required to possess any specific credentials. There is not even a consensus on the appropriate "training" for GALs. In most states, the way to get on the "list" for appointment is to attend a continuing education course, agree to accept assignments, and then continue accepting assignments. GALs become experts by default: "The more often a particular individual performs that role, the more likely that the trial court will rely on him [or her] as if he [or she] were an expert."[9]

States vary in how they define the role of a GAL and the duties attributed to that role. A state-by-state in-depth comparison of GALs and their respective roles is beyond the purview of this chapter, but it would help if we were to look at a few states and how they have defined the roles of a GAL. For instance, in Michigan, the term "'guardian ad litem' is considered a legal term of art and therefore, resort to a legal dictionary to determine its meaning is appropriate."[10] And while a GAL's role is to assist a Michigan family court in determining the child's best interests, he or she need not be an attorney.[11] In Ohio, a GAL "is appointed to protect and ensure that the children's best interests are represented throughout the divorce proceedings" and "this is accomplished by the GAL conducting an investigation of the child's situation and then making recommendations, written or oral, to the court as to what decisions would be in the child's best interest."[12] In Alabama, a GAL can play three possible roles in a custody case: as counsel, as an investigator and/or fact witness, and as an opinion witness.[13] When serving as counsel, the GAL "represents a child but owes a

---

8. Cecka, D. M. (2016). Inequity in private child custody litigation, *City University of New York L. Rev.*, 20, 203, 220–22 (footnotes omitted).

9. *Id.*

10. Farris v. McKaig, __ N.W.2d __ (2018), 2018 WL 2269775, *2 (Mich. App., May 17, 2018), citing King v. Emmons, 283 Mich. 116, 124-125, 277 N.W. 851 (1938); Ford Motor Co. v. City of Woodhaven, 475 Mich. 425, 440, 716 N.W.2d 247 (2006).

11. MCL 712A.13a(f).

12. Wilburn v. Wilburn, 169 Ohio App.3d 415 (2006), citing MacFarlane v. MacFarlane, 8th Dist. No. 86835, 2006-Ohio-3155, 2006 WL 1704531, Sabrina J. Robbin C., 6th Dist. No. L-00-1374, 2002-Ohio-2691, 2002 WL 1303148.

13. Rogers v. Rogers, ___ So.3d ___, *9 (2019).

duty to the appointing court."[14] Accordingly, a GAL acting in his or her role as counsel is not necessarily an advocate for a child's desires if those wishes are not in the child's best interests.[15]

At times, some jurisdictions, such as Connecticut, allow a GAL to serve in a dual capacity of GAL and counsel to the child *if* the court finds that there is no conflict of interest between the child's wishes and the best interests of the child.[16] In such instances, where one professional is appointed to serve "as guardian ad litem and counsel for the child," he or she is charged with "protecting the child's best interest as well as the child's legal rights in the process."[17] In cases where the GAL perceives that his or her obligation to advocate for the child's legal rights is in conflict with the child's actual best interest, the professional must bring that to the court's attention and the court, in turn, must appoint a separate guardian ad litem to protect and to promote the child's best interest.[18]

In other jurisdictions, such as Michigan, if the court determines that the minor's interests are inadequately represented, the court may appoint a lawyer, such as a lawyer-guardian ad litem (LGAL), to represent the minor.[19] The role of the LGAL is distinct from a GAL and is defined by the statute, which provides that the duty of the LGAL *is to the child and not to the court* and that the attorney-client privilege applies.[20] But while the LGAL's duty is to the child, it does not translate into the professional simply being a mouthpiece for the child's wishes. The LGAL has the duty to first determine and then advocate for the child's *best interests*.[21] And while the child's wishes are relevant to the determination of his or her best interests, they should be weighed according to the child's competence and maturity. When serving in this role, an LGAL functions as a "guardian" with the statutory authority and duty to care for the child by advocating for the child's best interests.[22]

However, the term "guardian" when applied to a counsel for the child could be misleading, because there are significant differences between a GAL and a counsel for the child. For instance, in Michigan, a GAL need not be an attorney, while an LGAL, as the term itself suggests, must be an attorney.[23] A GAL, after

---

14. *Id.*
15. *Id.*
16. Wilburn v. Wilburn, *supra; see also*: *In re* Tayquon H., 76 Conn.App. 693, 704 (2003) (Connecticut: The guardian ad litem "is not required to be an attorney-at-law but shall be knowledgeable about the needs and protection of children").
17. *In re* Tayquon H., 76 Conn.App. 693, 703 (2003).
18. *Id.*
19. MCL 700.5213(4).
20. MCL 712A.17d.
21. MCL 712A.17d(1)(h).
22. Farris v. McKaig, *supra*, *3. In fact, in child protective proceedings, the LGAL "satisfies the dictionary definition of 'guardian ad litem.'" *Id.*
23. MCL 712A.13a(1)(f) and (g). Also see *In re* Tayquon H., 76 Conn.App. 693, 704 (2003).

conducting an independent investigation, "shall make a report in open court or file a written report of the investigation and recommendations."[24] The GAL's report and any subsequent reports "may be received by the court and may be relied on to the extent of their probative value."[25] Parties have a right to "examine and controvert reports received into evidence" and can cross-examine the GAL who prepared the report.[26]

An LGAL, like a GAL, must conduct a diligent investigation, but unlike a GAL, "[t]he court or another party shall not call [an LGAL] as a witness to testify regarding matters related to the case."[27] Also, an LGAL's "file of the case is not discoverable."[28] And while the court must appoint an LGAL in a child protective proceeding, a court is not required to appoint a GAL in such proceedings.[29] The duties of an LGAL are far broader and more extensive than that of a GAL. And while a GAL owes his or her duty to the court and does not enjoy an attorney-client relationship with the child, an LGAL has an attorney-client relationship with the child and owes his or her duty to the child. Perhaps "the starkest difference between the two is that unlike an LGAL, appointment of GAL 'does not create an attorney-client relationship' and '[c]ommunications between that person and the guardian ad litem are not subject to the attorney-client privilege.'"[30]

Notwithstanding the differences between the two roles, when determining a child's best interests, there is an important overlap between the duties of the GAL and LGAL. "[A]n LGAL serves the same basic function as a GAL: independently investigating, determining, and representing the child's best interests."[31] But an LGAL must serve this purpose differently than a GAL. An LGAL is not tasked with simply assisting the court in determining the child's best interests, but rather is tasked with the duty to *make* "a determination regarding the child's best interests and advocate for those best interests."[32] And an LGAL is obligated to serve as the "independent representative for the child's best interests": he or she may advocate for a position, call witnesses, file all necessary pleadings and papers, attend hearings, and monitor the implementation of case plans and court orders and is otherwise "entitled to full and active participation in all aspects of the litigation."[33]

24. MCR 5.121(C).
25. MCR 5.121(D)(1).
26. MCR 5.121(D)(2)(a)–(c).
27. MCL 712A.17d(1)(b).
28. MCL 712A.17d(3).
29. MCL 712A.17c(7) and (10).
30. Farris v. McKaig, *supra*, *3, citing MCR 5.121(E)(1).
31. *Id.*, at *4.
32. MCL 712A.17d(1)(i).
33. MCL 712A.17d(1)(b) and (g) and (i).

Finally, an LGAL is not the child's attorney in a traditional sense; he or she is an *independent* representative of the child's best interests. Such professional would owe the child "the same duties of undivided loyalty, confidentiality, and zealous representation of the child's expressed wishes as the attorney would to an adult client."[34] And when a child's interests differ from the LGAL's determination of the child's best interests, the court has discretion to appoint an attorney—a traditional one—for the child.[35] Whether "such dual, conflicting advocacy" is in the best interests of the child is a decision that the court has the discretion to make on a case-by-case basis.[36] For a chart outlining different states' approach to defining the role of a minor's counsel and the professional's duty to advocate for the child's best interests, see Appendix E.

Parental Alienation and the Child's Preference

Both the "client centered" (LGAL / child representative) and the "best interests" (GAL) models assume that the child has the ability to consult with and provide voluntary, knowing, and intelligent input and/or directions to the attorney. The "client centered" model goes a step further and assumes that the child-client also has the ability to direct an attorney as to a specific course of action. In turn, the child representative must then advocate the child's articulated position—*if it is in the best interests of the child*—by first ascertaining the child's wishes and then making them known to the court.[37] Presence of parental alienation in a custodial dispute requires the professionals to acknowledge that children are susceptible to influence, intimidation, and manipulation, and the child's wishes may not reflect the child's actual position or best interests.[38] The National Association of Counsel for Children (NACC)—the largest child's attorney organization in the United States—defines the role of the attorney for the child as a zealous advocate unless one of two exceptions exists: the child lacks the capacity to make a reasoned choice or the child's stated preference is "considered to be seriously injurious to the child."[39] The child's "voice"—his or her right to express a reasonable preference in a custody setting—is attached to the best interests of the child and "not to the rights of the contestants in the

34. MCL 712A.13a(1)(c).

35. MCL 712A.17d(2). Of course, in an alienation setting, having two advocates represent the child (or one for the child and another for the child's best interests) might be more expensive and traumatic for the child rather than helpful. *See* Rosen, *supra*, at 335.

36. *In re* Tayquon H., 76 Conn.App. 693, 702 (2003).

37. Rosen, *supra*, at 333.

38. ABA Standards of Practice for Lawyers Who Represent Children in Abuse and Neglect Cases, Section A-1.

39. Rosen, *supra*, citing Patton, W. W. (2010). Viewing child witnesses through a child and adolescent psychiatric lens: How attorneys' ethical duties exacerbate children's psychopathology, *Widener L. Rev.*, 16, 369, 382.

custody battle."[40] And the child's preference always "exclude[s] those preferences that are arbitrary or inherently indefensible."[41]

Parental alienation is a result of indoctrination, manipulation, brainwashing, and programming of a child. And "[l]oss is the greatest, all-encompassing feature of programming and brainwashing. The effects of losing not only the intact family, but also a parent, hang heavily over children, touching them in ways that can wreak havoc in many realms of life, both in the present and future. . . . This loss cannot be undone. Childhood cannot be recaptured. Gone forever is that sense of history, intimacy, lost input of values and morals, self-awareness through knowing one's beginnings, love, contact with extended family, and much more. Virtually no child possesses the ability to protect himself or herself against such an undignified and total loss."[42] The wish or desire of an alienated child to not see or have a relationship with the target parent is not normal; it is a result of brainwashing and programming, inherently indefensible and not in the best interest of the child.[43] As a New York court held, "[t]he desires of young children, capable of distortive manipulation by a bitter, or perhaps even well-meaning, parent, do not always reflect the long-term best interest of the children."[44]

Consider this statement from a 15-year-old male adolescent whose maternal history was *replete* with breastfeeding and full care by his mother: "*My mother abandoned us and never did anything for me, so I don't need her now.*"[45] Or, "*[t]ell the judge I won't see my Dad again. That's that, I have legal rights you know. I'm 14.*"[46] Despite the fact that alienated children are so brainwashed and manipulated into rejecting the target parent, many professionals, including children's representatives and GALs, often give significant weight to the preferences of alienated children. Excuses to not abide by court-ordered visitation are not only tolerated but, in fact, the target parent is often advised to show "empathy"

---

40. Maeir v. Maier, 311 Mich. App. 218, 224; 874 N.W.2d 725 (2015); Rogers v. Rogers, ___ So.3d ___, *9 (2019).

41. *Id.*, citing Pierron v. Pierron, 282 Mich. App. 222, 259, 765 N.W.2d 345 (2009), aff'd by and quoted in Pierron, 486 Mich. At 92, 782 N.W.2d 480. Also see: *In re* Marriage of Milovich, 105 Ill.App.3d 596, 612 (1982), citing Patton v. Armstrong, 16 Ill.App.3d 881, 307 N.E.2d 178 (1974).

42. Clawar, S. & Rivlin, B. (2013). *Children Held Hostage: Identifying Brainwashed Children, Presenting a Case and Crafting Solutions* (2nd ed.), American Bar Association, 164.

43. O'Connor v. O'Connor, 146 A.D.2d 909, 911 (1989). (Court "determined that in view of defendant's conduct in alienating the children from plaintiff, and their young ages, custody should be given to plaintiff. The court thus properly based its decision on the children's ages and maturity and the potential for influence having been exerted over them.")

44. Young v. Young, 628 N.Y.S.2d 957 (1995). Also see: Price v. Price, 611 N.W.2d 425, 435 (S.D., 2000). (In reversing a trial court's award of physical custody to an alienating parent, the appellate court held: "The standard remains the best interest of [child] and an 11-year-old child can not always determine his own best interest."); Nehra v. Uhlar, 43 N.Y.2d 242, 401 N.Y.S.2d 168 (1977) ("The desires of young children, capable of distortive manipulation by a bitter, or perhaps even well-meaning, parent, do not always reflect the long-term best interest of the children.").

45. Clawar, S. & Rivlin, B., *supra*, at 1-26 (Brainwashing and Programming).

46. *Id.*, at 335.

by *not* seeking to enforce visitation. A target parent who has coached Little League sports teams and has been an active parent all his life is now asked to not show up at sporting events lest little Johnny get upset and walk off the field. In such instances, a child's representative or GAL's reliance on the alienated child's wishes in custody or parenting time disputes not only continues the child's exposure to parental alienation, but, in some cases, it solidifies it and leads to judicially enabled parental alienation as well.[47] The guardian becomes an *enabler* of alienation, creating a vicious cycle and nefarious incentives for the alienating parent to continue to manipulate and influence his or her child's position.[48] Moreover, now the alienating parent has an important ally: the child's representative, or the court's agent, the GAL. And if the child's representative or GAL advocates for the favored parent to have custody because the alienated child wants the professional to do so, the favored parent in effect has two lawyers in the courtroom: his or her own and the GAL or child's representative.[49] It is not uncommon to see alienated children threaten the targeted parents and defy their parenting by abusing the GAL's role and power. A legitimate parenting act—say, disciplining a child for rude behavior—is challenged and defied by an alienated child by having the GAL or minor's counsel intervene and rebuke the parent. Alienated children, who are typically over-empowered to begin with, get further over-empowered by the legal professionals in challenging and defying the targeted parent.

Parental Alienation, Diminished Capacity, and a Child's Best Interests

We generally do not trust children to make judgments in their best interests.[50] In an alienation situation, the need for caution is even greater. Under the influence of an alienator, the affected child may not be cognitively or psychologically able to make a judgment in his or her best interests.[51] Courts recognize

47. *See, e.g.*, Weiss, D. (2018). Appeals court criticizes "judicially created parental alienation" in case of baby with broken ribs, *ABA Journal*, May, at http://www.abajournal.com/news/article/appeals_court_criticizes_judicially_created_parental_alienation_in_case_of/.

48. House, B. (1998). Considering the child's preference in determining custody: Is it really in the child's best interest? *J. Juv. L.*, 19, 176, 181.

49. Rosen, *supra*, at 333.

50. Referee Kessler, M., Role of the Guardian ad Litem, Guardian ad Litem Handbook for Divorce Practice, State Bar of Michigan Family Law Section (Edited by Connie Thacker & Donna Mobilia), pg. 1 ("There is a myth in the family law arena that there is a magic age when the wishes of the child become all controlling and there is no further need to attempt to address the best interests of the child or even expect the child to follow the rules and wishes of his or her home let alone the court. . . . there is no such magic number.")

Bala, N. (2006). Child representation in Alberta: Role and responsibilities of counsel for the child in family proceedings, *Alta. L. Rev.*, 43, 845, 861.

51. *Id.*

that in an alienation setting, children "are impressionable, have social deficits, and could be manipulated."[52] The professional standards that apply to lawyers who represent children in such cases also underscore this concern:

> One of the most difficult ethical issues for lawyers representing children occurs when the child is able to express a position and does so, but the lawyer believes that the position chosen is wholly inappropriate or could result in serious injury to the child. . . . A child may desire to live in a dangerous situation because it is all he or she knows, because of a feeling of blame or . . . because of threats or other reasons to fear the parent.[53]

In an alienation case, a GAL or child's representative must strive to assess whether the child's wish is a result of brainwashing or programming by the alienating parent or his or her own independent judgment, prior to making a recommendation to the court or advocating in favor of the child's wish.[54] The professional must determine whether the child's preference is reasonable; whether the child is psychologically able to make a judgment; and whether the child is able to exercise his or her judgment without influence, coercion, manipulation, or exploitation.[55]

The Model Rules of Professional Conduct provide that when a client is not able to make adequately considered decisions as part of the attorney-client relationship, the client is said to be functioning "under a disability" and has diminished capacity.[56] While the child's representative may still owe the child-client with diminished capacity a duty of zealous advocacy, the attorney also has a duty to prevent the client from pursuing decisions that are potentially harmful.[57]

Courts too are required to take into consideration the child's reasonable preference when evaluating the best interest factors for custody determination.[58]

---

52. Harner v. Harner, 2018 WL 521863, (Mich., January 23, 2018). (Due to mother's alienating behavior, which included undue influence and coaching, the "moral fitness" factor under MCL 722.23(f) strongly favored father.)

53. Standards of Practice for Lawyers Representing Children in Custody Cases, ABA Section of Family Law, IV(C)(3), Commentary (2003).

54. Fidler, B. J. & Bala, N. (2010). Children resisting postseperation contact with a parent: Concepts, controversies, and conundrums, *Fam. Ct. Review*, 48, 10, 32. Also: MCL 712A.17d(1)(d) requires an LGAL to "assess" the child's needs and wishes, not just listen to the child's wishes or demands.

55. Rosen, *supra*, citing Bala, *supra* at 861; Thacker, C., The Child: Michigan Protocol, Guardian ad Litem Handbook for Divorce Practice, State Bar of Michigan Family Law Section (Edited by Connie Thacker & Donna Mobilia), 16.

56. Model Rules of Professional Conduct 1.14; also see, *e.g.*: Michigan Rules of Professional Conduct Rule 1.14; also see: Standards of Practice for Lawyers Representing Children in Custody Cases, ABA Section of Family Law (2003), IV(C)(1).

57. Fidler, B. J., Bala, N., & Saini, M. (2012). Children Who Resist Postseparation Parental Contact: A Differential Approach for Legal and Mental Health Professionals, Oxford Scholarship Online, doi: 10.1093/acprof:oso/9780199895496.001.0001, 4, 167. ("Advocating uncritically the influenced and manipulated views of children is unhelpful and irresponsible.").

58. MCL 722.23(i).

But the key word here is *reasonable*. It's the reasonable preference that's considered, not just a naked, biased, ill-conceived and absolute preference. What a minor child wants may not be what's in the child's best interests—especially in a case where the child has been manipulated, brainwashed, programmed, and alienated by a parent to reject the other parent. For instance, a North Dakota court reversed a modification that relied on the child's wishes instead of the child's best interests because "the court may not rely solely on the child's wishes in visitation enforcement and modification actions, but the child's wishes and evidence of parental alienation are factors that may be considered in the best interest of the child analysis."[59] Similarly, a Michigan Court of Appeals recently affirmed a trial court's disregard of the testimony of two alienated children when the court found that the children, having being manipulated and alienated, were unable to express a reasonable preference.[60]

Where a child expresses "strong and alarmingly negative opinions about [a parent] with little or no explanation" or cannot provide any concrete or consistent examples of bad conduct by a parent to justify his or her rejection of the parent, the child's preference is not reasonable.[61] And while a child over the age of six is presumed to be capable of forming a reasonable preference, "such presumed capacity can be compromised by surrounding circumstances."[62] Circumstances leading to compromising a child's presumed capacity could include undue influence, coaching, and manipulation—all typical tools of the trade of an alienating parent. In severe alienation cases, it is not uncommon to find the children saying the "right" words that suggest "abuse," but also demonstrating the appropriate affect (tears, grief, and/or anguish).[63]

In such circumstances, what constitutes the child's best interests is ultimately a "professional judgment call" made by the child's representative or GAL.[64] This "call" must be made independent of the child's wishes, although

---

59. Votava v. Votava, 2015 ND 171, ¶ 15, 865 N.W.2d 821, 825. *See also*: Lind v. Lind, 2014 ND 70, ¶ 14, 844 N.W.2d 907; Loll v. Loll, 1997 ND 51, ¶¶ 15–16, 561 N.W.2d 625; *see also* Milligan v. Milligan, 149 So.3d 623, 628 (Ala.Civ.App.2014) (holding that under the circumstances the trial court abused its discretion when it allowed teenage children to determine whether they would visit their father).

60. Brown v. Pentoney, No. 349532 LCNo. 12-108147-DM (Mich. Court of Appeals, May 7, 2020).

61. Harner v. Harner, *supra*, *7 (Mich., January 23, 2018).

62. *Id.*, citing Maeir v. Maier, 311 Mich. App. 218, 224-225; 874 N.W.2d 725 (2015).

63. *See* Prisk v. Prisk, 2017 WL 2131511, *5 (Mich. App., May 16, 2017) ("The trial court conducted an in-camera interview of [the child]. [The child] communicated to the court that [father] had sexually abused her when she was four and again when she was seven." After three separate CPS investigations into allegations of sexual abuse against the father, none of which were substantiated, the court found the child to have been "coached" and never asked her about her custodial preference during a best interests change of custody hearing). Note: Unpublished opinions are not precedentially binding. MCR 7.215(C). But they may be cited by a party if relevant to the issues presented. At times, published opinions on propositions of law, unique facts, and mental health issues involving parental alienation are just not available. In the author's experience, courts usually welcome not only unpublished opinions but also opinions from sister states if they are significantly pertinent to the issues presented before the court.

64. Farris v. McKaig, *supra*, *3.

those wishes could be considered as part of the GAL or child's representative's determination.[65] When required to make this "call," although a child's representative or LGAL functions like an attorney and his or her duties go beyond those of a GAL, their duties ultimately conform to those of a GAL: investigating and independently determining the child's best interests and then serving those interests.[66]

Even commentators who have raised concerns about a child's attorney advocating for a result "they themselves prefer" from a subjective standpoint rather than advocating what the child wants concede that "there are certain hierarchical needs which do not particularly involve the attorney's subjective values, the child's physical and emotional safety being chief among them."[67] Also included in these hierarchical needs are "freedom from abuse or neglect" and "retaining ties among siblings" and a parent.[68] And, these commentators also concede that a child "may not be able to appreciate that a 'preferred' parent is negligent, abusive, or irresponsible, and therefore an inappropriate physical custodian."[69]

How should a GAL or child representative "make the call" in order to determine whether the child has diminished capacity due to parental alienation?

Making the "Call": Determining Whether the Child Has Diminished Capacity

There is no exhaustive checklist of factors that must be satisfied before a child-client is determined to suffer from a disability or lack capacity to inform a GAL or instruct a child's representative.[70] Each decision is based on its own unique set of facts and circumstances. As a Michigan court acknowledged, "[j]ust as adults may lack the capacity to give competent testimony because of infirmity, disability, or other circumstances, so may a child's presumed capacity be compromised by circumstances peculiar to that child's life."[71]

Here's how the Supreme Court of Alaska opined on the issue:

> [A] guardian is not required to advocate whatever placement might seem preferable to a client of tender years. A young child may well prefer the less disciplined environment to the more disciplined one. He may pre-

---

65. In contrast, an attorney for the child, if appointed, advocates for the child's wishes or interests, regardless of what those interests are.

66. Farris v. McKaig, *supra*, at *5; Edone v. Edone, 1991 WL 11657831 (Supreme Court of Alaska), citing Veazey v. Veazey, 560 P.2d 382 (Alaska, 1977) (A GAL "is in every sense the child's attorney . . . He should exercise his judgment on what disposition would further the best interests of the child . . .").

67. *See* Haralambie, A., & Glaser, D. (1995). Practical and theoretical problems with the AAML Standards for Representing "Impaired" Children, *J. Am. Acad. Matrimonial Law*, 13, 57, 75.

68. *Id.*

69. *Id.*, at 89.

70. Model Rules of Professional Conduct ("MRPC"), Rule 1.14, comment 5.

71. Maeir v. Maier, 311 Mich. App. 218, 225; 874 N.W.2d 725, *5 (2015).

fer the parent who takes him on outings for recreational activities over the one who stays home to prepare his meals and keep home clean. But the guardian would be abdicating his responsibility to his client and the court to use his best professional judgment, were he to automatically recommend that young child's preference without further scrutiny. A child who has been living for some time with one parent might understandably select that parent, good or bad, because it represents the only home the child has ever known. . . . A child may have his thinking consciously or subconsciously colored by one parent against the other. The guardian ad litem must try to delve into this question and take all relevant factors into account regardless of what the child may or may not believe he "ought" to say.[72]

Here are some factors that could be considered by a guardian: the child's developmental stage, the child's expression of a relevant position, the child's individual decision-making process, the child's ability to understand consequences, the child's age, degree of maturity, intelligence, ability to communicate, the relationship that existed between the child and the target parent prior to separation or filing of divorce between the parents, and, finally, the expressed preference: the degree or magnitude of rejection of the target parent.[73]

As one legal commentator advocates:

The best way for an attorney to make the determination of whether or not the child client has diminished capacity is to use every tool available to him or her. In order to represent a client competently and diligently, the attorney must interview his or her client, as well as the parents and other family members, doctors, teachers, therapists, or friends as part of his or her initial investigation.[74]

Where a child has been subjected to coaching, manipulation, or emotional distress in going through unsubstantiated police or CPS investigations and traumatic visitation exchanges, it's likely that the child's "fragile emotional state" coupled with the alienation has "rendered him unable . . . to form a reasonable preference" and has thereby diminished his or her capacity.[75] If the child's representative or LGAL makes a determination that the child-client has diminished capacity, the attorney must decide what action to take as an advocate for the child's best interests. The professional should consider alerting the court of this issue and evaluate whether and to what extent to inform the court

72. Veazey v. Veazey, 560 P.2d 382, 390 (1977).

73. Rosen, *supra*; American Academy of Matrimonial Lawyers. (2009). Representing children: Standards for attorneys for children in custody or visitation proceedings with commentary, *J. Am. Acad. Matrimonial Law*, 22, 227, 239.

74. Rosen, *supra*, at 335.

75. Maeir v. Maier, 311 Mich. App. 218, 226; 874 N.W.2d 725 (2015).

as to the child's wishes and preferences in keeping with the law governing attorney-client privilege.[76] Alerting the court of the child's diminished capacity in a case of parental alienation helps avoid a situation where the court relies on a child's preference that has been influenced by an alienator and/or others and is not reflective of the child's independent judgment.[77]

The Model Rules of Professional Conduct, the American Bar Association, and the NCAA all agree that when the child lacks the capacity for knowing, voluntary, and considered judgment, or the child's expressed preference would place the child at risk of substantial harm, the attorney may substitute judgment.[78] The attorney should explain to the court that given the alienation, pathological alignment with one parent and alienation from the other strips the child of a "genuine voice"[79] and that the "child's voice," in reality, reflects "the words, attitudes, and beliefs of the parent who exercises the most influence over him or her."[80] The attorney should explain to the court what he or she is advocating for the child, even if the situation is painful and contentious and the child doesn't agree.[81]

Guardians and Immunity

GALs who handle contentious cases must be able to function without the worry of possible later harassment and intimidation from dissatisfied parents.[82] One court noted its concern that without immunity, GALs "would act like litigation lightning rods. Lawsuits would, in the words of Learned Hand, 'dampen the ardor of all but the most resolute, or the most irresponsible, in the unflinching discharge of their duties.'"[83] Also, courts have reasoned that the duty of the GALs to secure the best interests of the children places these professionals "squarely within the judicial process."[84] Accordingly, courts have almost

76. MCL 712A.17d(1)(i).

77. Garber, B., & Landerman-Garber, L. (2006). How should the child's voice be heard when parental rights and responsibilities are contested? *N.H.B.J.*, 47, 46, 47.

78. Rosen, *supra*, at 336, citing ABA Comm. on Ethics & Prof'l Responsibility, Formal Op. 96-404 (19960, Standards of Practice for Lawyers who Represent Children in Abuse and Neglect Cases, Section B-2).

79. Warshak, R. (2003). Bringing sense to parental alienation: A look at the disputes and the evidence, *Fam. L. Q.*, 37, 273, 375.

80. Gould, J., & Martindale, D. (2009). Including children in decision making about custodial placement, *J. Am. Acad. Matrimonial Law*, 22, 303, 310.

81. Fidler, B. J., Bala, N., & Saini, M. (2012). Children Who Resist Postseparation Parental Contact: A Differential Approach for Legal and Mental Health Professionals, Oxford Scholarship Online, doi: 10.1093/acprof:oso/9780199895496.001.0001, 4, 168; also see: Whitley v. Leonard, 772 N.Y.S.2d 620 (2004).

82. Kurzawa v. Mueller, 732 F.2d 1456, 1458 (6th Cir. 1984).

83. Short v. Short, 730 F.Supp. 1037, 1039 (D.Colo. 1990), citing Gregoire v. Biddle, 177 F.2d 579, 581 (2d Cir. 1949), cert. denied, 339 U.S. 949, 70 S.Ct. 803, 94 L.Ed. 1363 (1950).

84. Kurzawa v. Mueller, *supra*.

unanimously accorded GALs absolute immunity for their actions that are integral to the judicial process.[85]

Furthermore, courts have agreed that, in the performance of this function, for the purposes of an immunity analysis, a court-appointed attorney for the minor child closely resembles a GAL.[86] While such attorneys perform a hybrid role because of their simultaneous duty to function as an advocate for the child, that function, however, must always be subordinated to the attorney's duty to serve the best interests of the child.

> Even when an attorney for the minor child functions less as a guardian ad litem and more as an advocate because of factors such as the child's advanced age, maturity level and ability to articulate her preferences, the shifting of the balance from an objective evaluator of the child's best interests to personal advocate happens because those factors increase the likelihood that the child is able accurately to identify and to make choices to pursue her own best interests independently, without the aid of an objective assistant to the court.[87]

Therefore, even the advocacy role of the appointed attorney for the minor child may be reconciled with the attorney's primary duty—to assist the court in serving the best interests of the child. Accordingly, courts have accorded appointed attorneys for minor children a similar level of immunity that has been traditionally accorded to GALs, at least in the performance of those functions that are integral to the judicial process.[88]

For instance, in Michigan, LGALs, for purposes of immunity analysis, are considered a "subset" of GALs and, therefore, are entitled to governmental immunity as well.[89] And immunity serves a laudable intent: independent investigation and determination—free from outside influence—of the child's best interests. "Fear of liability to one of the parents can warp judgment that is crucial to vigilant loyalty for what is best for the child; the guardian's focus must not be diverted to appeasement of antagonistic parents."[90] But that doesn't mean that GALs or LGALs have blank checks to operate as to their whims and fancies with no oversight or accountability. While some courts have lamented

85. *See, e.g.*, Fleming v. Asbill, 42 F.3d 886, 889 (4th Cir.1994); Cok v. Cosentino, 876 F.2d 1, 3 (1st Cir. 1989); Gardner v. Parson, 874 F.2d 131, 146 (3d Cir. 1989); Myers v. Morris, 810 F.2d 1437, 1466–67 (8th Cir.), cert. denied, 484 U.S. 828, 108 S.Ct. 97, 98 L.Ed.2d 58 (1987); Kurzawa v. Mueller, 732 F.2d 1456, 1457–58 (6th Cir.1984); Babbe v. Peterson, 514 N.W.2d 726 (Iowa 1994); Tindell v. Rogosheske, 428 N.W.2d 386, 387 (Minn.1988); Billups v. Scott, 253 Neb. 287, 571 N.W.2d 603 (1997); Collins v. Tabet, 111 N.M. 391, 806 P.2d 40 (1991).

86. *See, e.g.*, Carrubba v. Moskowitz, 274 Conn. 533, 546 (2005).

87. *Id.*

88. *Id.*

89. Farris v. McKaig, __ N.W.2d __ (2018), 2018 WL 2269775 (Mich. App., May 17, 2018).

90. Farris, *supra*, citing Short by Oosterhous v. Short, 730 F.Supp. 1037, 1039 (D Colo, 1990).

the fact that "unlike the trial court who answers to the appellate courts and the electorate, a guardian ad litem in a domestic-relations proceeding is essentially accountable to no one,"[91] judicial mechanisms do remain in place to prevent abuse, misconduct, and irresponsibility of these professionals. First, a GAL or LGAL's immunity only attaches to conduct within the scope of the professional's duties, and a GAL acting outside his or her role can lose immunity.[92] Second, the court monitors a GAL or LGAL's performance and can remove a rogue or incompetent professional if necessary.[93] Third, a guardian is simply another advocate in our adversary system; whatever position a guardian takes during a proceeding can be addressed and rebutted by the other parties, "thereby ensuring that the trial court will be apprised of the facts and can issue an informed decision."[94] And finally, a GAL (if an attorney) and an LGAL may be subject to punishment by the Attorney Grievance Commission[95] if his or her conduct fails to meet the standards set forth in the Michigan Rules of Professional Conduct.

A Suggested Checklist of Best Practices

Below are some suggestions to the GALs and lawyers who represent children in a case involving parental alienation. These are not just "wouldn't it be nice in an ideal world" suggestions; rather these suggestions are in keeping with the important quasi-judicial functions that GALs discharge and children's representatives' obligation to function as competent, responsible officers of the court in advocating for the child/client's best interests:[96]

1. First, do no harm.[97] The first rule of the rules of professional conduct applicable to attorneys mandates "competent representation."[98] An attorney should not handle a legal matter that he or she knows (or should know) that he or she is not competent to handle without associating with a lawyer who is competent to handle it. Before accepting an appointment as a GAL or child's representative in a case involving allegations of parental alienation, ask yourself: Are you competent to

91. Ex Parte J.G. (*In re*: J.G. v. B.G.), 281 So.3d 371, 391 (Alabama 2019; Dissenting Opinion).

92. *See, e.g.*, Fleming v. Asbill, 42 F.3d 886, 889 (4th Cir. 1994); also see Michigan statute MCL 691.1407(6).

93. MCR 3.915(2), MCL 712A.17(c)(9).

94. Farris, *supra*, FN 4.

95. *See, e.g.*, Grievance Administrator v. Carson, Case No. 02-53-6A (September 5, 2002) (revocation of license to practice law for failure to visit child, consult with social worker, visit foster parent, establish a permanency plan for the child, or make reasonable efforts to expedite the proceedings).

96. *See* Martinson, Hon. D. J. (2010). One case–one specialized judge: Why courts have an obligation to manage alienation and other high-conflict cases, *Family Court Review*, 48(1), 181.

97. Miller, S. (2018). Why do specialists say that parental alienation is counterintuitive, Part 2, *PASG Newsletter*, 3(4), 17.

98. *See, e.g.*, MRPC Rule 1.1; also see Standards of Practice for Lawyers Representing Children in Custody Cases, ABA Section of Family Law (2003), III(A).

handle the assignment? Have you handled such cases before? Are you current on the professional literature on the topic? And, last but not least, are you willing to put in the significant time and effort that will undoubtedly be required on your part to do your job?

2. Fools rush in where angels fear to tread. Don't rush in with "solutions." For instance, judges who have wrestled with cases involving parental alienation have realized that giving a "speech" in an attempt to "get through" to an alienating parent will not result in an epiphany or help the situation.[99] Nor will sending off the kids to "therapy." In fact, it would be difficult to find a more common yet *egregious* blunder that GALs routinely commit than advocating for what amounts to traditional "reunification" therapy for parental alienation.[100] Not only are such therapies known to be ineffective, they are known to be potentially harmful—they "validate" an alienated child's distorted view of the world, encourage the child to express grievances, and give the child some "control" or choice while advising the rejected parent to "listen, empathize, validate, and apologize (or even to 'find something to apologize for')."[101] Traditional therapy is *contraindicated*[102] and typically makes things worse.[103] Even when provided under court order, such therapies are of little benefit.[104] In fact, if you are a GAL or a minor's counsel, you have a duty to *stop* such therapy if it is not accomplishing its intended purpose.[105]
3. Keep yourself abreast of the latest professional literature and case law. Parental alienation is a dynamic area and the research is constantly evolving. Also, it is *profoundly* counterintuitive.[106] This is not merely a warning to "be careful." Rather, professionals who have thoroughly studied this area caution us how everything about parental alienation

---

99. Lowrance, M. (2013). A judge's perspective on parental alienation. In Lorandos, D., Bernet, W., & Sauber, R. (Eds.), *Parental Alienation: The Handbook for Mental Health and Legal Professionals*, Charles C. Thomas, 502, 511.

100. Miller, S., *supra*, Part 2, at 17.

101. *Id.*

102. *Id.*, at 18 (". . . the word contraindicated does not mean 'not indicated.' It means forbidden. If a patient is allergic to penicillin, then penicillin is contraindicated. In the face of a penicillin allergy, it would not be proper to prescribe penicillin to see what happens.").

103. Clawar, S., & Rivlin, B., *supra;* also see Warshak, R. A. (2015). Ten parental alienation fallacies that compromise decisions in court and in therapy, *Prof'l Psychol.: Research & Practice*, 46.

104. Gould, J. et al. (2003). Is the child's therapist part of the problem? What judges, attorneys, and mental health professionals need to know about court-related treatment for children, *Family Law Quarterly*, 37(2). 241–271; also see Harner v. Harner, 2018 WL 521863, FN 4 (Mich., January 23, 2018) ("The therapist . . . adopted defendant's view of events and uncritically accepted every statement that the children made, regardless of the mountain of evidence suggesting that there was no sexual abuse.")

105. *See, e.g.*, MCL 712A.17(d)(1)(j).

106. Miller, S. (2018). Why do specialists say that parental alienation is counterintuitive, Part 1, *PASG Newsletter*, 3(3), 19.

is so counterintuitive—profoundly counterintuitive—that many professionals will almost always make major errors if they attempt to solve problems or make critical judgments using their usual professional intuition.[107] Using intuition to solve complex problems—"I've been doing this for a long time" or "have seen many cases"—is rarely, if ever, adequate.[108] In cases involving parental alienation, it can be downright disastrous. For instance, an alienated child could be very convincing of the "abuse" that he or she has allegedly suffered at the hands of the target parent. Before giving in to the child's demand of having no contact with the target parent, ask yourself: Has the target parent been found guilty of abusive conduct by a neutral agency? What was the parent-child relationship like prior to the divorce or separation of the parties? Is the child's response to the alleged abusive or inappropriate conduct proportionate?

4. Understand that parental alienation meets the criteria for child abuse: It poses severe risks to children in developing major physical and mental problems in adult life and can cause structural damage to their brain.[109] Also understand that "time is a major enemy" in alienation cases.[110] In cases involving parental alienation, the primary goal is *not* reunification or increasing visitation for the target parent. The top priority is to protect the child from further abuse. Focus on ensuring the child's safety and to protect him or her from ongoing alienation (instead of focusing on the child's relationship with the rejected parent). Once the child is protected from being subjected to ongoing alienating behaviors, the focus then can be shifted to remedial measures, including reunification.
5. Do not prejudge the case. Familiarize yourself with the *facts*. Thoroughly review court records; Friend of the Court records; police reports; child protective services reports; school records; and medical, mental health, and/or therapy records. These records are protected by both federal and state confidentiality laws that may need to be addressed before access is obtained. A detailed and thorough record review will help you get a sense of the people involved and the real issues in the case. A thorough record review will also provide you with a 360-degree view

107. *Id.*

108. *Id.* (". . . people who attempt to use intuition to solve counterintuitive problems tend to have great confidence in their conclusions, whether right or wrong.").

109. Miller, S., *supra*, Part 2, at 17; also see Anda, R. et al. (2006). The enduring effects of abuse and related adverse experiences in childhood, *European Archives of Psychiatry and Clinical Neuroscience*, 256(3), 174–186. The American Professional Society on the Abuse of Children (APSAC) has endorsed the premise that causing parental alienation is child abuse.

110. *See* Walters, M. G., & Friedlander, S. (2016). When a child rejects a parent: Working with the intractable resist/refuse dynamic, *Family Court Review*, 54(3), 6.

of the case and information from collateral sources, not just one or two sources of information.

6. Meet and assess the parties, the parents. Remember: "Alienating parents tend to present well; targeted parents tend to present poorly."[111] Generally, alienating parents present with the Four Cs: cool, calm, charming, and convincing.[112] That is because effective alienators tend to be master manipulators who are highly skilled at managing impressions, especially initial impressions. "These traits are usually related to an underlying personality disorder, typically of the borderline, narcissistic, and/or sociopathic types."[113] In contrast, targeted parents tend to present with the Four As: anxious, agitated, angry, and afraid.[114] That is because they are trauma victims, attempting to manage a horrific family crisis while being attacked by professionals who fail to recognize the counterintuitive issues.[115] The alienating parent believes that the child has no need for a relationship with the other parent. The alienating parent may have employed techniques such as badmouthing the target parent; limiting or interfering with parenting time, mail, or phone contact; interfering with information (e.g., school or medical records); fostering an unhealthy alliance with the child ("enmeshment"); and emotional manipulation.[116] The alienating parent may *say* the right words—*"Of course, I want my child to have a relationship with the other parent!"*—but their actions speak otherwise. The alienating parent will generally refuse to listen to positive remarks about the target parent and will quickly discount any happy memories or experiences as trivial and unimportant.[117] He or she will be quick to portray the target parent as dangerous and exaggerate negative attributes about the other parent, including unfounded, false or fabricated allegations of sexual, physical, and/or emotional abuse.[118] On the other hand, the targeted parent may be very frustrated with the alienating behaviors of the favored parent and the child's rejection, and his or her frustration is often misperceived as "anger issues" or emotional imbalances. Poor parenting abilities also contribute to the target parent's victimization.

---

111. Miller, S., *supra*, Part 1, at 19.
112. *Id.*
113. *Id.*, at 20.
114. *Id.*
115. *Id.*
116. Fidler, B., & Bala, N. (2010). Children resisting postseparation contact with a parent: Concepts, controversies, and conundrums, *Fam. Ct. Rev.*, 48, 10, 19.
117. Rosen, *supra*, at 332.
118. *Id.*

Consider suggesting a coach for the target parent and discuss this possibility with his or her attorney.[119]

7. Do not mistake pathological enmeshment between the favored parent and the child for healthy bonding. A pathologically dependent parent treats the child in a manner that is not age-appropriate, such as treating the child as a "friend" or companion, rather than as a child. This involves severe boundary violations of the child by the parent to the point that the parent not only violates the child's boundaries, but *erases* them.[120] Enmeshment is a form of child abuse.[121] What may appear as a "close" relationship—parent and child wearing matching outfits, finishing off each other's sentences, holding hands, being Facebook buddies, etc.—may indeed be a relationship that is too close and pathological.
8. Meet and *assess* the child. Don't just go by the child's words or wishes or even affect. In an alienation setting, the child accepts as true the "delusion of falsehood created by the alienating parent, leading to a belief that he or she cannot show or receive love from both parents."[122] The child's behavior consists of a campaign of unfair criticism towards the targeted parent; weak, irrational and at times downright ridiculous justifications for rejection; absence of guilt or remorse ("splitting"[123]); and the presence of borrowed scenarios. An alienated child will deny good or positive experiences with the targeted parent. And the only solution acceptable to the child is for the target parent to "leave him or her alone." In contrast, abused children develop and maintain attachment relationships with their abusive parents.[124]
9. Remember that in an alienation case, perception is not reality; perception is often a *distortion* of reality. "The single most important element in uncovering the content, intensity, and impact of programming-and-brainwashing in children is *researching the social history of the children*."[125] Conduct a series of interviews with people who have varying perspectives. Observe the child in the context of both parental environments for periods of time that would allow you to observe interaction that is

119. *See, e.g.*, Flood, R. (n.d.). How to Respond to Parental Alienation, at https://menscenter.org/respond-to-parental-alienation/

120. *Id.*

121. *See* Hart, S. et al. (2018). Psychological maltreatment of children. In *The APSAC Handbook on Child Maltreatment* (4th ed.), 145–162.

122. Fidler, B. J., & Bala, N., *supra*, at 15.

123. "Splitting" is a psychological phenomenon that is considered a hallmark behavioral symptom of parental alienation. Alienated children demonstrate splitting, i.e., the favored parent is presented as all good or "perfect" versus the target parent is presented as all bad or "horrible" in all respects. Splitting does not typically occur in children who have been abused, neglected, or otherwise mistreated.

124. *See* Baker, A. et al. (2016). Foster children's views of their birth parents: A review of literature, *Children and Youth Services Review*, 67, 177–183.

125. Clawar, S., & Rivlin, B., *supra*, at 321 (emphasis in original).

more than situational (as in a professional office) or momentary (this is called participant observation). You might be surprised to see the child who professes a fear of his father (the target parent) gravitate to him, laugh with him, sit on his lap, initiate activities and in other ways counter the assertion of fear and desire not to be with him. You may also be surprised to observe that upon returning to the mother (the alienating parent), the child would inform her that she "did not have a good time" or that she was just "faking it."[126] Your careful observation may reveal facts that are often different from what you hear or what you obtain from the child.

10. Watch out for alienating parent's repeated and constant interference in parenting time of the target parent. Interference could appear "innocent," such as sending gifts to the children during the other parent's visitation or frequent calls or texts to the children, or it may be more substantial interference, such as asking police officers to conduct "welfare checks." An alienating parent is "alarmist, overprotective, intrusive, controlling and [feels] compelled to check on the children whenever they [are]" in the target parent's care.[127] Attempts to "protect" the children from "domestic violence" or "sexual assault" could be a concerted and continued effort to alienate the children.[128] Also watch out for frequent and/or repeated allegations of abuse—emotional, physical and/or sexual—made by or orchestrated by the alienating parent against the target parent. If the allegations are found to be unsubstantiated by the CPS, think about obtaining appropriate court intervention.[129] Alienators have been found to abuse the court process and triangulate the professionals; don't get sucked into it.
11. If court ordered parenting time, visitation, or counseling is not followed by the target parent and/or the child, do not advocate a "cooling off" period. Rather, attempt to get appropriate court intervention to *enforce* court ordered parenting time, counseling, and other court orders. A parent's "parenting time rights might become meaningless if a court cannot enforce a visitation schedule through the use of its contempt powers."[130] Alienators tend to harbor and demonstrate low respect for the judicial system.[131] "They will, directly or indirectly, intentionally or

---

126. *Id.*
127. Harner v. Harner, 2018 WL 521863, (Mich., January 23, 2018).
128. *See* Prisk v. Prisk, 2017 WL 2131511, *5 (Mich. App., May 16, 2017).
129. Harner, *supra*, *1.
130. Porter v. Porter, 285 Mich. App. 450, 457; 776 NW2d 377 (2009). In fact, in a recent unpublished decision, the Court of Appeals found a trial court had abused its discretion when it refused to issue a finding of contempt and incarcerate a party who had refused to comply with a parenting time order. Magryta v. Magryta, unpublished per curiam opinion of the Court of Appeals (Docket No. 336433, June 20, 2017).
131. Clawar, S., & Rivlin, B., *supra*, at 335.

unintentionally, undermine any directive that prevents them from challenging or controlling the child's relationship with the target parent."[132] Court orders must have teeth and must be enforced; "vague warnings have virtually no impact" in an alienation case.[133] Court orders are enforceable through a variety of mechanisms, such as criminal sanctions, suspension of alimony or maintenance, tort action for custodial interference, and orders of protection.[134] Your job is not to be a spectator watching, from the sidelines, the repeated violations of court orders. If you are a GAL, your duty is to assist the court to protect the best interests of the child. If you happen to represent the child, your role is to serve as the independent representative for the child's best interests, not just advocate for the child's wishes, which in a case involving parental alienation will be to end the relationship with the target parent.

12. Challenge your assumptions and/or biases. Debunk the myths. It is a common myth that adolescents' stated preference should dominate custody decisions, even though the adolescent has been alienated.[135] It is also a common myth that courts cannot enforce orders for parent-child contact against an alienated teen's wishes.[136] Or that children who irrationally reject a parent but thrive in other respects (such as in school or with peers) need no intervention.[137] These common false beliefs —the *woozle* effect[138]—have been repeatedly debunked, and these assumptions have failed to hold up in the light of research, case law, or experience.
13. In a case of severe parental alienation, think about advocating change of custody or removing the child from the alienating parent's manipulation and control. Understand that the peer-reviewed research demonstrates that the risks of separating a severely alienated child from an alienating parent are very low, and the risks of permitting such a parent to remain in contact with such a child are very high.[139] Moreover, upon removal, the risks go down, not up. Don't buy into "sensational predictions lacking a basis in established scientific and professional knowledge" on what may happen if an alienated child is separated from the

132. *Id.*, at 336.

133. *Id.*

134. *See, e.g.*, Lauren R. v. Ted R., No 293699-02, slip op. (N.Y. Sup. Ct., May 25, 2010).

135. Warshak, R. (2015). Ten parental alienation fallacies that compromise decisions in court and in therapy, *Professional Psychology: Research and Practice*, 6–7.

136. *Id.*

137. *Id.*, at 7.

138. *Id.*, at 1. *See also* Milne, A. A. (1926). In which Pooh and Piglet go hunting and nearly catch a Woozle. In *Winnie The Pooh* (1st ed.), Methuen & Co.

139. *Id.*, at 10.

alienating parent.[140] Also acknowledge the fact that "sending a child for . . . 'reconciliation therapy' for an hour a week is never going to work if the child is then returned to the [alienating parent] for the other 167 hours in that week."[141] Educate yourself on psycho-educational programs that draw on social science research to help alienated children and adolescents adjust to court orders that place them with a parent they claim to fear or hate.[142]

GALs and children's representatives must realize that parental alienation calls for urgent and effective court intervention. Often it results in major life decisions for a child, such as those related to custody, parental access, child protection, and/or mental health treatment intervention. These decisions should not be advocated or made by those who lack adequate skill, experience, or expertise. "Those who attempt to manage such cases using intuition—even professional intuition—instead of a deep knowledge of the science are likely to make catastrophic errors."[143] A GAL's / child representative's failure to properly investigate the case and advocate for the child's best interests could result in significant harm and may constitute professional negligence.[144] On the other hand, a diligent, competent, skilled, and experienced GAL / child representative can make an enormous difference in helping the court understand the phenomenon of parental alienation and assist the court in crafting and enforcing appropriate remedies in the best interests of the child.

140. *Id.*

141. Clawar, S., & Rivlin, B., *supra*, pg. xx–xxi.

142. Warshak, R. (2010). Family Bridges: Using insights from social science to reconnect parents and alienated children, *Fam. Ct. Rev.*, 48; Sullivan, M. et al. (2010). Overcoming Barriers Family Camp: A program for high-conflict divorce families where a child is resisting contact with a parent, *Fam. Ct. Rev.*, 48, 116.

143. Miller, S., *supra*, Part 2, pg. 18–19.

144. *See* Haralambie, A., & Glaser, D. (1995). Practical and theoretical problems with the AAML Standards for Representing "Impaired" Children, *Journal of the American Academy of Matrimonial Lawyers*, 13, 57, 92; also see Snyder, L., & May, A. (2005). Guardian ad litem immunity revisited: Recent history, *Michigan Probate & Estate Planning Journal*, 24(3).

CHAPTER 6

Fallacies, False Positives, and Fake News: Misinformation about Parental Alienation

A legal professional—attorney or judge—faced with a case involving parental alienation should be prepared to devote significant time and effort to the case. Parental alienation cases are not only chock-full of allegations and accusations that require careful sifting through records and facts but also involve commonly held misconceptions about the theory of parental alienation and the underlying research in mental health and social sciences. Between 1990 and the writing of this chapter, there has been considerable discussion and debate regarding parental alienation and PAS in the mental health and legal professional literature. Most of the discussion regarding parental alienation has consisted of the typical dialogue among practitioners and scholars regarding any number of psychological disorders, for example: the criteria for diagnosing parental alienation, the pathways by which parental alienation comes about, the relative culpabilities of the favored and targeted parents, the prevalence of parental alienation in custody and parenting time litigation, appropriate and effective interventions, the roles of professionals, and preventive measures. However, the discussion of parental alienation has been a lightning rod for controversy, vitriol, and *ad hominem* attacks on professionals, and it has featured an unusual level of misinformation and deceptive propaganda.

An overwhelming majority of mental health and legal professionals accept the basic premise of the theory of parental alienation—that is, that some parents manipulate, brainwash, or indoctrinate their children to dislike or fear the other (targeted) parent. Similarly, an overwhelming number of court decisions around the country accept this fundamental premise. Nevertheless, misinformation about parental alienation is frequently presented in legal proceedings regarding divorce, custody, parenting time, and ancillary matters. For instance, when one side wants to present expert testimony on how a parent's alienating behaviors are harming the child's wellbeing and destroying the child's relationship with the other parent, the opposing side attempts to preclude or undermine such testimony by making one or more of the following arguments: the parental alienation theory has no scientific underpinnings, is not generally accepted by the scientific community, is not endorsed by professional organizations, is not included in DSM-5, and is "junk science." And so, the propaganda of misinformation begins. Sometimes the trial court conducts an elaborate *Daubert* or *Frye* hearing to discharge its gatekeeping obligation. On other occasions, the court may rule that it does not really care about the esoteric labels of "PAS" and "parental alienation," but would rather focus its attention on the behaviors of the parents and the best interests of the children.

Family law practitioners should be aware that blatantly false statements and misinformation regarding parental alienation regularly occur in professional literature, popular media, and court filings. For example, statements such as: "Parental alienation is a hoax, invented by Richard Gardner to enable abusive fathers to gain control of their children" or "There is no empirical evidence published in peer-reviewed journals to support the reality of parental alienation," are false.[1] This chapter attempts to address some common fallacies and misinformation regarding parental alienation that I have encountered in courtrooms across America.

At the outset, I would like to point out that the phenomenon of parental alienation is not nebulous, as many detractors make it appear. It can be identified with a careful, thoughtful, and methodical approach. As the Five-Factor Model teaches us, the key issue supporting the possible presence of parental alienation is a child's disproportionate rejection of a parent and an irrational motivation for such rejection. The next task is then to determine how the irrational motivation developed. Proper investigation and assessment are needed in all investigations, and an investigation focused on parental alienation is no exception to the rule. Utilizing good data and technique, incorporating various sources of information, considering bias, implementing psychological testing and psychometric tools, careful consideration of the baseline parent-child relationship, and following ethical principles and professional codes of conduct help evaluators formulate solid opinions that are based on facts and science.

One of the seminal peer-reviewed articles that has debunked parental alienation fallacies that compromise decisions in court and in therapy was published by the American Psychological Association. Dr. Richard Warshak,

1. Lorandos, D., & Bernet, W. (2020). Preface. In Lorandos, D., & Bernet, W. (Eds.), *Parental Alienation: Science and Law*, Charles C. Thomas, xvii.

a clinical professor of psychiatry at the UT Southwestern Medical Center and an internationally renowned scholar in the psychology of alienated children, wrote about the false beliefs about parental alienation that lead courts and professionals, both legal and mental health, astray in shaping judicial opinions and decisions that fail to meet children's needs.[2] Dr. Warshak's article examined ten fallacies or mistaken assumptions: (1) children never unreasonably reject the parent with whom they spend the most time; (2) children never unreasonably reject mothers; (3) each parent contributes equally to a child's alienation; (4) alienation is a child's transient, short-lived response to the parents' separation; (5) rejecting a parent is a short-term healthy coping mechanism; (6) young children living with an alienating parent need no intervention; (7) alienated adolescents' stated preferences should dominate custody decisions; (8) children who appear to function well outside the family need no intervention; (9) severely alienated children are best treated with traditional therapy techniques while living primarily with their favored parent; and (10) separating children from an alienating parent is traumatic.

Attorneys who represent targeted parents or assist the courts as guardians ad litem or represent the minor children would greatly benefit from reading this article and the professional literature cited therein. A big part of the battle in handling a parental alienation case is educating and empowering the court. "Common false beliefs about parental alienation lead therapists and lawyers to give bad advice to their clients, evaluators to give inadequate recommendations to courts, and judges to reach injudicious decisions."[3] Dr. Warshak's article provides the practitioners with tools to debunk fallacies about parental alienation that shortchange alienated children and targeted parents by supporting outcomes that fail to provide effective relief.

In addition to the fallacies discussed by Dr. Warshak, other commonly found fallacies, myths, and misinformation about parental alienation that I have encountered (and continue to do so) are as follows:

1. Parental Alienation Does Not Exist.

American family courts have finally exposed the myth of the much-dreaded *woozles* — the honey-stealing villains, living in cold, snowy places that Winnie-the-Pooh has long warned us about. The myth that the phenomenon of parental alienation doesn't exist, or has no underpinning in science, or is simply an ideology masquerading as science in the gender war over the children has so often been repeated that people assume it to be true. No more. A review of

2. Warshak, R. (2015). Ten parental alienation fallacies that compromise decisions in court and in therapy, *Professional Psychology: Research and Practice*, 46(4), 235.

3. *Id.*

recent legal opinions from the family courts around the country together with the professional, scientific literature debunks this myth. Family court judges have acknowledged that not only "there is no doubt that parental alienation exists," but that it is "not a new phenomenon," and that "[a]nybody old enough to drink coffee knows that embittered parties to divorce can and do manipulate their children."[4] So where does this myth come from?

A leading expert on parental alienation and a legal scholar, Dr. Demosthenes Lorandos, recently wrote:

> What about the meme that PA does not exist? Reviewing the 3,555 cases the query for this research found lends itself to new conclusions about PA misinformation. It appears that most of the misinformation about the construct PA comes from two sources: (1) legal professionals and law students without a scientific background challenging the validity of the science behind PA, and (2) other professionals and students, who lack a legal background, opining on evidence law. Together, they raise specious concerns about the materiality, relevancy, and admissibility of PA.[5]

Hacking away at the cobwebs of needless psychobabble, family courts have determined that "whether or not a psychological 'syndrome' exists, parental alienation clearly does."[6] Judges—the triers of facts in domestic relations litigation—have found that it is far more important and effective to focus on a parent's *behavior* rather than to go down the rabbit-hole chasing esoteric theories of a "syndrome" that may or may not exist. The devil is in the details, and "there is no reasonable dispute that high-conflict custody disputes frequently involve acts by one parent designed to obstruct or sabotage the opposing parent's relationship with the child."[7]

Mental health experts have used different terms to describe parental alienation. In their book, *Children Held Hostage*, published by the ABA Section of Family Law, Stanley Clawar, a sociologist, and Brynne Rivlin, a social worker, used the terms "programming," "brainwashing," and "indoctrination" when describing the behaviors that cause the children to reject a parent without a legitimate justification. There are two key features of the phenomenon of parental alienation. First, it can be conceptualized as a mental condition present in the *child*, i.e., the child has a distorted or false belief that the rejected or disfavored parent is "evil," "dangerous," or somehow unworthy of love or affection. Second, the child's rejection of the alienated or target parent is *without legitimate justification*. And this is the key distinction: If there is a documented

4. J.F. v. D.F., 61 Misc.3d 1226(A), 2018 N.Y. Slip Op. 51829(U), *8 (2018).

5. Lorandos, D. (2020). Parental alienation in U.S. Courts, 1985 to 2018. In Lorandos, D., & Bernet, W. (Eds.), *Parental Alienation: Science and Law*, Charles C. Thomas, 378.

6. *Id.*

7. Martin v. Martin, Michigan Court of Appeals No. 349261 (January 28, 2020), FN 2.

or objectively verifiable history of the rejected parent being abusive or severely neglectful, the child's rejection of that parent could be legitimate and, if so, it would not be a case of parental alienation.

As to *how* parental alienation takes place, the research conducted by Dr. Amy Baker and her colleagues describing the seventeen alienating strategies is widely used and accepted by the courts and the mental health community. They include badmouthing, limiting contact, confiding in the child, asking the child to spy on the target parent, referring to the target parent by first name, withholding important information from the target parent, and undermining the authority of the target parent. Take, for instance, the behavior of a father who was found to have engaged in severe parental alienation. His *modus operandi* included sending text messages to his son telling him that he had "a right to be ugly to [his] [Mother]," the mother was "mentally ill" and "can't help the way [she] [was] born and created by God," that he had to visit his mother "because the law forces you to go," and that he "will never like her. Nobody likes her. It is impossible."[8] Subjected to such indoctrination, children may turn on the targeted parents, vilify them, reject them, and show no ambivalence or guilt in treating them in a most cruel fashion. The trauma is suffered not just by the rejected parent; the brainwashed children too are robbed of "a normal childhood, normal sibling relationships, and a normal relationship with [the] [targeted] [parent]."[9]

It should not come as a surprise that courts have agreed that parental alienation "is a form of emotional abuse that should not be tolerated."[10] And to remedy such abuse, they have realized that it is necessary to jettison the "conservative" approach of taking baby steps and ordering traditional psychotherapy while keeping the abused child in the custody of the alienator. To do so will only result in a litigious "merry-go-round" that has neither worked in the past nor will it "work in the future."[11] Courts have increasingly taken seemingly drastic but ultimately necessary steps of changing custody, ordering psycho-educational counseling for the alienating parent, and ordering specialized reunification program for the targeted parent and the child, together with financial sanctions, reallocation of attorney fees and litigation costs, and, in severe cases, incarceration for repeated violation of court orders.

And this unfortunate phenomenon is by no means unique to America. Parental alienation has been described, discussed, and debated in the legal and scientific literature by numerous writers all over the world. It is addressed in thousands of court rulings in Canada, United Kingdom, Brazil, Mexico, Israel,

8. McClain v. McClain, 539 S.W.3d 170, 194-195 (Tenn.Ct.App. 2017).
9. Matter of Marriage of Reichert, 2 Wash.App.2d 1063, *2 (2018).
10. McClain v. McClain, *supra*, at 200.
11. *Id.*

France, Spain, India, Australia, New Zealand, Hong Kong, the European Court of Human Rights, and other jurisdictions around the world. This is not surprising as it is an expression of human behavior, albeit pathological, which occurs worldwide with similar patterns. A parent who violates the boundaries by treating the child as a weapon in a divorce or custody litigation undoubtedly causes his or her child serious emotional harm.

2. Parental Alienation Syndrome Is "Junk Science"

Critics and detractors have persistently used the "junk science" epithet to undermine the reality and credibility of the phenomenon of parental alienation. For instance, as Dr. William Bernet, a professor emeritus at Vanderbilt University School of Medicine, explains, there exists "a provocative, colorful meme states that PA and PAS are 'junk science' or 'pseudoscience.' A *meme* is a concept, image, catchphrase, or piece of media which spreads from person to person via social networks, news sources, or professional journals. Similar to a fad or craze, the meme takes on a life of its own."[12] The word "meme" was introduced by Richard Dawkins in his book, *The Selfish Gene*, as a way to explain how cultural information spreads:

> Just as genes propagate themselves in the gene pool by leaping from body to body via sperms or eggs, so memes propagate themselves in a meme pool by leaping from brain to brain via a process which, in the broad sense, can be called imitation.[13]

Lazy, incompetent, or unscrupulous practitioners have no qualms about putting forth an argument advocating this meme, and, unless confronted with swift and strong response (together with relevant and helpful caselaw and professional literature rebutting the meme), such fallacies risk distracting the court's focus and attention.

Some professionals have offered an opinion that Parental Alienation or PAS is "junk science" only for the media and other critics to jump on the bandwagon and fan the flames of such *ipse dixit* opinion. For example, a psychiatrist, Paul J. Fink, opined in 2003 that PAS constitutes "junk science."[14] Dr. Fink repeated his opinion many times and in turn, was quoted by other critics of PA and PAS. In a short amount of time, the phrase "PAS is junk science" became a fashionable catchphrase, or a meme. In 2010, Dr. Fink went a step further. He

12. Bernet, W. (2020). Introduction to parental alienation. In Lorandos, D., & Bernet, W. (Eds.), *Parental Alienation: Science and Law*, Charles C. Thomas, 31.

13. Bernet, W., *supra*, citing to Dawkins, R. (1976). *The Selfish Gene*, Oxford UP, 206.

14. Talan, J. (2003, July 1). The debate rages on . . . in death, can he survive? *Newsday*, at http://www.leadershipcouncil.org/1/pas/talan.html.

now opined—in his column in *Clinical Psychiatry News*—that PAS was "junk science invented by a psychiatrist."[15] This statement caused a furor amongst the experts and professionals who had spent decades studying the phenomenon of parental alienation. After receiving several letters objecting to Dr. Fink's statements, *Clinical Psychiatry News* arranged for him to issue an apology and a clarification. Dr. Fink then wrote, "I do not deny that parental alienation occurs and that a lot of people are hurt when there is an alienator."[16] This is one example of misinformation broadcasted in reputable publications only to be corrected, fortunately, by the person who issued it in the first place. But such misinformation is frequently repeated and recycled. As Dr. Bernet points out, "Fink's comments have frequently been recycled. For example, an article in *Newsweek* magazine said that the president of the Leadership Council on Child Abuse & Interpersonal Violence, Paul Fink, has called PAS 'junk science at its worst.'[17] A newspaper in Israel ran a headline regarding PAS, 'Junk science has its way in court,' and quoted Paul Fink."[18]

Dr. Fink was not the lone voice spreading misinformation about parental alienation. Several other authors have repeated and recycled the same false statements regarding parental alienation and PAS. In 2001, Carol S. Bruch published an article, "Parental Alienation Syndrome: Junk Science in Child Custody Determinations."[19] In 2015, Rebecca M. Thomas and James T. Richardson published an article, "Parental Alienation Syndrome: 30 Years On and Still Junk Science," in *The Judges Journal*.[20] The article by Thomas and Richardson was refuted by Dr. Bernet in the same issue of *The Judges Journal*.[21] In a 2016 law review article, student Holly Smith said, "This Note proposes that parties involved in child custody disputes should be educated on the junk science of parental alienation syndrome."[22]

It is astounding that such misinformation continues to spread in the face of legal decisions where the courts around the country have acknowledged parental alienation as emotional or psychological abuse and have intervened by providing the necessary measures. It is even more surprising that such misinformation exists when the family law professionals have access to sound

---

15. Bernet, W., *supra*, citing to Fink, P. J. (2010, March). Fink! Still at large, *Clinical Psychiatry News*, 6.

16. Fink, P. J., (2010, May). Letters, Dr. Fink replies, *Clinical Psychiatry News*, 10.

17. Bernet, W., *supra*, citing to Weller, C. (2014, July 18). Cut the baby in two: Parental alienation syndrome isn't in the DSM yet, but it's in plenty of arguments, *Newsweek*, 52, 53.

18. Bernet, W., *supra*, citing to Traubman, T. (2003, August 15). Junk science has its way in court, *Haaretz*, at https://www.haaretz.com/1.5351271.

19. Bruch, C. S. (2001). Parental Alienation Syndrome: Junk science in child custody determinations, *Eur. J. L. Reform*, 3, 383.

20. Thomas, R. M., & Richardson, J. T. (2015). Parental Alienation Syndrome: 30 years on and still junk science, *Judges J.*, 54, 22.

21. Bernet, W. (2015). Parental alienation: Misinformation versus facts, *Judges J.*, 54, 23.

22. Smith, H. (2016). Parental Alienation Syndrome: Fact or fiction? The problem with its use in child custody cases, *U. Mass. L. Rev.*, 11, 64, 64.

professional literature and solid research regarding PA. For instance, in 2013, the book *Parental Alienation: The Handbook for Mental Health and Legal Professionals* was released. The *Handbook* contained contributions from mental health and legal professionals and examined, in detail, the historical, scientific, and legal foundations of parental alienation. It contained a thorough review of North American caselaw on parental alienation together with a family law judge's perspective on parental alienation. With over 1000 bibliographic entries, 500 cases, and cites to peer-reviewed literature, the *Handbook* provides a slam-dunk rebuttal to the hypothesis that parental alienation or PAS is "junk science."

The year 2020 saw the release of another helpful book, *Parental Alienation—Science and Law*. The chapters in this book, taken together, explain how a family can be evaluated for the presence of PA in a methodical, professional manner; how testimony regarding PA passes both *Frye* and *Daubert* criteria; the research regarding treatments and interventions for PA; the qualitative and quantitative research in peer reviewed journals regarding parental alienation; how the phenomenon has been generally accepted by the relevant scientific community; and last, but not least, how expert testimony regarding parental alienation has been accepted in hundreds of courts in the United States.

Some ideologues have criticized the phenomenon of parental alienation as junk science, but readily endorsed the concept when it suited their purpose. For instance, Dr. Bernet found that some feminist writers, who sought to "debunk PAS" when mothers were accused of alienating their children, readily describe alienating behaviors when *fathers* are accused of causing parental alienation.[23] He cites as an example Phyllis Chesler, who wrote a provocative book, *Mothers on Trial*, which claims that family courts have been strongly biased against mothers. In her book, Chesler wrote, "['Parental Alienation Syndrome'], first pioneered by Dr. Richard Gardner and widely endorsed by fathers' rights groups, has been dismissed as junk science."[24] However, in another chapter, "Paternal Brainwashing," which is devoted to examples of alienating behaviors committed by fathers, Chesler wrote, "The paternal brainwashing of children is a conscious and systematic attempt to force children into rejecting their mothers—that is, into committing psychological matricide."[25] She went on to explain that one feature of psychological brainwashing is "the devaluation of the mother"—for example,

> A child who hates and rejects his or her maternal altruism. . . . Such a child has long been encouraged to criticize the mother in front of other

23. Bernet, W. (2020), *supra*, 32.
24. Chesler, P. (2011). *Mothers on Trial: The Battle for Children and Custody* (2d ed.), Lawrence Hill, xiv–xv.
25. *Id.*, at 130.

adults, to lie (or to "forget" the truth) in court, to run away from the mother's home, and ultimately to refuse to see the mother at all.[26]

Chesler, who strongly criticized PAS and "the misogynist rantings of one Dr. Richard Gardner,"[27] readily endorsed the concept of parental alienation, saying, "Alienation does exist. . . . Actual alienation is a very extreme phenomenon and one that is devastating to the alienated parent."[28]

3. Parental Alienation Has Been "Debunked."

Together with the fallacy that the theory of parental alienation is "junk science," we often hear an allegation that it has been debunked. In his recent book that he co-edited with Dr. Demosthenes Lorandos, Dr. William Bernet offers some examples of this allegation, which appears to have taken a life of its own:[29]

- In 2009, Neustein and Lesher wrote, "Parental Alienation Syndrome (PAS) is a hydra: chop off its head, and new ones sprout up to take its place. For 20 years, critics of PAS theory have debunked its flawed assumptions, its self-serving methodology, and its inadequacy to access allegations of child sexual abuse."[30]
- In 2014, law student Allison M. Nichols wrote in a Note, "The controversy surrounding allegations of parental alienation is multifaceted. On the one hand, various debunked mental health theories continue to exert inappropriate influence over the decisions of family courts. . . . Part I of this Note addresses the admissibility issue and concludes that testimony regarding PAS and related theories is inadmissible under the relevant evidentiary standards."[31]
- In 2016, a Michigan attorney wrote in her blog, "There is no such thing as 'Parental Alienation Syndrome.' It is a widely debunked pseudoscientific theory that, depending on what state litigants live in, is not infrequently promoted in contentious custody proceedings. It is not an accepted scientific theory in Michigan."[32]

---

26. *Id.*, at 135.
27. *Id.*, at 321.
28. *Id.*, at 325.
29. Bernet, W. (2020), *supra*, 33–34.
30. Neustein, A., & Lesher, M. (2009). Evaluating PAS: A critique of Elizabeth Ellis's "A Stepwise Approach to Evaluating Children for PAS." *J. Child Custody*, 6, 322.
31. Nichols, A. M. (2014). Toward a child-centered approach to evaluating claims of alienation in high-conflict custody disputes, *Mich. L. Rev.*, 112, 663, 665.
32. Stuart-Fink, L. (2016, March 21). Parental alienation–Fact and myth, The Law Offices of Laurel Stuart-Fink, P.L.L.C., at http://www.laurelfink.com/uncategorized/parental-alienation-fact-and-myth/.

And perhaps the most egregious one:

- "Parental Alienation Syndrome is a thoroughly debunked theory by Dr. Richard Gardner, a psychiatrist who really wanted to make it easier and acceptable for adults to have sex with children. We don't know he invented PAS, but that certainly has been the effect."[33]

Dr. Bernet goes on to explain that it is no doubt true that there has been a heated debate over, controversy surrounding, and *attempts* at debunking PAS and parental alienation. For example, in 1998, social work professor Kathleen Faller wrote an article, "The Parental Alienation Syndrome: What Is It and What Data Support It?"[34] The article strongly criticized child psychiatrist Richard Gardner, who published a detailed rebuttal as a letter to the editor of the journal, *Child Maltreatment*.[35] Faller then published a "Response to Gardner" in the same issue of *Child Maltreatment*.[36]

Thereafter, in 2001, attorney Carol Bruch published "Parental Alienation Syndrome and Parental Alienation: Getting It Wrong in Child Custody Cases."[37] Bruch relied on newspaper articles and internet web sites, among other sources, to make five primary criticisms of Richard Gardner, the person who originally introduced the term "Parental Alienation Syndrome":

- "First, Gardner confounds a child's developmentally related reaction to divorce and high parental conflict (including violence) with psychosis.
- Second . . . , Gardner vastly overstates the frequency of cases in which children and custodial parents manufacture false allegations or collude to destroy the parent-child relationship.
- Third . . . , PAS shifts attention away from the perhaps dangerous behavior of the parent seeking custody to that of the custodial parent. This person, which may be attempting to protect the child, is instead presumed to be lying and poisoning the child.
- Fourth, Gardner believes that, particularly in serious cases, the relationship of an alienated child with the rejected parent will be irreparably damaged, probably ending for all time, unless imme-

---

33. Stop Abuse Campaign (n.d.). What is a Parental Alienation Syndrome, at http://stopabuse campaign.org/adverse-childhood-experiences-study/preventing-trauma/safe-child-act-a/parental -alienation-syndrome/

34. Faller, K. C. (1998). The Parental Alienation Syndrome: What is it and what data support it? *Child Maltreatment*, 3, 100.

35. Gardner, R. A. (1998). Letter to the Editor, *Child Maltreatment*, 3, 309.

36. Faller, K. C. (1998). Response to Gardner, Child Maltreatment, 3, 312.

37. Bruch, C. S. (2001). Parental Alienation Syndrome and Parental alienation: Getting it wrong in child custody cases, *Fam. L. Q.*, 35, 527. This article was republished, largely intact, as Bruch, C. S. (2002). Parental Alienation Syndrome and alienated children–Getting it wrong in child custody cases, *Child & Fam. L. Q.*, 14, 381.

diate, drastic measures (custody transfer, isolation from the loved parent, and deprogramming) are taken.

- Fifth . . . , Gardner's proposed remedy for extreme cases is unsupported and endangers children."[38]

Since Bruch primarily criticized Gardner rather than the many other authors who have published articles about PAS and parental alienation in peer-reviewed journals, Drs. Lorandos and Bernet chose to let Gardner himself provide the "Rebuttal to Carol S. Bruch's Article."[39] For example, when Bruch alleged, "Gardner confounds a child's developmentally related reaction to divorce and high parental conflict (including violence) with psychosis," Gardner described that statement as a "gross misrepresentation." He explained,

> What I do state is that my experience has been that severe PAS represents about ten percent of the cases I have personally seen. Furthermore, I state that in some of those cases we do see paranoia in the accusing parent, which is a form of psychosis.[40]

Also, when Bruch criticized Gardner's estimate of the frequency with which "children and custodial parents manufacture false allegations" of abuse, Gardner responded,

> From the vantage point of the innocent victim, it does not matter whether he (she) is in the one-percent group, the twenty-percent group, or any other percent group; that individual is still being falsely accused and may very well be sentenced to jail.[41]

At the end of her article, Bruch proposed recommendations for the future, saying, "The first question is whether scientific sufficiency has been indicated by respected professional vetting, for example, inclusion in the American Psychiatric Association's DSM-5 or the World Health Organization's ICD-10."[42] Lorandos and Bernet explain in detail in Chapter 6 of their new book, *Parental Alienation—Science and Law,* that "the *concept* PA is clearly stated in DSM-5, although the actual words are not; and that the words "parental alienation" and "parental estrangement" are introduced in ICD-11 as index terms for the diagnosis, caregiver-child relationship problem."[43]

---

38. Bernet, W. (2020), *supra,* 34, citing to Bruch, *supra* at 530–533 (2001).
39. Gardner, R. A., Rebuttal to Carol S. Bruch's Article, "Parental Alienation Syndrome and Parental Alienation: Getting it Wrong in Child Custody Cases, at http://www.pas-kon-ferenz.de/e/dok/gardnerbruch_e.doc. Gardner explained at the top of this unpublished article that the acting editor-in-chief of *Family Law Quarterly* declined to publish his rebuttal of Bruch's article.
40. *Id.*
41. *Id.*
42. Bruch, C. S., *supra* note 37, at 550–551 (2001).
43. Bernet, W., *supra,* 35.

While some professionals continue to debate and even reject the concept of PAS as defined by Richard Gardner, almost all mental health and legal professionals accept the general definition of the phenomenon of parental alienation. That is, almost all mental health and legal professionals agree that *some* children, whose parents are engaged in a high-conflict separation or divorce, align strongly with one parent and reject a relationship with the other parent—and that they do so without legitimate justification. Courts have followed suit. In *Martin v. Martin,* the Michigan Court of Appeals, similar to several other courts around the country, refused to get drawn into the meaningless controversy surrounding the "Parental Alienation Syndrome" and instead focused its attention on the alienating parent's *behaviors*:

> [Mother] . . . essentially contends that "parental alienation" is junk science. While there may be a dispute in the scientific community about whether there is diagnosable, pathological condition called parental alienation syndrome . . . there is no reasonable dispute that high-conflict custody disputes frequently involve acts by one parent designed to obstruct or sabotage the opposing parent's relationship with the child.[44]

At the 2010 annual meeting of the Association of Family and Conciliation Courts (AFCC), about 300 attendees completed a brief survey regarding parental alienation. Dr. Amy J. L. Baker and her colleagues reported:

> Nearly all of the respondents to the survey (98 percent) endorsed the question, 'Do you think that some children are manipulated by one parent to irrationally and unjustifiably reject the other parent?'. . . The survey results were overwhelming in support of the basic tenet of parental alienation.[45]

Contrary to the myth, Dr. Bernet reports that individual writers and researchers have endorsed the premise that the concept of parental alienation has not been debunked but has been accepted by the wide community of mental health and legal professionals. In his new book, he provides three specific examples:

- In 2000, Elizabeth Ellis, the author of *Divorce Wars: Interventions with Families in Conflict,* explained that the concept of parental alienation has "come to be accepted by clinicians working with families involved in post-divorce conflict."[46]

---

44. Martin v. Martin, Michigan Court of Appeals No. 349261 (January 28, 2020), FN 2.
45. Baker, A., Jaffe, P., Bernet, W., & Johnston, J. (2011, May 5). Brief report on parental alienation survey, AFCC ENEWS, at https://www.afccnet.org/Portals/0/PublicDocuments/2011_may.pdf?ver=2015-08-04-134136-377.
46. Ellis, E. (2000). *Divorce Wars: Interventions with Families in Conflict,* APA, 227.

- In 2010, Joan Kelly stated that there was "broad consensus among the mental health and family law community that the risk of child alienation is increased in highly conflicted separations accompanied by protracted adversarial child custody disputes."[47]
- In 2016, Michael Saini and his colleagues reported on their review of 58 research studies regarding parental alienation. Finding that the quantitative research is relatively strong regarding the identification and assessment of parental alienation, they wrote, "There is remarkable agreement about the behavioral strategies parents can use to potentially manipulate their children's feelings, attitudes, and beliefs in ways that may interfere with their relationship with the other parent. The cluster of symptoms or behaviors indicating the presence of alienation in the child can also be reliably identified."[48]

Finally, Lorandos and Bernet's 2020 book leaves no doubt that to say that parental alienation has been debunked is to spread misinformation and fake news. Chapter 6 of their book, "Recognition of Parental Alienation by Professional Organizations," demonstrates how the concept of parental alienation has been accepted by numerous professional organizations in the U.S. and other countries. Chapter 5, "Parental Alienation in U.S. Courts, 1985 to 2018," and the associated appendix identify more than one thousand trials in the United States in which the court accepted the concept of parental alienation.

To paraphrase Mark Twain, the reports of the debunking of the theory of parental alienation are greatly exaggerated.

4. Domestic Violence or Abuse Must Be Ruled Out before Considering Parental Alienation

Some commentators suggest that parental alienation should not be even considered until the presence of domestic violence or abuse is effectively ruled out. For instance, the American Professional Society on the Abuse of Children published a position paper that stated:

> In situations of marital/relationship dissolution, the allegation of interpersonal violence needs to be addressed before issues of custody and visitation can be addressed. . . . If interpersonal violence is determined to be

47. Kelly, J. B. (2010). Commentary on "Family Bridges: Using Insights from Social Science to Reconnect Parents and Alienated Children" (Warshak 2010), *Fam. CT. Rev.*, 48(1), 81.

48. Saini, M., Johnston, J. R., Fidler, B. J., & Bala, N. (2016). Empirical studies of alienation. In Drozd, L., Saini, M., & Olesen, N. (Eds.), *Parenting Plan Evaluation: Applied Research for the Family Court* (2nd ed.), 374, 423.

unlikely, the best interest of the child in case specific factors should determine the custody and visitation arrangement.[49]

It would be a mistake to put on the blinders and be willfully blind to the evidence of parental alienation simply because the possibility of domestic violence or abuse, however small, has not been completely ruled out. Dr. Bradley W. Freeman, an associate clinical professor in the Department of Psychiatry and Behavioral Sciences, Vanderbilt University Medical Center, is board certified in general, child and adolescent, and forensic psychiatry. Dr. Freeman writes:

> While being vigilant about interpersonal violence is necessary in conducting parenting time evaluations, this can be accomplished in parallel to the overall evaluation. Proving something does not exist asserts the need to investigate and definitively determine the absence in all its forms, no matter how small or unlikely. A realistic approach to arriving at a conclusion regarding the presence or absence of domestic violence is being methodical and thorough. The evaluator should request and review police reports, court documents, medical documentation (psychological and physical), interview the parties, speak with collateral sources who know the parties in question, and review other pieces of information made available to them by the parties themselves.[50]

An evaluator should give more weight to *data*, which is less subjective and less likely to be biased. The methodical approach that Dr. Freeman recommends can help to uncover hidden patterns of abuse together with evidence of alienating behaviors or signs of alienation present in the children. Generating different and even conflicting hypotheses can be done in parallel by evaluators undertaking custody or visitation evaluations. The evaluator can thereby explore the possibility of domestic violence as well as gather information about alienating behaviors or signs of alienation present in the children *simultaneously*. Of course, the evaluator must come to a decision about the presence of domestic violence or abuse and the related safety factors before generating her final opinion concerning parental alienation. Experienced evaluators and professionals know that domestic violence or abuse can be difficult to discern yet can have a strong impact regarding the presence or absence of parental alienation.

---

49. American Professional Society on the Abuse of Children. (2016). Position Paper on Allegations of Child Maltreatment and Intimate Partner Violence in Divorce/Parental Relationship Dissolution, 2, 4.

50. Freeman, B. W. (2020). The psychosocial assessment of contact refusal. In Lorandos, D., & Bernet, W. (Eds.), *Parental Alienation: Science and Law*, Charles C. Thomas, 75, citing Jaffe, P. G., Johnston, J. R., Crooks, C. V., & Bala, N. (2008). Custody disputes involving allegations of domestic violence: Toward a differential approach to parenting plans, *Fam. CT. Rev.*, 46, 500.

5. It Is Not Possible to Distinguish Alienation from Estrangement

Another common false belief about parental alienation is that some professionals argue that alienation cannot be effectively distinguished from estrangement. For instance, one legal commentator argues:

> My experience tells me that some extremely angry parents alienate children from their other parent. My experience also tells me that some self-absorbed parents use accusations of alienation to blame their former partner and excuse their selfish disregard of their children. . . . [However,] I do not have confidence in my own, or anyone else's, ability to discern truth in divisive divorces . . . and I would be greatly impressed if some investigator could punch a hole in my skepticism with research demonstrating reliable and valid discriminations between accurate and inaccurate accounts of his or her divorce.[51]

It is not overly difficult, much less impossible, to tell the difference between parental alienation and estrangement. As Dr. Bradley W. Freeman explains:

> The difference is straightforward: estrangement is a rational rejection of a parent while PA is based on an irrational rejection. For an experienced MHP [Mental Health Professional], the process of differentiating alienation from estrangement is analogous to diagnosing delusional disorder (i.e., distinguishing a rational from an irrational opinion) or a specific phobia (i.e., distinguishing a rational from an irrational fear). For example, one of the DSM-5 criteria for specific phobia is, "The fear or anxiety is out of proportion to the actual danger posed by the specific object or situation and to the sociocultural context."[52] Similarly, the basic premise of PA is that the child's rejection of the alienated parent is out of proportion to anything that parent has done.[53]

Family courts have distinguished alienation from estrangement. As a Tennessee court held:

> Alienation and estrangement, as psychological terms of art that may describe some of these family dynamics, are not interchangeable or synonymous concepts. The difference between estrangement and alienation resides in the presence vs absence of a reasonable objective basis for a child's severe and persistent rejection and denigration of a parent. Rejection and denigration of a parent with a reasonable objective basis is

51. Emery, R. E. (2005). Proponents bear the burden of proof, *Fam. CT. Rev.*, 43, 8, 9.

52. American Psychiatric Association. (2013). *Diagnostic and Statistical Manual of Mental Disorders* (5th ed.) (DSM-5), Author.

53. Freeman, B. W., *supra*, 76.

estrangement; rejection and denigration without such a basis is parental alienation.[54]

Let's remember, the key issue supporting the possible presence of parental alienation is an irrational or frivolous excuse for the rejection of a parent. For instance, a teenager stating to an evaluator: "I refuse to see my father because he never listens to me." The task for the evaluator then is to determine how the irrational motivation developed. To identify the presence of parental alienation, the Five-Factor Model described earlier in this book provides the evaluator with a reasonable methodology to follow. Once rejection of the parent or contact refusal is ruled in and maltreatment by the rejected parent is ruled out, the evaluator needs to identify three other factors. These include a history of a previously positive relationship between the child and rejected parent, the exhibition of alienating behaviors by the preferred or favored parent, and the common symptoms of parental alienation in the child. It is not only possible to distinguish alienation from estrangement; it is critical to do so because the effective therapeutic or mental health intervention differs greatly in cases involving alienation compared to those of estrangement.

6. Parental Alienation Cannot Be Diagnosed or Identified Because It Is Not in DSM-5

This fallacy comes up often in litigating cases involving parental alienation. Stealing a page from Tom Cruise's JAG Lt. Daniel Kaffee in the movie *A Few Good Men*, attorneys attempt to cross-examine experts propounding the theory of parental alienation by handing them a copy of DSM-5 and asking: "Dr. Smith, would you turn to the page in this book that defines the term "parental alienation," please?" These lawyers argue that parental alienation is not specifically mentioned or recognized in the DSM-5. Therefore, the argument goes, parental alienation is not a legitimate phenomenon, let alone a diagnosis. For example, in 2016, O'Donoghue and his colleagues stated, "[PAS] has not been accepted by any official organization. It is not in the American Psychiatric Association's DSM (not DSM-IV nor in the more recently published DSM-V); not in the International Classification of Diseases, nor is it adopted by any organization (e.g., the American Psychological Association)."[55]

It's not just the detractors and opponents who make this incorrect argument. Even professionals who accept the concept of parental alienation commonly make this mistake. Dr. William Bernet provides us with an illustration

54. McClain v. McClain, 539 S.W.3d 170, 182 (2017).

55. O'Donohue, W., Benuto, L. T., & Bennett, N. (2016). Examining the validity of Parental Alienation Syndrome, *J. Child Custody*, 13, 113, 120.

of writers who are friendly to the concept of parental alienation making this mistake:

> For example, chapter authors of the *Principles and Practice of Forensic Psychiatry*, a book that is often considered comprehensive and authoritative, made incorrect statements regarding PA. In 2017, Ciric and Billick published a chapter on "Role of the Psychiatric Evaluator in Child Custody Disputes." They referred to "the controversial Parental Alienation Syndrome (PAS)," and then said, "PAS was ultimately not included as a mental disorder in the DSM-5, because it has never been shown to be both reliable and valid."[56] That statement was incorrect because the authors of DSM-5 never expressed doubt regarding the reliability and validity of PAS/PA. They simply said that PA should be considered a "mental condition," not a "mental disorder." When contacted about this error, the editors of *Principles and Practice of Forensic Psychiatry* readily agreed to correct it when the book is reprinted.[57]

The place of parental alienation in DSM-5 is commonly misunderstood and misrepresented. The editors and authors of DSM-5 have *never* stated that they doubted the reality or importance of parental alienation.[58] Rather, they have explained that the phenomenon of parental alienation does meet their criteria for a "mental disorder" (the term used for diagnostic entities in the DSM-5 chapter, "Other Conditions That May Be a Focus of Clinical Attention"). Although parental alienation is not a codified diagnosis, the DSM-5 includes three diagnoses that can be used in classifying cases of parental alienation: Child affected by parental relationship distress; Parent-child relational problem; and Child psychological abuse. As Dr. Bernet explains,

> [t]he clinician should select one or more of those DSM-5 diagnoses, depending on the focus of the practitioner's evaluation. If the focus is on the condition of the child, the clinician could use child affected by parental relationship distress; if the focus is on the relationship between the child and the rejected parent, they could use parent-child relational problem; if the focus is on the activities of the alienating parent, they could use child psychological abuse.[59]

Additionally, medical and psychiatric diagnoses are evolutionary and diagnoses in DSM can be transformed, modified, added, and removed over time due to expansion of knowledge and research on parental alienation,

56. Ciric, S. J., & Billick, S. B. (2017). Role of the psychiatric evaluator in child custody disputes. In Rosner, R., & Scott, C. L. (Eds.), *Principles and Practice of Forensic Psychiatry* (3rd ed.), 366.

57. Bernet, W. (2020), *supra*, 275 (internal citations omitted).

58. *Id.*, at 275.

59. *Id.*, at 276.

which may lead to better recognition of symptomatology. The fact that the precise term "parental alienation" is not currently included in DSM-5 does not mean that the concept lacks scientific underpinning. As an illustration, the word "psychopathy" is not in DSM (the official term is "antisocial"). However, the term psychopathy is commonly used in professional and legal literature and there exists a validated checklist for the identification of psychopathy. No professional would be criticized for making a "diagnosis" of "psychopathy" on the ground that the term is not to be found in the DSM. The phenomenon of parental alienation has been accepted by psychologists, psychiatrists, attorneys, and judges in not just the United States, but all over the world. The idea that a child's affection for a parent can be deliberately disrupted and manipulated by the other parent in a contentious custody litigation is neither novel nor bizarre. Unfortunately, as many practitioners who practice family law can aver, it is pathetically common.

7. Parental Alienation Is Not Supported by Empirical Research

One of the commonly advanced excuses for rejecting the theory of parental alienation is that it lacks empirical support. Almost from its inception, the theory of parental alienation has been criticized as lacking scientific or empirical support. And these criticisms persist to this day. It is not uncommon for an attorney representing the favored parent or for a guardian ad litem or the counsel for a minor (alienated) child to put forward this argument. Some do it as a deliberate and calculative strategy in order distract the court from the real issue at hand, i.e., child psychological abuse. Others do it out of blissful ignorance. Regardless, this red herring of an argument continues to distract the courts. At the outset, it is important to note that the vast majority of these arguments are focused on PAS, as opposed to the parental alienation theory.

For example, as one legal commentator wrote in 2013, "While Gardener and PAS have had many adherents, particularly among forensic evaluators and litigants, there is actually no empirical research validating the existence of PAS. And there is extensive empirical proof that the assumptions underlying the theory are false."[60] A similar sentiment has been echoed by others.[61]

The argument that parental alienation lacks empirical support has no merit. Recently, in the book, *Parental Alienation—Science and Law*, Dr. Amy J. L. Baker wrote an entire chapter on parental alienation and empirical research. In her chapter, Dr. Baker describes numerous studies on parental alienation, which

60. Meier, J. S. (2013). Parental Alienation Syndrome and Parental alienation: A research review, Vawnet, at https://vawnet.org/sites/default/files/materials/files/2016-09/AR_PASUpdate.pdf

61. *See, e.g.*, Benjamin, G., Andrew H., Beck, C. J., Shaw, M., & Geffner, R. (2018). *Family Evaluation in Custody Litigation: Promoting Optimal Outcomes and Reducing Ethical Risks* (2nd ed.), 34.

refute the argument that the theory lacks empirical support. As Dr. Baker explains:

> The numerous studies described in this chapter are offered as counter evidence. That is, in each study the measures of PA behaviors in the child and ABs [Alienating Behaviors] by the alienating parent were reliable and valid; objective, reliable and valid measures of other constructs were included (for example, measures of psychological maltreatment, parenting, depression, anxiety, and so forth); sample sizes were adequate; response rates were high; and statistically significant effects were found that support the foundational concept of PA theory: that exposure of children to ABs on the part of one parent are damaging to children and can interfere in their relationship with the other parent.[62]

Opponents to parental alienation often cite to a book chapter authored by Michael Saini and his colleagues in support of their argument challenging the scientific validity of the parental alienation theory.[63] However, the chapter and its findings are often distorted and misrepresented in litigation, and it is worthwhile to briefly discuss the chapter here. As Dr. Baker points out in her chapter on parental alienation and its empirical support, there are two notable problems with the Saini chapter.[64]

First, the authors reviewed and evaluated parental alienation research studies using what is known as the GRADE system, which stands for Grading of Recommendations Assessment, Development, and Evaluation.[65] However, the GRADE system was developed for a particular kind of medical research study known as a PICO study (Patient, Intervention, Comparator, Outcome). This means that the GRADE system was developed specifically to evaluate the quality of evidence in a *very specific type of study*, one in which patients with known medical conditions receive one of two comparable interventions, and outcomes are assessed as a way to determine the relative effectiveness of each intervention. The GRADE system is not an appropriate tool to evaluate all types of parental alienation research studies. As Dr. Baker explains:

> If a study in the field of PA were conducted to address a question about the comparative effectiveness of two interventions, then the GRADE system would be appropriate for the evaluation of the quality of that study. However, that is not the type of research that Saini et al. applied the GRADE

62. Baker, A. J. L. (2020). Parental Alienation and Empirical Research. In Lorandos, D., & Bernet, W. (Eds.), *Parental Alienation: Science and Law*, Charles C. Thomas, 244.

63. Saini, M., Johnston, J. R., Fidler, B. J. & Bala, N. (2016). Empirical studies of alienation. In Drozd, L. et al. (Eds.) *Parenting Plan Evaluations: Applied Research for the Family Court* (2nd ed.), Oxford UP, 374 .

64. Baker, A. J. L., *supra*, 244–245.

65. Atkins, D. et al. (2004). Systems for grading the quality of evidence and the strength of recommendations I: Critical appraisal of existing approaches, *BMC Health Serv. Res.*, 4, 38.

system to. They applied the GRADE system to a variety of other types of PA research studies and unsurprisingly concluded that the study fell short. This is comparable to evaluating an apple to see if it has the qualities of a good orange and concluding that it does not. Thus, while some of their criticisms of the PA studies they reviewed in their chapter were valid, many were not. For example, most studies are given low marks because the samples were not randomly drawn from the population. However, most social science research employs samples of convenience and the ability to generalize is not considered compromised unless there is a specific reason to believe that the characteristics of the sample are different from the population in a way that would be related to the variables studied.[66]

The second problem with the Saini et al. chapter is that "the authors fail to provide information about inter-rater reliability in their coding of the studies reviewed. This is a notable problem because not only is it standard practice in the field to provide the reader of a review article with information about the extent to which the reviewers agreed with their evaluations ofthe studies, but the GRADE system in particular has been difficult for coders to use reliably."[67] Even the creators of the GRADE system admitted having difficulty achieving reliability using their own system. Therefore, it would be even more important for Saini and his colleagues to provide that information about their coding of the parental alienation studies that they reviewed and evaluated.[68]

The numerous studies described by Dr. Baker in her aforementioned chapter provide evidence that the theory of parental alienation has a solid empirical support. It has been validated by using objective, reliable, and valid scientific measures.

8. Parental Alienation Does Not Pass the *Daubert/Frye* Gatekeeping

Family court judges often are asked to preclude all expert testimony on the issue of parental alienation on the ground that the testimony does not meet the *Frye* or *Daubert* standard of admissibility and should not be permitted in court. More often than not, a straw-man argument is put forward challenging the validity and reliability of PAS (even though the issue before the court may concern a parent's alienating *behaviors* or symptoms of alienation manifested by the child without any reference to the "syndrome"). And thereafter the attack attempts to paint the controversy with the broadest possible brush

66. Baker, A. J. L., *supra*, 245.
67. Baker, A. J. L., *supra*, 245
68. Baker, A. J. L., *supra*, 245–246.

strokes, equating PAS with PA, and asking the court to rule that any all evidence related to parental alienation be ruled inadmissible.

For example, a publication of the National Council of Juvenile and Family Court Judges incorrectly states, "The theory positing the existence of 'PAS' has been discredited by the scientific community."[69] The argument is advanced further by arguing that Parental Alienation Syndrome does not pass *Daubert* criteria, so, "Any testimony that a party to a custody case suffers from the syndrome or 'parental alienation' should therefore be ruled inadmissible and/or stricken from the evaluation report."[70] Also, some professionals have argued that "parental alienation syndrome should not be recognized in . . . child custody disputes because it is not a medically recognized syndrome, nor does it pass either of the evidentiary reliability standards."[71]

Like many deceptive arguments, absent a thorough understanding of the parental alienation construct together with a solid knowledge of the *Frye* and *Daubert* progeny of cases, it is easy to be deceived and buy into the propaganda. The rules for admissibility of expert evidence vary among jurisdictions, although they share the common goal that such evidence be useful and reliable.[72] See Appendix D for a chart outlining different states' rules regarding admissibility of expert testimony. The prevailing standards for admissibility of expert evidence have been articulated in two federal cases, *Frye* and *Daubert*, from which the states have derived their own variations. The majority of jurisdictions today follow a *Daubert*-leaning standard, while others lag behind with a *Frye*-leaning standard.[73]

Daubert bestows the gatekeeping obligation on a trial court and identifies the judge as the gatekeeper, who, prior to admitting expert testimony, must determine that the evidence is not only relevant and helpful to the controversy at hand but that the expert's methodology is based on the scientific method, "meaning that (1) hypotheses have been formulated and tested, (2) the results were subjected to peer review and published, (3) there is a known error rate, and (4) the methods in theory are generally accepted in the scientific community."[74]

In addition to the material covered in this book, proponents of the parental alienation theory facing a *Daubert* or *Frye* challenge would do well in reviewing Dr. Demosthenes Lorandos's chapter "Admissibility of the Construct-Parental

---

69. Dalton, C., Drozd, L. M., & Wong, F. Q. F. (2006). *Navigating Custody & Visitation Evaluations in Cases with Domestic Violence: A Judge's Guide*, SJI, NCJFCJ, 24.

70. *Id.*

71. Smith, H. (2016). Parental Alienation Syndrome: Fact or fiction? The problem with its use in child custody cases, *U. Mass. L. R.*, 11, 64.

72. Daubert v. Merrell Dow Pharmaceuticals, Inc., 509 U.S. 579, 589 (1993).

73. Lorandos, D. (2020). Admissibility of the construct—parental alienation. In Lorandos, D., & Bernet, W. (Eds.), *Parental Alienation: Science and Law*, Charles C. Thomas, 326.

74. Baker, A. J. L. (2020). Parental alienation and empirical research. In Lorandos, D., & Bernet, W. (Eds.), *Parental Alienation: Science and Law*, Charles C. Thomas, 246.

Alienation" in the recently published book, *Parental Alienation: Science and Law.*[75] These materials examine the application of *Daubert / Frye* criteria to the parental alienation theory in greater detail, but suffice it to say here that the following points are established from the review of case law and professional literature.

First, Dr. Lorandos's research has found more than one thousand cases addressing parental alienation from 1985 to 2018, which clearly demonstrates that the courts have found the construct of parental alienation useful, reliable, and admissible.[76] Second, there is a plethora of scientific or medical literature, including peer-reviewed literature, to support parental alienation theory. Vanderbilt University's Center for Knowledge Management database contains citations to over one thousand treatises relevant to the parental alienation construct.[77] Third, hypotheses relevant to alienating behaviors have been generated and tested, which means that the theory is falsifiable.[78] Fourth, the results of the research on parental alienation have been repeatedly subjected to peer review and have been published in renowned peer-review journals.[79] Fifth, with respect to error rate—known or potential rate of error is an important factor in *Daubert* gatekeeping—both the qualitative and quantitative research housed at the Vanderbilt University's database demonstrates that all measures used in parental alienation research have known error rates. This demonstrates more than adequate reliability.[80] Finally, while there is a dispute amongst experts as to whether parental alienation should be considered a syndrome that resides within the child, there is widespread acceptance of the core concepts of the parental alienation theory, to wit: parents can engage in behaviors that can adversely affect a child's relationship with the other parent.

The essential elements of the *Daubert* and *Frye* standards are met by the body of research in the field of parental alienation. The scientific basis underlying parental alienation theory is sound.

9. Men Do Not Alienate; Only Women Do (Or Vice Versa)

The theory of parental alienation is often misrepresented—at times, deliberately, to create an unwarranted controversy—as a weapon to fan the flames of the

75. Lorandos, D. (2020). Admissibility of the construct—parental alienation. In Lorandos, D., & Bernet, W. (Eds.), *Parental Alienation: Science and Law,* Charles C. Thomas, 324–364.

76. Lorandos, D. (2020). Parental alienation in U.S. Courts, 1985 to 2018. In Lorandos, D., & Bernet, W. (Eds.), *Parental Alienation: Science and Law,* Charles C. Thomas, 365–38.

77. *See* www.mc.vanderbilt.edu/pasg.

78. Baker, A. J. L., *supra,* 246.

79. *Id.;* also see Lorandos, D., Bernet, W., & Sauber, R. (Eds.), *Parental Alienation: The Handbook for Mental Health and Legal Professionals,* Charles C. Thomas, which contains a bibliography with hundreds of peer-reviewed articles regarding the topic of parental alienation from more than thirty countries.

80. Baker, A. J. L., *supra,* 247.

gender war over children: Dads versus Moms. On one end of the spectrum, it is argued that alienation is a choice weapon of women to "get even" against men. At the other end of the spectrum, an argument is made that men accuse women of parental alienation in order to excuse or distract from their abusive conduct that is the root cause of the children's rejection.[81] Both arguments are ideologies masquerading as science. As shown in this book, before diagnosing parental alienation, an evaluator has to methodically go through the Five-Factor Model. The model is gender blind. An intellectually honest evaluation and application of the model will preclude a finding of parental alienation if there's evidence of bona fide abuse or neglect on the part of the now rejected parent.

Courts have acknowledged that the theory of parental alienation does not lend itself to a "simplistic analysis," where it is portrayed as a "gender war over the children."[82] However, statistics aren't sexist, and we do have to reckon with some interesting data. In 2010, Canadian law professor Nicholas Bala and his colleagues published a paper that studied all reported Canadian cases between 1989 and 2008 that dealt with claims of parental alienation.[83] The study found that between 1989 and 2008, alienation was found by Canadian courts in 106 out of 175 cases raising the issue. And the mother was the alienating parent in 72 cases (68 percent), and the father was the alienating parent in 33 cases (31 percent). The Canadian study is not alone in finding mothers significantly more as the alienating parent. In the United States too, the statistics do indicate that percentage of women who have been found or identified to have engaged in alienating behaviors outnumber men by 3 to 1 ratio. The results of Dr. Demosthenes Lorandos's research project, wherein he and his team analyzed over one thousand cases involving parental alienation, demonstrated "that during 1985–2018, about 75% of the identified alienators were female and 25% were male. This proportion has remained approximately the same over the years."[84] However, to simply consider this statistic in vacuum and rush to a conclusion that women alienate significantly more than men would not be appropriate. As Dr. Lorandos explains,

> the residual effects of patriarchy may account for some of the skew in the numbers of male to female alienators. According to a Pew Research Center, analysis of median hourly earnings of both full-and part-time workers in the United States, women earned 82% of what men earned. Based on this estimate, it would take an extra 47 days of work each year for women

81. *See, e.g.*, Drew, M. (2017). Collaboration and intention: Making the collaborative family law process safe(r), *Ohio St. J. On Disp. Resol.*, 32, 373n.

82. J.F. v. D.F., 61 Misc.3d 1226(A), 2018 N.Y.Slip Op. 51829(U).

83. Bala, N. et al., (2010, January). Parental alienation: Canadian court cases 1989–2008, *Family Court Review*, 48(1), 164–179.

84. Lorandos, D. (2020). Parental alienation in U.S. Courts, 1985–2018. In Lorandos, D., & Bernet, W. (Eds.), *Parental Alienation: Science and Law*, Charles C. Thomas, 371–372.

to earn what men do. And in the process of a marital breakup, working males may have more access to ready cash. These differentials should be considered when reviewing the gender difference found in this research.[85]

In other words, men, having more financial resources, may have been more willing to litigate cases involving parental alienation, using skilled legal representation and top-notch experts, as compared to women.

Keeping the gender disparity data aside, when we review the pertinent case law—judicial opinions from family courts around the country where courts have found parental alienation to exist—we find that neither gender has a monopoly on engaging in alienating behaviors. We find dads behaving badly as well as moms.[86]

10. Bad Behavior Equals Parental Alienation: The Risk of False Positives

On occasions, evaluators—even the good, competent ones—may get it wrong. Concluding that parental alienation exists in a case where it really does not results in false positive identifications and fuels concerns about the application of the parental alienation theory in family law cases.[87] "False positive identifications of parental alienation can occur with respect to a parent's alienating behaviors, a child's alienation from a parent, or both."[88] For example, false positive identifications of a parent's alienating behaviors can occur when the parent's behavior is mistakenly interpreted as undermining or potentially undermining a child's positive regard for the other parent. For instance, Dr. Richard Warshak provides an example of a situation where a simplistic understanding of a specific behavior may result in false positive conclusion about alienating behavior: A parent giving a child a cell phone and instructing the child to call when he or she feels like speaking.[89] The significance of this behavior depends on the context in which it occurs and how the child subsequently uses the phone given by the parent. For example, has the parent who provided the phone planted in the child a false belief that the other parent is dangerous? Has the parent instructed the child to call 911 if the other parent did anything that the child did not like, such as disciplining the child for rude

---

85. *Id.*, at 373–374, citing Graf, N. et al. (2018, April 9). The narrowing, but persistent, gender gap in pay, *Facttank: News in the Numbers*, at http://www.pewresearch.org/fact-tank/2018/04/09/gender-pay-gap-facts/.

86. *See* (2020). Appendix C, Cases illustrative of alienating behaviors. In Lorandos, D., & Bernet, W. (Eds.), *Parental Alienation: Science and Law*, Charles C. Thomas, 603–634.

87. Warshak, R. A. (2019). When evaluators get it wrong: False positive IDs and parental alienation, *Psychology, Public Policy, and Law*, 26(1), 54–68.

88. *Id.*, at 54.

89. *Id.*, at 63.

or disrespectful behavior? Has the parent instructed the child to use the phone to record the other parent? Has the parent repeatedly encroached on the child's time with the other parent by frequently calling and texting the child? Has the parent attempted to undermine the child's relationship with the other parent? If so, these would be the examples of alienating behaviors and, in that context, providing the phone to the child would a continuation of the pattern of alienating behaviors.[90] But if all that the parent did was to provide a cell phone to the child and instruct the child to call when he or she felt like speaking to the parent, that behavior by itself would not rise to the level of being an alienating behavior.

It is important to note that the term "parental alienation refers either to the state of the relationship between a child and a parent whom the child rejects without good cause or to the child's attitudes and behaviors that reflect an unreasonable aversion to a parent with whom he or she formerly enjoyed normal relations."[91] However, it is possible that a parent can engage in negative, alienating behaviors—for example, persistently disparaging the other parent—without the child becoming alienated from the parent who is the target of such negative behavior. Alienating behaviors do not *always* result in parental alienation. For instance, in a New York case, even though three experienced experts concluded that the mother had alienated the children, the court, rejecting the experts' conclusions, opined, "There is not an iota of evidence that any one of three daughters are alienated from their father."[92] By the same token, another court in New York concluded that a child's rejection of a parent was a justified response and not due to alienation.[93]

A child's alienation from a parent can arise from factors independent of, or in combination with, the favored parent's behavior. For instance, the child could be reacting to abuse, gross mistreatment, severe mental illness, witnessing domestic violence, or substance abuse.[94] Further, negative behavior towards a parent, such as denigrating, complaining, and resisting contact, is insufficient by itself to identify a child as "alienated."[95] Experts identify seven criteria that distinguish negative behaviors of moderately or severely alienated children from negative behavior that does not indicate moderate or severe levels of parental alienation. A child with moderate or severe parental alienation displays negative behavior that meets all of the following criteria:[96]

90. *See, e.g.,* McRoberts v. Superior Court of Los Angeles County, B234877 (Cal. Ct. App. Jun. 19, 2012).
91. Warshak, R. A. (2019), *supra*, 57.
92. J.F. v. D.F., 61 Misc.3d 1226(A), 2018 N.Y.Slip Op. 51829(U).
93. A.E. v. S.E., NY Law Journal, Dec. 11, 1990 (No. O-1433-90, Fam. Ct. N.Y. Westchester County, Nov 19, 1990).
94. Warshak, R. A. (2019), *supra*, 57.
95. *Id.*, at 58.
96. *Id.*

(a) The behavior is chronic rather than temporary and short-lived;
(b) The behavior is frequent rather than occasional;
(c) The behavior occurs in most situations rather than only in certain situations;
(d) The behavior occurs without displays of genuine love and affection toward the rejected parent;
(e) The behavior is directed at only one parent;
(f) The behavior does not reflect typical dynamics for the child's state of development;
(g) The behavior is disproportionate to, and not justified by the rejected parent's past or current behavior.

11. Professional or Clinical Intuition Is Sufficient to Resolve Parental Alienation

Parental alienation is a nuanced field of expertise and specialization. It is also profoundly counterintuitive.[97] Professionals who rely on their personal experiences or intuition ("gut") are highly vulnerable to making catastrophic mistakes. Intuition, clinical or professional—*I've been doing this for a long time, and I know exactly what's required here*—is rarely adequate to solve complex, counterintuitive problems. And using intuition in cases involving parental alienation can be downright disastrous.

For starters, it is well known how mental health professionals, especially psychologists, fail to "use the interventions for which there is the strongest evidence of efficacy" and "give more weight to their personal experiences than to science."[98] In parental alienation context, this could result in a serious error, such as the professionals rejecting evidence-based interventions (which they, not having the benefit of being trained or educated on, consider "drastic") and instead giving more weight to conventional therapy with local therapists with whom they have personal experience or affinity. "'The disconnect between what clinicians do and what science has discovered is an unconscionable embarrassment' [and] . . . there is a 'widening gulf between clinical practice and science.'"[99]

Professionals should recognize that children are susceptible to influence, intimidation, and manipulation, and, in a case involving parental alienation, the child's "voice" may neither reflect the child's actual position nor her best

97. Miller, S. G. (2018). Why do specialists say that parental alienation is counterintuitive, Part 1, *Parental Alienation International*, 3(3), 19.

98. Begley, S. (2009, October 1) Why psychologists reject science, *Newsweek*, at https://www.newsweek.com/why-psychologists-reject-science-begley-81063.

99. *Id.*

interests.[100] But time and again, when we review family court cases, we see professionals—guardians ad litem, minors' counsel, parenting coordinators, evaluators—give significant weight to preferences of alienated children. We observe that alienated children's rejection of the targeted parent and their excuses to not abide by court-ordered parenting time are not only condoned—rather, the professionals recommend that the target parents show "empathy" and *not* seek enforcement with court orders. We frequently see the well-meaning professionals attempt to manage these cases by relying on their intuition and make recommendations along the lines of: *Your child needs some space. By attempting to enforce your parenting time, you will only succeed in driving her farther away. Just be patient.*

Such professionals *enable* alienation by valuing personal opinion, ideology, or experience over research evidence and create a vicious cycle and nefarious incentives for the alienating parent to continue to manipulate and influence his or her child's position. Moreover, now the alienating parent has an important ally: the professional, who may be a quasi-judicial authority such as the guardian ad litem or a court-appointed evaluator. And if this professional advocates for the favored parent to have custody because the "voice" of the alienated child must be heard and respected, the alienating parent in effect has two lawyers in the courtroom—his or her own and the professional.

We generally do not trust children to make judgments in their best interests. In an alienation situation, the need for caution is even greater as the affected child may not be cognitively or psychologically capable to make a decision in her best interests.[101] The professional standards that apply to lawyers who represent children in such scenarios underscore this concern: "One of the most difficult ethical issues for lawyers representing children occurs when the child is able to express a position and does so, but the lawyer believes that the position chosen is wholly inappropriate or could result in serious injury to the child."[102]

It is important that the professionals study the *science*—research and findings on parental alienation, the empirical studies on parental alienation, the phenomenon of pathological enmeshment of the child with the alienator parent, Adverse Childhood Experiences studies that outline the significant cognitive and psychological harm to the child, and success outcomes of specialized intervention programs to remedy parental alienation. If they do, they will realize that the alienated child has been stripped of a "genuine voice."[103] Rather,

100. Standards of Practice for Lawyers Representing Children in Custody Cases, ABA Section of Family Law, A-1.

101. Rosen, J. (2013). The child's attorney and the alienated child: Approaches to resolving the ethical dilemma of diminished capacity, *Family Court Review*, 51(2), 330.

102. Standards of Practice for Lawyers Representing Children in Custody Cases, *supra*, IV(C)(3), Commentary (2003).

103. Warshak, R. (2003). Bringing sense to parental alienation: A look at the disputes and the evidence, *Fam. L. Q.*, 37, 273, 375.

the child's voice reflects the words, attitudes, and beliefs of the alienator, who exercises a nefarious influence over the child. But without proper training, it is very difficult, if not impossible, for professionals and clinicians to make well-reasoned, professional judgment calls. And those professionals and clinicians who are ambivalent about the role of science usually fall back on their personal experience in resolving the cases involving parental alienation and, in doing so, often find it very difficult to navigate these turbulent waters. The two most glaring pitfalls—the Scylla and Charybdis of parental alienation cases—that confront the professionals are: Enmeshment and Traditional Therapy.

For an untrained professional or clinician, it is easy to mistake the phenomenon of enmeshment between an alienator and the child for a close relationship: *Certainly, the mother and the son appear to be very close and bonded with each other. They are buddies!* What appears to be a close relationship on a superficial level may actually be a pathologically enmeshed relationship. A pathologically dependent parent *adultifies* the child—treats the child in a manner that is not age-appropriate, such as treating the child as a "friend," rather than as a child. This involves severe boundary violations of the child by the parent to the point that the parent not only violates the child's boundaries but *erases* them. Enmeshment is a form of child abuse and the professionals and clinicians who work on such cases should be trained to look for signs of enmeshment. Also, they should not hesitate to ask the court for additional resources, such as a psychological evaluation, to analyze the issue further if needed.

Another snare that untrained professionals risk falling into is traditional therapy. Fools rush in where angels fear to tread; sending off a target parent and the children to traditional therapy in a case involving parental alienation is a recipe for disaster. It would be difficult to find a more common yet egregious blunder that professionals and clinicians routinely commit than advocating for what amounts to traditional "reunification" therapy in alienation cases. It is important that the professionals be trained to understand the difference between traditional therapy and specialized intervention programs. They should be trained to appreciate the fact that not only traditional therapy is known to be ineffective, it is also known to be potentially devastating—such "therapy" validates an alienated child's distorted view of the world, encourages the child to express grievances, and gives an already-over-empowered child more control while advising the disempowered-target-parent to "listen," show empathy, and apologize (or even to find something to apologize for).[104] In alienation cases, traditional therapy is *contraindicated*[105] and typically makes

104. Miller, S. G. (2018). Why do specialists say that parental alienation is counterintuitive, Part 2, *PASG Newsletter*, 3(4), 17.

105. *Id.*, at 18 (". . . the word *contraindicated* does not mean 'not indicated.' It means forbidden. If a patient is allergic to penicillin, then penicillin is contraindicated. In the face of a penicillin allergy, it would not be proper to prescribe penicillin to see what happens.").

things worse. And even when provided under a court order, such therapy is of little benefit.

As this chapter shows, litigation landscape of parental alienation resembles the wild west where fallacies and myths abound. Lawyers who accept cases involving allegations of parental alienation or accept court-appointed assignments in such cases must realize that these cases often call for an urgent and effective intervention. Often it results in major life decisions for a child, such as those related to custody, parental access, child protection and/or mental health treatment intervention. These decisions, if advocated or made by those lacking proper training and relying on their personal experiences than science, can lead to catastrophic errors. It is paramount that the legal practitioner handling these cases is familiar with the professional literature and relevant caselaw pertaining to parental alienation.

CHAPTER 7

Parental Alienation and Domestic Violence

Child abuse and domestic violence come in many forms—physical, social, sexual, and emotional. There is often an interplay between the claims of parental alienation and the claims of domestic violence or abuse. The issue of domestic violence and abuse is the 800-pound gorilla in the courtroom when it is raised to either detract, defend against, or justify claims of parental alienation. The fundamental concept of the parental alienation theory is that children who are alienated reject a parent because they have been brainwashed, programmed, or manipulated by the other parent to hold false beliefs and distorted perceptions about the rejected parent. It is important to remember that the theory of parental alienation does not state that *all* children who reject a parent are alienated. It is also important to acknowledge the fact that the theory does not assume that any child who is rejecting a parent *must* be an alienated child. The phenomenon of parental alienation is only applicable to a situation "when the target parent has not exhibited anything close to the degree of alienating behavior that might warrant the campaign of vilification exhibited by the child."[1] The child's resistance to or rejection of the parent is always disproportional to anything that the parent is alleged to have done.

The detractors of the parental alienation theory often put up a strawman argument and claim that the parental alienation theory *assumes* that any child who rejects a parent must be alienated. For instance, some professionals have argued: "Parental alienation syndrome further assumes that a child's strong

1. Gardner, R. A. (1998). *The Parental Alienation Syndrome: A Guide for Mental Health and Legal Professionals*, Creative Therapeutics, xx.

alignment with one parent while rejecting a relationship with the other parent is without legitimate justification, including situations in which there is child abuse."[2] The theory of parental alienation "assumes" no such thing. It is important to debunk this strawman argument and explicitly acknowledge that not only is this argument false, but it deliberately distorts the theory of parental alienation. In responding to such strawman argument, it is also important for a practitioner to educate the court that it is not possible to determine based solely on the rejecting behavior of a child whether that child is alienated or estranged. An evaluator or clinician who claims that all children who reject a parent are alienated or claims that it is possible to make a determination regarding whether a child is alienated *solely based on the child's behavior* is making a fundamental clinical error. While a child's polarized view of his or her parents and absolute rejection of a parent may generate a hypothesis of parental alienation, an evaluator or clinician must consider the total clinical picture before making a determination of whether parental alienation exists. Such determination cannot be made without considering the attitudes, perceptions, actions, and omissions of all the parties—the child, the rejected parent, and the favored parent.

Further, parental alienation is the result associated with alienating behaviors that are manifested by a parent (or a third party). While alienating behaviors may not always result in severe parental alienation—an absolute and complete rejection of a parent—they still impact the child and the targeted parent in many negative ways. Even "mild" parental alienation could lead to outcomes that include the child feeling abandoned and experiencing anger against or rejection of the targeted parent for unjustifiable reasons; the child suffering from depression; academic decline; and physical ill effects, such as high blood pressure.[3]

Applying the Tools: Using the Five-Factor Model to Rule Out Abuse

As discussed *supra,* Dr. Amy J. L. Baker and her colleagues have come up with the Five-Factor Model as a methodology to determine whether a child who is aligned with one parent while rejecting the other has been alienated.[4] It is only when *all* five factors are present that an evaluator or clinician (or a

2. Benjamin, G. et. al. (2018). *Family Evaluation in Custody Litigation: Promoting Optimal Outcomes and Reducing Ethical Risks* (2nd ed.), APA, 34.

3. Harman, J., & Biringen, Z. (2016). *Parents Acting Badly: How Institutions and Societies Promote the Alienation of Children from their Loving Families,* CreateSpace Independent Publishing Platform.

4. Baker, A. J. L. (2020). Parental alienation and empirical research. In Lorandos, D., & Bernet, W. (Eds.), *Parental Alienation: Science and Law,* Charles C. Thomas, 209.

factfinder, e.g., the court) should conclude that the child is alienated as opposed to estranged, which refers to warranted or justified rejection of a parent.

For the purposes of this chapter, we will explore Factor Three of the Five-Factor Model in detail. Factor Three states that the now rejected parent did not engage in abuse, neglect, or demonstrate seriously deficient parenting of the type and magnitude that could reasonably be expected to cause a child to reject a parent. It bears repeating that in keeping with the premise of the theory of parental alienation, Factor Three requires that the child's rejection of the target parent is far out of proportion to anything that parent has done to justify the rejection. This requires a factfinder to investigate what exactly the rejected parent is alleged to have done to the child and whether such action (or omission) justifies the child's rejection of the parent.

Cases involving allegations of parental alienation often involve allegations of abuse as well. It is often alleged by the favored parent that the rejected parent "deserves" being rejected or that the child's rejection of the parent is justified.[5] It is very important that allegations of abuse—physical, psychological, or sexual—and neglect are properly and thoroughly investigated at the outset. If not, it may be difficult if not impossible to later investigate and adjudicate such allegations with the passage of time and the deterioration of the strength and quality of available evidence. Further, unsubstantiated allegations take on a life of their own and continue to haunt the targeted parent and confound the court professionals who may be unable to investigate such allegations long after they were first made. As Dr. Baker explains, for purposes of the Five-Factor Model, "it is important to determine whether formal child abuse investigations concluded that the rejected parent had in fact engaged in any form of maltreatment."[6] This is important for several reasons.

Firstly, domestic violence is a serious matter and such abusive behavior should neither be ignored nor condoned. A parent who is a victim of domestic violence may attempt to limit the contact between the abusive spouse or partner and the child not with an intention to alienate the child, but to protect the child from the violent or abusive behavior. Similarly, a child who has been subjected to severe abuse or neglect or who has witnessed a persistent pattern of domestic violence may reject the abusive parent not because of any indoctrination by the other parent, but because of the psychological and cognitive harm that such abusive behavior wreaks on the child's psyche. Consider for instance, the case of *Jillian EE v. Kane FF7*, where a New York appellate court affirmed a trial court's rejection of a father's allegations of parental alienation.

5. Kopetski, L. et al. (2006). Incidence, gender and false allegations of child abuse: Data on 84 parental alienation cases. In Gardner, R. A., Sauber, S. R., & Lorandos, D. (Eds.), *The International Handbook of Parental Alienation Syndrome: Conceptual, Clinical and Legal Considerations*, Charles C. Thomas, 65.

6. Baker, A. J. L., *supra*, 212.

7. Jillian EE. v. Kane FF., 165 A.D.3d 1407 (2018).

The trial court also awarded custody to the mother because of a documented history of domestic violence, which explained and justified the mother's efforts to keep the child away to protect him from the father's violent behavior. Upon a full evidentiary hearing, the trial court found that the mother and the child were subjected to domestic violence by the father, and the child, who exhibited bruises, clearly stated that the father had squeezed, punched, and hit him. The court determined that while the mother had made some efforts in driving the father away from the child, she did it for "a valid reason—to protect him from the father's violent behavior." Importantly, she had never previously prevented the father from spending time with or contacting the child and never talked poorly about the father to him. Given these facts, the court rejected the father's argument that the mother had engaged in parental alienation.

Secondly, not all conduct that is alleged to be abusive rises to the level of domestic violence. If the acts complained of do not rise to the level of domestic violence or domestic abuse, as the term is defined under a relevant state's statute, they cannot be considered as such. Further, if such acts do not fit squarely within the statutory definition of domestic violence, they should not be considered for the purposes of rebuttable presumption that many states have in favor of the victim and against the abuser for an award of custody.[8] In addition, the term "abuse" has different thresholds and connotations in different cultures. While some cultures consider spanking to be an "abusive" act, in other cultures, *not* spanking a child is considered a dereliction of parenting. Physical differences in child discipline vary by countries, and it is important to remember this fact, especially when evaluating the family dynamics involving first or second-generation immigrant family members. For instance, in a peer-reviewed study, a team of international researchers conducted interviews with 336 mother-child dyads (children's ages ranged from 6 to 17 years; mothers' ages ranged from 20 to 59 years) in China, India, Italy, Kenya, the Philippines, and Thailand to examine the link between mothers' use of physical discipline and children's adjustment.[9] The researchers found that the mothers and children in Kenya and Italy generally reported more frequent use and more normative use of physical discipline than did mothers and children in other countries, mothers and children in China and Thailand generally reported less frequent and less normative use of physical discipline, and mothers and children in India and the Philippines reported moderate levels of frequency and normativeness of use of physical discipline.[10]

---

8. *See, e.g.*, Oates v. Oates, 2010 Ark.App. 346 ("our statute requires that a person engage in a pattern of domestic abuse; if the acts did not rise to the definition of domestic abuse, they cannot be considered for purposes of the presumption").

9. Lansford, J. E. et al. (2005). Physical discipline and children's adjustment: Cultural normativeness as a moderator, *Child Dev.*, 76(6), 1234–1246, at https://www.ncbi.nlm.nih.gov/pmc/articles/PMC2766084/.

10. *Id.*

In some cultures, child nudity, even into the teen years, is considered normal and healthy. A forensic sociologist's cautionary tale comes to the mind to exemplify this point:

> A story comes to mind of a father, some years ago, who was waiting to have his pictures developed at a K-Mart (pre-cell phone era) when he found himself being approached by police. He was handcuffed and taken into custody as the clerk, who saw the pictures, called the police. The pictures showed his son bouncing on a bed in different positions and degrees of undress along with a buddy. This was identified as "pedophilia-type photography." This was used as incriminating information in the (family) court along with his practice of kissing his son on his mouth, squeezing his cheeks, and hugging him regularly and in a very robust fashion. It became my task to explain to the court that he was a first generation Italian male and that he had done nothing culturally inappropriate. Nudity, and pictures thereof; kissing on the lips; and extensive physical contact, including hugging, kissing, and patting children were all appropriate behaviors within segments of this first generation Italian family (ethnic) culture.[11]

Therefore, real abuse must be sorted out from abuse allegations that may either be unfounded or false or made out of cultural ignorance. Cultural knowledge is imperative, and practitioners, when in doubt, should consult a cultural anthropologist or a clinical sociologist to ascertain whether the behavior that is alleged to be abusive has alternative explanations. In addition, allegations of domestic violence or abuse must be specific and supported by evidence, especially if the alleged victim is seeking orders of protection that may curtail a parent's access to his or her child. Allegations of abusive behavior that are inconsistent or those that do not demonstrate knowing and intentional behavior on the part of the alleged perpetrator may result in dismissal of allegations or vacation of protective orders, if such were issued on an *ex parte* basis.[12]

Thirdly, false allegations of abuse and domestic violence are not uncommon in contentious and high-conflict divorce and child-custody proceedings. It is important to investigate the allegations of domestic violence or abuse to ensure that the allegations have merit. As a Family Court of Delaware[13] noted in a difficult case that it presided over:

> Mother has made numerous allegations of physical abuse by Father against [child] and testified graphically as to her allegations of abuse at the hand

11. Clawar, S. S. (2020). *Parent-Child Reunification: A Guide to Legal and Forensic Strategies*, American Bar Association, 60.
12. *See, e.g., In re* the Matter of Cusick v. Gerth, 2020 WL 1527913 (Ariz.Ct.App.).
13. T.C.C. v. M.L.C., 2004 WL 3245937.

> of Father. The allegations of abuse . . . were determined to be unfounded and, in fact, caused DFS to have concerns about Mother and her parenting ability. . . . This series of unfounded domestic abuse allegations does not demonstrate a pattern of domestic violence by Father, rather a pattern of histrionic and self-serving behavior by Mother.

Not only did the mother here make unfounded allegations of domestic violence, but having made these allegations, she thereafter leveraged the family court system to undermine the father's relationship with the children:

> The Court also notes Mother's frequent attempts at parental alienation, which include the Criminal No Contact Order and refusal to visit at the [visitation center], which led to no visitation between Father and the children for four months. In addition, this Court notes the DFS testimony that Mother tended to file these and similar charges right before scheduled court hearings. These actions speak to Mother's credibility, which was a significant consideration for the Court in reviewing the testimony of the parties."

Acknowledging the grievous harm caused to the children due to the mother's behaviors, the court awarded the father sole custody of the children and ordered supervised visitation for the mother.

On the other hand, as the Five-Factor Model demonstrates, if the rejected parent has indeed abused or neglected the child, the case should not be considered a pure alienation case. And this would be true regardless of the behaviors of the favored parent and the child. This is not to say that evidence of abuse or neglect negates any finding of parental alienation or that findings of abuse or neglect and parental alienation are mutually exclusive. One could have a situation where the rejected parent engaged in abusive behavior together with the favored parent having engaged in alienating behaviors. But the devil is in the detail, and the factfinder will have to carefully undertake the causation analysis—the cause or explanation for the parent-child broken bond or relationship. Suffice it to say, however, that in such scenarios, it is highly unlikely that the case would be considered as a pure alienation case. As noted by Dr. Richard Gardner, who put forward the theory of Parental Alienation Syndrome, "I am referring here to those who are truly innocent of any behavior that warrants the degree of victimization visited upon them by their PAS children."[14] If the rejected parent has indeed abused or neglected the child—in keeping with the definition of child maltreatment, which varies from state to state[15]—the

14. Gardner, R., *supra*, at 209.

15. The federal child abuse law, the Child Abuse Prevention and Treatment Act, allows states to define specific types of child maltreatment in their own statutes. *See* Child Abuse Prevention and Treatment Act (CAPTA) of 1974, 42 U.S.C. §§ 5101-5116i (2019).

case could be a "hybrid" case (having shades of alienation and estrangement) or it might be a case of estrangement (some professionals term it as "realistic estrangement"), but it cannot be a case of pure parental alienation. Such abusive or neglectful behavior on the part of the rejected parent would provide an alternative explanation for why a child would reject the parent and would challenge the validity of an alienation hypothesis as the only explanation for the child's rejection.

For instance, consider the facts in the Connecticut case of *Sylvain v. Krajewski*.[16] The court was faced with dueling claims: mother claimed physical abuse of the children by the father and the father claimed that he was the victim of parental alienation. After considering all the evidence and testimony that was presented at the trial, the court concluded that parental alienation was *not* present in the case. Rather, the father had self-diagnosed the family dynamics as alienation dynamics with a granite-like certainty while remaining willfully blind to his own behavior. As the court noted:

> The father persists in and pursues his claim that he is the victim of parental alienation. To that end he has created a foundation for victims of parental alienation. His telephone is answered by a recording regarding the foundation, he has attempted to force the children to wear purple wrist bracelets supporting his cause and posted photographs of his children, against their wishes, on his website. . . . [Father] had attended a rally in Washington, D.C. in support of parents claiming parental alienation rather than attend his own trial. [Father] has had little respect for the orders of the court regarding therapeutic intervention: Choosing to seek visitation and access on his terms rather than those recommended by the children's therapists and the guardian ad litem and ordered by the court. To that end, for almost a year, [Father] did not participate in non-relative supervised visitation. By the final hearing date, [Father] had not seen his children for almost two years.

The court carefully evaluated the father's claim that the mother engaged in parental alienation by not promoting visitation between him and the children. The court found some merit to this claim, but explained why the mother's refusal to promote visitation was justified:

> The mother clearly would not go out of her way to promote visitation between the father and the children. She dislikes [Father], his family and friends. They have assailed her character and parental skills. They have made derogatory comments about her to the children and attempted to make contact with the children against her wishes. She has seen her

16. Sylvain v. Krajewski, 2009 WL 2231223.

> children's privacy violated by the posting of their photographs and claims of parental alienation posted on the father's website. She is vilified as the cause of the children's lack of interest in visiting with their father. Based on the court's observations, [Mother], although her claims of physical and mental abuse toward the children are exaggerated, she is a concerned, protective, and loving parent. She has the best interests of her children as her main objective. She attended her court-ordered individual therapy. She dutifully takes her children to their counseling sessions, meetings, and evaluations. She makes every effort to comply with court rules. She is respectful to the court's authority. She has complied with every recommendation of therapists and the guardian ad litem.

In contrast, the court found the father to be so blinded by his hate of the mother and obsessed with proving parental alienation that he became "a self-centered, egotist who cannot accept the fact his own behavior has destroyed and jeopardized any future attempts to correct his relationship with his children." Lamenting that "if there ever was a person who fits the description of 'not being able to see the forest for the tree,'" the court found that the father was that person. The court ultimately awarded sole custody to the mother.

In another case, a highly contested matter of *Hrabovsky v. Axley*[17], an Ohio court rejected the findings of a guardian ad litem and a court-appointed mental health professional, both of whom had raised concerns of parental alienation by the father against the mother. Instead, the court found that the children were estranged from the mother because of the mother's actions—her cohabitation with her paramour, who had a criminal record; her conviction for domestic violence (punching the father in the face); and her possession of drugs and drug paraphernalia in her home. The court, being the ultimate factfinder and issue resolver, chose not to believe the testimony of the GAL and the expert because, in its opinion, "the evidence presented demonstrated Mother's conduct could be a source of the children's strained relationship with Mother, as opposed to Father's conduct as the sole reason for the children to feel negatively about Mother." The court found that the determination of parental alienation was not supported by the evidence on the record.

Therefore, it is important to thoroughly investigate and determine the cause of the child's rejection of a parent. Without undertaking such causation analysis, a court cannot fashion the appropriate remedy, to wit: legal and mental health intervention necessary to repair the broken relationship between the parent and the child. While it is rare to come across a situation where a hybrid case

---

17. Hrabovsky v. Axley, 2014 WL 1340768 (Ohio.Ct.App.).

of alienation and estrangement turns into a pure alienation, it is by no means impossible. Consider, for example, the Michigan case of *Martin v. Martin*.[18]

Martin v. Martin exemplified the high-conflict, post-judgment divorce litigation that spanned over several years and presented complex family dynamics, with several mental health professionals involved in the litigation. Writing in January of 2020, the Michigan Court of Appeals found that since 2010, the mother had denigrated the father to their three children. The mother's alienating behaviors included telling the children that "daddy doesn't care about you" and giving them permission to call their father names and otherwise disrespect him because "he deserve[d] it." The mother undermined the father and the children learned at a young age that a "no" from their father could easily be changed into a "yes" by their mother, and the consequences imposed by their father would not be enforced or would be undermined by their mother. During the first round of litigation, in 2012, the trial court found that the father was not blameless and that he was controlling and misused corporal punishment in times of anger. The court found evidence of *both* alienation and estrangement—referring to a breach in a parent-child relationship from the words and conduct of the affected parent as "estrangement," and a breach in the parent-child relationship resulting from the words and conduct of the other parent as "alienation." In 2012, the trial court awarded sole legal and physical custody of the children to the mother, with parenting time with the father to take place under therapeutic supervision. The therapy didn't work out, the father exercised no parenting time, and neither party took any further action for the next three-and-a-half years.

During that period, however, father participated in extensive individual and group therapy including completing a "Nurturing Dads" curriculum. In 2016, father sought court intervention to get parenting time and for a proper reunification with his children. The trial court referred the matter to the friend of the court for an investigation and recommendation. Similar to the trial court's earlier finding, the friend of the court found the case to be a hybrid case of both alienation and estrangement and proposed a team of therapists to work on reunification. The trial court adopted the recommendations and ordered counseling to commence with a team of mental health professionals, each with a different role to play. The parties returned to court for a review hearing in early 2017, where the trial court took testimony from the parties and the mental health counselors and interviewed the minor children *in camera*. Thereafter, the court held mother in contempt of court, sentenced her to 45 days in jail (41 days of which were suspended), and awarded father 30 days of continuous make-up parenting time. The court also scheduled multiple review hearings through

18. Martin v. Martin, 2020 WL 448325 (Mich. Court of Appeals, January 28, 2020); also see Martin v. Martin, Circuit Court of Ottawa County File No. 10-68039-DM, Opinion dated May 28, 2019.

the year, the father retained exclusive parenting time during this time with ongoing counseling, and the mother saw the minor children only in sessions with the reunification counselor. Litigation continued, and, ultimately, in May of 2019, the trial court, in keeping with the best interests of the minor children, awarded the father sole legal and physical custody of the remaining minor child (other children having reached the age of emancipation) and ordered the mother to exercise her parenting time only under therapeutic supervision.

The unusual feature of the *Martin* case is the court's finding that a hybrid case of estrangement and alienation, in time and with change in one parent's behavior, transformed into a *pure* alienation case. As the trial court found:

> In 2012, the court concluded that the parties' respective capacities to provide love, affection, and guidance to the children had been negatively affected by their own behavior. [Father] was found to be "strict, too often angry, and sometimes vindictive." . . . [T]rend in mother's behavior has continued and worsened. Her capacity and disposition to provide proper guidance is worse now than it was a year ago, as her deliberate undermining of the court's orders and the counseling process is even more obvious. . . . At the same time, [Father's] behavior has improved significantly due to his long participation in counseling and group therapy, and his great patience and consistency over the past year-and-a-half shows that he has made a much more substantial and effective effort to improve his capacity and disposition to provide appropriate love, affection, and guidance.
>
> . . .
>
> In 2012, the court concluded that this case involved mutual hostility and a 'moderate-to-severe' level of parental alienation. . . . The situation is now one of 'severe' alienation, while [Father's] contribution to the hostility has significantly abated with the assistance of several years of counseling.

Martin is not the only case where a trial court took note of a parent's remorse for the past behavior or his or her attempts to change the negative behavior that was at issue. For example, in *Dean v. Valinho*, a Connecticut court found that while both parents had engaged in being "emotionally abusive" of their son, "a major distinction for the court" was that the Father had "shown regret for his behavior; [while] [Mother] does not accept or even recognize her own abusive conduct."[19] In a yet another case, a North Dakota court[20] found that while both parents were guilty of parental alienation, the father's attitude

19. Dean v. Valinho, Superior Court of Connecticut (Judicial Dist. Of Middlesex, No. FA044012513, July 6, 2011).
20. *In re* T.T., 681 N.W.2d 779 (2004).

was more cooperative compared to the mother, who the court found to be an "obsessed alienator." The court described the severe psychological and emotional harm caused to the child due to the parents' parental alienating behaviors and ordered the child to be placed in the care, custody, and control of the Department of Human Services.

Interestingly, while some acts of abuse or violence are perceived as inexcusable and unjustifiable (e.g., choking a spouse or a romantic partner or a child), other abusive acts are sometimes perceived as more "socially acceptable." In a study conducted by Dr. Jennifer Harman and her colleagues, they found that although parental alienating behaviors are perceived negatively by adults, they are somehow more "acceptable" when mothers do them than when fathers do them.[21] Other commentators have argued that parental alienating behaviors are "justifiable" when the other (targeted) parent is abusive, mentally ill, or dangerous. The term "justified estrangement" has been used by some professionals to imply that the child's rejection of the targeted parent is justified because the parent is abusive or "bad," and that the alienating behaviors, if manifested by the other parent, are acceptable in that scenario. Equating parental alienation with "justified estrangement" (or subsuming parental alienation within the umbrella of "justified estrangement) reflects a misunderstanding of the difference between parental alienation and *self*-estrangement.[22] Self-estrangement behaviors, as the term implies, are those that a parent does to damage their relationship with their own child, either due to the parent's own shortcomings (e.g., parenting skills) or abusive behavior. In contrast, parental alienating behaviors are those behaviors that are committed by the alienating parent against the targeted parent to hurt the targeted parent and to damage or destroy the relationship between the targeted parent and the child.[23] Equating self-estrangement with parental alienation (or subsuming the latter phenomenon within the former) implies that the actions or behaviors of the alienating parent are the targeted parent's fault, which blames the victim.

No doubt claims of abuse or domestic violence should be investigated (and thoroughly investigated at that) in order to protect the well-being of the child and the family members. But claims of parental alienation should be considered with the same gravity and shown similar concern. As discussed ahead, these claims, similar to claims of abuse and domestic violence, involve psychologically (and at times, physically) aggressive behaviors and cause substantial harm to the child and the targeted parent subjected to such alienating behaviors. Like other forms of family violence, parental alienating behaviors

21. Harman, J. et al. Parents Behaving Badly: Gender Biases in the Perception of Parental Alienating Behaviors, *Journal of Family Psychology*, 30, 866–874.

22. Harman, Jennifer, et. al. (2018). Parental alienating behaviors are family violence, *Psychological Bulletin*, 144(12), 1275–1299, 1289.

23. *Id.*

are never justified—they are abusive to both the child and the targeted parent.[24] As a society we do not condone domestic violence or family violence by blaming the victim. Similarly, parental alienating behaviors should not be overlooked—neither socially not legally. There is no legal or psychological justification for parental alienating behaviors and these behaviors should be seen and dealt with as a child protection issue.[25]

Fourthly, treatment interventions differ when comparing cases involving parental alienation with those involving abuse or neglect, and it is important to rule out child maltreatment on the part of the rejected parent before making a decision of the treatment intervention. The mental health treatment should be tailored to the cause of the ruptured or damaged parent-child relationship. If the rejected parent *actually* engaged in abuse or neglect of the child (not just alleged by the favored parent and/or child) then the appropriate treatment in such circumstances would be the one designed for abusive parents, not alienated parents. For instance, "abuse-specific treatment models," such as Alternatives for Families: A Cognitive Behavioral Therapy (AF-CBT)

> are designed to decrease the reliance on punitive parenting styles of an abusive parent and increase the use of non-punitive behavior management strategies on the part of the parent, while simultaneously helping the child process the trauma from the abuse.[26]

But such abuse-specific treatment model would be ill suited, if not catastrophically counter-productive, for alienation cases. An alienation-specific treatment is designed to gently but firmly confront the child's false beliefs and distorted perceptions about the rejected parent and to provide him or her with tools and opportunities to correct such false and distorted thoughts and feelings. Such treatment attempts to provide experiential opportunities for the alienated parent to once again function as a safe, loving, and available attachment figure for the child.[27] It would be contraindicated to put an abused child in an alienation-specific treatment or vice versa, and, therefore, it is essential to determine the cause of the parent-child dysfunction prior to designing the treatment intervention.

Finally, in cases involving parental alienation, allegations of domestic violence or abuse are likely to continue to be made by the favored parent or the child as an excuse for the child's resistance to or rejection of the rejected parent.

---

24. *Id.*

25. *Id.*, 1290.

26. Baker, A. J. L., *supra*, 213, citing Kolko, D., & Swenson, C. (2002). *Assessing and Treating Physically Abused Children and Their Families: A Cognitive Behavioral Approach*, Sage.

27. Gottlieb, L. (2013). The application of structural family systems therapy to the treatment of Parental Alienation Syndrome. In Baker, A. J. L., & Sauber, S. R. (Eds.), *Working With Alienated Children and Families: A Clinical Guidebook*, 209–210; Warshak, R. A., & Otis, M. (2010). Helping alienated children with Family Bridges: Practice, research and the pursuit of "humbition," *Fam. Ct. Rev.*, 48, 91.

It is important that the court and the court-involved professionals fully address this issue at an earliest opportunity to make findings of fact and resolve it one way or the other. Often, a trial court is faced with conflicting versions of the events relating to the alleged abuse, and it is important to remember that in a family law setting, the goal behind the consideration of the domestic violence factor is to evaluate parental fitness, protect the children, and to protect and aid victims of domestic violence by providing an immediate and effective remedy. The primary goals are preventive, protective, and remedial, *not* punitive—and certainly not imposing punishment for past conduct where doing so would infringe upon a parent's relationship or access to his or her child.[28] And often, due to parental alienation or an enmeshed relationship between a parent and the child, allegations of domestic violence are made in support of obtaining "protective orders," only to be found upon investigation by the court to have no factual support.[29]

Also, context and timing of the alleged acts of domestic violence or abuse are important considerations when evaluating allegations of domestic violence. When the alleged incidents of "domestic violence" or abusive conduct took place several years prior to the divorce, a court is well within its discretion in concluding that such incidents do not establish a "history of acts of domestic violence."[30] The broad discretion that family trial courts enjoy is due to the court's unique opportunity to observe the parties, interview the children, and listen to the testimonies of collateral witnesses to determine witness credibility and to sort out conflicting evidence. Inappropriate or suboptimal behavior of a parent, such as ranting, raving, gesturing, or property damage, while concerning to courts, may not rise to the severity of domestic violence and the courts may view it as boorish or "juvenile and not dissimilar to the usual bickering and hostility that [a court] frequently sees when a marriage breaks down."[31] In such scenarios, presence of parental alienating behaviors may raise a "much greater concern" for the court if a parent is misusing allegations of domestic violence to sabotage the parent-child relationship, indoctrinate the children about the false ideas and beliefs about the other parent, and keep the children away from the parent who is accused of bad behavior.[32]

Even in cases where there is bona fide evidence of domestic violence, it is not *fait accompli* that a court will see this evidence as a danger to the child and therefore award primary custody to the victim of such domestic violence. For instance, a Washington court acknowledged that though the father had

---

28. *See* Barton v. Hirshberg, 137 Md.App. 1 (2001); Coburn v. Coburn, 342 Md. 244, 252, 674 A.2d 951 (1996).
29. Barton v. Hirshberg, *supra.*
30. *In re* Davis, 107 Wash.App. 1047 (2001); also see Oates v. Oates, 2010 Ark.App.346.
31. *In re* Marriage of Sheridan, 2013 IL App (4th) 130394-U.
32. *Id.*

admitted assaulting the mother during the marriage, the father did not pose a danger to the parties' daughter and declined to grant the mother's request that the father undergo a certified domestic violence program prior to visitation with his daughter.[33] The court evaluated the matter and considered the totality of circumstances: the father's proactive efforts to undergo psychiatric treatment for domestic violence counseling for over a year prior to trial, the signs of parental alienation in the child, and the mother's harassment of the father by sending letters to his friends which included allegations against the father.

Similarly, the Supreme Court of Alaska affirmed a trial court's ruling that awarded the father sole legal and primary custody of child and awarded the mother supervised visitation despite the father having a history of domestic violence.[34] The evidence supported finding that the father successfully rebutted Alaska's statutory presumption that a parent with a history of perpetrating domestic violence should not be awarded sole legal or sole physical custody. And it was also determined by the trial court that it was in the child's best interest to be in the father's sole custody. The court determined that the father's acts, though problematic, were "situational" and that he posed no threat of committing future acts of domestic violence. Nor did he pose a danger to the child. On the other hand, the court was alarmed by the mother's behaviors that demonstrated parental alienation and how her behavior interfered with the relationship between the father and the child:

> the record presents a mound of evidence from which the [c]ourt can fairly easily draw conclusions about the relationship that are characteristic of the parental alienation dynamic. The court cited the facts that [mother] "has prevented and frustrated [father's] visitation in the past"; that she "has been controlling of how visits with [father] occur," limiting contact to "email, not phone or video [S]kype"; that she "sees her relationship with [father] as a package deal, i.e., 'If you want me, you get son too, if you don't want me, then you don't get son either'"; that "numerous texts and emails" indicate her "angry view of [father]" and her negative comments about his contact with the child; and that despite "her [expressed] desire to foster a relationship between father and son, [she] effectively makes visitation and interactions between father and son difficult."

These decisions are not gender specific. Evidence of severe parental alienation behaviors have raised more alarm for courts than evidence of domestic violence or abusive conduct in the remote past—irrespective of gender. For instance, a Washington court of appeals affirmed the trial court's decision to modify the parenting plan and make the mother the primary residential parent

---

33. *In re* the Marriage of Henry John Shen, 11 Wash.App. 1046 (2002).
34. Joy B. v. Everett B., 451 P.3d 365 (2019).

where the court found that the father had made repeated allegations of abuse, none of which were substantiated.[35] The court found that while the mother had engaged in domestic violence in the past, there was no recent evidence of domestic violence. Instead, the court was more concerned with the father's unfounded concerns about the mother, his "abusive use of conflict," and having "engaged in parental alienation which has created a danger of serious damage to the child's psychological development."

Unless a court or an independent trier-of-fact thoroughly investigates allegations of abuse, such allegations may continue to be made in court, in therapy, to court-involved professionals (such as the friend of the court or guardian ad litem), and so forth. Such allegations, if not properly investigated and adjudicated at the trial level, may be difficult to assess at the appellate level. As a panel of the Court of Appeals of Minnesota found:

> The issue of domestic violence has been difficult to assess. On the one hand, the Court did not make a finding of domestic abuse. On the other hand, [mother] had documented bruising on her face. [Father] denied physically assaulting [mother]. He has no known history of violence and [his previous wife] denies that violence occurred in their marriage. [Mother] reports that [his previous wife] told her about [father's] violence but that [his previous wife] is too scared to tell publicly. The evaluator could not substantiate this concern.[36]

The appellate court ultimately affirmed the trial court's decision which did not find the allegations of domestic violence to be credible, especially in light of its finding that the Mother demonstrated a "pattern of making vague reports of abuse and neglect and then denying responsibility for the subsequent Child Protection investigations"—"a pattern often . . . associated with parental alienation dynamics as the child gets older and can voice his 'wishes.'"[37]

Yet another reason to properly investigate allegations of domestic violence or abuse at the earliest opportunity is that such allegations may also continue to be made as an excuse to justify violation of court-ordered parenting time or visitation orders. And the more such allegations are repeated, the higher the risk that "it may become a truth in the mind of the child (as well as in the belief systems of the legal and mental health professionals) even if it never actually happened."[38]

Some children may "cross over," meaning that they never want to have contact with the parent again who had engaged in severe abuse or neglect

35. Matter of Marriage of Reichert, 2 Wash.App.2d 1063 (2018).
36. Breitenfeldt v. Nickles-Breitenfeldt, 2003 WL 1908070 (Minn.Ct.App).
37. *Id.*
38. Baker, A. J. L., *supra*, 213.

"because of experiences that have induced fear, anxiety, suicidal thoughts / actions, other types of self-harm, self-esteem depletion and a whole host of other negative consequences."[39] As one child put it, "Just the thought of seeing him made me feel scared and like a bad person all over again."[40] But child abuse claims in divorce cases are relatively common and a significant number of these accusations come up as "unfounded." A study from 1990 in which 9,000 divorces across twelve states were studied revealed the following results:[41]

- In 48 percent of cases, mothers accused fathers
- In 19 percent of cases, mother accused stepfathers or others
- In 6 percent of cases, fathers accused mothers
- In 16 percent of cases, fathers accused stepfathers or others
- In 11 percent of cases, third parties accused fathers, mother, or others

Out of all the cases in the study, 5 percent to 8 percent of the accusations were deemed intentionally false reports. For instance, in *Delekta v. Delekta*, the Michigan Court of Appeals affirmed a trial court's denial to grant a mother's motion to change the custody of the parties' two children because, as the mother alleged, the father had "physically and emotionally abused them."[42] The Court found that the mother had "called in 17 complaints [to the Child Protective Services] between April of 2009 and April of 2018," "making false accusations" against the father, that "no evidence substantiated [mother's] . . . allegations of domestic violence or abuse," and that it was logical for the trial court to consider the presence of parental alienation.[43]

In his recent book on parent-child reunification, Dr. Stanley S. Clawar, a certified clinical sociologist, discusses two cases that exemplify intentionally false reports of abuse in divorce cases:[44]

> a father . . . had been accused of serially molesting his daughters. Each time he was exonerated only to be followed by another abuse accusation, facilitated by the mother. One of the suggestions that I made in this case was for him to install cameras in different locations within his home, as serial accusers usually continue that behavior. Sure enough, the mother re-accused the father of molesting the children again. The mother was asked for the day and approximate time when this alleged incident

---

39. Clawar, S. S. (2020). *Parent-Child Reunification: A Guide to Legal and Forensic Strategies*, American Bar Association, 58.

40. *Id.*; also see, e.g., T.G.G. v. C.G.G., 2020 WL 261701 (Superior Court of 58 (Pennsylvania) on children's rejection of their father due to father's persistent abusive behaviors.

41. *Id.*, 59, citing Editorial Staff (Ed.), Child Sexual Abuse and Divorce (July 20, 2016), at https://www.divorcesource.com/blog/child-sexual-and-divorce

42. Delekta v. Delekta, 2019 WL 2711294 (Mich.Ct.App.).

43. *Id.*

44. *Id.*

> occurred. She issued the requested time and day information only to find out that the video camera, which had a timestamp, revealed that the father was at bedside reading storybooks to his daughters. All of the time before and after that was also accounted for. Unfortunately, children can actually "report" abuse when it didn't occur or they can expand a non-abusive incident to a bigger-than-life occurrence. This may not be the norm, but forensic experts must be aware of the possibility. . . . In another case, a mother had filed 15 accusations—all came back "unfounded." Custody was finally shifted to the father, but it was too late—the father had committed suicide.

Counterintuitive Feature of Abused Children: They *Want* a Relationship with the Abuser

When evaluating a case for the presence of parental alienation, it is important to note the strength or magnitude of the child's rejection of a parent. Generally speaking, the more adamantly a child rejects a relationship with a parent, the more likely it is that the child is alienated, not estranged—which is counterintuitive and the reverse of what most people would predict. A highly counterintuitive feature of parental alienation is that most abused children continue to seek a relationship with their abusive parent. On the other hand, alienated children (who were never abused) strongly reject a relationship with the targeted parent. How does one address this apparent conundrum? Some experts suggest that one way to address this conundrum is to acknowledge just how rare and unusual it is for a child to actually reject a parent, especially in a vehement manner, without any ambivalence, as typically occurs in cases involving parental alienation.[45] As Dr. Baker clarifies:

> Even children who have been beaten, molested, and abandoned by a parent generally do not behave in a callous and extreme manner when dealing with an abusive parent. It is well known among those in the field of child maltreatment that despite the abuse and neglect experienced at the hand of a parent, most children want to maintain a relationship with the abuser.[46]

This counterintuitive phenomenon of abused children wanting to maintain a relationship with their abuser is referred to as "bonded to the abuser" by the researchers. And there are at least six sources of evidence for this phenomenon,

45. Baker, A. J. L., *supra*, 213.

46. *Id.*, citing Baker, A. J. L., & Schneiderman, M. (2015). *Bonded to the Abuser: How Victims Make Sense of Childhood Abuse*, Rowman & Littlefield.

including clinical observations, animal studies, findings from attachment research, studies of youth in the foster care system, and memoirs written by survivors of childhood maltreatment.[47] When we consider these six separate sources of evidence, they strongly support the premise that children form and maintain attachment relationships with their caregivers, even abusive caregivers. Why? "They cannot help but do so because they are hard-wired to form a preferential relationship with a caregiving adult who is likely to protect them from danger."[48] The abusive caregiver's maltreatment does affect the bond between the caregiver (parent) and the child, but what is affected is the *quality* of the attachment, not its existence. An understanding of this counterintuitive feature of parental alienation is essential for any mental health or legal professional who is tasked with the duty to evaluate a case for the presence of parental alienation. This can counter the false but commonly held beliefs that children typically reject "bad" parents or that if a child is rejecting a parent it *must* be because the parent did something to "deserve" it. As important it is to remember that just because a child rejects a parent does not mean that the child is alienated, it is equally important to acknowledge and remember how aberrant and rare it is for a child to truly reject a parent.

Parental Alienation *Is* Family Violence

In the preceding discussion, we explored how the Five-Factor Model requires an evaluator or clinician to ensure that there is an absence of abuse or neglect or seriously deficient parenting on the part of the now rejected parent when evaluating a case of parental alienation. Apart from this, the concepts of violence and parental alienation also interact in another manner: Causing parental alienation may be a form of domestic violence. The abuser—the alienating parent—continues to control the children post-divorce or separation and alienate them from the ex-spouse as a way to punish the former partner. Parental alienation causes significant psychological and emotional harm to children. Domestic violence encompasses acts or behaviors that cause mental or emotional or psychological injury. A child who suffers a "mental injury"—"any behavioral, cognitive, emotional, or mental disorder in a child by an act or omission that is described [in the statute] . . . and is committed by the parent or other person responsible for the child's care"—is included in the definition of an abused child.[49]

Dr. Jennifer Harman and her colleagues, who have extensively explored this interplay between parental alienation and family violence, found that "[t]his

47. Baker, A. J. L., *supra*, 213–214.
48. *Id.*, 215.
49. Schottenstein v. Schottenstein, 2003 Ohio 5032; 2003 WL 22176786 (Ohio.Ct.App.).

complex form of aggression entails a parental figure engaging in the long-term use of a variety of aggressive behaviors to harm the relationship between their child and another parental figure, and/or to hurt the other parental figure directly because of their relationship with their child."[50] The link between perpetrators of domestic violence and parental alienation has been studied by several mental health experts. Experts have found that

> abusive ex-partners are likely to attempt to alienate the children from the other parent's affection (by asserting blame for the dissolution of the family and telling negative stories), sabotage family plans (by continuing criticism or competitive bribes), and undermine parental authority (by explicitly instructing the children not to listen or obey).[51]

Dr. Harman and her colleagues have conceptualized alienating behaviors as a form of family violence, both as child abuse and intimate partner violence, because the ultimate alienation of a child is primarily a result of abusive behaviors of an alienating parent.[52] In doing so, it is important to define and understand the definition of family violence. On an international front, the World Health Organization has defined violence as "the intentional use of physical force or power, threatened or actual, against oneself, another person, or against a group or community, that either results in or has a high likelihood of resulting in injury, death, psychological harm, maldevelopment or deprivation."[53] The Organization for Economic Cooperation and Development (OECD) defines family violence (also known as "domestic violence") as "any violent act inflicted by one family member onto another," a term that would encompass both child abuse and intimate partner violence. And the term "violence" here includes physical, sexual, emotional, and economic violence, as well as neglect.[54] On the domestic front, definitions of family violence have included several different types of behaviors. For instance, the U. S. Department of Justice identifies physical, sexual, emotional, economic, or psychological actions or threats of actions as forms of violence that can intimidate, manipulate, humiliate, isolate, frighten, terrorize, coerce, threaten, blame, hurt, injure, or wound someone.[55] On a state level, individual states define what violence or domestic violence is, and the majority of the states have codified the definition of family or domestic

---

50. Harman, J. et al. (2018). Parental alienating behaviors are family violence, *Psychological Bulletin*, 144(12), 1275–1299, 1275.

51. Jaffe, P. G. et al., (2008). Custody disputes involving allegations of domestic violence: Toward a differentiated approach to parenting plans, *Fam. Ct. Rev.*, 46, 500, 503.

52. Harman, J., & Matthewson, M. (2020). Parental alienating behaviors. In Lorandos, D., & Bernet, W. (Eds.), *Parental Alienation: Science and Law*, Charles C. Thomas, 82.

53. Harman, J. (2018), *supra*, 1276, citing Krug et al. (2002). *World Report on Violence and Health: Summary.*

54. *Id.*, 1277, citing Organization for Economic Cooperation and Development. (2013). SF3.4: Family Violence.

55. Office of Violence Against Women, U.S. Department of Justice (2017), Domestic Violence.

violence and include within the definition acts that cause emotional or mental or psychological harm.

Parental alienation specialists have argued that severe alienating behaviors are a form of family violence—these behaviors constitute a form of child abuse resulting in a psychiatric disorder (CARPD) and "parent-child relationship problem" as described in DSM-5.[56] As we attempt to understand the pathology and sequalae of parental alienating behaviors, it would be helpful to examine the power and control wheels used in the Duluth Model, which is the most widely known protocol for intervening in cases of domestic violence.[57] The power and control wheel is a well-known measure used by domestic violence advocates and clinicians to conceptualize the behaviors used by perpetrators of domestic violence or intimate partner violence. The Duluth Model has its roots in feminist theory and contributed a great deal to the understanding of family violence in both research and practice.[58] Dr. Jennifer Harman and Dr. Mandy Matthewson have adapted the Duluth Model in a gender-neutral manner to conceptualize and present parental alienating behaviors.[59]

The figure[60] titled "Parental Alienating Behaviors," a gender-neutral Harman-Matthewson adaptation of the Duluth power and control wheel, illustrates the power and control aspects of the parental alienating behaviors. The researchers combined the *post-separation power and control wheel*, the *abuse of children wheel*, and the *power and control wheel* from the Duluth Model because the behaviors used by alienating parents are represented in all of them. As these researchers explain:

> The wheels were designed to depict violence between two adults, but A[lienating] B[ehaviors] are more complicated due to the children also being victims and, oftentimes, the weapons used against the alienated parent. As a consequence, this form of family violence can be very complicated due to the number of people who can be involved; it is not just two parents because it often involves children as well as extended family members (e.g., grandparents) and other third parties (e.g., teachers, family friends).[61]

The category of parental alienating behaviors is classified into emotional abuse; coercion; threats and intimidation; physical and sexual abuse; using isolation,

56. Bernet, W. et al. (2016, July). Child affected by parental relationship distress, *Journal of American Academy of Child & Adolescent Psychiatry*, 55(7).

57. Pence, E. et al. (1993). *Education Groups for Men Who Batter: The Duluth Model*, Springer.

58. Harman, J. (2018), *supra*, citing Young, C. et al. (2007). Domestic violence: New visions, new solutions. In Hamel, & Nicholls (Eds.), *Family Interventions in Domestic Violence: A Handbook of Gender-Inclusive Theory and Treatment*, 602.

59. Harman, J., & Matthewson, M., (2020), *supra*, 83–84.

60. *Id.*, 84.

61. *Id.*, 83.

minimizing, denying, and blaming; using privilege; using economic abuse; and using children.

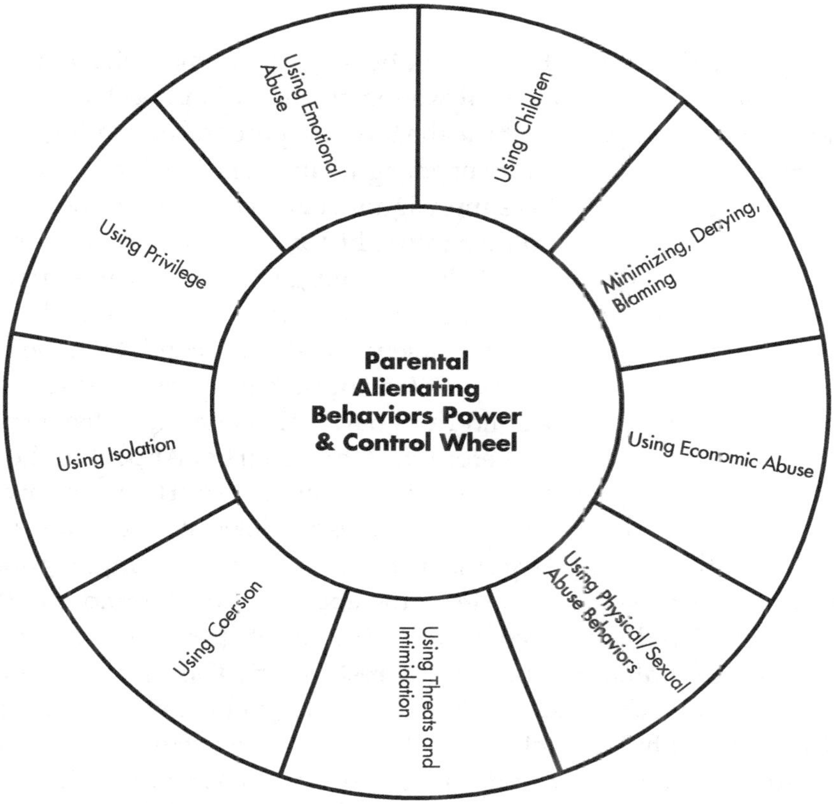

It can be argued that parental alienating behaviors are tantamount to child abuse. Child abuse is a broad and amorphous term, but is generally defined as a specific form of harm to children that is *significant* and may be attributed to *human agency* that is proscribed, proximate, and preventable.[62] Child maltreatment is an even broader term than child abuse and incorporates both abuse and neglect—behaviors that a caregiver manifests that result in a child feeling worthless, unloved, and only valued for meeting the caregiver's needs.[63] Family courts have viewed parental alienating behaviors as a form of "emotional abuse that should not be tolerated."[64] Courts have also acknowledged that such behaviors can cause "a child lifelong suffering."[65] Many mental health professionals agree that using parental alienating behaviors to cause

62. Harman, J., (2018), *supra*, 1278.
63. *See*: The American Professional Society on the Abuse of Children. (1995). *Guidelines for the Psychosocial Evaluation of Suspected Psychological Maltreatment in Children and Adolescents*.
64. McClain v. McClain, 539 S.W.3d 170 (2017) (Court of Appeals of Tennessee).
65. *In re* H.M., 2019 WL 3522043 (Court of Appeal, California) (Unpublished).

parental alienation is a form of child psychological abuse.[66] Indeed, mental health experts have found that the tactics used by alienating parents in alienating the child are often tantamount to extreme psychological maltreatment of children.[67]

So severe are the parental alienating behaviors and their effect on the children's emotional and psychological wellbeing that it is plausible that a court may grant custody to a parent who is the target of parental alienating behaviors even if that parent was once guilty of engaging in abusive behavior or domestic violence. It is not that the courts simply ignore evidence of domestic violence or abusive behavior. They duly note a parent's history of or convictions for domestic violence or otherwise abusive behavior and give this evidence appropriate consideration when evaluating the best interest factors. However, where a parent who has been guilty of domestic violence or abusive conduct in the past has not engaged in similar conduct thereafter, courts have given greater weight to the concern for protecting the child from parental alienating behaviors.[68]

Consider the dreadful facts before the Ohio Court of Appeal in the case of *Habo v. Khattab*.[69] The appellate court affirmed the trial court's award of custody to the father despite his conviction for domestic violence. The appellate court disagreed with the mother's argument that the trial judge simply ignored the evidence of domestic violence. Instead, the appellate court found that the trial judge duly considered father's conviction and gave it appropriate consideration and weight when evaluating the best interest factors. The trial judge, however, was more concerned about the mother's alienating behaviors, which were abusive in their own right and included calling the police alleging she was abused by father (the police did not find any abuse) and locking the children in her bedroom because she was, unreasonably, afraid that the father would kidnap them. Particularly troubling to the trial court was an incident that was tape recorded by the mother and which she put forward as evidence of the father's "abusive" behavior:

> [Contrary to the mother's characterization of the incident], the tape showed the mother being "hysterical and screaming at father in front of the children, 'Don't hurt my kids' over and over again. At one point, mother yelled 'Don't hurt my kids' 12 times in a row . . . while mother was engaging in these histrionics, father could be heard in the background calmly telling

66. Verrocchio, M. et al. (2016). Associations between exposure to parental alienating behaviors, anxiety, and depression in an italian sample of adults, *Journal of Forensic Sciences*, 61, 692–698.

67. Baker, A. L. J. (2010). Even when you win you lose: Targeted parents' perceptions of their attorneys, *American Journal of Family Therapy*, 38, 292–309. Also see Schottenstein v. Schottenstein, 2003 Ohio 5032; 2003 WL 22176786 (Ohio.Ct.App.) (parental alienating behaviors together with other pathological behavior, including Fictitious Disorder by Proxy / Munchausen).

68. *See, e.g.*, Horning v. Wolff, 2006 WL 3505864 (Ohio.Ct.App.).

69. Habo v. Khattab, 2013 WL 6869804.

the children to 'get in the car' and telling mother, 'I will take the children to school. You will see them after school.' . . . [T]he tape actually showed it was mother's 'hysteria' that caused the children to become upset and to resist being put in the car by father. After father was struggling to get the children in the car for about 20 minutes, mother called the police reporting domestic violence. The trial court found mother's actions that day were further evidence of her efforts to alienate the children from father."[70]

The trial court was especially alarmed at how the mother's alienating behaviors were causing the children to reject their father and significantly harming the children's relationship with the father. The court first considered the baseline relationship between the father and the children, which was healthy and loving, and found that all three children "were affectionate with father and eager to spend time with him." But in a matter of months, the court found that the children's attitude towards their father changed drastically. When the father arrived to pick the children up for his visitation, the oldest child, in their mother's presence, became "hysterical, crying, and screaming that she was not going with father and that he would hurt her." The court noted that the mother did nothing to stop their outbursts. Instead, the mother told the children that they had to visit their father or she would be arrested. Also, she told the children that "she did not blame them if they did not want to see father and that she [mother] would go to the Supreme Court to keep them from ever having to live with [the father]." The court found that the children's refusal to visit with father was not due to fear of him, but, instead "was a 'game' to them" and the children were observed "smiling and smirking while screaming that father had abused them, which the trial court had also seen during its in-camera interviews." In granting custody to the father, the court found the mother's actions rose to the level of "extreme parental alienation."

Emotional abuse—psychological aggression using verbal and non-verbal communication—is the most common form of child maltreatment found in parental alienating behaviors. Such behavior attacks a child's emotional and social well-being, and can include spurning, terrorizing, isolating, corrupting or exploiting, and denying emotional responsiveness.[71] Despite being one of the more challenging behaviors to observe directly (because they often occur in privacy), researchers have extensively documented alienating parents engaging in such aggressive behavior.[72] Dr. Jennifer Harman and her colleagues describe how alienating parents have been documented to engage in emotionally abusive and psychologically aggressive behaviors such as:[73]

70. *Id.*
71. Harman, J. et al. (2018), *supra*, 1279.
72. *Id.*
73. *Id.* (internal citations omitted).

- Terrorizing the children by derogating the targeted parent and creating fear in children that the targeted parent might be dangerous or unstable;
- Reject, shame, or make the child feel guilty for showing any loyalty or warmth towards the targeted parent or the targeted parent's extended family;
- Ridicule them for showing the targeted parent affection;
- Withdraw love and affection when the child talks positively about the targeted parent;
- Reward the child for rejecting the targeted parent (e.g., not saying hello at a sporting event);
- Encouraging the child to use the same derogatory label that the alienating parent uses to describe the targeted parent; and
- Making the children throw away all clothing, gifts, or reminders of the targeted parent after they return from visits with them.

In an extreme example of shocking emotional abuse, two mental health professionals reported an alienating parent as having conducted a "burial ceremony" with the children to symbolically "bury" their living father in order to start their "new" family.[74] Yet another common tactic utilized by alienating parents that is tantamount to emotional abuse is gaslighting. Gaslighting

> refers to the presentation of false information to the victim with the intent of making them doubt their own memory or perception. Alienating parents will rewrite history, or use events that the child recalls and then exaggerate or fill in with details that never happened in an attempt to distort the child's memory about the [targeted parent] and the [targeted parent's] relationship with them and/or the [alienating parent] (e.g., brainwashing).[75]

They will send e-mails or written correspondence that rewrite past events in order to create a new version of reality that is self-serving and geared towards their goals. They will create a paper trail of "proof" to support their version of reality and for future use in litigation.

Consider the Florida case of *Schumaker v. Schumaker*, where the father, who had committed child abuse and domestic violence, turned around and accused the mother of engaging in domestic violence.[76] The court found that the father had filed false and misleading domestic violence allegations against the mother and had attempted to mislead the court in an attempt to gain custody

74. Dunne, J., & Hedrick, M. (1994). The Parental Alienation Syndrome: An analysis of sixteen selected cases, *Journal of Remarriage and Divorce*, 21, 21–38.
75. Harman, J. et al. (2018), *supra*, 1279.
76. Schumaker v. Schumaker, 931 So.2d 271 (2006).

of the children. Not only did the father make false and fabricated allegations of domestic violence against the mother, he also engaged in severe parental alienating behaviors:

> The Father has throughout these proceedings attempted to partially alienate the minor children and the Court has grave concerns about the children having primary residence ever with the Father. The Father has consistently made degrading and obscene comments about the Mother. The Mother had a previous child out of wedlock prior to this marriage and the Father has made sure the minor children of this marriage know the circumstances of their half-sister's . . . out of wedlock birth and routinely refers to the Mother in derogatory terms. The Father has told the minor son . . . that he does not have to listen to his mother and made derogatory statements about . . . half-sister.

Concluding that the father was in need of "in-depth parental alienation counseling," and needs to "clean up his act," the trial court awarded the residential custody of the children to the mother and gave the father a very limited visitation.

Another gaslighting strategy is for the alienating parents to accompany the child to his or her medical appointments and to provide inaccurate information about the targeted parent so that the information is recorded in the medical records—e.g., claims of drug abuse, sex abuse, alcoholism, domestic violence, pornography addiction, etc. The goal is to have third parties (who for all ostensible purposes are professional, neutral, and have no stake in the underlying divorce or custody litigation) memorialize the allegations in their records. Also, if such third parties happen to be school teachers or counselors or health care providers, they are mandated to report any and all reasonable suspicions of child abuse. Having been informed of a parent's alleged abusive conduct towards his or her child may lead to a professional making a report of suspected child abuse to a child protective agency. Once such report is made, the alienating parent can "cooperate" with the investigation and make additional allegations. Unfortunately, such gaslighting behaviors can be very effective and can work for the alienating parents to not only hoodwink professionals but to also turn them into unwitting, but powerful, allies:

> Representatives from social systems, such as social workers, mental health professionals, guardian ad litems [sic], teachers, medical providers, and police officers, can be 'blinded' by the A[lienating] P[arent]'s stories and engage in legal and administrative aggression against the [targeted parent] on behalf of them. Social system representatives often have negative biases about the [targeted parent] (e.g., gender or racial biases), poor training in the identification of parental alienation and/or human development

> (e.g., a belief that children never lie), and will often stop at nothing to limit or interfere with contact or a relationship between the [targeted parent] and the child.[77]

Parental alienating behaviors are not just tantamount to child abuse; they are also attacks—direct and indirect—on the targeted parent that have a lot in common with behaviors manifested by a domestic violence perpetrator or perpetrator of intimate partner violence. The most commonly used form of intimate partner violence by alienating parents is psychological aggression. And most parental alienating behaviors directed at the targeted parent are examples of psychological aggression that attempts to control the targeted parent, demonstrate power, or damage the targeted parent's sense of self. Humiliation, especially in front of the children, is a commonly utilized alienating tool:

> The [Alienating Parent] will also use humiliation to hurt the [Targeted Parent], such as mocking their hobbies, personality, job, friends, or family, and focusing the child and others on the [Targeted Parent's] flaws and mistakes they have made. For example, a [Targeted Parent] reported to one of the authors that the [Alienating Parent] in his life put him on speakerphone when he called to speak with this children, and the [Alienating Parent] mocked him during calls to make the children see him as a joke.[78]

It is not just psychological aggression or coercive controlling behaviors; some parental alienating behaviors are downright physical violence or threats. An example was documented in a case where an alienating father blocked the targeted mother's car in his driveway so that she was unable to leave his property while he read the mother's court motion to the children out loud.[79]

Outcomes of Family Violence

Parental alienation, similar to domestic violence or intimate partner violence, leaves scars. Most of time, the damage caused by parental alienating behaviors fall under the category of psychological injury. In forensic settings, such injuries are classified in three categories: chronic pain, traumatic brain injury, and posttraumatic stress or distress.[80] In addition, victims of parental alienation, both the children and the targeted parents, experience other negative outcomes associated with family violence, such as anxiety and depression. For

---

77. *Id.*, 1284.
78. *Id.*, 1281 (internal citations omitted).
79. Lorandos, D. (2013). Parental alienation and North American law. In Lorandos, D., Bernet, W., & Sauber, R. (Eds.), *Parental Alienation: The Handbook for Mental Health and Legal Professionals*, Charles C. Thomas, 348–424.
80. Harman, J. et al. (2018), *supra*, 1286.

the children, the consequences of parental alienation, which is a form of child maltreatment, are severe and lifelong. A concern over such severe and long-lasting consequences has led the United Nations to call for action to eliminate violence against children due to many personal, community, and societal-level costs associated with it.[81] Children subjected to parental alienating behaviors have been subjected to or have witnessed abuse, and these children are at risk for a host of negative outcomes, such as having shorter lifespans; developing internalizing behavior problems, such as depression, anxiety, and social withdrawal; developing externalizing behaviors, such as aggression and acting out; poorer academic performance and physical health; neurological damage; physical health problems, including cancer, cardiac disease, and asthma; and other mental problems.[82] These outcomes are not just limited to a particular country or culture; they are evident across different countries and cultures.[83]

Often, courts show unwillingness to take action when presented with evidence of what they consider, rightly or wrongly, to be a case of "mild" parental alienation. Parental alienation has been described as ranging from mild to severe. In mild cases, the alienated child criticizes the targeted parent and, on occasions, resists contact but still goes on visitation / parenting time and even enjoys the company of the targeted parent when away from the influence of and interference by the alienating parent. In such scenarios, courts and professionals sometimes fail to see the urgency of intervention and advise "patience," "empathy," or other well-intended but ultimately ineffective measures to counter alienation. In such circumstances, the attorney representing the targeted parent would do well to educate the court that although not all children who are exposed to alienating behaviors become severely alienated,[84] the court should not wait to take proper steps to address alienating behaviors. To wait until the alienation progresses to a "moderate" or "severe" level would be a catastrophic mistake and often an irreparable one. For the child, being subjected to parental alienating behaviors—mild, moderate, or severe—is a serious mental health issue that implants and encourages a false belief that the targeted parent is a dangerous and unworthy parent. As a society, we do not condone "mild," "moderate," or "severe" sexual abuse of a child; parental alienation, which is a form of psychological abuse, should be viewed on the same level. Even "mild" and "moderate" harms to children that result from

81. *Id.*, citing Hillis, S. et al. (2017). The enduring impact of violence against children, *Psychology Health and Medicine*, 22, 393–405.

82. *Id.*, 1286.

83. Fry, D. et al. (2012). The consequences of maltreatment on children's lives: A systematic review of data from the East Asia and Pacific region, *Trauma, Violence & Abuse*, 13, 209--33.

84. Baker, A. J. L., & Darnall, D. (2006). Behaviors and strategies of parental alienation: A survey of parental experiences, *Journal of Divorce & Remarriage*, 45, 97--24.

the alienating parent's behaviors are devastating and no different from other forms of child abuse.

Self-hatred is particularly disturbing among children affected by parental alienation, as children internalize the hatred towards the targeted parent, who, after all, is part of their own identity. Alienated children are brainwashed and indoctrinated to believe that the targeted parent does not love or want them, and, therefore, they are unlovable or unworthy of the parent's affection.[85] These children's "depression is rooted in feelings of abandonment, being unloved by the [targeted parent], and being denied the opportunity to mourn their loss"—all of which increases the risk of the children engaging in self-destructive behaviors.[86] Even if "mildly" alienated children appear on the surface to be "normal," such as excelling in school or sports, they fall short of their optimal development in other areas, such as psychological or emotional domains. Finally, it would be important to note that the parental alienating behaviors are transmitted intergenerationally, just like other types of family violence.[87] A child whose parent has demonstrated alienating behaviors—mild, moderate, or severe—is at high risk of becoming alienated from their own children, just as children who are victims of other forms of child abuse are more likely to become abusers as well.[88] Therefore, a court, when faced with evidence of parental alienation—whether mild, moderate, or severe—should act with alacrity.

The harm of parental alienation to a targeted parent is no different than other forms of intimate partner violence. Targeted parents have reported being diagnosed with posttraumatic stress disorder due to the behaviors of the alienating parent, depression, anxiety, loss of employment, homelessness, inability to form new relationships, and suicidality.[89] The rejection from your flesh and blood and the ensuing fight in courts to save their children and the parent-child relationship take a heavy emotional, physical, and financial toll on the targeted parents. Mental health professionals have coined the term "ambiguous loss" to refer to incomplete or uncertain loss, such as when a loved one is physically present but psychologically absent (e.g., a parent with Alzheimer's disease), or when someone is physically absent but psychologically present (e.g., kidnapped children).[90] Targeted parents experience such ambiguous loss for their alienated children—these children may be physically present during their parenting time but may be psychologically unavailable or even be hostile

85. Reay, K. (2011). *Toxic Divorce: A Workbook for Alienated Parents*, Author.

86. Harman, J. et al. (2018), *supra*, 1287.

87. Baker, A. J. L. (2005). The long-term effects of parental alienation: A qualitative research study, *American Journal of Family Therapy*, 33, 289–302.

88. Baker, A. J. L., & Eichler, A. (2016). The linkage between parental alienation behaviors and child alienation, *Journal of Divorce & Remarriage*, 57, 475–484.

89. Harman, J. et al. (2018), *supra*, 1288 (internal citations omitted).

90. *Id.*

or downright cruel to their targeted parent. And of course, in cases of severe parental alienation, targeted parents have been completely denied access to their children. This ambiguous loss goes largely unrecognized by society and is not acknowledged as a significant loss, resulting in what is termed as "disenfranchised grief."[91] Dr. Jennifer Harman describes the heart-wrenching grief of a targeted parent caught in the tentacles of the alienation monster:

> The [Targeted Parent] is unable to mourn for their children publicly, they are often told by others that it will get "better" when the children get older, or are encouraged to just "move on." As a consequence, [Targeted Parents] are often unable to formally process their grief and loss, and have problems moving on with their lives. Indeed, mental health professionals who have worked with [Targeted Parents] have reported feelings of rejection, depression, disbelief, anger, guilt, and loss, and often, the [Targeted Parents] are isolated from others due to other people's ignorance and negative judgments about what they are experiencing.[92]

When we add the detractors' cruel denial that parental alienation is even a real phenomenon, the disenfranchised grief experienced by targeted parents is all the more severe. It should come as no surprise that researchers have found a "suicide epidemic" among targeted parents, particularly fathers.[93] To make matters worse, it is extremely challenging for a targeted parent to be emotionally available to the alienated child and to parent the child who is hostile, brainwashed, and indoctrinated to hold false beliefs about the parent. In such situations, targeted parents may unwittingly contribute to the child's alienation—for instance, by allowing the child to make decisions as to when he will have contact with the targeted parent and on what terms or by being far too passive and conflict avoidant, allowing the situation to continue.[94] Alternatively, a targeted parent might inadvertently and out of frustration manifest suboptimal parenting behaviors that may confirm what the child falsely believes and can be used by the alienating parent (or a guardian ad litem or child's attorney who is not knowledgeable or trained in the area of parental alienation) to justify the child's rejection of the parent and to further cut down

---

91. *Id.*, citing Attig, T. (2004). Disenfranchised grief revisited: Discounting hope and love, *Omega: Journal of Death and Dying*, 49, 197–215; Doka, K. J. (1989). Disenfranchised grief. In Doka, K. J. (Ed.), *Disenfranchised Grief: Recognizing Hidden Sorrow*, 3–11.

92. *Id.*, 1288 (internal citations omitted).

93. Kposowa, A. J. (2003). Divorce and suicide risk, *Journal of Epidemiology and Community Health*, 57, 993–995.

94. Dean v. Valinho, Superior Court of Connecticut (Judicial Dist. Of Middlesex, No. FA044012513, July 6, 2011).

on the parent-child contact.[95] This is a toxic and vicious cycle that plays out in family courts around the country to no end.

Agenda of the Advocacy Groups

There are groups of activists that have persistently claimed that the phenomenon of parental alienation simply does not exist and the whole idea of parental alienation is a hoax. Perhaps the Supreme Court of Vermont provided the best rejoinder to such detractors when it held that

> [a]cross the country, the great weight of authority holds that conduct by one parent that tends to alienate the child's affections from the other is so inimical to the child's welfare as to be grounds for a denial of custody to, or a change of custody from, the parent guilty of such conduct.[96]

Such decriers of "fake news" allege that the child psychiatrist Richard Gardner "invented" the theory of parental alienation as a way to help abusive fathers take their children away from protective mothers[97] or that the parental alienation theory assumes that a mother who communicates child abuse allegations is malicious or psychologically disturbed and therefore an unfit parent. Debunking this propaganda of misleading and false information, Dr. William Bernet has written: "To my knowledge, no writer in the entire history of [Parental Alienation] *assumes* that mothers who report [child abuse] allegations are malicious or mentally disturbed."[98]

These activists, who claim themselves as advocates for victims of domestic violence, allege that the reason children do not want to have a relationship with their father is simply because the father has abused the children and/or the mother, even in cases where there have been no independent substantiation of abuse or where independent investigation (e.g., child protective services) has failed to substantiate abuse. Some have argued that men who successfully win custody after their ex-wives make abuse allegations are "batterers" and "abusers with custody."[99] Not only is such argument wholly belied by the facts reported in court opinions and peer-reviewed research, it assumes that *all* reports of abuse are valid and that "no one ever, intentionally or unintentionally, makes a

95. Stahl, P. (2004). Understanding and evaluating alienation in high conflict custody cases, *Wisconsin Journal of Family Law*, 24.

96. Renaud v. Renaud, 168 Vt. 306, 309, 721 A.2d 463, 465-66 (1998); also see Spaulding v. Butler, 172 Vt. 467 (2001).

97. Bernet, W. (2020). Introduction to parental alienation. In Lorandos, D., & Bernet, W. (Eds.), *Parental Alienation: Science and Law*, Charles C. Thomas, 18.

98. Bernet, W. (2020, May). Message from William Bernet (President of PASG) to David Corwin (President of APSAC) and Christopher Greeley (Editor of APSAC Advisor), *Parental Alienation International*, 21.

99. Meier, J. (2009). A historical perspective on Parental Alienation Syndrome and parental alienation, *J. Child Custody*, 6, 232, 234.

false abuse report. This is absurd."[100] As Dr. Demosthenes Lorandos points out in his critique of the detractors' propaganda of misinformation about parental alienation, a majority of states employ rather low standards of proof to "substantiate" or "indicate" an allegation of child abuse.[101] Despite this, a recent report of the U.S. Department of Health and Human Services Children's Bureau regarding child abuse allegations reveals that "more than 4 out of every 5 abuse reports are so lacking in any verifiable support, they cannot reach the typically low evidentiary standards most states use when 'substantiating' a child abuse allegation."[102] This tells us a lot about the quality and veracity of most abuse allegations, especially in cases involving parental alienation, "where false allegations often fly like swarms of locusts."[103] Clearly, these detractors' claims that *all* allegations of abuse are valid and *all* men accused are batterers are fantastical and lack evidentiary support.

Courts too have criticized this ideology-driven argument when it masks the true underlying facts. For instance, a Washington Court of Appeals found a mother's appeal brief challenging the trial court decision awarding custody to the father "unhelpful," when the brief failed to reference the underlying facts—the trial court's rejection of claims of "domestic violence" and making findings of parental alienation—and instead focused on literature warning of the injustice of custodial arrangements that favor "an abusive father over a battered and fearful mother."[104] The Court was so displeased with the mother's "one-sided presentation of the evidence, lack of citation to relevant authority," and failure to acknowledge the trial court's significant findings of parental alienation that it found the appeal to be frivolous and granted the father's request for attorney fees.[105] Family courts have seen through the ruse of allegations of "domestic violence" when such allegations are made to cover up or "justify" parental alienating behaviors. For instance, as this Connecticut court found:

> The court agrees with the evaluator in rejecting the view that the alienation of the child from the father results from the father being abusive to either the child or the mother. There is simply no evidence before the court to show he was abusive toward the child. The evaluator's information gathering regarding the mother's claim of abuse by the father supported no instances of abuse other than, inconclusively, one claim that he shoved her. The mother presented in court as one who would never tolerate physical abuse from anyone.

---

100. Lorandos, D. (2020). Admissibility of the construct–parental alienation. In Lorandos, D., & Bernet, W. (Eds.), *Parental Alienation: Science and Law*, Charles C. Thomas, 342.
101. *Id.*
102. *Id.*, 342–343.
103. *Id.*, 343.
104. *In re* Davis, 107 Wash.App. 1047 (2001).
105. *Id.*

. . .

[Domestic violence] simply was not present . . . it is crucial for the court to act now because [child] should not be entering his adolescence with views of his father that do not comport with reality.[106]

Despite the fact that courts around the country have unequivocally recognized the phenomenon of parental alienation and its deleterious effect on the children and the targeted parent's emotional and mental health, a small band of activists persistently refuse to consider the possibility that a parent could indoctrinate the child to fear or dislike the other parent. Such a polemical and absurd position is not only negated by empirical science—which has shown support for the alienating behaviors leading to child's indoctrination—but also by case law from family courts around the country that demonstrates that not only do the courts acknowledge the phenomenon of parental alienation, they consider it to be very harmful to the parent-child relationship. As the trial court in the earlier-referred Connecticut decision wrote: The alienating mother's "bitterness and distrust, while valid emotions for herself as an adult, have never been held in check as she has undermined her son's relationship with his father, which has caused the child grave harm."[107]

Dr. William Bernet summarized the situation aptly when he wrote: Domestic violence is real, although there have been false allegations of domestic violence; similarly, parental alienation is real, although there have been false allegations of parental alienation. "The solution is not to argue one extreme or the other, but to find ways to distinguish real domestic violence from real PA."[108] Denial of parental alienation "is reminiscent of the societal-level denial of the existence and prevalence of domestic violence and the abuse of children in the United States and Canada at the start of and throughout the 20th century."[109] Such baseless denial detracts attention away from a serious public health crisis that is affecting an estimated 22 million or more fathers and mothers and their children in the U.S. and millions more across the world.[110]

---

106. Dean v. Valinho, Superior Court of Connecticut (Judicial Dist. Of Middlesex, No. FA044012513, July 6, 2011).

107. *Id.*

108. Bernet, W. (2020). Introduction to parental alienation. In Lorandos, D., & Bernet, W. (Eds.), *Parental Alienation: Science and Law*, Charles C. Thomas, 19.

109. Harman, J. et. al. (2018). Parental alienating behaviors are family violence, *Psychological Bulletin*, 144(12), 1275–1299, 1277.

110. *Id.*

CHAPTER 8

Parental Alienation Around the World[1]

Parental alienation has been described, discussed, and debated in the legal and scientific literature all over the world. Thousands of court rulings address the phenomenon in the United States and in other jurisdictions globally. This is not a surprise. Parental alienation, while pathological, is, after all, an expression of human behavior occurring worldwide with similar patterns.

Different terms have been used to describe the phenomenon throughout the legal and scientific communities. The terms are associated with either the condition of alienation (the symptoms observed in children) or the alienating behaviors (the behaviors or tactics of the preferred or alienating parents). These processes have been referred to as: "aligned children," "Parental Alienation Syndrome (PAS)," "Medea syndrome," "programming and brainwashing," "not-based-on-actual-interaction," "divorce-related malicious parent syndrome," "pathological alienation," "attachment-based 'parental alienation,'" and "resist/refuse dynamic."[2]

It is a mistake to dismiss the phenomenon of parental alienation as Richard Gardner's theory or an American invention. Doing so would require turning a blind eye toward the voluminous, peer-reviewed literature published

1. This chapter has been adapted from the author's 2020 chapter, "Parental Alienation: An International Perspective," in Lorandos, D., & Bernet, W. (Eds.), *Parental Alienation: Science and Law,* Charles C. Thomas.

2. *See* Appendix A, "Terminology and Definitions," citing mental health literature where the phenomenon of "parental alienation" has been referred to using various terms, in Lorandos, D., & Bernet, W. (Eds.), *Parental Alienation: Science and Law,* Charles C. Thomas, 547.

on parental alienation as well as initiatives and interventions that are being undertaken by courts, legislatures, professional groups, and grass-roots organizations the world over.

As discussed previously in this book, parental alienation arises out of "parental alienation theory," which "is a psychosocial principle that posits that some children who reject a parent do so because they have been manipulated by the other parent to hold false and distorted thoughts and feelings about the rejected parent."[3] "The psychological foundation of parental alienation—lack of empathy and the inability to tolerate the child's separate needs and perception—is also the foundation of psychological maltreatment."[4]

So, what then is the reaction to parental alienation on the international stage? How do different legal systems around the world attempt to intervene and provide remedial measures to counter this form of psychological maltreatment? Which jurisdictions have been successful? How do different jurisdictions react to the scientific literature? As we journey on this world tour of parental alienation, it is helpful to understand the two major legal systems that exist in the world—at least in the jurisdictions that follow the rule of law.

The world is divided between countries that follow the common law system and those that follow the civil law system. Although there is a trend toward convergence between the two systems, they are nevertheless distinct. The distinction is summed up in the somewhat simplistic, unfortunate, and, at times, confusing labels given to these two systems: "adversarial," as the common law system is often called, versus the civil law system's "inquisitorial."

Let's look at how countries around the world have addressed parental alienation. But first, a disclaimer. This by no means is an exhaustive survey of all the countries that have dealt with the phenomenon of alienation. Rather, it's a generalized summary of different countries'—with their different legal systems, legislatures, courts, and organizations—attempts to tackle the problem of parental alienation. The information presented for these selected countries is not exhaustive. Each country has a long and nuanced history—legislative, judicial, and political—of how it has come to the point where it currently stands on the issue of parental alienation. To peel this onion, in all its layers of information, is well beyond the scope of this chapter. With that caveat in mind, let us begin our journey and start with countries in the common law system.

---

3. *Id.*, at 548.

4. Baker, A. J. L., & Ben-Ami, N. (2011). To turn a child against a parent is to turn a child against himself: The direct and indirect effects of exposure to parental alienation strategies on self-esteem and well-being, *J. of Divorce & Remarriage*, 52 472–489.

The Common Law System

Common law was adopted in England after the Anglo-Saxons settled there in the 5th century.[5] It was derived from Germanic trial law, with its central concept relying on "precedent." Under common law, previous decisions by judges can be cited as authority to obtain a similar result in future cases. Over time, the body of judicial rulings becomes the law. Common law is used in England and most former English colonies that adopted the English institutions, jurisprudence, and procedure. Common law posits that the best way of learning the "truth," when two parties have vastly different positions, is for each to present his or her position or case before an impartial decision maker, which could be a judge or a jury.[6]

In a common law system, a judge moderates and arbitrates between presentations on law and facts made by rival advocates. While the judge is tasked with ensuring that courtroom decorum, procedural formalities, and rules of evidence are complied with, the fundamental responsibility for identifying the legal contentions, the evidence to be considered, and witnesses to be presented remains with the lawyers.

This adversarial system resembles the old trial-by-combat system in England that was abolished around 1819. The traditional proxies are now lawyers speaking words instead of brandishing swords. While swords have been exchanged for words, "[I]t is still very much a 'bloody battle.' Many lives have been destroyed by the system. Many have been drained of all financial resources. Many have suffered irreparable psychological damage over the course of protracted litigation."[7] In fact, "The practice of ending the battle at sunset, and making a decision then, is in a sense more humane than the system today where litigation can go on for years."[8]

The countries that have adopted a common law system acknowledge the construct of parental alienation yet have different approaches on how to remediate alienation allegations in court. For instance, in Canada,[9] courts acknowledge that "alienation is a serious allegation . . . [and] should be proved" in a court of law.[10] Parental alienation is defined by Canadian family law judges as a situation "where one parent, consciously or unconsciously, attempts to keep the children from the other."[11] This can occur where one parent has a negative

---

5. International Divorce, Custody, and Child Support Systems, Real World Divorce, at http://www.realworlddivorce.com/International [hereinafter International Divorce].

6. Gardner, R. A. (1998). *The Parental Alienation Syndrome: A Guide for Mental Health and Legal Professionals*, Creative Therapeutics.

7. *Id.*, at 10.

8. *Id.*

9. Canadian court decisions are published, detailed, and demonstrate the "decision calculus." Canlii, at www.canlii.org.

10. Williamson v. Williamson, 2016 BCCA 87, 395 DLR (4th) 510.

11. Mungal v. Mungal, 2013 ONCJ 71, at para. 68.

or unsupportive attitude toward the other. This can also occur where one's conduct and words in the presence of the children demonstrates one's anger and bitterness toward the other.

The method Canadian jurists use in order to make a finding of parental alienation is succinct: First, a court must examine the threshold admissibility of alienation evidence in accordance with the *Mohan*[12] factors (relevance, necessity, absence of an exclusionary rule, and a properly qualified expert). If the evidence meets the threshold requirements of admissibility, then the court must exercise its gatekeeping function and balance the potential risks and benefits of admitting the evidence.[13] But similar to the American courts, parental alienation has had a controversial history in Canadian courts. Family judges have recognized that while parental alienation may not be readily identified as a "diagnosis" or "syndrome" in a clinical setting, that "does not mean that it does not exist, nor that it is not a seriously regarded problem in the field of psychology or family law."[14] Also like the American courts, Canadian judges have seen parental alienation to constitute child abuse.[15] And Canadian courts "almost in all jurisdictions have the power to order all members of a family to participate in therapy," including customized intervention that is specifically tailored to remedy alienation.[16]

On occasions, North American (as well as English) judges have lamented and criticized a parent's scorched-earth tactics to prove "parental alienation" in a court of law, where none exists in fact. What often emerges in this scenario is "a picture of two parents constantly in court over issues involving the children"[17] and a never-ending attempt by one to take the other down. These unfortunate cases involve an intractable parent who, having "read a lot" on parental alienation, maintains "with granite like certainty" that "it was quite simply a case of alienation," that the professionals and/or judges who don't "get it" are either untrained or incompetent, and the only person on whose shoulder the blame rests is the "alienator."[18]

These Dickensian, draining, and devastating courtroom battles demonstrate that not only is the term "parental alienation" vulnerable to abuse and misuse, but also that "alienation can be a two-way street. Excessive litigation based on a flimsy theory can be as alienating as any other strategy."[19] Aggressive use of

12. In Canada, the relevant test for admissibility of expert testimony was laid down in the case of R v. Mohan [1994]. 2 SCR 9, 114 DLR (4th) 419.

13. Williamson, 2016 BCCA 87.

14. M.L.S. v. N.E.D., 2017 SKQB 183 at para. 172.

15. L.M.A.M. v. C.P.M., 2012 MBQB 311 at para. 62.

16. Ludmer, B. (2018, November). Structured intervention trumps therapy in child contact refusal cases, *Parental Alienation Int'l*, 13.

17. Mastrangelo v. Mastrangelo, No. FA054012782S, 2017 WL 951087, at *2 (Conn. Super. Ct. Feb. 1, 2017).

18. B (A 14-Year-Old Boy) [2017] EWFC B28 ¶¶ 24, 77, Family Law Hub, at https://www.familylawhub.co.uk/default.aspx?i=ce5891.

19. J.F. v. D.F., 61 Misc. 3d 1226(A), 2018 WL 6530810, at *7 (Monroe Co., N.Y. Sup. Ct. Dec. 6, 2018).

expert witnesses in an attempt to fit a square peg of case-specific facts into a round hole of the alienation theory has led some courts to express frustration at "an unwarranted attempt to make an alienation mountain out of a series of irritating molehills" and at the same time, express skepticism that "the parental alienation theory is a new tool in the 'para-psychology-in-the-courtroom complex,' as part of a strategy to upend negotiated parenting agreements by the more aggressive and more moneyed spouse."[20]

On the other side of the pond, England's judicial system has come far from where it was in its approach towards PA. In 2016, the country's Child and Family Court Advisory and Support Service (CAFCASS), a public body set up to promote the welfare of children and families involved in U.K.'s family courts, warned that "parental alienation is responsible for around 80% of the most intransigent cases that come before the family courts."[21] This was followed by CAFCASS CEO, Sir Anthony Douglas, determining that PA is "undoubtedly a form of . . . child abuse."[22] In a fiery address before the House of Commons in March 2017, UK's Attorney General spoke of how "children struggle to reach their full potential" because "judges and social workers turn a blind eye to parental alienation."[23]

English courts have recognized that parental alienation is real and requires proper and timely intervention.[24] At times, courts interchange the term "parental alienation," with other phrases, such as "implacable hostility" or "parental hostility," but the message is not lost and English courts have long recognized the harmful effects of the alienating behaviors[25] regardless of the nomenclature. English courts have also weighed the wishes and feelings of children with an eye on the impact upon a child being manipulated, consciously or unconsciously, through alienation.[26] More importantly—and this is in contrast to many American family courts' approach—English judges have criticized

---

20. *Id.*, at *7, 35.

21. Hill, A. (2016, July 14). Programme aims to help people affected by "parental alienation," *The Guardian*, at http://www.theguardian.com/society/2016/jul/14/programme-aims-to-help-people-affected-by-parental-alienation.

22. Finnigan, L. (2017, February 12). Divorced parents who pit children against former partners "guilty of abuse," *The Telegraph*, at http://www.telegraph.co.uk/news/2017/02/12/divorced-parents-pit-children-against-former-partners-guilty/.

23. The UK Parental Alienation Study (2020), at www.parentalalienationuk.info.

24. *See*, generally, Re L and M (Children: Private Law) [2014] EWHC 939 (Fam), Family Law Hub, at https://www.familylawhub.co.uk/default.aspx?i=ce3916; Re S (A Child) [2010] EWHC 3721 (Fam); Re S (A Child) [2010] EWHC 192 (Fam); Re A (A Child) [2007] EWCA Civ; Re L-W [2010] EWCA Civ 1253; Re C (Children) (Prohibition on Further Applications) [2002] EWCA Civ 292; Re T (A Child) (Contact: Alienation: Permission to Appeal) [2002] EWCA Civ 1736; Re M (Intractable Contact Dispute: Interim Care Order) [2003] EWHC 1024 (Fam).

25. *See, e.g.*, Re J (A Child – Intractable Contact) [2017] EWFC B103, Family Law Hub, at https://www.familylawhub.co.uk/default.aspx?i=ce6253; Re B (A Minor) (Access) [1984] FLR 648; In the Matter of Lancashire CC v Z (Parental Hostility).

26. Re H (Children) [2014] EWCA Civ 733, Family Law Hub, at https://www.familylawhub.co.uk/default.aspx?i=ce4074; Re K (Abduction: case management) [2011] 1 FLR 1268; S (Children) [2010] EWCA Civ 447.

the "softly, softly" approach by social workers when, even after a target parent is exonerated of false allegations (which were a likely result of alienation), the social workers and guardians *ad litem* have suggested taking "baby steps" towards re-establishing contact.[27]

While it may have been controversial at one time, "the concept of alienation . . . may today be regarded as mainstream" in the U.K. courts.[28] The British Psychological Society has now approved accreditation—Continuing Professional Development (CPD)—in parental alienation.[29]

In Ireland, there does not appear to be a consistent method in place to define, detect, or resolve parental alienation,[30] perhaps partly due to the rapid changes to the family structure in Ireland and the overwhelming need of family law court reform. Divorce was not introduced in Ireland's courts until 1996. "As a result of the law and culture in Ireland, our divorce rate remains low at 0.6% out of 1,000."[31] Getting a divorce in Ireland requires the parties to live apart for four years; a contested divorce may take another two years.[32] When custody is contested, Ireland's courts tend to give more weight to the voice of the child.[33] This is problematic if the child is under the influence of an alienating parent. Often, critics claim that the dynamics of parental alienation are not recognized by Irish courts or literature. However, as previously noted, parental alienation has been documented in the empirical psychiatric and psychological literature since the early 1950s.With no system in place, Irish courts are limited in what they can do about it.[34] The lack of a system may contribute to the breakdown of the relationship between one parent and a child.[35] A recent research

27. *In re* K [2016] EWCA Civ 99, Family Law Hub, at https://www.familylawhub.co.uk/default.aspx?i=ce5052.

28. Re S (A Child – Transfer of Residence) [2011] 1 FLR 1789.

29. Whitcombe, S. (2017, July). Making progress in the UK and Wales, *PASG Newsletter*, 11–12.

30. Conneely, S., & O'Shea, R. (2019). Innovative family mediation research initiative embedded in the community in Ireland, *Fam. Ct. Rev.*, 57, 342.

31. *Id.; see also* Family Law (Divorce) Act (1996) (Ir.).

32. *Id.; see also* O'Shea, R. (2014). Judicial Separation and Divorce in the Circuit Court: Headline Findings, 296 (where the Northern Circuit had the highest rate of "old" cases yet to come to court for a substantive hearing, with several cases waiting ten years or more for a decree of divorce). *See also* A Private Members Bill, introduced in April 2017 by Minister Josepha Madigan, proposed to reduce waiting time for divorce from four years to two. *See* Thirty-fifth Amendment of the Constitution (Divorce) Act 2016 (Act No. 57/2016) (Ir.), at https://data.oireachtas.ie/ie/oireachtas/bill/2016/57/eng/initiated/b5716d.pdf.

33. O'Sullivan, B. (2013). *The Irish Journal of Family Law*, 16(1), 20–25.

34. O'Shea, R., *supra. See also* The Law Reform Commission, Report on Family Courts (1996), LRC 52-1996, ii, at https://www.lawreform.ie/_fileupload/Reports/rFamilyCourts.htm. (The failings of the system have continued to be highlighted by the Law Reform Commission in the intervening years.). See, also, Shatter, A. J. (1997). *Shatter's Family Law* (4th ed.). (Alan Shatter as a minister was responsible for the development and implementation of far-reaching legislative changes beginning with the Judicial Separation Act in 1989.). See, also, Dr. Róisín O'Shea, Judicial Separation and Divorce in the Circuit Court (2013) (unpublished thesis), at https://repository.wit.ie/2825/1/thesis_ROS_WITLIB_201405final.pdf (The same issues identified by the Law Reform Commission in 1996 were found to still exist in the Irish courts.).

35. O'Shea, R., *supra.*

project conducted by Dr. Roisin O'Shea and Dr. Sinead Conneely[36] at Waterford Institute of Technology observed 360 family law cases over a period of 14 days. Notably, "in the majority of cases that the rulings were in favor of the wife in terms of property orders, primary care of the children, and custody of the children, and no sanction was ordered for unilateral withholding of access by the mother, in breach of court orders."[37] The study also described the difference in how courts dealt with violations of court orders. In access violations, fewer than 30 percent of applications resulted in jail time, whereas on support violations almost half of the applications were issued summonses.[38]

Moreover, the researchers point out the availability of enforcement procedures written out in Sec. 60 of the Children and Relationships Act,[39] under which a judge may order parenting time, costs for the parent denied time with their child, attendance at mediation, a parenting program, or counselling.[40]

Moving south of Europe, alienation allegations are commonly found in high-conflict divorces. In Israel—which has two parallel court systems, Civil Family Courts and Rabbinical Courts—considerable time, energy and resources are spent addressing the construct of parental alienation.[41] [42] In 2018, Israel's Nazareth Family Court found that a nine-year-old child was alienated from his mother, the primary custodial parent.[43] The father asked for sole custody due to the very problematic connection between mother and son. The son expressed a strong desire to live with the father. The court ruled, after an extensive review of the PA literature, that there was clear evidence of alienating behaviors on the father's part which could, if not addressed, reach the pathological stage. The court denied the father's petition and ordered mental health intervention.

In a different case involving two young children, the appellate court upheld the trial court's decision of change of custody to the target parent.[44] The trial court found that the mother was responsible for the existence of PA, which resulted in the complete refusal of the children to have contact with the father. The mother relocated with the children without permission during the custody proceedings to a place 72 miles away from their prior residence. Social

---

36. O'Shea, R., *supra.*
37. O'Shea, R., *supra.*
38. *Ibid.*
39. Child and Family Relationships Act 2015 (Act No. 9/2015)(Ir.), at http://www.irishstatutebook.ie/eli/2015/act/9/section/60/enacted/en/html.
40. *Id.*
41. Gottlieb, D. (2006). Parental Alienation Syndrome—An Israeli perspective: Reflections and recommendations. In Gardner, R. A. et al. (Eds.) *The International Handbook of Parental Alienation Syndrome,* Charles C. Thomas, 105.
42. Dum, C. T. (2013). Parental alienation initiatives around the world, In Gardner, R. A. et al. (Eds.) (2006). *The International Handbook of Parental Alienation Syndrome,* Charles C. Thomas, 426.
43. Anonymous vs. Anonymous, No. 5075-04-15 (Nazareth Family Court May 23, 2018).
44. K.L. vs Y.P., No. 60592-03-15 (Tel Aviv Dist. Ct. June 8, 2015).

Services recommended that custody be transferred to the father. The trial court accepted the recommendation and ordered the immediate change of custody to the father. The appellate court affirmed the trial court's decision but gave the mother two months to prepare the children for the change.

In India, in 2017, the Supreme Court addressed the term "Parental Alienation Syndrome" and discussed its "at least two psychological destructive effects."[45] India's Supreme Court decision was a victory for the grassroots awareness campaign of the phenomenon of PA that was spearheaded by the Children's Rights Initiative for Shared Parenting (CRISP). In 2008, CRISP was created in India by people who recognized the serious effects of parental alienation on children due to single parent families on account of divorce or separation. CRISP is focusing on furthering the rights of children to remain connected with both parents.[46]

After the 2017 Supreme Court decision, the Child Rights Foundation (CRF) filed a Writ Petition[47] before the Court urging it to declare PA as child abuse and in violation of Article 21[48] of the Constitution of India.[49] The Petition also asks that the Court issue guidelines to the Family Courts (trial courts) across the country to change custody to target parents upon a finding of PA.[50] India's Family Court Act, 1984, only allows for primary custody with one parent and very limited access or visitation rights to the noncustodial parent. The law pits divorcing spouses against each other, incentivizing PA. As a result, hundreds of thousands of noncustodial parents have been cut off from their children without justification. In support of its Petition, CRF has also provided the Supreme Court with a survey of international court cases involving PA from the courts in the United States, Canada, and Australia and the ECtHR.[51]

As in India, parental alienation is also found in Malaysia, which is a multiethnic society but with Islam as the dominant religion.[52] The awareness also exists in the Philippines, "where to date no legal divorce is possible, only legal separation under rather stringent circumstances."[53] The Philippines Supreme Court Justice Roberto Abad specifically mentioned PA, albeit as "paternal alienation,"

45. Singh v. Singh, No. 3962 of 2016 (Supreme Ct. of India Feb. 13, 2017), at https://indiankanoon.org/doc/48721287/?type=print.

46. Home, Children's Rights Initiative for Shared Parenting (CRISP), at www.crisp-india.org/.

47. Writ Petition, In the Matter of Child Rights Foundation (CRF) v. Union of India, No. 1031 of 2018.

48. Constitution of India art. 21 ("No person shall be deprived of his life or personal liberty except according to a procedure established by law.") Indian courts have ruled that the protection of family is an integral part of right to "life."

49. Joshi, A. (2018, November). India's Supreme Court petitioned to end state-sponsored parental alienation and "Santa parenting," *Parental Alienation Int'l*, 3, 22–23.

50. Child Rights Foundation, at http://childrightsfoundation.com/.

51. Joshi, A., *supra*.

52. Dum, C. T., *supra*, at 427 (citing the website www.pemalik.org and other resources in Malaysia).

53. Dum, C. T., *supra* note 29, at 426.

when he criticized the country's civil code which mandates sole maternal custody for children under seven years of age barring compelling reasons.[54]

In Hong Kong, Family Court decisions show that the construct of parental alienation is regularly addressed by the courts. In *CLL and SW,*[55] a high-conflict case involving parental alienation allegations, the judge found the mother had fabricated sex abuse allegations against the father to obtain the custody of their seven-year-old daughter. The father alleged that the mother was "brainwashing" the child and engaging in "parental alienating" behaviors. After reviewing an "unusually voluminous amount of materials" in a case that the Court characterized as "one of the most difficult and emotive . . . ever," the Court ordered that the child be returned to the care and control of the father.

Traveling further south and east, Australian family courts have rejected "parental alienation syndrome."[56] Instead, the courts, similar to many American family court judges, recognize alienating *behaviors* and have ordered remedial measures in appropriate circumstances.[57] In one such case, the Australian Family Court made a finding that the mother engaged in alienating behaviors that led to the father's complete estrangement from his children.[58] However, given the ages of the children—twelve and seventeen years old—the court was unwilling to change the residency of the children.[59]

This approach was not in line with what Australian researchers have determined. After reviewing scientific papers from English-speaking countries from the years 1990 through 2015 in a meta-analysis on the scientific literature concerning parental alienation, the authors found that a change in custody or residence of the child in favor of the target parent is an effective remedial measure in alienation cases together with psychoeducation and specialized systemic family therapy.[60] The authors also discussed a coordinated approach for mental health interventions and court action (with sanctions against alienators and uncooperative parents) in order to resolve parental alienation. The authors

54. Dacasin v. Dacasin, G.R. No. 168785 (Supreme Ct. of the Philippines Feb. 5, 2010)(Abad J. concurring), at http://www.lawphil.net.

55. CLL v. SW, [2013] HKEC 38, 2013 WL 6842 (Dist. Ct. Matrimoial Causes Dec. 17, 2012).

56. *See* Goudarzi and Bagheri [2018] FamCA 217 ¶¶ 146-147, 2018 WL 1904903 (Apr. 13, 2018); Cambridge and Walter [2010] FCWA 30; Udall and Oaks [2010] FamCA 1482, 2010 WL 5880096 (Oct. 22, 2010); P and P [2004] FCWA 150; O and O [2005] FCWA 20; T and B [2006] FCWA 37; Matthews and Bender [2015] FamCA 654, 2015 WL 5257188 (June 11, 2015).

57. An example of some cases where Australian judges have rejected PAS or not accepted it as a scientific concept: C and C [2004] FamCA 708; Lane and Arthurs [2006] FamCA 87; Parker and Elliott [2003] FamCA 990; SS and AH [2005] FamCA 481; Summers and Nathan [2005] FamCA 1406. Note: Australian commentators use pseudonyms to protect the identity of the parties. *See* http://www.australiandivorce.com.au/parental-alienation-in-australia/.

58. Goudarzi [2018] FamCA 217.

59. *Id.*

60. Templar, K., Matthewson, M., Haines, J., & Cox, G. (2016). Recommendations for best practice in response to parental alienation: Findings from a systematic review, *J. Fam. Therapy,* 39 103–122, at https://doi.org/10.1111/1467-6427.12137.

also found that it was less harmful for children to be separated from the alienating parent than to allow the alienation process to continue unaffected. None of the studies that were reviewed by this team of researchers recommended waiting for the alienation to resolve itself or having the children decide which parent should have custody or where to live. Australia continues to host international conferences on the exchange of ideas and cutting-edge research in the field of PA.[61]

New Zealand courts, like those in many other parts of the world, have focused on alienating behaviors rather than on defining the word "syndrome."[62] Here, the courts occasionally have used the term "pathological alienation" instead of parental alienation.[63] Additionally, in New Zealand, courts have found that a parent who has made false allegations against another parent and portrayed the other parent as "dangerous" or "abusive"—sexually, physically, or psychologically—may have demonstrated an alienating behavior.[64]

Overall, judicial interventions have had different results.[65] In some instances, judges' warnings regarding continued alienating behavior have led to cessation of alienating behaviors. In other instances, the court's warnings fell on deaf ears and the alienating parent refused to change the bad behavior.[66] Also, more stringent, proactive measures—fines, bond, intensive counseling, and threats to make the children wards of the court—have worked in some instances and offered enough deterrent for all but the most unrelenting of alienators.[67]

The Civil Law System

The civil law system evolved on the European continent. It was derived from the Justinian Code, issued by the Roman emperor in A.D. 529, and was substantially updated in 1804 as the Napoleonic Code.[68] Unlike the common law system, in a civil law system, judges are not supposed to make law. Instead, they are supposed to work from the law—the statutory framework—which is more precise than in a common law jurisdiction. Precedent does not hold bar in

61. *See, e.g.*, Parental Alienation: Family Violence Lost in the Fog, Parental Alienation Conference 2018 (Hobart, Tasmania Oct. 17–19, 2018) at https://parentalalienation.org.au/conference

62. *See, e.g.*, ASM v DSM [2016] NZHC 137; Gebrien v. Todd [2015] NZFC 4949; Belford v Belford [2014] NZFC 4530; Secrest v Axley [2014] NZFC 493; Palmer v Holm [2014] NZHC 2268; McInnes v McInnes [2014] NZHC 2822.

63. Gebrien,[2015] NZFC 4949.

64. *See, e.g.*, *Id.*; Belford, [2014] NZFC 4530.

65. *See* ALZ v. FLZ [2013] NZFLR 145.

66. Secrest v Axley [2014] NZFC 493.

67. Garrett v. Garrett [2013] NZFC 6314; F v. F High Court, Invercargill, Fogarty J, 11 February 2011, CIV 2010-425-000440; M v. N [2017] NZFC 2358.

68. International Divorce, *supra* note 5.

a civil law system. Any previous decisions and/or interpretations of the law by other judges are not binding. Germans, who developed common law, now use civil law, as do nearly all other European countries, nearly all Latin American countries, China, Japan, Turkey, and some Arab countries.

The civil law system relies on active and robust inquiry by the judge to uncover the truth. Unlike the common law system, here the judge wields great power, which is restricted by evidentiary requirements."[69] In civil law systems, cases are directed by the judge; participation by the parties' advocates is passive. Traditionally, it is up to the judge to determine the matters in dispute, identify the necessary evidence, schedule the necessary intermediate and final hearings, and eventually formulate the judgment according to the law and the proof.[70] The judge in the inquisitorial system is a very active factfinder who controls the mechanisms of inquiry.[71] He has the affirmative responsibility for establishing the truth of the case. The lawyers' role here is passive, residual, and deferential.[72]

In the civil law system, the judge calls in the witnesses and interviews them in the presence of the attorneys and the clients. Comparatively, witnesses are allowed great leeway with their testimony.[73] With the judge questioning, the witness provides narrative that will enable the judge to discover the truth. Also, there is only a court-appointed expert—not one for either party. The court generally will rely heavily on the opinion of the appointed expert.[74] Thereafter, counsel may supplement the opinion of the court-appointed expert with that of experts of their own choosing; the testimony of the latter is likely to be accorded considerably less weight, and, in many jurisdictions, such as Germany, the practice is rare and frowned upon.

The first civil law system we approach is the Federal District of Mexico, the first jurisdiction to adopt a reference to parental alienation in its civil code in 2004: "each parent must avoid any act of manipulation, parental alienation aimed at producing in the child resentment or rejection of the other parent."[75] The reference was eliminated in 2006, however, after lobbying by special interest groups, which included *ad hominem* attacks on Richard Gardner.[76] The state

---

69. Gardner, R., *supra* note 6, at 13 ("Torture came to be viewed as an excellent and reliable method of finding out 'the truth.'")

70. Hazard, G., & Dondi, A. (2006). Responsibilities of judges and advocates in civil and common law: Some lingering misconceptions concerning civil lawsuits, *Cornell Int'l. J.*. 39, 59, 60–62.

71. *See, e.g.*, Gardner, R., *supra*, at 15.

72. Hazard, G., & Dondi, A., *supra*, at 61.

73. Gardner, R., *supra*, at 15.

74. *Id.*

75. Dum, C. T., *supra*, at 425, 445.

76. *Id.* (citing Diario de los debates de la Asamblea Legislative del Distrito Federal, Num. 40, 28 de diciembre de 2006).

of Morelos, Mexico, adopted the same article into its civil code as Article 224.[77] From there, the state of Aguascalientes, Mexico, modified the civil code in 2007 by adding language that prohibited parents from engaging in PA, empowered courts, and mandated that the courts order "therapeutic measures necessary . . . in order to restore healthy contact with both parents." Doing so, the law in Aguascalientes authorized "enforcement measures" to be used by courts, including, but not limited to, "suspension of . . . custody or contact," if necessary.[78]

Next, the state of Queretaro, Mexico, approved the inclusion of parental alienation in its civil code, Articles 443 to 449, in June 2011, acknowledging that the behavior is "a form of abuse of minors."[79] Like Aguascalientes, Queretaro's Civil Code Article 443 allows parental authority to be suspended for "engaging in behaviors of parental alienation."[80] Similarly, parliamentary proposals for including definitions of PA in the Civil Code have been made in Mexican states of Michoacán de Ocampo, Chihuahua, and Morelos.[81]

The Supreme Court of Mexico finally ruled on the constitutionality of the articles 336 Bis B, 429 Bis A and 459, fraction IV, and Decree 1380 of the Civil Code for the State of Oaxaca, which outlawed PA on May 16, 2018. The Court found the language of the original Act to be too punitive toward alienating parents because the Act violated "the principle of proportionality" by threatening to revoke parental authority entirely in cases of alienation.[82] The original statute did not give judges the ability to weigh the "best interest" of the child when considering the remedy to PA. Nevertheless, the Supreme Court upheld the concept of parental alienation and ruled in favor of editing the legislation.

Further south, Brazil became the first country to adopt national legislation regarding parental alienation. Judge Elizio Luiz Perez drafted the first legislation incorporating parental alienation in May 2008.[83] The legislation was

---

77. Dum, C. T., *supra*, at 445 (citing Ikeda, J. K. (2008). Legislative proposal for the state of Morelos on shared custody and parental alienation. Thesis. Available from Lulu.com).

78. Dum, C. T., *supra*, at 445.

79. *Id.*, at 445–447.

80. *Id. See also* José Francisco Coronato Rodriguez, Initiative That Reforms the Article 343 Bis of the Federal Penal Code, in Charge of the Deputy José Francisco Coronato Rodríguez, of the Parliamentary Group of the Citizen Movement, Gaceta Parlamentaria (2015), at gaceta.diputados.gob.mx/Black/Gaceta/Anteriores/62/2015/mar/20150305-IV/Iniciativa-6.html.

81. *Id. See also* José Francisco Coronato Rodriguez, Initiative That Reforms the Article 343 Bis of the Federal Penal Code, in Charge of the Deputy José Francisco Coronato Rodríguez, of the Parliamentary Group of the Citizen Movement, Gaceta Parlamentaria (2015), at gaceta.diputados.gob.mx/Black/Gaceta/Anteriores/62/2015/mar/20150305-IV/Iniciativa-6.html.

82. Norma Lucia Piña Hernández, Judgment Issued by the Full Court of the Supreme Court of Justice of the Nation in the Unconstitutionality Action 11/2016, as Well as the Concurring Opinion Formulated by the Minister Luis María Aguilar Morales, Diario Oficial De La Federacion (2017), dof.gob.mx/nota_to_doc.php?codnota=5522808.

83. Brockhausen, T. (2013). Parental alienation and the new Brazilian law. In Lorandos, D., Bernet, W., & Sauber, R. (Eds.), *Parental Alienation: The Handbook for Mental Health and Legal Professionals*, Charles C. Thomas, 466.

introduced after Brazilian researchers published psychological studies on children who have been victims of alienation. The research indicated that these children are more likely to develop psychological disorders, such as chronic depression, social phobias, identity and self-image distortions, and, in extreme cases, suicidal tendencies.[84] As the former Public Prosecutor in Rio de Janeiro explains, in Brazil, parental alienation is considered "an unethical behavior adopted by someone who takes care of a child or adolescent to disqualify the children's mother or father in order to make the child hate them or to damage their relationship."[85]

Brazilian law applies alienation broadly to inappropriate actions and/or omissions of parents, grandparents, and third parties. The law describes alienating or inappropriate behaviors and does not require that the child be alienated from a parent or even exhibit symptoms of alienation.[86] The law is intended to promote equal access to both custodial and non-custodial parents.[87] Brazil's social context, with its long history of mothers receiving exclusive legal and physical custody of children upon separation or divorce, pressed for a more balanced coexistence of children with both parents and for legal mechanisms to counter abuse of parental authority.[88]

Brazil's law not only defined parental alienation and alienating behaviors, but also armed its judges with powerful remedies to assist target parents and alienated children.[89] The law defined an act of parental alienation as "the interference in a child's or adolescent's psychological training promoted or induced by either parent, by grandparents, or by those who hold the child or adolescent under their authority, guardianship, or surveillance to reject one of the parents, or that hampers building or maintaining bonds with them."[90] The statute declared the practice of parental alienation as infringing on the "fundamental right the child or adolescent has in having a healthy family life." As such, specific civil remedies that courts can use to address the problem were also provided.[91]

---

84. Denise Maria Perissini Da Silva, Psicologia Juridica No Processo Civil Brasileiro 86 (2003).

85. Ramos, P. P. C., Parental Alienation in Brazilian Law, at http://p-web01.mp.rj.gov.br/Informativos/cao_civel/2017/abr_mai_jun/parental_alienation_law.pdf; also see Brockhausen, T., *supra* note 42, at 475–476 ("Contrary to the interventional model proposed by Gardner, Richard, however, the model proposed by Lei 12.318 does not require for the child to show signs of PAS for which measures are applied. That is, the child does not need to reject the parent for legal action to be undertaken." In this sense, the Brazilian law departs from a psychologizing and pathologizing notion found in Gardner's model and extends the concept of PA to milder family dynamics and family conflicts.)

86. Brockhausen, T., *supra*, at 480.

87. Gomide, P. I. C., Camargo, E. B., & Fernandes, M. G. (2016). Analysis of the psychometric properties of a parental alienation scale, *Paidéia*, 26(65), 291.

88. Brockhausen, T., *supra*, at 463–465.

89. Taking Parental Alienation Seriously – Brazil's New Law, Warshak, Dr. Richard A., at http://warshak.com/blog/?s=brazil

90. *Id.*

91. Ramos, P. P. C., *supra*.

A Brazilian judge has several remedial options when parental alienation is identified, such as increased or reparative parenting time for the alienated parent, levying financial sanctions on the alienating parent, change of custody, and/or suspension of the parental rights/responsibilities. Courts began making decisions regarding compliance with visitation in alienation cases under penalty of criminal contempt and condemnation.[92] After the new legislation on parental alienation, Brazilian courts began finding both parents guilty of engaging in alienating behaviors, giving warnings to a variety of family members who acted in conjunction with an alienating parent, enforcing compliance with visitations under penalty of criminal contempt and condemnation, and ordering prosecution for parental alienation with a possible change of custody and fines.[93] Forensic tools, such as The Parental Alienation Scale, were also developed to help the courts make objective decisions free from procedural biases.[94]

Earlier, parental alienation was considered an "administrative infraction," which can be punished by a fine determined by the judge; it was not considered a "crime."[95] In April 2017, this changed. Brazil passed a new law that classifies parental alienation as "criminal conduct" in the form of "psychological violence" (Lei 13.431, April 4, 2017).[96] While there has been an increase in Brazilian scientific literature regarding parental alienation, there appears to be a dearth of quantitative research in this area.[97] Also, critics of Brazil's law say the law pathologizes and criminalizes the phenomena of typical post-divorce behavior, effectively dehumanizing the child.[98]

In continental Europe's civil law systems, the construct of parental alienation is often challenged. Let's consider France. The earliest mention of PAS—called *Syndrome Alienation Parentale* (SAP)—in French-language literature was published in the 1990s.[99] The Supreme Court of France (*Cour de Cassation*) has recognized parental alienation as a "change of circumstances" (*un element*

92. *See* Brockhausen, T., *supra*, for a summary of the cases and Brazilian jurisprudence before and after Lei 12.318.

93. *Id.*, citing R.C.D.C. and D.B.S. (2011), A.C.F. and C.R.D.M. (2011), W.R. and S.B. (2011), R.C.D.S.T. and E.L.D.S. (2011).

94. Gomide, P. I. C., et al., *supra*.

95. *Id.*

96. Presidência da República, Casa Civil, Subchefia para Assuntos Jurídicos, LEI N° 13.431, 2017 at www.planalto.gov.br/ccivil_03/_Ato2015-2018/2017/Lei/L13431.htm.

97. Soma, S. M. P., de Castro, M. S. B. L., Williams, L. Cavalcanti de Albuquerque, & Tannús, P. M. Parental Alienation in Brazil: A Review of Scientific Publications, *Psicologia Em Estudo*, 21, 377, at http://www.redalyc.org/articulo.oa?id=287148579003; *see also* Brockhausen, T., *supra* note 83, at 466.

98. *See, e.g.*, Mendez, J., & Bucher-Maluschke, J. (2017). Destructive divorce in the family life cycle and its implications: Criticisms of parental alienation, *Psicologia: Teoria E Pesquisa*, 33, 1, 6.

99. *See* Anne-France Goldwater, « Le Syndrome d'Aliénation Parentale », In Développements récents en droit familial, Les Éditions Yvon Blais, 1991, 121–145; Paule Lamontagne, « Syndrome d'Aliénation Parentale: Contexte et pièges de l'intervention », in : Us et abus de la mise en mots en matière d'abus sexuel, sous la direction de Hubert Van Gijseghem, Les Éditions du Méridien, 1999.

nouveau) justifying revisiting issues related to custody and/or parenting time. In the case before the French Supreme Court, the existence of parental alienation justified transfer of custody from mother to father.[100] But despite the awareness regarding parental alienation or SAP in France, it remains a controversial topic.

In late 2016, the French Ministry of Family, Children, and Women's Rights attempted to prohibit the use of SAP.[101] In doing so, the Ministry published the assessment of its fourth plan of prevention and fight against violence against women (2014–2016).[102] This report contains an action item: "Action 58: To inform about the medically unfounded nature of the 'parental alienation syndrome.'"[103] It reads:

> In cases of domestic violence or violence against children, the allegation of "parental alienation syndrome" raises real difficulties. It leads to discrediting the word of the mother, exceptionally the father or the child and therefore to deny the status of victim by reversing responsibilities. However, no scientific authority has ever recognized such a "syndrome" and the scientific consensus underlines the unreliability of this notion. It is not recognized by the *Diagnostic and Statistical Manual of Mental Disorders* (DSM5) . . . or by the *International Classification of Diseases* published by the World Health Organization (WHO). This is why a communication to outlaw the use of this concept will be made, via the publication of a sheet on this topic, on the website of the Ministry of Justice.[104]

Because of intense and relentless anti-SAP propaganda unleashed on the Ministry (especially the former minister, Senator Laurence Rossignol) by women's groups, children's groups, and other social organizations in France, the Ministry of Justice published instructions to the judges for family matters to inform them "of the controversial and unrecognized nature of the parental alienation syndrome, to encourage them to look with caution this means when raised in defense and remind them that other tools are available to them in

---

100. Cour de cassation, civile, Chambre civile 1, 26 juin 2013, 12-14-392.

101. Gryson-Dejehansart, M.-C., [Tribune] Justice 2018: Proscription du Syndrome D'Aliénation Parentale (SAP), C'est Officiel [Prohibition of Parental Alienation Syndrome (SAP), It's Official], Village De La Justice (Dec. 5, 2016), at https://www.village-justice.com/articles/Expertises-Judiciaires-recours-SAP-Syndrome-Alienation-Parentale-proscrit-tant,23689.html.

102. Bilan du 4eme Plan de prevention et de Lutte Contre les Violences Faites Aux Femmes (2014-2016) [Review of the 4th Plan of Preention and Fight Against Violence Against Women (2014-2016)], in 5EME Plan De Mobilisation Et De Lutte Contre Toutes Les Violences Faites Aux Femmes 2017-2019, Republique Francaise, at www.egalite-femmes-hommes.gouv.fr/wp-content/uploads/2016/11/5e-plan-de-lutte-contre-toutes-les-violences-faites-aux-femmes.pdf.

103. Gryson-Dejehansart, M.-C., *supra* note 101.

104. *Id.*

civil matters to deal with the sometimes real situations of a parent who would try to gradually move the child away from the other parent."[105]

The French Ministry's position was misinformed and inaccurate. While the actual words "parental alienation" are not used in DSM-5, the concept of PA is expressed in at least three mental conditions that are mentioned in DSM-5:[106]

- *Child affected by parental relationship distress:* defined as "negative effects of parental relationship discord (e.g., high levels of conflict, distress, or disparagement) on a child in the family."
- *Parent–child relational problem*: defined as "negative attributions of the other's intentions, hostility toward the other, and unwarranted feelings of estrangement."
- *Child psychological abuse*: defined as "harming/abandoning people or things that the child cares about."

Moreover, the *International Classification of Diseases* (ICD-11) is considering including the term "parental alienation" where it is considered a synonym or an index term for a specific diagnosis—that is, *caregiver–child relationship problem* (QE52.0).[107] Further, the Vanderbilt University School of Medicine at Nashville, Tennessee, in the U.S. lists around 1200 publications of scientific relevance from about 40 countries worldwide about parental alienation and related topics.

The French Ministry's view that the construct of parental alienation or SAP is not supported by science or recognized by other researchers or professional organizations is myopic and incorrect. The concept of parental alienation has been accepted by the following professional organizations in the United States:[108]

- In 1991 (and again in 2013), the American Bar Association published the seminal book by Clawar and Rivlin, *Children Held Hostage*, which extensively discusses PA.
- In 1997, the American Academy of Child and Adolescent Psychiatry published Practice Parameters for Child Custody Evaluation, an "AACAP Official Action," which contains a section on "Parental Alienation."

105. *Id. See also* The French Minister of Families Tries to Delete "PAS" and "PA" Before its Term Expires in May 2017, at http://jm2p.e-monsite.com/medias/files/attack-against-pas-and-pa-by-the-french-minister-of-families...-jm2p-responds....pdf [hereinafter French Minister of Families].

106. Bernet, W., Wamboldt, M. Z., & Narrow, W. E. (2016). Child affected by parental relationship distress, *J. Am. Acad. Child & Adolescent Psychiatry*, 55, 571. *See also* von Boch-Galhau, W. (2018). Parental Alienation (Syndrome) – A serious form of child mental abuse, *Neuropsychiatrie*, 32, 133 ("Parental alienation is a type of child mental abuse disorder diagnosed in DSM-5 . . . under the diagnostic code V 995.51 [where] child psychological abuse is located.").

107. Bernet, W. (2018, July). ICD-11 includes parental alienation, *Parental Alienation Int'l*.

108. Bernet, W. (2020). Recognition of parental alienation by professional organizations. In Lorandos, D., & Bernet, W. (Eds.), *Parental Alienation: Science and Law*, Charles C. Thomas, 254–281.

- In 2006, the Association of Family and Conciliation Courts published Model Standards of Practice for Child Custody Evaluations, which refers to "attempts to alienate children from a parent."
- In 2012, the American Psychological Association published Guidelines for the Practice of Parenting Coordination, which refers to "the dynamics of complex postseparation situations, such as refusal to visit a parent, parental undermining of the child's relationships with the other parent."
- In 2015, the American Psychological Association published the *APA Handbook of Forensic Psychology,* which contains a section on "Child Alienation."
- In 2015, the American Academy of Matrimonial Lawyers published Child Centered Residential Guidelines, which says, "A child may also resist parenting due to contrived or magnified concerns regarding a parent that may be supported by the non-rejected parent."
- In 2016, the American Academy of Pediatrics published a clinical report called "Helping Children and Families Deal with Divorce and Separation," which cites publications regarding PA.
- In 2016, the American Professional Society on the Abuse of Children published a Position Paper on Allegations of Child Maltreatment and Intimate Partner Violence in Divorce/Parental Relationship Dissolution, which refers to "an attempt to alienate the child from a parent. . . . Such indoctrination is a form of psychological maltreatment."
- In 2017, the American Professional Society on the Abuse of Children published The Investigation and Determination of Suspected Psychological Maltreatment of Children and Adolescents, which says that "restricting or interfering with or directly undermining the child's important relationships" is a form of psychological abuse.

Still another example of France's ideological groups' attempts to smother any discussion or publication of parental alienation literature is seen in the fiasco involving the esteemed French psychiatrist Paul Bensussan. Bensussan, who has been honored by the French government for his work as a forensic psychiatrist, was appointed a National Psychiatric Expert by the French Supreme Court.[109] In 2016, Dr. Bensussan was invited to contribute an article regarding alienation by the editors of the French medical encyclopedia *Encyclopedie medico-chirurgicale*. Dr. Bensussan did, and, after a "reading committee" of peer reviewers made some suggestions, submitted a revised article that was accepted for publication. Bensussan's article was published in the online version of the *Encyclopedie* in March 2017; however, a few days later, the

109. (2018, January). A tale of two editors, *Parental Alienation Int'l*, 10.

article was removed. Apparently, "a female psychologist and her colleagues had complained to the editorial board of *Encyclopedie*, and the editors immediately conceded to the protesters without informing [Bensussan] or giving him any chance of reply."[110] Ultimately, the French journal of psychiatry *L'Encephale* published Bensussan's article, along with an editorial from William Bernet (Emeritus Professor of Psychiatry & Behavioral Sciences, Vanderbilt University) in its December 2017 issue.[111]

Critics of the French Ministry's negative stance against parental alienation have complained that the Ministry's view is willfully blind to the research of "hundreds and thousands of researchers" from around the world.[112] They also point out that the Ministry refuses to acknowledge the well-established fact that while the term "parental alienation" does not appear in the DSM-5, the concept and its psychiatric sequalae are included in the treatise.[113] Given the French courts' acceptance of SAP, the French ministry's position is retrograde and contrary to other European countries' view and treatment of parental alienation, including the European Court of Human Rights.

But there is hope. The French Ministry's position on PA is refuted by publications that investigate the dynamics of parental alienation.[114] Also, the *Association Contre L'aliénation Parentale pour le Maintien de Lien Familial* (ACALPA) (Association against Parental Alienation and for the Maintenance of Family Ties), founded by Olga Odinetz in 2004, brings together people, parents, and professionals; provides cutting-edge research and information about parental alienation; interacts with the media; participates in related conferences; and has even trained police about parental alienation in order to aid in their duty to enforce parenting time orders.[115] ACALPA is registered by the French Ministry of the Interior as an association of aid and support to victims of child abduction and parental abductions.

Despite the vehement attempts by France's ideological groups, it appears that the construct of SAP is recognized in France. The release of [Psychiatrist] Marie France Hirigoyen's 2012 book devotes 43 pages to the topic of PA and

---

110. *Id.*

111. *Id.*

112. *See* French Minister of Families, *supra*.

113. *Id.*

114. *See, e.g.*, Broca, R., & Odinetz, O. (2016). *Separations Conflictuelles Et Alienation Parentale*. This book, published in French, does an excellent job in exploring the dynamics of parental alienation and provides specific examples provided by adults who had been alienated as children about the ongoing effects of the alienation. The author was provided with an unofficial English translation of Chapter 1 (The Concept of Alienation and Its Recognition in France).

115. Association Against Parental Alienation and for the Maintenance of Family Ties (ACALPA), at www.acalpa.org.

considers the phenomenon as child abuse.[116] Also, the publication of the book *The International Convention on the Rights of the Child: A Special Convention* in 2014 was a decisive turning point in recognition of SAP in the French-speaking world.[117] The book contained a chapter on SAP and its damaging effect on the alienated child and discussed the jurisprudence from the European Court of Human Rights condemning the phenomenon. Despite the controversy surrounding SAP, French courts continue to crack down on alienating behaviors. In September 2015, the Criminal Court of Lyon, after presiding over a trial wherein an expert psychiatrist testified about SAP and a father's manipulation of the children, convicted the father of "psychological violence against his children" and sentenced him to five months of imprisonment.[118]

Traveling across the Rhine, it is notable to mention Germany's good beginning. The German organization Väter für Kinder (Fathers for Children), founded in 1988, was a positive one. The organization puts out information on psychological and legal aspects of custody. Its web site (www.beideeltern.de) is frequently consulted by parents, professionals, students, and the media. Germany's Federal Ministry of Justice regularly asks for comments on any new law drafts related to family law, and sometimes the German Supreme Court does as well, prior to making custody-related decisions.[119]

> An important conclusion to draw from this experience, which applies also to other web sites that report on developments from other countries and also to translations in print, is that only if these reports closely relate to the situation in their own country will there be a significant resonance.[120]

There was a major breakthrough in Germany in the late 1990s when a team of researchers wrote about the existing German family law and what they called "*Leuchtturmurteile*" (lighthouse judgments) that had described, independently, the alienating behavioral patterns that Richard Gardner wrote about in his work.[121] This work led to publication of more papers, seminars, media reports, and new judgments explicitly referring to the phenomenon of parental alienation.[122]

---

116. Broca, R., & Odinetz, O., *supra* (citing Hirigoyen, M.-F., Abus De Faiblesse Et Autres Manipulations (J - C. Lattès, 2012)). (Chapitre 1 "Emergence du concept d'alienation parentale et sa reconnaissance en France"). Also, telephone correspondence with Odinetz, Olga (Feb. 2, 2019) (with author).

117. *Id.*, Footnote 54 (citing Neirinck, Claire & Bruggeman, Maryline, La Convention Internationale Des Droits De L'enfant, Une Convention Particuliere, (Dalloz-Sirey 2014).

118. Broca, R., & Odinetz, O., *supra*.

119. Dum, C. T., *supra*.

120. *Id.*, at 428.

121. Kodjoe, U., & Koeppel, P. (1998). The Parental Alienation Syndrom (PAS) I, *Der Amtsvormund*, 72, 9.

122. Stadler, M., & Salzgeber, J. (1999). Parental Alienation Syndrom (PAS)—alter Wein in neuen Schläuchen? [Parental Alienation Syndrome (PAS)—Old Wine in New Skins?], 4 Familie, Partnerschaft Und Recht 231.

While the discussion on the topic of parental alienation was enthusiastic and in the popular domain, it was not followed up by original, empirically based research. Most of the "research" consisted of the exchange of opinions, rehashing the all-too-well-known controversies. This was not surprising. Peer review as a fair and effective tool for quality assurance in the field of psychology and behavioral sciences is largely unknown in Germany, although it has been a standard practice in the German academe's approach in natural sciences such as biology or physics.[123] Consequently, very few scientific papers on parental alienation from Germany have undergone peer review and made it into the largest psychological database, PsycINFO, of the American Psychological Association.[124] PsycINFO otherwise contains hundreds of peer-reviewed papers, currently some 360, with the key words "parental alienation."[125]

Further, what little did get published in Germany was not helpful. In 2001, a translated version of a polemical article was published in a widely circulated German family law journal.[126] This article, which criticized the phenomenon of parental alienation (syndrome), served as the key reference on this topic and was published in a prestigious, yearly handbook on German case law, the *Palandt*, "which is on practically every lawyer's and judge's desk."[127] This polemical article was cited by some German courts in rejecting parental alienation as a scientific theory. In 2006, due to the perseverance of some German experts, the *Palandt* replaced the polemical article with an article by

123. Dum, C. T. Begutachtete Aufsätze in Fachzeitschriften und das Parental Alienation Syndrom [Peer-reviewed Articles in Professional Journals and the Parental Alienation Syndrome], in Das Parental Alienation Syndrome: Eine Interdisziplinäre Herausforderung Für Scheidungsbegleitende Berufe [The Parental Alienation Syndrome: An Interdisciplinary Challenge for Professionals Involved with Divorce] 384 (von Boch-Galhau, Wilfrid, et al., eds., 2003).

124. *Id.* (citing Anneke Napp-Peters, Mehrelternfamilien als "Normal"-Familien – Ausgrenzung und Eltern-Kind-Entfremdung nach Trennung und Scheidung [Multi-parent families as "normal" families: Segregation and parent-child alienation after separation and divorce], 54 Praxis Der Kinderpsychologie und Kinderpsychiatrie, 792–801 (2005).

125. Dum, C. T., *supra*.

126. Bruch, C. S. (2001). Parental Alienation Syndrome and parental alienation: Getting it wrong in child custody cases, *Fam. L. Q.*, 35, 550. It is interesting to note that at the time of publication of her article, Bruch criticized the PA/PAS phenomenon as not having "scientific sufficiency" on the ground that it wasn't included in DSM-5 or ICD-10. Fast forward fifteen years and now we find that the concept of PA is included in DSM-5 and the term "parental alienation" is included in ICD-11. *See* Bernet, W., Wamboldt, M. Z., & Narrow, W. E. (2016). Child affected by parental relationship distress, *J. Am. Acad. Child & Adolescent Psychiatry*, 55, 571. Bernet, W. (2018, July). ICD-11 includes parental alienation, *PASG Newsletter*, 3. In addition, in 2006, Bruch's article was thoroughly debunked as "junk science." *See* Lorandos, D. (2006). Parental Alienation Syndrome: Detractors and the junk science vacuum. In Gardner, R. A. et al. (Eds.), *The International Handbook of Parental Alienation Syndrome*, Charles C. Thomas, 403–406.

127. Dum, C. T., *supra*, at 429.

Richard Warshak,[128] translated by Dr. Christian Dum and commented jointly by Dr. Wilfrid von Boch-Galhau.[129]

Difficulties associated with "lost in translation" and lack of publication of scientific papers in the German language has created an unfortunate situation. In 2007, an article appeared in a German family law journal with an arbitrarily altered title, "Entfremdete Scheidungskinder?" ("Alienated Children of Divorce?").[130] In a flawed, but also slanted translation, a researcher's characterization of the author of the polemical article against parental alienation as a "women's advocate" became the German equivalent of "attorney for women."[131] Difficulties in translation led to some other anomalies, some funny (the colloquial "goodies" for enticements was translated as the equivalent of "sweets"), other not so much ("role-reversal" became the equivalent of "overidentification").[132] In the end, due to a lack of German publications (not even in translated versions), starting with the 2010 edition of *Palandt*, the handbook only contains a reference to a court decision of 2005 which rejected parental alienation based on the earlier-mentioned polemical article.[133]

Also, the tradition of training on issues related to alienation that we see in other European countries, organized by professional organizations and in part also sponsored by government agencies, is absent in Germany.[134] Professionals, lawyers, and judges tend to avoid mentioning the term "parental alienation" or "Parental Alienation Syndrome." And it is difficult, if not impossible, for German courts to order any kind of involuntary counseling, mediation, or therapy in family court cases. Such orders, if made, are coercive and regularly quashed by the appeals courts.

Adding to these problems in Germany are two other problems. The first is "the all-powerful role of the expert," in Germany's civil law system, whose opinion is not only unquestioned by courts but who is usually not subjected to a thorough cross-examination or rebuttal testimony as is typically found

---

128. Warshak, R. A., Eltern-Kind-Entfremdung und Sozialwissenschaften-Sachlichheit statt Polemik [Parent-child-alienation and social sciences-objectivity instead of polemics], 92 Zentralblatt für Jugendrecht, no. 5, 186-200 (2005).

129. Palandt, O., Bassenge, P., & Brudermüller, G. (2006). Gesetzbuch, Bürgerliches, [German Civil Code] (65th ed. Beck Juristischer Verlag).

130. Johnston, J. R. (2007). Entfremdete Scheidungskinder? [Alienated children of divorce?], Kindschaftsrecht und Jugendhilfe, no. 6, 218–224. Based on children of divorce who reject a parent and refuse visitation. Johnston, J. R. (2005). Recent research and social policy implications for the alienated child, *Fam. L. Q.*, 38, 757–775.

131. Dum, C. T., *supra*.

132. *Id.*

133. Bruch, C. S., *supra*, at 527–552.

134. For example, in London, U.K., a clinic run by Karen and Nick Woodall, in cooperation with the "Child and Youth Protection Center" of Zagreb, Croatia, undertakes serious and competent work in the area of Parental Alienation. *See* Family Separation Clinic, at https://www.familyseparationclinic.com.

in the common law systems.[135] The second is the "cultural" issue that gives a significant deference to the "voice of the child"—even if that child happens to be alienated and giving voice to "the expectations of the custodial parent."[136] Many cases end with the "patent solution" of suspending all contact between the child and the alienated parent—"child has to come to rest"—often until the child reaches maturity. Sometimes, a case ends up in the European Court of Human Rights, but often there is no intervention. In the infamous case of *Buchleither*,[137] for example, the Applicant/Father alleged that the indefinite suspension of contact between him and his daughter had violated his right to respect for his family life under Article 8 of the Convention for the Protection of Human Rights and Fundamental Freedoms. At the heart of the controversy was the German courts' exclusion of the father from contact with his daughter, and the baffling rationale of the German Court of Appeal, which held: "It is up to the mother to overcome her aversion to the father, and up to the father to learn that contact can only be reinstated through patience, restraint and understanding of both the mother's and child's feelings."

The case was closed at the end of a very tortuous and litigious history, making the following notations: "1. Seen. Nothing to be done. 2. To be stored."[138] The majority (four versus three) opinion of the European Court of Human Rights held that the German court, in suspending the father's contact with his daughter, did "not overstep the margin of appreciation afforded to the domestic courts in matters concerning a parent's contact with his or her minor child, and can still be regarded as having been 'necessary' in a democratic society."[139] Hence, the Court ruled, there was no violation of Article 8 of the Convention. But the dissenting judges disagreed. They held that the child was "in a loyalty conflict" with her mother and the German courts were not justified to suspend contact without a time-limit and "without counterbalancing the serious impact of this decision."[140] The dissent also pointed out, "The problem did not seem primarily to lie with the father but with the mother and her aversion to the father" (as is typical in cases involving parental alienation).[141] The dissent wrote about the German court's "positive obligation," i.e., "the national courts are under a positive and ongoing obligation to reassess the situation and to try to overcome any of the obstacles which might hinder the granting of even very

---

135. Kaul, J. (2018, May). German case study: Consequences of legal failures concerning parental alienation, *PASG Newsletter*, 24-26. (Ms. Kaul is quoting from an article by Dr. Michael O. Heuchemer, Kardinalfehler der Rechtsprechung im Umgangsrecht, Familie und Recht 368–372 (2017), at http://www.fur.luchterhand.de/.

136. Kaul, J., *supra* note 122.

137. Application No. 20106/13, Buchleither v. Germany, [2016] Eur. Ct. H.R. 399.

138. *Id.*, at 5.

139. *Id.*, at 11.

140. *Id.*, at 13.

141. *Id.*, at 14.

limited contact."[142] "The [German] authorities should have actively taken measures in order for the father to see his daughter and, even more importantly, for the daughter to see her father." Given the German court's lack of action, the dissent believed that there most certainly was a violation of Article 8 of the Convention.

While many German courts remain skeptical of parental alienation, a form of interdisciplinary cooperation successfully practiced since 1993 in the German province of Cochem, Rhineland-Palatinate, appears to be an effective way in dealing with PA cases. The "Cochem practice," as it is known in Germany, attempts to address PA and prevent its associated social, medical-psychological, and economic consequences.[143] The Cochem method de-escalates the parents' conflict by

> changing the 'winner-loser' attitude of parents and professionals and restor[es] parent-autonomy and responsibility based on protecting both children's rights and parents' rights. It requires a high degree of experience and qualification of the interdisciplinary professional groups involved in working with high [conflict] divorce families.[144]

Now German organizations and professionals are working together to develop a better understanding of parental alienation. In September 2016, *Deutsche Kinderhilfe*, an independent, non-partisan organization that works for children's rights and child protection, supported a workshop on parental alienation.[145] Then, in September 2016, the German "Kindergerechte Justiz" conference was held in the House of the Federal Press Conference in Berlin, which included a workshop titled, "Parent–Child Alienation: Identification, Understanding and Assessment."[146]

In German-speaking countries—especially Austria and Switzerland—a similar practice consisting of a cooperative procedure of psychology and law has been offered for some years.[147] Also, there appears to have been limited research on parental alienation in Austria. Despite strident complaints of how Austrian mothers have significant power to alienate the children against their

---

142. *Id.*

143. Boch-Galhau, W., *supra.*

144. *Id.* (citing Jürgen Rudolph. You are my child—The "Cochem practice"—Ways to a human family law. Berlin: Schwarzkopf & Schwarzkopf; 2007), at http://scholar.google.com/scholar_lookup?title=Du bist mein Kind—Die „Cochemer Praxis"—Wege zu einem menschlichen Familienrecht&author=J.Rudolph&publication_year=2007.

145. Foerster, C. (2017, March). Developing better understanding of parental alienation in Germany, *PASG Newsletter*, 8–9.

146. *Id.*

147. Boch-Galhau, W., *supra.*

father and abuse the court system, not much has been done about it.[148] Austrian courts seem to severely limit or outright suspend fathers' access to children based on manipulation, misperception, and a lack of understanding of the theory of parental alienation.[149] And, even though Austria has codified joint custody into law, in practice, it is done only when the mother agrees to it.[150]

Further north, in Sweden and Norway, the phenomenon of parental alienation remains controversial. Despite the Scandinavian policy trend toward equality between parents, the rate of children's loss of their contact with mothers has risen but not the number of children losing their fathers after separation or divorce.[151] On the other hand, Swedish and Norwegian courts have challenged the existence of parental alienation and with some very few exceptions refused to give any weight to expert testimony on this issue.[152] The documented existence of parental alienation has not found acceptance in the Nordic mental health community—perhaps due to the fact that little has been done in terms of publication and awareness of parental alienation in the Swedish or Norwegian languages.[153] The classic book by Lena Hellblom Sjögren, *Barnets rätt till familjeliv: 25 svenska fall av föräldraalienation (The Child´s Right to Family Life. 25 Swedish Cases of Parental Alienation*) was published in 2012 by a large Swedish academic publishing house. However, protests from a loud group of women defining themselves as child and women protectors caused that company to withdraw the book from publication, so it was published privately in 2013. Very recently, in 2019, a journalist, Anna Lytsy, and a lawyer, Christina Bergenstein, published *Barn som tvingas välja bort en förälder: föräldraalienation i Sverige: fakta, rättsregler, erfarenheter (Children Who are Forced to Reject a Parent: Parental Alienation in Sweden: Facts, Legal Rules, Experiences*). The authors emphasize that parents, mental health professionals, social service workers, and the judiciary need to be educated regarding the alienation phenomenon, which they define as psychological child abuse.

Further south, in Italy, there are two different kinds of professional interventions that are designed to assist and support parents through the separation and divorce process: family mediation and child custody evaluation practices.

---

148. Franklin, R. (2012, July 20). Austria: Unmarried Fathers to Get Parental Rights, National Parents Organization, at https://nationalparentsorganization.org/blog/20651-austria-unmarried-fathers-to-get-parental-rights.

149. Blesch, A. (2013, October 28). Parental Alienation Syndrome: Austrian case studies, Academia, at http://www.academia.edu/10328727/Parental_Alienation_Syndrome_Austrian_Case_Studies.

150. *Id.* (citing Franklin, *supra*).

151. Areskoug, N.-G. (2019, January). Parental slienation: A Swedish perspective: Introduction to a transgenerational case study with policy recommendations: Towards a Resolution of the controversy in science and society on parental alienation, Book I (2013), *Parental Alienation Int'l*, 15, 1.

152. *See, e.g.*, Family Law Matter, No. T 8831-16 (Goteborgs Tingsratt Nov. 16, 2017).

153. *See* Sjogren, L. H. (2002, October 18–19). Presentation at Interdisciplinary Challenge for Professionals Involved in Divorce, International Conference: Making a parent dangerous: PAS in Sweden and Norway (Frankfurt, Germany).

Mediation is voluntary and a matter of choice, whereas child custody evaluations are imposed by a judge.[154] Since 2006, a new law has been introduced in Italy regarding divorce and child custody.[155] The new law recognizes joint legal custody as the "privileged and customary form of parenthood exercise."[156] This law preserves not only the "best interests of children," allowing them access to both parents, but also preserves and protects each parent's right and duty to exercise the parental function after the breakup of the marriage or relationship.[157]

Italian courts have addressed the construct of parental alienation and have not hesitated to take the necessary remedial action.[158] One of the early cases dealing with parental alienation arose out of Milan and involved a child of divorced parents who wanted to live with his father.[159] However, the court found that the father was paranoid about the mother's intentions to "kidnap" their son and he repeatedly attempted to isolate the child from the mother. The court explicitly referred to the father's behavior as constituting parental alienation and ultimately awarded custody to the mother.[160]

In another case, the court found that the mother had alienated the daughter from the father by telling her he was going to take her away from her mother and instilling a false fear in her mind, which led the daughter to refuse to visit her father. The court recognized that the daughter's fears and negative opinion of her father were unfounded and derived from the mother's ill will. The court fined the mother and ordered more frequent and longer visitation with the father.[161]

Italy has also demonstrated a robust professional and research-backed approach to combat alienation. The Italian Society of Neuropsychiatry of Childhood and Adolescence (SINPIA) has described parental alienation as psychological abuse in its official guidelines.[162] Another organization, REFARE (Reconnecting Family Relationships) is the first Italian healthcare treatment on parental alienation. Based in Cosenza, Calabria, the program was created by

---

154. Ranieri, S. et.al. (2016). Promoting coparenting after divorce: A relational perspective on child custody evaluations in Italy, *J. of Divorce & Remarriage*, 57, 361, 362.

155. Law 54/2006; also see Ranieri, et. al., *supra* note 141, at 361–373.

156. Ranieri, S., *supra*, at 362.

157. *Id.*

158. *See* Giurisprudenza, Alienazione Parentale.It, at https://www.alienazioneparentale.it/giurisprudenza/ for Italian decisions on parental alienation.

159. Un'ordinanza del Tribunale per I Minorenni di Milano, No. 1652 / E / 97 (ord. 19/6/1998).

160. *Id.*; also see Lubrano Lavadera, A. et al. (2012). Parental Alienation Syndrome in Italian legal judgments: An exploratory study, *Int'l J. of L. and Psychiatry*, 35, 334–342, at www.sciencedirect.com/science/article/pii/S0160252712000477.

161. Decree, Family Law Matter at 9 (Trib. Milano Section IX Civ. 2017), at www.crdf.it/Upload/636264831729976633_decreto_tribunalemilano_marzo2017_alienazioneparentale.pdf.

162. Linee Guida Anno 2018 [2018 Guidelines], Societa' Italiana Di Neuropsichiatria Dell'infanzia E Dell'adolescenza (SINPIA) [The Italian Society of Neuropsychiatry of Childhood and Adolescence (SINPIA)] (30 Aug. 2018), at www.sinpia.eu/linee-guida/linee-guida-anno-2018/.

Marco Pingitore, a psychologist and psychotherapist, along with Alessia Mirabelli, a psychologist.[163] The REFARE program is provided only after a court decision and is based on various preconditions.

Further, Italy has formed an umbrella organization, Adiantum, consisting of various parent–child organizations to represent their agenda more effectively.[164] In a hearing by the Italian Senate in July 2011, Adiantum advocated the inclusion of parental alienation in the current shared custody reform project. Unlike France and Germany, Italy has a tradition of awareness of parental alienation connected to academic teaching and research. Also, several comprehensive books on the construct of parental alienation are available in Italian. They are complemented by peer-reviewed articles that have appeared mostly in the journal *Maltrattamento e Abuso all'Infanzia*, with special editions focusing on parental alienation in 2005 and 2009.

By way of illustration, in 2015, Italian psychologist Maria Christina Verrocchio and the well-known American researcher and author Amy J. L. Baker published a paper on Italian adults' recall of childhood exposure to parental loyalty conflicts.[165] Their surveyed 739 adults in Chieti, Italy, regarding their childhood exposure to twenty "parental loyalty conflict behaviors," "psychological maltreatment," and "measures of current functioning."[166] The loyalty conflict behaviors that were surveyed (one parent making untrue or disparaging statements about the other parent, one parent asking the child to keep secrets from the other parent, etc.) are commonly recognized as alienating behaviors by experts[167] and also by judges in the United States, United Kingdom, Canada, and elsewhere. Verrocchio and Baker's findings support the theory that children's exposure to parental conflict has detrimental effects on their long-term functioning and poses a significant risk factor for adult well-being.[168] Earlier, in 2013, in another paper, the same team of researchers surveyed 257 undergraduate psychology students in Italy regarding their childhood exposure to parental alienating behaviors and found "high levels of reported exposure" to such behaviors.[169] The study also found that "those with any exposure to parental alienation reported higher rates of parental psychological maltreatment, lower rates of parental caring, as well as poor functioning with respect to

163. REFARE—Reconnecting Family Relationships Program: Trattamento Psicologico Alienazione Parentale, Marco Pingitore, Psicologo-Psicoterapeuta, at www.marcopingitore.it/refare-program-alienazione-parentale/2203.

164. *See* Associazione Di Aderenti Nazionali Per La Tutela Dei Minori, www.adiantum.it.

165. Verrocchio, M. C., & Baker, A. J. L. (2015). Italian adults' recall of childhood exposure to parental loyalty conflicts, *J. Child Fam. Stud.*, 24, 95–105.

166. *Id.*, at 95.

167. Baker, A. J. L. (2007). ***Adult Children of Parental Alienation Syndrome***, W.W. Norton & Company.

168. Verrocchio, M. C., & Baker, A. J. L., *supra*, at 95.

169. Baker, A. J. L., & Verrocchio, M. C. (2013). Italian college student-reported childhood exposure to parental alienation: Correlates with wellbeing, *J. of Divorce & Remarriage*, 54, 609–628.

self-esteem, depression, adult attachment styles, alcohol abuse, self-direction, and cooperation."[170] These findings support the theory that parental alienation represents a risk factor for compromised outcomes across the life span.[171]

In Spain, the construct of parental alienation has generated robust scientific discussions and publications amongst the country's mental health professionals.[172] By 2005, Spanish Provincial Courts had rendered several judgments that contained an indication of parental alienation.[173] Spanish law prohibits one parent from interfering in the other parent's exercise of parental authority,[174] a behavior typically found in cases of parental alienation. If the target parent is vigilant and reacts to the early signs of alienation, Spanish courts will intervene, and the alienating parent may face sanctions.[175] In Spain, repeated interference or infringement on the rights of the target parent may even result in a change of custody.[176]

A group of researchers investigated 783 divorce and separation judicial decisions in Spain, most of which were approved without considering the concept or presence of parental alienation. The review found that in Spain, there is a preference in most families to opt for maternal custody in cases of divorce and separation.[177] Also, Spanish judges grant custody more frequently to mothers because of their belief that the mothers have more time available to care for children.[178] Further, only in cases where mothers presented severe behavior was custody assigned to fathers.[179] A different researcher analyzed divorce decisions from Spanish courts from 2008 and 2011 in which parental alienation was mentioned as grounds for appeal.[180] The researcher found that, despite the different reasons presented by the parents for initiating the process—parental authority, custody change, etc.—accusations of parental alienation permeated most pleas.[181]

On the heels of significant research on the importance of the child's maintaining a relationship with both parents after divorce and separation, in 2005 a

170. *Id.*, at 609.

171. *Id.*

172. Gaffal, M. (2012). Parental alienation in divorce judgments, *InDret*, 4 (citing to the research papers that were published in Spain, at http://dx.sdoi.org/10.2139/ssrn.2182523.

173. *Id.*

174. *Id.*

175. *Id.*

176. *Id.* (citing Spanish Law on Civil Procedure (Art. 776.3 LEC)).

177. Gaffal, M., *supra* note 172.

178. Kelly, R. F., Redenbach, L., & Rinamon, W. C. (2005). Determinants of custody arrangements in a national sample of divorces, *Am. J. of Fam L.*, 25–43.

179. Gomide, P. I. C., et al., *supra* note 87, at 291–298 (citing Arce, R., Farina, F., & Seijo, D. (2005). Razonamientos judiciales en procesos de separacion [Judicial reasoning in parental separation and divorce proceedings: Content and cognitive analysis of judicial reasoning], *Psicothema*, 17, 57–63, at http://www.psicothema.com/pdf/3064.pdf

180. Gomide, P. I. C. et al., *supra* (citing Gaffal, M., *supra* note 172, at 1–23).

181. Gomide, P. I. C. et al., *supra*.

new law was introduced to facilitate joint custody as a preferred post-divorce parenting option.[182] The motivation for the new law was an emphasis on the principle of parental co-responsibility. However, a 2013 study investigated the knowledge of court professionals (judges, lawyers, technicians) concerning the phenomenon of parental alienation and found a lack of knowledge and, worse, misconceptions regarding the construct, suggesting that there is a need for training.[183]

The first National Symposium on Parental Alienation in Spain took place in 2006, organized by the Official College of Physicians of Madrid. It was followed by other conferences by professional organizations with broad participation by experts from Spain and abroad. In 2011, the Center for Domestic Violence and Gender, part of the Ministry of Health, Social Policy, and Equality, issued a report that warned that parental alienation represented "dangerous consequences for mothers and children."[184] On the other hand, the governing body of Multidisciplinary Spanish Association for the Investigation of Parental Interference (ASEMIP) has endorsed the inclusion of parental alienation in DSM-5 and ICD-11 and has issued a comprehensive report on this topic.[185]

Spanish judges, however, have routinely adjudicated claims of parental alienation. In a case where a psychological evaluation found no evidence of alienation and the mother refused to accept the results and asked the Court to repeat testing, the Spanish family judge held that "specialization in PAS [is] not a necessary condition for the psychologists to render an expert assessment."[186] The Court instead found the mother's authoritarian style and domineering behavior to be the source of the daughters' rejection. In another case where the mother was found to have repeatedly violated the visitation agreement, the Court intervened and sanctioned the mother to pay a fine.[187]

There are provisions of the Spanish Civil Code which have enough teeth to prevent parental alienation. If a parent repeatedly interferes with the other parent's right to visitation with the children, the Spanish Criminal Code provides

---

182. *See* Act 15/2005 on the Modification of the Civil Code and the Law of Civil Procedure in the Field of Separation and Divorce.

183. Gomide, P. I. C. et al., *supra* (citing Saldaña, Angela Cristina Tapias, Bobadilla, Lizzette Alejandra Sánchez & Torres, Sandra Teresa Torres, (2013). Reconocimiento de indicadores de alienacion parental en operadores de justicia de Bogota [Recognition of parental alienation indicators in Bogota operators of justice], 20 Suma Psicologia, no. 1, 111–120, at http://publicaciones.konradlorenz.edu.co/index.php/sumapsi/article/view/1354 and http://www.redalyc.org/articulo.oa?id=134229197010.

184. Nafs, A. E. et al. (2010). Report by the Research Task Force on Parental Alienation Syndrome, at https://bit.ly/2Ov0Oiv.

185. Fariña , F. et al. (2010). Separación y Divorcio: Interferencias Parentales, Asociacion Espanola Multidisciplinar De Investigacion Sobre Interferencias Parentales (ASEMIP), at www.usc.es/export9/sites/webinstitucional/gl/servizos/uforense/descargas/Separacixn_y_Divorcio._Interferencias_parentales.pdf.

186. Gaffal, M., *supra* (citing to SAP Albacete 12.12.2007 (JUR 2008\101505; MP: Rodriguez, Manuel Mateos).

187. Gaffal, M., *supra* (citing SAP Toledo 23.3.2011 (JUR 2011\189719; MP: Urbano Suárez Sánchez).

more stringent measures to deal with the behavior.[188] Further, Spanish law provides necessary tools to family judges to take counter-measures against parental alienating behaviors.[189] There are three effective ways to do it. First, the judge can extend the target parent's visitation and grant him or her more time with the child. Second, if the alienating behaviors continue, the judge can change custody in favor of the target parent. And third, in severe cases, the judge can invoke the provisions of the criminal code against the alienator to seek an appropriate and effective remedy.[190]

Regarding other European countries, a committee in The Netherlands, appointed by the government has "for the first time, acknowledged parental alienation" after receiving input from parents and others.[191] In December 2017, there was an article published in a Slovenian professional journal that provided a general overview of parental alienation.[192]

Meanwhile, the construct of parental alienation is not only recognized in Romania, but in 2016 was recognized as a form of psychological violence against children under Directive No. 2/2016.[193] The Romanian law defines abuse in Article 94 par. (1) of Law no. 272/2004 as

> any deliberate action of a person who is in a relation of responsibility, trust or authority towards this, through which there are jeopardized the life, physical, mental, spiritual, moral or social development, bodily integrity, mental or physical health of the child.[194]

In Romania, parental alienation is defined in the scientific literature as a form of severe emotional abuse that is committed against children.[195] More specifically, according to the definition specified in Romanian law, Article. 1 para. (1) of the Directive No. 2/2016, this form of abuse signifies the "activity of systematic denigration of one parent by the other parent, with the intention of the child's alienation by the other parent."[196]

The recognition and legal acknowledgment of parental alienation as emotional abuse intensified the need of education on the construct and how to deal with it in courts. The ARPCC (The Romanian Association for Common Custody) is a non-governmental organization that assists actors in the family legal system of common custody provisions in Romania. The organization claims to

---

188. Gaffal, M., *supra* (citing Art. 618.2 CP).
189. Gaffal, M., *supra*.
190. *Id.*
191. PA Gains Recognition in the Netherlands, PASG Newsletter at 3 (Mar. 2008).
192. *See* (2018, January). Breaking news from Slovenia, *PASG Newsletter*, 4 (citing to Matej Zaplotnik's article Starsevsko Odtujevanje, Pravosodni Bilten).
193. Matic, A., & Mirica, S. (2016). *Perspectives of Business Law Journal*, 5(1) 94–100.
194. *Id.*
195. *Id.*
196. *Id.*

"work with Romanian courts to compile a collection of good jurisprudential practices regarding the application of common parental authority."[197] The organization also distributes brochures and provides access to scholarly research databases to attorneys, judges, and other interested parties on a plethora of custody issues, including parental alienation.[198]

An allegation of parental alienation must be proven in Romanian court for that court to find a parent guilty of inflicting emotional abuse upon a child.[199] According to Article 331 of the Romanian Code of Civil Procedure, an expert will be appointed and will issue a report. Additionally, the Court will hear the minor child pursuant to Article 226 of the Criminal Procedure Code.[200] Overall, Romanian commentators agree that to resolve parental alienation will involve a holistic approach, taking into consideration the people whose relationships are affected, the underlying stresses they are subject to, and the consequences the proposed solutions will have on their lives.[201]

Conclusion

Many questions remain unanswered. Is one system or jurisdiction better than the other in addressing parental alienation? Is the civil law system more likely than the common law system to accept the reality of the phenomenon? Is it easier to prove a case of parental alienation under one system more than the other? Some experts believe that the civil law system, which allows "free rein" in presenting testimony, is superior to the common law system, which provides for checks and balances before expert testimony is presented to a trier of fact.[202] While this may be true in some instances, overall, in the civil law system it is up to the judges to determine the matters in dispute, identify the necessary evidence, and control the mechanisms of inquiry, thereby concentrating great power in the hands of judges. The risk with this approach is—as we saw in Germany, Sweden, and Norway—that civil law judges and their experts could prevent a robust presentation and examination of scientific theories along with their empirical support if these theories do not pass muster with some special-interests groups or are politically incorrect. While it is encouraging to see Brazil and Mexico's legislation that has codified the construct of parental alienation and also provided concrete remedial interventions (in Brazil's case,

---

197. The Romanian Association for Common Custody, at http://www.arpcc.ro/rapoarte.
198. *Id.*
199. Matic, A., *supra* at 98.
200. Matic, A., *supra* at 99.
201. Ibid.
202. Lorandos, D. (2013). Parental alienation and North American Law. In Lorandos, D., Bernet, W., & Sauber, R. (Eds.), *Parental Alienation: The Handbook for Mental Health and Legal Professionals*, Charles C. Thomas, 348.

criminal sanctions as well), generally speaking, civil law systems fall short of demonstrating a solid understanding and acceptance of the reality of parental alienation and, more importantly, the necessary remedial interventions. Common law systems on the other hand have been criticized for their scorched-earth litigation tactics and never-ending, intractable court cases. In addition, it takes a long time for court interventions to extricate the child victims from the clutches of alienators—sometimes years.[203] Nevertheless, in reviewing judicial opinions from Canada, United States, Australia, England—the common law systems—it is abundantly clear that the judges in these jurisdictions, for the most part, "get it." The trial-by-combat tradition allows the target-parent-party-litigant and his or her lawyer to identify the appropriate legal issues, select the evidence to be presented, and, more importantly, produce expert witnesses to present the evidence. With an opportunity to identify the proper legal issue, there also exists an opportunity to persuade the factfinder in crafting the appropriate remedy. In reviewing the common law system's court decisions, it becomes apparent that the dogged lawyers in these adversarial systems "understood that, for the most part, their judges tended to emphasize logic and linear thinking rather than express concern for emotional suffering or for feelings of others."[204] As these judges made decisions and wrote the judicial opinions—essentially, created "common law"—they left a trail for others to follow. As awareness builds, professionals, researchers, and clinicians come together and engage in an exchange of ideas and cutting-edge research in the field of parental alienation.

But human behavior and conflict has common denominators. In the end, whether we look at the civil law systems or those following the common law, parents who are implacably hostile toward each other leave a wake of destruction, often through litigation. Parents who continue to be at loggerheads and, following divorce or separation, continue to fight the battles of the past, show each other no respect, and engage in winner-takes-all mode of litigation undoubtedly cause their children serious emotional harm.

203. Lorandos, D., *supra*, at 420–421.
204. *Id.*

CHAPTER 9

Litigating Parental Alienation: Tips for Practitioners

The American Bar Association reports that family law is one of the top three highest risk areas of practice for attorneys in terms of malpractice exposure.[1] Within family law, cases involving parental alienation and related issues are some of the most challenging matters for a lawyer to handle.

In 2010, Dr. Amy J. L. Baker published a peer-reviewed paper containing the results of a survey involving parents who were targets of parental alienation. Dr. Baker's survey, published in her paper—"Even When You Win You Lose: Targeted Parents' Perceptions of Their Attorneys"[2]—focused primarily on client perceptions of key components of the attorney-client relationship as outlined in the American Bar Association's model rules of professional conduct, specifically: caring, competence, diligence, communication, advocacy, and advertising. The results of Dr. Baker's study highlighted the twin themes of frustration and powerlessness on part of the targeted parent-litigants. Their "narratives portray the chronic frustration, intense and overwhelming sense of helplessness and/or rage at the ongoing interference; and the nearly constant dread that as bad as things are, they will probably get worse."[3] The survey asked each participant targeted parent about his/her experience with his/her attorney(s). The questions covered areas related to lawyers' competence,

1. *See, e.g.*, https://www.americanbar.org/news/abanews/publications/youraba/2018/april-2018/why-every-lawyer-needs-malpractice-insurance/.

2. Baker, A. J. L. (2010). Even when you win you lose: Targeted parents' perceptions of their attorneys, *The American Journal of Family Therapy*, 38, 292–309.

3. *Id.*, 293.

diligence, and communication; them caring about the case; and their advisory role. The results of Dr. Baker's survey speak volumes about targeted parents' view of their attorneys and present a dismal picture of how attorneys typically handle cases involving parental alienation.

For instance, lawyers received a very low rating on the topic of attorneys caring about the client and the case. One targeted parent reported:

> The second attorney didn't care about my case. . . . She left the country to adopt a baby for an extended period of time, was completely unreachable and didn't have someone to cover her work for her. After about a year with her and many mistakes on her part (untimely responses to judge, etc.), we met with her in a last attempt to salvage the relationship. She told me, "No-one cares about your case . . . not even me, except that I represent you."

Other targeted parents reported that the lawyers were "in it" only for the money and lacked "any compassion or concern for the clients." One parent reported, "I feel like he couldn't care less about custody/access/visitation/parenting time. All he wanted to do was his paralegals and himself bill as many hours as possible." Yet another reported that the lawyer "told me to give up fighting for custody" and "tried to convince me to settle before all of my concerns were heard."

On the issue of competence, 60 percent of the targeted parents that were interviewed reported that "not one attorney understood parental alienation." The parents complained that apart from not understanding parental alienation, the lawyers who represent targeted parents did not understand the factual details of the case, were not familiar with the concerns of the client, and failed to file motions that were responsive to the clients' concerns. The parents' grievances against their lawyers had three main themes: bad advice, errors in fact or judgment, and lack of familiarity with parental alienation. Dr. Baker describes some examples of these parents' frustration with their lawyers:

> He guaranteed me if I did what he suggested it would look good to the court but in the end, it cost me my son.
>
> First attorney responded to first motion with gross errors in the document. She did not forward it to me for review prior to submission. This mistake damaged my credibility from the very start.
>
> I had a final male lawyer who said that even though he wasn't a divorce attorney it was "all the same." He thought I was owed child support and subpoenaed the tax consultant without asking me . . .
>
> None of the attorneys involved in my custody case understood the impact of PAS, how it doesn't go away as the children get older! They kept

telling me, "Once the divorce is over, they will come back to you" . . . they had NO IDEA!

My first attorney did not understand PAS at all and actually called Dr. Gardner a quack. I should have fired her at that time. She convinced me to follow the GALs recommendation and not fight for custody although the GAL clearly stated the father's actions were the cause of the estrangement the kids and I suffered.

I feel that both attorneys were not fully supportive of PAS issue . . . so I was treading on thin ice when I argued it to them which made me feel a lack of validation.

The vast majority of attorneys who represented the targeted parents were perceived as not preparing their clients for the myriad of professionals that become involved in cases involving parental alienation, including guardians ad litem, forensic evaluators, court-appointed therapists, psychological evaluators, and child protective service workers. As Dr. Baker reported, "around half of the sample reported that their attorney did not at all help them prepare for most of the professional interfaces involved in custody disputes." Adding to the targeted parents' frustration was their outrage that their lawyers did nothing to enforce their rights or to hold the alienating parent accountable:

My ex-spouse has currently over 50 violations of the current order within the past 1.5 years and NOTHING has been done about it.

The orders mean very little.

You can barely read a single paragraph of my final decree without running into an issue of non-compliance by my ex-wife.

A lawyer who takes on the challenge of representing a targeted parent must understand that the task requires thorough knowledge of the subject, enormous preparation, foresight, self-control, creativity, and energy. In addition, one can imagine the stress, anxiety, and horror of a parent who, along with the child, is clutched in the tentacles of the parental alienation monster and sees the life of the parent-child relationship slowly ebbing away. Such parents may come across as unreasonably demanding, overbearing, poor listeners, highly irritating, and entirely self-absorbed. It is fair to assume that clients who are going through parental alienation "are probably not any attorney's favorite client."[4] Additionally, this dynamic has the potential to cause a vicious downward spiral: the *more* the client shows her frustration and outrage at the "system," the *less* the attorney makes himself available or shows that he cares,

---

4. *Id.*, 306.

which further increases the feelings of helplessness and hopelessness of the client . . . and so on the downward spiral continues.

Family law lawyers taking on parental alienation cases can vastly benefit from proper training and education. Parental alienation has been observed and written about extensively for the last twenty to thirty years and has produced a wealth of information: books, articles in legal journals, articles in professional and clinical literature, peer-reviewed articles, research studies, continuing legal education programs, webcasts, podcasts, etc. It is imperative that lawyers who handle these cases take the time to thoroughly study the phenomenon of parental alienation, carefully evaluate the facts of the case for evidence of alienation, and discuss with the client (if necessary, with input from experts in the area of behavioral sciences) the appropriate legal and mental health interventions to remedy the situation.

Having represented targeted parents and litigated cases involving parental alienation and ancillary issues in a variety of jurisdictions all over the United States (and having consulted with clients, lawyers, and experts internationally), I have following tips to offer to my professional colleagues.

1. One of the oldest heuristics in medicine is *primum non nocere*: "First, to do no harm."

This maxim applies squarely to legal practitioners who are thinking of taking on a case involving parental alienation. Parental alienation cases are not only notoriously difficult but *profoundly* counterintuitive.[5] They require a tremendous amount of time, energy, patience, and an ability and willingness to delve into the behavioral sciences literature to learn the fundamentals. A lawyer who is asked to represent a targeted parent in a case involving parental alienation should first determine whether he is competent to take on such a case. The ABA Model Rules of Professional Conduct Rule 1.1. requires competence. "A lawyer shall provide competent representation to a client. Competent representation requires the legal knowledge, skill, thoroughness and preparation reasonably necessary for the representation."[6] No lawyer would take on a case involving a complex medical or psychiatric issue without ensuring that she possesses the required specialized knowledge, skill, and experience, together with the willingness to invest the time necessary for proper preparation, in order to provide a competent representation to the client. For example, an attorney who

5. Miller, S. (2018, July). Why do specialists say that parental alienation is counterintuitive, Part 2, *PASG Newsletter*, 3(4), 17.

6. *See* https://www.americanbar.org/groups/professional_responsibility/publications/model_rules_of_professional_conduct/rule_1_1_competence; also see Standards of Practice for Lawyers Representing Children in Custody Cases, ABA Section of Family Law (2003), III(A).

agrees to represent a client accused of severely injuring or killing an infant in a case involving diagnosis of Shaken Baby Syndrome would be expected to have basic knowledge of the concepts of *encephalopathy*, or brain swelling; *subdural hemorrhage*, or bleeding in the brain; and *retinal hemorrhage*, or bleeding in a part of the eye called the retina. On top of it, the attorney would be expected to "read," understand, and be able to explain to the court or jury, the intricacies contained in the results of an MRI scan, CT scan, skeletal X-ray, autopsy report, and ophthalmic exam. No lawyer would (or should) expect to take on such case involving a highly specialized topic and "wing it." But we routinely see family law practitioners who have little or no knowledge of the phenomenon of parental alienation, estrangement, enmeshment, or child alignment and, without any special training, representing targeted parents or alienated children in family courts. It is not surprising then how cases involving parental alienation not only get a bad reputation; are seen as "career killers" by lawyers and judges; and end up causing immense frustration for the lawyer, judge, and the parties involved.

Before accepting a client who complains of being a target of parental alienation (or a client who is accused of perpetrating parental alienation), a lawyer should go through a mental checklist. Ask yourself: Are you competent to handle the assignment? Do you have a solid understanding of the theory of parental alienation? Do you understand the difference between parental alienation and Parental Alienation Syndrome? Are you familiar with the myths and fallacies of the parental alienation theory? Are you prepared to debunk these myths and fallacies in court? Have you handled such cases before? What was the result? If permissible, would you be comfortable in allowing the potential client to speak with previous client(s) whom you represented in a case involving parental alienation? Do you keep up with the legal and mental health literature on the topic? And, last but not least, are you willing to put in the *significant* time and energy that will undoubtedly be required on your part to competently represent your client in such cases?

Severe parental alienation cases involve child psychological abuse and they take enormous toll on a targeted parent who is fighting hard to save the parent-child relationship while undergoing the trauma of being rejected by her flesh and blood. A lawyer should think hard and carefully before taking on a case involving parental alienation.

2. Check for and challenge your biases.

Cases of severe parental alienation tend to involve clinical—in a *medical* sense of the word—issues, such as psychopathology, cognitive distortions, emotional dysregulation, and bizarre behavior. These cases are not for a novice. This is not simply another facet of divorce litigation to make a lawyer think, "Why not give it a try?" Lawyers who do not understand the phenomenon of parental alienation often rely on intuition, which can often be misleading. Legal professionals—lawyers, judges, guardians ad litem, minors' counsel—like any other professionals, are susceptible to cognitive biases that can compromise deliberate, analytical thinking. The term *bias*, when used in a scientific sense of the word, refers to an error in reasoning. Dr. Steven G. Miller, one of the well-regarded experts on parental alienation, has described the interplay between parental alienation and the issues of heuristics (rules of thumb), biases, and metacognition.[7] It is critical to be aware of cognitive heuristics or biases and how they affect a lawyer's perception, thinking, and thereby his ability to frame and present a case.

As Dr. Miller explains:

> Human thought is not always analytical. For the most part, people do not make decisions by carefully weighing (or weighting) evidence and processing it in accordance with the laws of logic, probability, and statistics. The human brain is not well wired for that. Rather, they draw conclusions based on intuitive judgments. Such judgments rely on cognitive templates that permit humans to make quick, efficient, reasonably accurate decisions . . . these templates are known as cognitive heuristics.

For instance, consider the heuristic of the Fundamental Attribution Error: concluding that a behavior is dispositional when in fact is situational. Your client, a targeted parent / mother, sits before you. As her lawyer, you can clearly see that your client is angry. Very angry. She is angry about how her children mistreat her and disrespect her. She is angry about her ex, the father of the children, consistently undermining her as a parent, badmouthing and ridiculing her in front of the children. She is angry about how her parenting time is repeatedly violated, with zero consequences for such violations. She is angry about how no one "gets it." As an observer, it is quite likely that you, the lawyer, may think that your client has a characterological or dispositional flaw rather than looking at her behavior as situational. That is, you may think, "*I can see how angry she is in general. No wonder she is having problems with her kids and her ex. Perhaps, therapy can help her deal with her anger. In fact, I know just the right therapist who can help her.*" But just because a person is angry about a *specific* situation does not mean she is an angry person in *general*. However, because the human brain is hard-wired to give too much weight to dispositional factors and not enough to situational factors, it feels confident making seemingly natural (but ultimately, incorrect) judgments about people's dispositions and

---

7. Miller, S. G. (2013). Clinical reasoning and decision-making. In Baker, A. J. L., & Sauber, S. R. (Eds.), *Working with Alienated Children and Families: A Clinical Guidebook*, Routledge, 25–26.

characters.[8] Another cognitive heuristic or bias is the Affect Heuristic: engaging in "emotional reasoning" by making a judgment based on an emotion or feeling. Continuing with the example of the angry-mother-client, a lawyer could find the rejected parent off-putting because she is anxious or assertive. Such a lawyer would be more open to an argument of estrangement or a hybrid theory (i.e., both parents are at fault theory) from the opposing counsel, a guardian ad litem, or a minor's counsel, without looking at what the facts demonstrate. The lawyer, engaging in emotional reasoning, decides the case to be a hybrid case (instead of parental alienation), and accordingly frames the case as such before the court. Such a framing error, in turn, leads the court to a different conclusion and incorrect ordering of priorities (for example, focusing primarily on "reunification therapy," instead of protecting the children from abuse by the alienating parent). So, it is important to check for and challenge one's biases before framing a case involving allegations of parental alienation. A lawyer should ask herself, am I stereotyping? Do I find the rejected parent off-putting because he is anxious, agitated, and assertive? Could it be because he is actually afraid of losing his relationship with his child? Am I engaging in emotional reasoning? Have I been paying too much attention to information that supports my initial impressions and neglecting evidence that might refute those impressions? In other words, have I fallen prey to Confirmatory Bias? Unless the lawyer checks for and challenges her biases, she runs the risk of relying on her intuition and making a cognitive error.

3. Keep yourself abreast of the latest research, publications, and peer-reviewed literature.[9]

Parental alienation is a dynamic area and the research is constantly evolving. Also, it is *profoundly* counterintuitive.[10] And this is not merely a warning to "be careful"; rather, professionals who have thoroughly studied this area caution us how everything about parental alienation is so counterintuitive—*profoundly* counterintuitive—that many professionals, legal and mental health, will almost always make major errors if they attempt to solve problems or make critical judgments using their usual professional or clinical intuition.[11] Using intuition to solve complex problems—"I've been doing this for a long time"

8. *Id.*, 29.

9. The bibliography provided at the end of this book offers suggestions about books that I have found very helpful in litigating cases involving parental alienation.

10. Miller, S. (2018), *supra*.

11. *Id.*

or "have seen many cases"—is rarely, if ever, adequate.[12] In cases involving parental alienation, it can be downright disastrous. Be prepared to challenge your assumptions or biases. Get ready to debunk the myths and fallacies that surround the theory of parental alienation. Be prepared to educate the court that, despite the commonly held belief, it is a myth that adolescents' stated preference should dominate custody decisions, especially if the adolescent has been alienated.[13] It is also a commonly held but false belief that courts cannot enforce orders for parent-child contact against an alienated teen's wishes.[14] Or that children who irrationally reject a parent but thrive in other respects (such as in school or with peers) need no intervention.[15] These common false beliefs have been repeatedly debunked in professional literature and judicial opinions. Nor have these assumptions held up when evaluated in the light of research, case law, or experience. Be prepared to get in the "hot seat." You may face criticism, even hostility, from your fellow professionals or court for being "aggressive." Be calm but firm, persistent but professional. It is a mistake to slide into complacency and think that the court or a court-appointed professional would eventually "see" what's going. Unless you present a strong, robust, and irrefutable case of parental alienation using a blend of science and law, there is a high likelihood that a court or court-appointed professionals may succumb to the fallacy of the "high conflict" model.

Aside from the books that I list in the Bibliography at the end of this book, I have found the following journals and periodicals helpful in my career of litigating cases involving parental alienation:

- *Litigation*
- *Family Advocate*
- *Journal of Divorce*
- *Journal of Marriage & Family*
- *Journal of Family Law Review*
- *Family Law Quarterly*
- *Family Court Review: An Interdisciplinary Journal*
- *Journal of Family Issues*
- *Journal of Child and Family Studies*

Don't be afraid of reaching out to experts who contribute to these and other journals on the topic of parental alienation. In my experience, I have found professionals to be patient and extremely generous with their knowledge and

12. *Id.* (". . . people who attempt to use intuition to solve counterintuitive problems tend to have great confidence in their conclusions, whether right or wrong.").

13. Warshak, R. (2015). Ten parental alienation fallacies that compromise decisions in court and in therapy, *Professional Psychology: Research and Practice*, 6–7.

14. *Id.*

15. *Id.*, at 7.

time when discussing the subject. Show your interest; be curious; ask questions. As you learn more and discuss the topic with the experts, you will build your confidence.

4. Frame the case properly.

Don't frame a case of child abuse as a child custody and visitation case. Professional literature makes it clear that causing severe parental alienation is a form of child psychological abuse. Therefore, it is critical that the number one priority in such cases is to protect the child from further abuse. Instead, more often than not, lawyers and mental health professionals ignore and downplay the abuse issue and, instead, focus on the child's relationship with the rejected parent. A leading forensic psychologist, Dr. Robert A. Evans, writes:

> Attorneys need to fully understand the dire consequences to children as a function of being alienated from a parent. The more an attorney appreciates how parental alienation is an adverse childhood experience, a clear form of child abuse, the more passionate they will pursue direct and cross examinations. The Court has to fully understand how this phenomenon is destroying our next generations and treat these cases as if the children's lives are at state, which they are![16]

The failure to properly frame the case shifts the focus from child protection to getting more parenting time for the rejected parent. Instead of taking urgent and appropriate measures to ensure the child's safety and mental health, courts and professionals soon begin discussing "reunification therapy." This is a striking example of a misunderstanding of legal and clinical priorities. As an analogy, given evidence of physical or sexual abuse, *no* professional—legal or mental health—would choose to focus on remedial measures *without first ensuring that the child is out of danger* and is no longer at risk of further abuse. Failure to do so would not only be absurd but endanger a child's physical and emotional well-being. Psychological abuse, including parental alienation, is no different from physical or sexual abuse when one considers the sequalae of such abuse. And in such scenarios, the primary goal must be to protect the child from further abuse.

---

16. Correspondence between Ashish Joshi and Dr. Robert A. Evans, on file with the author.

5. Get ready to debunk the most commonly held fallacy of parental alienation cases—the "high conflict" model.

The high conflict model *assumes* that both parents are equally or significantly responsible for the family dynamics. It also *assumes* that a child's rejection of or resistance to one parent cannot be traced to primary contributions from the other parent. It is, of course, plausible that this indeed may be the case—that upon a forensic evaluation, one could determine that the case is "hybrid"—with both parents contributing to the family dynamics and the child's rejection of or resistance to a parent. But it would be a mistake, and a huge one at that, to simply *assume* from the outset that a case is a "high conflict" case simply because the parties appear to be hostile to each other or because one party (or both) has been aggressively filing motions with the court seeking relief. It would be no more fitting to assume that a rejected mother is equally or substantially responsible for her child's rejection of her than it would be to hold a mother equally or substantially responsible for her husband's physical abuse of the children without first undertaking an investigation. The high conflict model fails to consider the possibility that one parent might be the alienator or aggressor and the other might be in a defense mode, trying to manage a horrific family crisis and to save the parent-child relationship.

It is possible that, in some cases, the rejected parent's behavior can add to or worsen the family dysfunction. But this does not mean that the rejected parent is equally responsible for a child's *alienation*, which was formed due to the alienating parent's psychological abuse and through use of specific alienating behaviors. From both clinical and legal perspectives, the assumption and use of the high conflict model in a case of parental alienation is one of the worst mistakes a professional can make. Operating under this fallacy, professionals (and court) turn a blind eye to the history of the now rejected parent's relationship with the child, the "baseline" relationship. Succumbing to cognitive errors, such as Fundamental Attribution Error or Confirmatory Bias, professionals start citing aspects of the rejected parent's personality or behavior that the children complain about, such as being too strict about homework or not giving enough attention to the child's extracurricular activities, without considering that this parenting behavior had not previously undermined the child's love, affection, and respect for the parent. Operating under the high conflict model—holding both parents equally culpable for the child's rejection of one parent—mental health professionals are likely to avoid making recommendations that they believe would take the children out of their comfort zone. The much-dreaded words, "baby steps," are used in making recommendations that typically require that the child remain with the favored parent while undergoing "therapy" to overcome his or her negative perception of the other parent.

This "therapy" proceeds in an unproductive manner and take a life of its own. The therapists advise the rejected parent to "show empathy" and to modify his or her behavior, not realizing that the child's complaint about the parent's behavior is simply a pretext and not the reason for the child's rejection of the parent. The more the process validates the child's complaints (which have no basis in reality) as legitimate, the more frustration is caused to the targeted parent who sees herself caught in this nightmarish Groundhog Day of a situation. Unless a proper forensic evaluation, done by a competent professional, has determined a case to be a hybrid case that shows how both parents have contributed to the child's rejection, it is a mistake to label the case as a "high conflict" case.

6. Don't use the term "parental alienation" lightly.

Understand that it took many years for parental alienation to be accepted as a legitimate process or theory by the courts. Now that we find almost universal acceptance by American family courts of parental alienating behaviors that can cause severe harm to a parent-child relationship, parental alienation has entered into an "overkill zone."[17] Lawyers and litigants appear to allege alienation at the drop of the hat. Inappropriate or bad parenting is equated with "parental alienation." Conclusory, even diagnostic, assertions are made without evidence, and terms such as "narcissist," "sociopath," "alienator," are thrown around in court filings. A practitioner should be careful in how he chooses to present a case of parental alienation. The last thing you want is to lose credibility in the court's eyes or desensitize a court towards the issue by overusing or misusing the term "parental alienation." Just because a child is resisting contact with or has rejected a parent, doesn't make it a case of parental alienation. Courts have thrown out allegations of "parental alienation" where they have found no evidence of alienation.[18] And expert testimony alone will not save the day. It is critical that an expert opinion is supported and substantiated by *evidence* of parental alienation.

17. Clawar, S. S. (2020). *Parent-Child Reunification: A Guide to Legal and Forensic Strategies*, American Bar Association, 25.

18. *See, e.g.*, Moir v. Moir, No. 323725, 2016 WL 555838, at *11 (Mich. Ct. App. Feb. 11, 2016), appeal denied, 500 Mich. 881 (2016); *In re* Marriage of Daniel, No. B174755, 2005 WL 1515414, at *4 (Cal. Ct. App. June 28, 2005); Maxwell v. Maxwell, 2008-Ohio-1324, 2008 WL 754861, at *5 (Ohio Ct. App. March 24, 2008).

7. Parental alienation cases are "won" (if that's the right word for these heart-wrenching cases) through meticulous and careful preparation.

It is critical to provide the tools to the trier of fact (forensic evaluator, custody evaluator, judge, or jury) to get the appropriate intervention and remedy. One of the effective ways to prove a case of parental alienation in a court is to present evidence using the Five-Factor Model. Remember, the Five-Factor Model requires that we consider the following factors in determining whether parental alienation is present in a particular case: (1) the child actively avoids, resists, or refuses a relationship with a parent; (2) presence of a prior positive relationship between the child and the now rejected parent; (3) absence of abuse or neglect or seriously deficient parenting on the part of the now rejected parent; (4) use of multiple alienating behaviors on the part of the favored parent; and (5) exhibition of many of the eight behavioral manifestations of alienation by the child.

Envisage each factor as an empty bucket and start filling up the "buckets" with evidence—photographs, video recordings, audio recordings, greeting cards, emails, voicemails, letters, eyewitnesses, records, etc. Conduct proper and thorough discovery. If there has been involvement of child protective services or law enforcement, get copies of every child protective services or police report. Protective services workers and police officers record witness statements when conducting an investigation. Such statements may provide you with proof of an alienating parent's campaign of denigration, badmouthing, false accusations, boundary violations, and triangulation. For instance, a police report may show that the father disparaged and bad mouthed the mother to the police officer while the child was present in the room. These reports may reveal an alienating parent's triangulation of other professionals to act as her allies in her campaign of destroying the other parent's relationship with the child.

For example, child protective services reports may reveal that a parent provided specific details to the protective services worker that the parent knew (or should have known) were false. Or the report may unravel a scheme whereby an alienating parent takes the child to a healthcare worker (who is a mandated reporter) where the child makes an accusation against the other parent that the professional is duty bound to report to the protective services. Once the investigation is commenced, the alienating parent then "suggests" to the protective services worker to contact the professional who recorded or memorialized what the child had alleged, thereby providing "corroboration" of the allegation. These reports may also reveal inconsistency in witness statements or statements earlier made in court filings that may prove invaluable for cross examination at a later stage.

Similarly, get hold of the child's medical and mental health records. In most states, a parent has a statutory right to obtain his or her child's records.[19] These records may reveal a pattern of alienating behaviors. For example, the records may show an alienating parent taking the child to a routine medical appointment and then using the occasion to make allegations against the other parent of inappropriate behavior. Sometimes this is done in front of the child; at other times, it may be done in a private session with the clinician or healthcare provider. No matter how it is done, the goal of the alienating parent is to get the professional to "record" this allegation in the child's medical record, which is later used as proof of the rejected parent's inappropriate behavior. So, a routine dental checkup record could reveal an accusation about the rejected parent's "alcohol addiction" or "pornography addiction" and may provide evidence of an alienating strategy or behaviors. In one instance, I found a child's therapist, who had been triangulated by the alienating parent, to have paid a personal visit to the child's pediatrician to discuss the complaints made by the child and the alienating parent against the rejected parent, without the rejected parent's knowledge or consent. The ensuing deposition of the therapist revealed a lot of other alienating behaviors.

Consider requesting the court to compel the alienating parent and the children to produce their electronic devices for a forensic examination. In this day and age of text messaging and social media, electronic devices, especially smart phones, can provide a goldmine of relevant and material information. Such an examination may expose an alienating parent who pretends to encourage and facilitate a relationship between the other parent and the child but, in reality, is indoctrinating and brainwashing the child into rejecting the other parent. For instance, a Tennessee court found a father to be an alienator and a "passive/aggressive liar" when the text messages between the father and the son were examined and which revealed the father indoctrinating the son by telling him that he had "a right to be ugly" to his mother, that his mother was "mentally

19. *See, e.g.,* Michigan statute, MCL 722.30. "Access to records or information by parents. Notwithstanding any other provision of law, a parent shall not be denied access to records or information concerning his or her child because the parent is not the child's custodial parent, unless the parent is prohibited from having access to the records or information by a protective order. As used in this section, 'records or information' includes, but is not limited to, medical, dental, and school records, daycare provider's records, and notification of meetings regarding the child's education." Also, parents have a constitutional right to the record and/or information of their children pursuant; *see* Troxel v. Granville, 530 U.S. 57, 66 (2000), "[I]t cannot now be doubted that the Due Process Clause of the Fourteenth Amendment protects the fundamental right of parents to make decisions concerning the care, custody, and control of their children."

ill," that "the bible tells us clearly that mental illness is a spiritual problem," and that the son "will never like her [since] nobody likes her."[20]

8. Build a detailed chronology.

When gathering, selecting, and organizing years' worth of convoluted facts involving different kinds of proofs, I like to use the "Clancy Method" of organization. I learned this method from my mentor and former law partner, Dr. Demosthenes Lorandos. The Clancy Method is a trial planning and presentation methodology developed by Dr. Lorandos and attorney Patrick Clancy of The Innocence Legal Team. Here is what you do:[21] First, create a master document file, by scanning into an Adobe Acrobat (.pdf) file, every document, picture, witness statement, report, or transcript. The clients (and their family and friends) should be involved in scouring their memories, photographs, greeting cards, emails, letters, reports, old transcripts, school records—whatever they can get their hands on that goes to show either the alienating parent's behavior, or the sign of alienation in the child, or both. Second, create a master chronology of three columns in a program such as Excel or Word. In column 1, write the date of each event of significance to the case; in column 2, the who, what, where, how, and why do we care details about each significant event. The columns 1 and 2 encapsulate the factors (4) and (5) and contain details regarding an alienating parent's behaviors and signs of alienation present in the child. If required, the chronology could be expanded to cover other factors as well. For example, columns 1 and 2 could offer details about the factor (2), information supporting the "baseline" relationship between the now rejected parent and the child from a historical perspective. Finally, in column 3, I include "the how do we prove" information about the event or behavior. Column 3 holds the exact location of the proof needed for trial—the exact page, paragraph and line number of the relevant record which is cross-referenced with the master document file. Thus prepared, the detailed chronology provides a blueprint for discovery strategy, trial preparation, and, ultimately, presenting evidence supporting a case of parental alienation.

20. McClain v. McClain, 539 S.W.3d 170, 189 (2017).
21. Lorandos, D. (2013). Managing clients in life-threatening litigation, *Litigation*, 39(3), 46–51.

For instance, here's what an excerpt of a typical chronology would look like:

Date	Event	How Do We Prove
August 1, 2019	Parental Alienation Strategy #1 – Badmouthing Father badmouthed the mother in front of the children. Called her "retarded," "alcoholic," and a "slut."	Police Report dated August 1, 2019, page 13, para 2 Witness: Officer John Doe [Note: Need to depose the witness]
August 25, 2019	Behaviors of Alienated Children #3 – Lack of Ambivalence & #6 – Absence of Guilt Little Jack told his school counselor that he wishes his father were dead. That he would rather kill himself than go visit his dad. That his family is his mom and her boyfriend, who are perfect. That his father is a "loser" who never pays child support and should be in jail.	School Counseling Notes dated August 25, 2019, page 2, para 1 Witness: Ms. Jane Doe Also see: Deposition of Jane Doe, page 24, lines 2–22

Once a detailed chronology is prepared, mini-chronologies could be culled from the master chronology which would help the lawyer prepare for a deposition, witness examination, or preparing court filings. For instance, you could pull out all evidence of parental alienating behaviors from a master chronology and prepare a mini-chronology or timeline of alienating behaviors. Ditto for alienation symptoms present in the child. Such data could be very useful in educating the court and court-appointed professionals; preparing your expert; cross-examining the opposing expert; preparing your client to testify in court; and in presenting a coherent, robust case of parental alienation in the court.

9. Learn to manage the clients.

Parental alienation cases are notoriously difficult and extremely stressful to litigate. Often, they produce an alarming number of false allegations of physical, emotional, or sexual abuse by alienating fathers or mothers manipulating and indoctrinating their children into believing false ideas and allegations. A targeted parent-client may be involved in a "three-ring circus": a family court proceeding where she is attempting to see the children who are strongly resisting contact, a criminal court or investigation where she is defending against false allegations of abuse, and, on occasions, a licensing proceeding to defend against false allegations made or orchestrated by the alienating parent alleging violations of professional ethics or code of conduct. Such clients experience a host of emotions, including frustration, outrage, bewilderment, anxiety, and fear, caused by being falsely accused of heinous crimes or terrible behaviors, on one hand, and being rejected by their children, on the other. They suffer from what psychologists call "ego-dystonic incongruity, a life-threatening form of stress with physical and psychological ramifications. Clients undergoing it can become so overwhelmed by cascades of repeated stress that they cannot sleep, think, or aid counsel."[22] Think about getting professional help to manage such clients.

Stress management professionals (SMPs) can help lawyers to help clients navigate and survive the stress of contentious and protracted litigation. Such professionals can be experienced mental health professionals, such as psychologists, social workers, or licensed counselors. In one of our cases, our client, a targeted mother, was a teacher in the rural South. She was accused by her ex of sexually assaulting their daughter. As the ex / father developed the case, he was joined by several mothers in the community. Soon the mob hysteria kicked in and our client was facing the possibility of life in prison after being charged with 22 felony counts alleging abuse of three little girls. The client could neither sleep nor eat; she was frantically seeking confidants, talking to way too many people, and desperate for help. We retained an SMP "to channel her manic energy into developing the science and the facts for her defense."[23] Following a tense three-week trial, our client was found not guilty on all 22 counts. Consider including SMPs as a part of the legal team, but prior to doing so, check the applicable jurisdiction's case law on confidentiality and attorney-client privilege. A handy reference for this issue is the indispensable work on attorney-client privilege and work product doctrine by Edna Selan Epstein.[24]

10. Think about using a parenting coach to help the client.

One of the top experts on parental alienation, Dr. Amy J. L. Baker, offers this advice:

> One piece of advice I have for legal professionals is to not provide parenting advice to their targeted parent clients—unless the advice directly

22. Lorandos, Demosthenes (2013), *supra*, 46
23. *Id.* (Lorandos, Demosthenes is the former law partner of the author)
24. Epstein, E. S. (2017). *The Attorney-Client Privilege and the Work Product Doctrine* (6th ed.), American Bar Association.

> impacts on the legal case. For example, it is helpful for an attorney to explain to a parent that s/he must always show up for parenting time even if the parent and child claim that the child will not be available because not showing up can create a negative impression on a custody evaluator or a judge. However, advice about how/whether to discipline a child is, in my opinion, outside the scope of what a legal professional should be discussing with a client. Another point I would like to make is that many targeted parents feel unprepared for custody evaluations and often make mistakes in that setting by doing and saying things that create a negative impression. I suggest that legal professionals advise parents to consult with a mental health professional about how to approach that situation in order to avoid what could be a catastrophic outcome for the client.[25]

Dr. Baker's advice is right on the money. Children are precious to their parents. They remain so even during terrible arguments between the parents. They remain so when parents separate and divorce, and when parents embark upon life after divorce. So, what happens when suddenly your child is "terrified" to be alone with you? What do you do if your beloved daughter, whom you tucked in every night and read a bedtime story, falsely accuses you of being "abusive"? What do you do when your teenage son accuses you of being a "narcissist" and a "jerk"? How does one manage the irrational, unjustified rejection of one as a parent? How does one counter the visceral, hateful falsehoods and distortions that are thrown against one during visitations and parenting time with the children (if the children are seeing the parent at all; many times, such accusations are made by text messages):

> "You were never there for us!"
> "You are an alcoholic!"
> "You are a narcissist!"
> "You cheated on dad/mom and abandoned your family!"
> "We hate you! I wish you were dead."

It is incredibly painful for rejected parents to experience their children—their own flesh and blood—resisting contact with or rejecting them. Alienated children or children who have been subjected to alienating behaviors are not easy to parent. As one parent described her children, "I no longer recognize my kids. It's like the spark has gone out of their lives. They are little zombies. As soon as they see me, they put in their earphones on or go into their room and close the door. No hi, no hello. . . . nothing." The targeted parent faces a dilemma: If he "truly" loves the children, he should, as the children (and the alienating parent) asks, "leave them alone" and "walk away." If he does that,

25. Correspondence between Ashish Joshi and Dr. Amy J. L. Baker, on file with the author.

the children may be alienated for good and the relationship gone. If he refuses to "walk away," the children retort, "You don't get it! It's all about you." It's the classic damned-if-you-do, damned-if-you-don't conundrum. As one expert put it, the targeted parent remains "the monster in the horror show you can't escape from."[26]

In such scenarios, there is a danger of the targeted parent's frustration boiling over and engaging in behaviors that essentially play into the hands of the alienating parent. As one parental alienation expert, Randy Flood, writes:

> Over time, you grow angry—angry at your ex-partner, angry at the counselors, and maybe even angry with your children. The hurt is too painful, the fear is too overwhelming. . . . You know it isn't [the children's] fault, but you've grown weary and impatient of their rejection and increasingly angry at their flagrant rudeness and hostility, seemingly encouraged by your co-parent and enabled by the silence of professionals. As you continue to tread water, you become more and more pissed and eventually find yourself ready to either give up or go down fighting. In this surge of anger, you might begin to confront your children, the professionals, even speak out of turn in court. And what happens? You unwittingly begin to follow the script of the antagonist—the monster you were cast as. No one is helping, so you turn into a warrior, fighting to win each battle so you can restore order, civility, and sanity back into your life and your children's lives.[27]

The scenario that Mr. Flood describes far too often plays out in parental alienation cases. The targeted parent's frustration at the underlying family dynamics boils over and s/he attempts to "take charge" of the situation. In doing so, the parent may vent his or her frustration and make sub-optimal parenting decisions. An attempt to discipline and ground a child for rude and disrespectful behavior may lead to a 911 call or a complaint to the protective services for "abusive" behavior on the part of the parent. The alienating parent then leverages such incidents and complains about the targeted parent's "abusive" or "authoritarian" parenting, which has led to the children rejecting the parent. Professionals, who are not trained in the parental alienation dynamic, mistake reactionary behavior (to alienation) for causation (the targeted parent did not cause the children's rejection; s/he was merely reacting, perhaps sub-optimally, to such rejection). To avoid such situations, a lawyer should act proactively and consider recommending that the client retain the services of a parenting coach.

---

26. *See* Randy Flood's suggestions at https://menscenter.org/respond-to-parental-alienation/; also see https://www.amyjlbaker.com/coaching.html.

27. Flood, R., *supra.*

As Dr. Baker explains, coaching for targeted parents is designed to help the parent be a more effective parent while contending with an alienating parent and with an alienated child.[28] The goal here is to prevent the targeted parent from engaging in behaviors that are likely to exacerbate the alienation dynamic and increase the rift in the relationship between that parent and his/her child. Coaching is not therapy. It is solution-focused as well as present and future oriented. There is no discussion of the childhood of the targeted parent or their current mental health except as it affects or impinges on parenting. Such coaching can be done via remote means, e.g., over Skype or Zoom video calls or phone calls.

Parental coaching is a valuable tool in a litigator's toolbox. Not only does it prevent the lawyer getting burned out by getting numerous calls from a client who is trying to manage a very difficult situation at home, but it also helps the lawyer stay in her lane and focus on legal issues, instead of giving parenting advice. Further, if necessary, the targeted parent and/or the coach could later provide information to a court-appointed professional or testify in court about the efforts made by the parent to manage a tough situation. A court would certainly take into consideration the proactive and sincere efforts made by a parent in dealing with the parental alienation dynamic. However, the primary goal of seeking out the services of a parental coach is *not* to enlist an ally in the underlying litigation. Rather, it is to help the client, a targeted/rejected parent, be a more effective and empathetic parent without unwittingly adding to the alienation dynamic.

11. Select the right expert.

If a trial is in the cards—and in parental alienation cases, it almost always is—you will need a proper expert to help present a case of parental alienation. Dr. Lorandos drilled into me that expert testimony in cases involving parental alienation should cover the three "Ss" of parental alienation: symptoms of alienation, behavioral strategies of alienators, and the sequelae of parental alienation in the lives of the children affected.

When making a decision on using an expert, a lawyer will need to decide whether such expert should function as a "general," education-only expert or as a "specific," education-and-case-specific expert. The former expert would not be privy to the underlying facts of the case and would not offer an opinion as to whether parental alienation is present in that particular case. Such an expert would, however, describe the phenomenon of parental alienation, the peer-reviewed scientific literature in support of the condition, the Five-Factor

28. Baker, A. J. L. at https://www.amyjlbaker.com/coaching.html.

model for determining whether parental alienation is present, typical behaviors of an alienating parent, typical symptoms of an alienated child, short-term and long-term sequalae of parental alienation, and, last but not least, why the court should intervene in cases involving parental alienation, and intervene early rather than late. Such general expert can also answer hypothetical questions from attorneys and/or judge, which can help link the educational testimony to the facts of the case. In contrast, the case-specific expert would be familiar with the underlying facts of the case, having conducted a detailed review of the pertinent records of the case, and would proffer an opinion as to whether parental alienation exists and, if so, what evidence supports such a finding. The case-specific expert would also offer the educational or instructional testimony as to the phenomenon of parental alienation and all other related topics that a general expert would testify to. But with this latter kind of expert, the attorney need not ask hypothetical questions. Rather, the attorney can direct the examination into specific facts or issues present in the case, which lead the expert to opine on the existence of parental alienation. As discussed in the earlier chapter on presenting a case of parental alienation in court, there are pros and cons associated with each kind of expert, and a lawyer should weigh these carefully before making a decision on which kind of expert to use in a particular case or jurisdiction. Regardless of the kind of expert that a lawyer ends up retaining on a case—general or case-specific—it is important to do due diligence in finding the right individual for the job.

Also, ensure that you have set aside adequate time to work with and prepare your expert. Dr. Jennifer J. Harman, a well-regarded expert in the area of parental alienation and family violence, offers some words of advice:

> Don't be afraid to consult with attorneys who have effectively litigated cases of parental alienation. Family law practitioners can be likened to family medicine practitioners. If a patient presents with a specific medical concern that requires specialized assessment / treatment, they will be referred to a specialist or two for several opinions. This same approach can be very effective in parental alienation litigation, which requires a very specific set of data and skills to litigate effectively. I have seen so many cases fail because an attorney ignored my advice on consulting with a parental alienation litigation specialist. They were not prepared on how to build their case in court and use my testimony effectively. And they failed to recognize that they had several legal strategies that they could have considered. An hour or two with a more experienced parental alienation attorney can make a huge difference in the case.[29]

29. Correspondence between Ashish Joshi and Dr. Jennifer J. Harman, on file with the author.

Remember that, although there is considerable research and empirical studies in support of parental alienation theory, it still is an emerging field. On top of it, the field is rife with propaganda of misinformation—both deliberate and out of ignorance—and fallacies. It is not uncommon to come across "experts" who are well-credentialed but woefully ignorant of the basic literature, empirical studies, and research underlying the theory of parental alienation. Worse still, I have found professionals who routinely handle court-appointed assignments subscribe to the fallacy that parental alienation is not "real," or that it has been "debunked." Such "experts" refuse or fail to learn the fundamental research in the field, much less keeping up with the cutting-edge professional literature that is published on the topic by leading experts around the world. Not infrequently, when questioned about their knowledge of parental alienation, these "experts" retort: "Oh, I have done some reading."

Below are some tips in finding a good expert.[30]

(a) Ensure that the expert has an advanced degree (masters or doctoral) from an accredited educational institution in a relevant discipline or field (preferably psychology, psychiatry, or social work). This is not to discount the importance of lay counselors or coaches who, through their skill and experience, may have much to offer. However, parental alienation is a complex area that requires substantial understanding and professional expertise in behavioral sciences, and it is important to ensure that the expert has a solid educational background.

(b) Test the expert's knowledge of clinical literature. It is critical that the expert have a solid, extensive knowledge of the clinical literature regarding pathological alignment, alienation, estrangement, and enmeshment, together with an understanding of personality disorders such as borderline, narcissistic, and sociopathic personality disorders. Personality disorders are common among alienating parents but are often missed by non-specialists.

(c) Test the expert's knowledge of peer-reviewed literature. There is extensive peer-reviewed literature on parental alienation. Results of parental alienation have been subjected to peer review and have been published in peer-reviewed journals.[31] A comprehensive book on parental alienation, *Parental Alienation: The Handbook for Mental Health and Legal Professionals*, includes a bibliography with hundreds of peer-reviewed

---

30. Adapted from Baker, A. J. L., "How To Find an Expert in Parental Alienation," at https://www.amyjlbaker.com/index.html

31. *See e.g.*, Baker, A. J. L. (2020). Parental alienation and empirical research. In Lorandos, D., & Bernet, W. (Eds.), *Parental Alienation: Science and Law*, Charles C. Thomas, 247.

articles on the topic of parental alienation from more than thirty countries.[32]

(d) Test the expert's knowledge of legal literature on parental alienation. A mental health expert of course is not expected to know the intricacies of legal literature on parental alienation and how courts around the country have ruled on this issue. However, the expert should have a basic, jurisdiction-specific understanding of how family courts view the theory of parental alienation in that jurisdiction and the different kinds of interventions that courts have provided when confronted with evidence of parental alienation.

(e) Check for authored or co-authored published works regarding parental alienation, preferably in peer-reviewed publications. However, be judicious. An otherwise excellent clinician or forensic expert might not have published any scientific or peer-reviewed papers.

(f) Check whether the expert has completed continuing educational or training programs on parental alienation by qualified experts.

(g) Check whether the expert has taught or presented at continuing educational or training seminars before other mental health or legal professionals.

Check whether the expert has been qualified as an expert in the area of parental alienation or related issues by a court. Also check whether the expert was precluded from offering expert testimony or whether the expert's testimony was excluded by a court. If this is the case, explore, in detail, the facts of such preclusion or exclusion of the expert's testimony and give it careful consideration. Such exclusion or preclusion may not be the expert's fault, but you should nevertheless evaluate the risk with an eye towards your jurisdiction and the orientation of your court.

12. Consider the necessity and helpfulness of a forensic evaluation.

When confronted with allegations of parental alienation or related issues, some lawyers reflexively ask for (or agree to) a "psychological evaluation." The term "psychological evaluation" is a nebulous term and leaves a lot of room for confusion. Ask yourself: *Why* do you need a "psychological evaluation"? What purpose will it serve? What are you trying to get out of it? Are you trying to rule in or rule out parental alienation? Then say so! A court order

32. Bernet, W. (2013). References in the professional literature. In Lorandos, D., Bernet, W., & Sauber, R. (Eds.), *Parental Alienation: The Handbook for Mental Health and Legal Professionals*, Charles C. Thomas.

for a generic "psychological evaluation" is different from that which orders a court-appointed professional to conduct a forensic evaluation to check for the presence of parental alienation in a particular case. A forensic evaluation is geared towards assisting a trier of fact—a court—by formulating opinions that can responsibly be expressed with a reasonably degree of professional certainty. The sufficiency of information, both from a qualitative and quantitative perspective, is judged by a higher standard in a forensic evaluation than that might be applicable to a clinical or treatment evaluation.[33] A forensic evaluation places responsibility on the evaluator to employ forensic methods and procedures, requires the professional to conduct him/herself in a manner consistent with that of a forensic specialist and in keeping with the applicable guidelines.[34]

Further, undertake proper diligence in finding the right professional to conduct the forensic evaluation. Don't assume that, simply because a suggested professional is a psychologist, he or she will be knowledgeable on the topic of parental alienation. Psychologists are assumed to be experts in areas of psychological science due to their education, training, and experience. However, not every psychologist is expert in all areas of psychology, and even experts within a specialized field are likely not to be familiar with everything that is relevant and material and that has been published in that field unless that expert happens to be a specialist. Learn the difference between an expert and a specialist. An expert is a person who has special skill or knowledge in some particular field, whereas a specialist is a person who devotes herself to one subject or to one particular branch of a subject or pursuit. Before proposing a name of an evaluator (or agreeing to one), inquire of the professional as to whether she has evaluated cases involving parental alienation. Ask the professional about the methodology employed to conduct such an evaluation. Ask the professional whether she has ever found parental alienation to exist in a case that she evaluated. If so, was it mild, moderate, or severe? How did she come to that conclusion? What recommendations did the professional put forward to remedy alienation? Did the professional suggest any specialized intervention programs for the alienated child and the targeted parent to attend? Which ones? How do we know which programs work? Is there any data available?

Choosing an evaluator is perhaps the single most important thing in a case involving parental alienation. Courts give a lot of weight to an independent, court-appointed forensic evaluation. It is imperative that the lawyer exercises due diligence to ensure that the professional chosen to perform this evaluation

33. *See* Gould, J. W., & Martindale, D. A. (2007). *The Art and Science of Child Custody Evaluations*, Guilford, 19.

34. For example, in the case of psychology, the evaluator should be aware of the specialty guidelines for forensic psychologists, the guidelines for child custody evaluations in divorce proceedings, and the ethical principles of psychologists and code of conduct. Gould, J. W., & Martindale, D. A., *supra*.

has the proper educational background, knowledge, training, skill, and experience in evaluating family dynamics for the presence of parental alienation.

13. Prepare the client for the forensic evaluation.

A forensic evaluation is an investigation, not *therapy*. One of the sure-fire ways to tank a forensic evaluation is for a lawyer to counsel his client "to be him/herself" when meeting with the evaluator. Remember the Snickers commercial where a belligerent Joe Pesci turns into an affable young man after taking a bite of the candy bar? Sending an unprepared targeted parent-client is like sending in Joe Pesci to a forensic evaluation. A targeted parent who is distressed by his or her children's rejection, who is outraged by the repeated violations of his/her court-ordered parenting time, who is frustrated having been through several baffling and infuriating "therapy" sessions with his/her children, is a person who has undergone trauma. Without proper preparation, such person, typically, is ill-equipped to present a coherent picture of the family dynamics to an evaluator. On top of it, experts have found that alienating parents tend to present well, whereas targeted parents tend to present poorly. As Dr. Steven G. Miller writes,

> [a]s a rule, alienating parents present with the Four C's. They are cool, calm, charming, and convincing. That is because effective alienators tend to be master manipulators who are highly skilled at managing impressions, especially initial impressions. . . . In contrast, targeted parents tend to present with the Four A's. They are anxious, agitated, angry, and afraid. That is because they are trauma victims. They are attempting to manage a horrific family crisis, usually without success, often while being attacked by professionals who fail to recognize the counterintuitive issues. Indeed, non-specialists often get these cases backwards—they conclude that the alienating parent is the more competent parent. That is likely to be catastrophic error . . .[35]

Unless a lawyer takes the time to ensure that the targeted-parent-client understands the dynamics of a forensic evaluation, there is a high risk that the client will rush in and regurgitate the pent-up complaints and frustration and simply trash the alienating parent. The client risks playing into the hands of the alienating parent who has or will portray the client as "abusive," "angry," "authoritarian," "devoid of empathy," or simply difficult to deal with.

35. Miller, S. G. (2018). Why do specialists say that parental alienation is counterintuitive? Part 1, *Parental Alienation International*, 3(3), 20.

It is important for a lawyer to carefully explain to the client the workings of a forensic evaluation.

For starters, understand (and explain to the client) that the targeted parent is neither the "client" nor the "patient" of the evaluator. The evaluator is assigned a job by the court and is acting as the court's agent or as an arm of the court. There is neither confidentiality nor privilege in a forensic evaluation. There is no patient and no therapist. There is no "off the record" or "between us" chats. The evaluator's role is to interview the parents and the children, obtain third-party information in the form of collateral interviews, review the relevant documents and records, undertake psychological testing if necessary, and provide an opinion on particular issues with a reasonable degree of professional certainty. To put it simply, in a case involving parental alienation, the evaluator's job is to rule in or rule out parental alienation (of course, there may be other dynamics involved such as estrangement). The evaluator is not providing treatment of anyone for anything.

In a case involving parental alienation, a forensic evaluator's job is to peel the onion of facts and allegations. An evaluator generates multiple hypotheses. For example, hypothesis #1 could be that the children have rejected the mother because the father has alienated the children against the mother. Hypothesis #2 could be that the mother's own behavior has led to the children's rejection. Hypothesis #3 could be that the case is "hybrid," which includes bad behavior on the part of both parents. And so on. An evaluator collects data through interviews, record review, and psychological testing and attempts to prove or disprove the hypotheses. It's a structured process.

Help the client prepare for the meeting with the evaluator. The primary goal is for the client to be honest, appear credible, and be likeable. Too many evaluations have gone sideways when a targeted parent walks in with the zeal of a crusader with binders full of documents to "prove" parental alienation to an evaluator. Go back to the Five-Factor Model. Put the chronology that you painstakingly prepared, with the help of the client, to a good use. Put forward the F-A-C-T-S, not opinions. Avoid using terms "parental alienation," or "Parental Alienation Syndrome," or "pathological enmeshment." Avoid referring to the alienating parent as a "narcissist," or "sociopath," or worse. Using pejorative epithets and diagnostic labels will not help your client. Leave the diagnoses and findings to the evaluator. Instead, have the client tell his/her story and provide the facts.

Forensic evaluators follow a structured process, and it usually starts with interviewing the parties. Follow the lead of the evaluator. S/he is the one who has (should have) questions for the client. Help the client practice listening to the questions asked and answering *those* questions, not the information that the client is desperate "to get on the record." It does not help when the evaluator asks: *Tell me about your relationship with your children before the separation?* And the client answers: *What relationship? Their psycho father/mother has completely destroyed my relationship with the kids! Wait till you hear what happened just this last weekend . . .*

It would be helpful to orient the client to present the facts of the case in keeping with the Five-Factor Model. Start by discussing the relationship with the ex-spouse or ex-partner. What was it like prior to the separation or divorce? What attracted them to each other? Explain the highs and lows of the relationship. Talk about the birth of the children. Was your client present at the birth? What was the client's role as a parent during the children's early years? Was the client the primary caregiver? If not, it's okay—there's no need to panic and invent facts. It's common for one parent to be the primary caregiver and the other to focus more on meeting the family's needs, at least during the children's infancy. But provide details of the parenting roles. Talk about the parent-child relationship prior to the separation or break-up of the marriage. If the children now have specific complaints against the rejected parent, were these issues present before? For instance, if a child is accusing the mother of having "abandoned" him or "never being there" when the child was young, talk about all the events that the parent planned, put together, and participated in, such as birthday parties, Halloween parties, picnics, soccer games, vacations, school trips, etc. This information would help the evaluator assess whether the children's complaints have any merit or are a product of distorted reality and indoctrination. Was the client an involved parent? Did s/he attend parent-teacher conferences? Coach or attend children's extra-curricular sport activities? Volunteer at the school's fundraisers, picnics, drama competitions, etc.? Talk about it. Also, many clients walk into an evaluation with nothing but bitterness or contempt for the other parent. This is understandable, given that the now rejected parent is humiliated, embarrassed, hurt, angry, and afraid, with everything that's going on with his/her relationship with the children. But if things were different "back then," and the other parent was co-parenting willingly without any complaints or accusations, talk about those times. Don't be afraid to share strengths of the other, now alienating parent. If the father, who now is an alienating parent, took time to help the children with their math homework, share the information with the evaluator. Alienated children and alienating parents have polarized view of the targeted parent—there is nothing good or positive about the targeted parent; there never was. Don't return the favor and offer a similar polarized view of the other parent. The goal here is to help the evaluator open a window into the "normal," healthy, and loving relationship that the now rejected parent enjoyed with the children prior to the separation or filing of the divorce. Remember, parental alienation involves disproportionate rejection of a parent by the child—the child's rejection of the parent is *far out of proportion* to anything that the rejected parent is alleged to have done. It is important for to provide information about the "baseline" relationship so that the evaluator can juxtapose the "then" relationship with the "now" scenario and assess the magnitude of the child's rejection.

Next, address the allegations made against the client. I find it helpful to ask clients to make a list of all the things they have been accused of. How is the client being portrayed by the alienating parent or the children? Is the portrayal accurate? Why not? How do we prove it? For instance, if the rejected parent is being portrayed as an "alcoholic," is there any truth to it? Has the client ever had problems with alcohol abuse? Any episodes of arrests or convictions related to alcohol consumption? Problems at work? Any embarrassing incidents at work or social gatherings? More importantly, was this rationale for rejecting a parent an issue before? Did the *child* have any complaints about the parent's behavior—true or not—prior to the separation or filing of divorce? Was the child even aware of the issue (if there is/was such a problem)? If there are allegations of abuse or domestic violence, address them. If there was an episode of inappropriate behavior, explain what happened (if the incident is subject to criminal investigation, the client should discuss the matter with his or her criminal defense attorney prior to discussing the issue with the forensic evaluator because there is no confidentiality or privilege attached to the evaluation). Was such an incident a one-off incident? An unfortunate, but situational episode? Or were there others? This is one of the most important areas of a forensic or custody evaluation, and the lawyer must help the client address the issues of abuse or domestic violence. Ignoring the issue or downplaying it will not help. If the client is ashamed of how he or she behaved during the incident, talk about it. If the client was made to attend any classes (or chose to do so proactively), such as anger management or group therapy, discuss it. It is important to help the evaluator see that if there was inappropriate behavior, marital or parental, the client has admitted the wrongdoing, has sought professional help, and is unlikely to behave in that manner again.

Be prepared to discuss the alienating behaviors on the part of the alienating parent. But don't "lecture" the evaluator. One of the pet peeves of forensic evaluators is a parent bringing in books or professional literature, flagged or highlighted, and explaining to the evaluator how their case is a "textbook case of parental alienation." *I mean, how can you not see it? It's evident!* Don't do it. Instead, again, provide the facts to the evaluator. Instead of saying, "my ex, the mother, has alienated the children," tell the evaluator if the mother has undermined the client's parental role. Provide examples of the alienating parent badmouthing the targeted parent in front of the child, at school, with the neighbors, at workplace, with friends, with family members. Instead of saying, "the father interferes with my parenting time," talk about how the father repeatedly and consistently texts or calls the children when they are with their mother. Discuss how this affects the children. Don't rush. Take your time to provide the details and examples. The evaluator may have to have more than one meeting with the client to get all of the facts. Similarly, discuss the signs or symptoms of alienation present in the children. Again, the client does not need to use the labels or jargon used in the professional literature. Instead of saying, "My children show a lack of ambivalence," discuss how the children portray the client as all bad. Instead of saying, "My child uses Borrowed Scenarios," talk about how the child has accused the targeted parent of things using words and expressions that are identical to those used by the alienated parent. Keep in mind that forensic evaluators are not passive recipients of offered information; the client is not sitting down in front of a scribe who simply takes down what's said. Evaluators will pose questions—to the parties, children, and collateral sources—they will attempt to confirm or disconfirm data and their working hypotheses and maintain their overall investigative mindset. The overall objective when meeting with the forensic evaluator is to provide the facts in a clear, cogent, and concise manner.

I believe that preparing the client for a forensic evaluation is a critical part of litigating parental alienation cases. If a lawyer does not believe that this is within the scope of the attorney-client relationship, he should alert the client to the need for preparation and make referrals or suggestions for such preparation. But "no attorney should remain silent on this matter as it could result in clients doing harm to their case by not understanding the purpose and nature of these interactions and evaluations."[36]

14. Help the client prepare a package of well-organized documents for the evaluator's review.

Forensic evaluators' findings, recommendations, and opinions are only as good as the data that they are based on. An experienced forensic evaluator is always prepared to meet an examining lawyer's (or judge's) question, "*Where'd you get that?*" and explain her analysis. Record review is an important part of the forensic evaluation process. Evaluators review a wide variety of records—photographs, videos, audio recordings, letters, emails, greeting cards, affidavits, transcripts, court pleadings, school records, therapy notes, medical records, police reports, child protective services reports, and a host of other kinds of materials. Again, when reviewing the records, the evaluators are operating from an investigative mindset and are trying to confirm or disconfirm data or information provided to them or the hypotheses generated by them.

---

36. Baker, A. J. L. (2010), *supra*, 308.

For instance, when attempting to investigate the allegations of a mother who now alleges that her marriage was plagued by persistent domestic violence and abuse, an evaluator may look at the divorce complaint and filings to see if the mother made allegations of abuse and whether such allegations were investigated by an independent, neutral party. The evaluator may check for the issuance of any personal protection orders by a court. He may review the police reports for allegations of abusive conduct and for any admissions of such behavior from the parent accused of such behavior. To investigate an allegation from a father who now alleges that the reason the child refuses to see her mother is because the mother "was never around" when the child was growing up, she/he would look to photographs, videos, school records, medical records, etc., to confirm or disconfirm this allegation.

It is important that the lawyer assist the client in putting together a package of documents and materials for the evaluator's review. Once such package is assembled, the lawyer should carefully go through it to ensure that the materials therein are relevant and material, properly organized, and do not contain any privileged material (such as attorney-client correspondence). Keep in mind that when information obtained by an evaluator casts a parent in a negative light, the evaluator will afford that parent an opportunity to offer a denial, an explanation, or a rebuttal. So, strive to present an accurate and complete picture to the evaluator. When submitting email correspondence, do not simply cherry-pick the emails that support the client's version of events. If the other parent sent email that refutes or otherwise negates the client's characterization of events, include the entire chain of email correspondence. If the evaluator ultimately finds the "missing" version (which she probably will), it will not help your client's credibility. It's better to present the complete facts, the first time.

Some evaluators may not accept documents offered by litigants but only from the attorneys. Most will insist that any documents forwarded to them should also be provided to the other side. When reviewing the list of documents or records provided to the evaluator by the other side, pay careful attention. If you find a document or record listed therein that you or the client are not aware of, ask to see a copy. There may be an opportunity to demonstrate to the evaluator that the alienating parent continues to portray the targeted parent in an inaccurate, false, or distorted manner. If so, take the opportunity. For instance, if the alienating parent argues that the targeted parent is abusive and provides old orders of protection that were later set aside by the court, but omits to provide the later orders, take the opportunity to educate the evaluator.

The exercise of putting together a package of materials for a forensic evaluator should be done carefully and with diligence. This is not a data dump. Do not expect an evaluator to comb through a mountain of haphazard documents and materials and find corroborating evidence to support the client's narrative.

It's the lawyer's job to help the client present an accurate, complete, and organized narrative to a forensic evaluator. Connect the dots for the evaluator. One way to do this would be to create a well-organized and tabulated binder of documents and materials. Prepare a table of contents listing every document or material (e.g., a flash drive or a CD containing audio recordings), preferably organized in a chronological or some other manner. It would be helpful if the table of contents provided the following detail: (1) exhibit tab number, (2) date relevant to the document or material, (3) a brief description of the document or material, (4) the relevance of the document or material. Think about submitting the binder together with a cover letter that briefly explains what is being submitted, when, the manner of delivery, and for what purpose. Providing relevant information in a detail-oriented and well organized manner makes the task easier for the evaluator. It also helps the lawyer later to effectively cross-examine the evaluator in an unlikely event where the evaluator goes rogue or ignores the information provided to come up with unhelpful findings and opinions.

15. Counsel the client to follow court orders and show respect towards the court and the legal process.

Targeted parents typically suffer from chronic frustration and an overwhelming sense of helplessness. When no relief is in sight and the interference with their relationship with the children continues (often with impunity), there is a risk that the parent may want to "shake the things up." Often, a lawyer's refusal or failure to seek timely action adds to the parent's frustration and outrage. A frustrated client is likely to express her frustration in an unhelpful manner. She may speak out of turn at a court hearing, refuse to make a child support or alimony payment, vent her frustration at the court or court-appointed professionals by writing letters or posting comments on social media, write letters or emails to the children explaining why she thinks they are "brainwashed," or refuse to see the children in a supervised capacity because "she has done nothing wrong." When faced with such a client, the lawyer should first ensure that the client knows and sees that the lawyer cares about the case. Take time to explain to the client the legal strategy and game plan. How do you plan on addressing the family dynamics including parental alienation? How do you plan on countering the other parent's violations of court orders? How do you plan on educating the court as to what's going on? A client who knows that her lawyer not only cares about the case but is also working diligently to execute a plan of action will not only be easier to deal with but will be an important ally in preparing the case for litigation. Some of my best outcomes in litigating parental alienation cases have been when the clients undertook the task of gathering and organizing a mountain of information for use in litigation. Encourage and empower the clients to help you help them.

Help the client understand that it's important that she/he not fall into the trap of not being able to see the forest for the tree. It is important to understand that judges, guardians ad litem, evaluators, parenting coordinators, and other family court professionals are human beings susceptible to impressions and bias. It is important to maintain professional decorum as well as credibility before the court. A client who is on a crusade to prove parental alienation "beyond a reasonable doubt" may be oblivious to his behavior, both in and out of court. For example, a father who is so obsessed with proving parental alienation that he chooses to attend an out-of-state rally instead of attending his own trial is neither going to invoke sympathy nor earn credibility with the court.[37] Similarly, a parent who chooses not to see his children rather than see them in supervised visitation risks a finding by a court that such a parent attempts to "seek visitation and access on his terms rather than those recommended by the children's therapists and the guardian ad litem and ordered by the court."[38] This does not mean that the lawyer asks the client to simply comply with whatever is asked of the client without a protest. By all means, object to the supervised visitation if such a limitation on a parent's visitation has no merit. But if one is ordered by the court despite your objection, it's better to follow the court order and see the children than go without seeing the children.

16. Understand that time is the enemy.

Dr. Richard A. Warshak, author of *Divorce Poison*, and Past Clinical Professor of Psychiatry at the University of Texas Southwestern Medical Center, recommends lawyers to:

> Prioritize getting the case before the court quickly. Swift action is key to successful outcomes because the effects of toxic parenting spread rapidly. Secure detailed orders for parent-child contacts with penalties for noncompliance and move quickly for sanctions when the orders are violated. Your clients want their case treated with the urgency given to cases with missing children because, for them, their children are missing.[39]

In cases involving parental alienation, the lawyer needs to move as quickly as possible, avoiding any delays in litigation. Delays in these cases only serve

37. Sylvain v. Krajewski, 2009 WL 2231223.
38. *Id.*
39. Correspondence between Ashish Joshi and Dr. Richard A. Warshak, on file with the author.

the favored/alienating parent and can frequently allow the child to "age out" and be beyond the court intervention. Even if children don't reach majority, they frequently come of an age where judges simply assume that any decision related to reunification will be fruitless, or it's simply too late, or the children will reunite "on their own" as they get older. Dr. Robert A. Evans, a forensic psychologist, writes: "The research is perfectly clear that children do not simply reunite as they get older, in fact the research suggests that the time span for the alienation can be as long as 22 years."[40]

In any case involving parental alienation—mild, moderate, or severe—it is important "that the alienating behavior [is] rather quickly arrested."[41] In fact, a "mild" case of parental alienation provides a unique opportunity to arrest the progress of alienation and to stop the case from becoming a "moderate" or "severe" case. And often, the first red flags to go up are violations of court-ordered parenting time of the targeted parents. Lawyers representing targeted parents have to be diligent and ensure that such violations are immediately and effectively addressed. Appellate courts have instructed trial courts to enforce the court orders and especially in cases where one parent flagrantly disobeys the court's parenting time orders. For instance, an Indiana Court of Appeals reversed and remanded a trial court's failure to find a mother in contempt for her repeated violations of the father's court-ordered parenting time:

> [W]e are at loss as to why the trial court found that Mother was not in contempt. She has, over the past several years, repeatedly and flagrantly disobeyed the trial court's parenting time orders, orders that have affirmed on appeal by this court. Under these facts and circumstances, we have little choice but to conclude that the trial court abused its discretion when it concluded that Mother was not in contempt for failing to abide by the trial court's previous parenting time and reunification orders. On remand, the trial court should determine what sanction is appropriate to remedy Mother's obstinate disregard for the trial court's authority.[42]

Often, an alienating parent (or an unsuspecting guardian ad litem or minor's counsel who may be innocently ignorant of the phenomenon of parental alienation) will argue that it is the minor child who doesn't want see the targeted parent and that the alienating parent cannot make the child comply with the court-ordered parenting time schedule. When faced with such an argument, the lawyer for the targeted parent should first remind the court that over-empowering the child to make decisions on parenting time is a type of

---

40. Correspondence between Ashish Joshi and Dr. Robert A. Evans, on file with the author.

41. Hulsing, Hon. J. (2020). Parental alienation is one thing, but what are you going to do when they come for you? *Litigation*, 46(4), 6.

42. *In re* Paternity of P.B., 60 N.E.3d 1092, 1099 (2016).

alienating behavior and is tantamount to psychological maltreatment of the child (*parentification* or *adultification* of the child). In addition, the law is clear that in such situations, the proper solution is not to wring hands and concede defeat, but rather ensure compliance with the court orders:

> While we sympathize with the dilemma with which the trial court was faced, the proper solution was not to refuse to enforce its orders. Instead, the trial court should have used its authority to ensure that its orders are obeyed and not disregarded as mere suggestions. No one, especially not a parent, should be under the impression that compliance with the trial court's parenting time order is optional.[43]

If a parent is to be deprived of his right to parenting time with his child, the law requires a finding that such parenting time would endanger the child's physical health or significantly impair his emotional development; absent such finding, parenting time must be enforced.[44] When appropriate, judicious use of contempt power can be helpful in not only arresting alienating behavior but sending a clear message to targeted parents (and their allies) that such behavior will have consequences. I learned a long time ago that while a lawyer cannot do much about changing the pathological mindset or perceptions of an alienating parent, he can certainly address the *behaviors* of an alienating parent. For example, when a parent interferes with the other parent's parenting time, a court, upon receiving an appropriate motion for contempt, can impose "a five-day suspended jail sentence" together with giving the errant parent an opportunity to purge the contempt by giving the affected parent make-up parenting time "and paying $500 of his attorney fees plus administrative fees."[45] Further, it is important to remember that in cases of civil contempt proceedings, it is not required that the alleged violation of a court order be "purposeful, willful, or intentional." Once a violation is established, the parent guilty of such violation bears the burden to prove an inability to comply with the court order. Absent such proof, a civil contempt finding is appropriate.[46]

It is a mistake on the part of some lawyers to think that filing motions seeking enforcement of court-ordered parenting time or asking the court to hold the alienating parents in contempt for violation of court orders may be perceived as "aggressive" by courts. It is not "aggressive" to stand up for your client's constitutionally protected and court-ordered parenting rights; it's simply a duty of competent representation that a lawyer owes to her client. Lawyers who fail or refuse to act appropriately and in a timely manner end up causing

---

43. *Id.*
44. *Id.*, 1100.
45. Burks v. Burks, 2019 WL 5295571, 2019-Ohio-4292.
46. *Id.*

a lot of frustration and harm, sometimes irreparable, to the clients and their relationship with their children. Targeted parents frequently lament how their attorneys lack knowledge about parental alienation and accordingly, fail to prioritize getting the case before the court quickly;

> None of the attorneys involved in my custody case understood the impact of PAS, how it doesn't go away as the children get older! They kept telling me, 'Once the divorce is over, they will come back to you' . . . they had NO IDEA![47]

17. Be mindful of the unjust criticism of the judiciary in cases involving parental alienation.

Parental alienation cases often demand hard-hitting decisions. A trial judge, after reviewing the record and weighing admissible evidence produced at a trial, may be required to fashion an appropriate remedy. Depending on the circumstances of the case, the remedy could be reunification therapy, change of custody, and/or jail time for violation of court orders. When faced with an adverse ruling, it's not uncommon for an alienating parent to disparage the court and the professionals involved by attacking, lampooning, and criticizing the court's ruling outside the confines of appellate process. In this day and age of Twitter mania and social media obsession, lines are blurred between free speech and cyber-bullying or harassment.[48] It is not uncommon to find judges to be accused of incompetence or bias, even labeled as a "total disgrace."[49] And when it happens on social media, the mob mentality takes over and things have a tendency to go "crazy."[50] The accused judges, of course, have to remain silent. Under the ABA's Model Code of Judicial Conduct, Rule 2.10(A), "a judge shall not make any public statement that might reasonably be expected to affect the outcome or impair the fairness of a matter pending or impending in any court. . . ."[51]

A lawyer who handles cases of parental alienation should be mindful of the scurrilous attacks that alienating parents launch on judges who are not afraid do the right thing and hold parents accountable for their actions. For instance, consider Hon. Jon Hulsing's eye-opening article in *Litigation*, the

47. Baker, A. J. L. (2010). Even when you win you lose: Targeted parents' perceptions of their attorneys, *American Journal of Family Therapy*, 38, 292–309.

48. Hulsing, Hon. J. (2020). Parental alienation is one thing, but what are you going to do when they come for you? *Litigation*, 46(4).

49. Pulgram, L. (2016, Fall). When attacks on judges go beyond the pale, 4–5, *Litigation*, 43, 1.

50. *Id.*

51. *Id.*

journal published by the ABA's Section of Litigation.[52] Judge Hulsing—a judge for the 20th Circuit Court in Ottawa County, Michigan—wrote about how alienators, upon being held accountable in court, enlist the help of special interests groups in pushing a false narrative to accuse judges and family courts of "corruption," "with the desire to take down judges." Judge Hulsing speaks of a case where the mother "had sown the seeds of parental alienation," in "a campaign to drive the children away from their father." In addition to her alienating behaviors, the court found that the mother "lacked the ability to tell the truth or discern fact from fiction" (according to the mother's emails that she sent to friends, "god directed her to flee" with the children and that "Jesus was sitting in the seat next to her and providing encouragement for her to abandon her husband."). After "six days of trial, 18 witnesses, and 64 exhibits," the court issued an opinion explaining in depth why the court awarded primary physical custody of the minor children to the father. The court's opinion went on at length to memorialize the mother's deception and manipulative behavior and "her campaign to damage, distance, or demonize all who opposed her version of reality." After the trial, the mother "dropped a nuclear bomb," and went on to file numerous complaints in two different states falsely alleging that the father had sexually abused the children. As Judge Hulsing put it, "How better to alienate a parent?" Engaging in an attempt to forum shop, kidnapping and secreting the children, dyeing their hair and limiting the children's ability to go outdoors, the mother spent some time in hiding. Ultimately, she was arrested and the children were reunited with their father.

Concurrent with the mother's attempts to alienate the children from their father, she and her allies "attempted to intimidate the judiciary" by filing groundless motions alleging bias on the part of the court, filing complaints with the Michigan Judicial Tenure Commission alleging bias and corruption, and enlisting help from a nationally known author in the area of domestic violence, who upon listening to the mother's "tale of woe, . . . immediately concluded that whatever the [mother] said was reality." The author began to blog and post comments regarding the case; criticized the court's evidentiary rulings; and began scurrilous, *ad hominem* attacks on the court alleging that the court had "declared war on mothers" and was "corrupt." Eventually, the children continued to reside with their father, even after becoming adults, and maintain a strong bond with their father. The father allowed the children to visit the mother and repair that relationship. Living through this nightmare of a case, Judge Hulsing notes:

> It can be unnerving for a judge to be the recipient of negative comments or publicity. Let's face it, most state judges are elected and there may be the

52. Hulsing, J., *supra*.

concern about the next election. This is particularly true because judges cannot tailor their decisions to appease the public. Rather, decisions must be based on the rule of law and sometimes those decisions are unpopular.

Judge Hulsing goes on to offer some suggestions to his judicial colleagues on what can judges do when faced with unjustified criticism. But it is not fair to ask judges to make tough, unpopular decisions and then abandon them when they are unfairly and unjustly attacked for doing so. Judges cannot fight back these unjustified attacks, especially when done through a campaign of denigration via traditional media, social media, or blogs. "That leaves to us, the lawyers, the task to speak up on behalf of judges unfairly accused."[53] To assist the state and local bar associations in coordinating responses to inaccurate and unjust criticisms, the ABA has prepared a guide called *Rapid Response to Unfair and Unjust Criticism of Judges*.[54] The guide, written by the prior Standing Committee on Judicial Independence, emphasizes the critical need to respond to attacks in a timely manner and appropriate manner.

The ABA's goal is:

> To provide a mechanism through which a bar association and members of other constituencies can provide timely responses to the serious, unjust criticisms of judges and the judiciary or to misunderstandings about the role of a judge or the judicial system. The focus of these responses is to provide the public with information to help them better understand the legal issues related to a specific situation, including the role of judges, the application of the law, and the restrictions and responsibilities placed on judges in the canons and rules.[55]

When confronted with such ugly, unjust, and unfair attacks against court and court-involved professionals, a lawyer representing targeted parents should not hesitate to reach out to the ABA and her state or local bar association to request an investigation. It's not for the lawyer to come to the rescue of the judge who is being attacked—doing so may violate rules of professional conduct and make the matters worse. It's ultimately for the judge to decide whether a public response is necessary and whether to avail of the resources offered by the ABA and the state and local bar associations. As Justice Sandra Day O'Connor reminded us, where democracy depends on the separation of powers and vital and independent judiciary, "[c]riticism is fine; retaliation and intimidation are not."[56]

---

53. Pulgram, L., *supra*.

54. *See* www.americanbar.org/content/dam/aba/administrative/judicial_independence/rapid_response_pamphlet.pdf.

55. *Id.*

56. Pulgram, L., *supra* (citing O'Connor, S. D. (2008, February). A fair, impartial and independent judiciary, *Nat'l Voter*, 8).

Litigating cases involving parental alienation is challenging, often frustrating, and, on occasions, painful. No matter how many cases I litigate, how many "wins" I accumulate, it's only a matter of time before a parent, once again, loses in court where I, as his or her lawyer, have failed to persuade the court to provide an appropriate intervention. On these occasions, it's gut-wrenching to observe a targeted parent's grief over the loss of a child—a child who is biologically alive, but emotionally and psychologically dead to the parent. And on these occasions, I go through my mental checklist. Where did I go wrong? Did I succumb to a cognitive bias? Was I wrong in how I framed the case for the court? Did I fail to properly prepare the client for her forensic evaluation? Was there something lacking in my choice of and presentation of expert evidence? Of course, there is no one right answer and one can only engage in "what if" and "if only" speculations. I will never know what exactly went wrong. But this I know. I will pick myself up, dust off the loss, and with a silent prayer to the universe to heal the parent's grief, continue my work to save the next parent-child relationship. Every case is unique. Each parent-child relationship precious. It has been my privilege to represent targeted parents and every case that I have litigated has made me more appreciative of the joys and frustrations that parenthood entails.

APPENDIX A

Bibliography

American Psychiatric Association. (2013). *Diagnostic and Statistical Manual of Mental Disorders* (DSM-5) (5th ed.). Washington, DC: American Psychiatric Association.

Baker, A. J. L. (2007). *Adult Children of Parental Alienation Syndrome: Breaking the Ties That Bind*. New York, NY: W.W. Norton & Company, Inc.

Baker, A. J. L. (2020). Parental alienation and empirical research. In Lorandos, D., & Bernet, W. (Eds.), *Parental Alienation: Science and Law*. Springfield, IL: Charles C. Thomas.

Baker, A. J. L., Bone, J. M., & Ludmer, B. (2014). *The High-Conflict Custody Battle: Protect Yourself & Your Kids from a Toxic Divorce, False Accusations & Parental Alienation*. Oakland, CA: New Harbinger Publications, Inc.

Baker, A. J. L., & Fine, P. R. (2014). *Surviving Parental Alienation: A Journey of Hope and Healing*. Lanham, MD: Rowman & Littlefield.

Baker, A. J. L., & Sauber, S. R. (2013). *Working with Alienated Children and Families: A Clinical Guidebook*. New York, NY & Hove, East Sussex: Routledge, Taylor & Francis Group.

Baldwin, A. (2008). A *Promise to Ourselves: A Journey Through Fatherhood and Divorce*. New York, NY: Author.

Bernet, W. (2013). References in the Professional Literature. In Bernet, W., Lorandos, D., & Sauber, S. R. (Eds.), *Parental Alienation: The Handbook for Mental Health and Legal Professionals*. Springfield, IL: Charles C. Thomas.

Bernet, W. (2020). Introduction to Parental Alienation. In Lorandos, D., & Bernet, W. (Eds.), *Parental Alienation: Science and Law*. Springfield, IL: Charles C. Thomas.

Broun, K. S. et al. (2006). *McCormick on Evidence* (6th ed.). Eagan, MN: Thomson, West Group.

Campbell, T., & Lorandos, D. (2001). *Cross Examining Experts in the Behavioral Sciences—Vol 1 & 2* (with yearly supplements). Eagan, MN: Thomson Reuters.

Ceci, S. J., & Bruck, M. (1995). *Jeopardy in the Courtroom: A Scientific Analysis of Children's Testimony*. Washington, DC: American Psychological Evaluation.

Ciric, S. J., & Billick, S. B. (2017). Role of the Psychiatric Evaluator in Child Custody Disputes. In Rosner, R., & Scott, C. L. (Eds.), *Principles and Practice of Forensic Psychiatry* (3rd ed.). Boca Raton, FL: Taylor & Francis Group.

Clawar, S. (2020). *Parent-Child Reunification: A Guide to Legal and Forensic Strategies*. Chicago, IL: American Bar Association.

Clawar, S., & Rivlin, B. (2013). *Children Held Hostage: Identifying Brainwashed Children, Presenting a Case and Crafting Solutions* (2nd ed.). Chicago, IL: American Bar Association.
Dalton, C., Drozd, L. M., & Wong, F. Q. F. (2006). *Navigating Custody & Visitation Evaluations in Cases with Domestic Violence: A Judge's Guide*. Reno, NV: National Counsel of Juvenile and Family Court Judges.
Darnall, D. (1998). *Divorce Casualties: Protecting Your Children from Parental Alienation*. Dallas, TX: Taylor Publishing.
Darnall, D. (2008). *Divorce Casualties: Understanding Parental Alienation*. Lanham, MD: Taylor Pub.
Darnall, D. (2010). *Beyond Divorce Casualties: Reunifying the Alienated Family*. Taylor, MD: Taylor Trade Pub.
Drozd, L., Saini, M., & Olesen, N. (2016). *Parenting Plan Evaluations: Applied Research for the Family Court* (2nd ed.). New York, NY: Oxford University Press.
Ellis, E. M. (2000). *Divorce Wars: Interventions with Families in Conflict*. Washington, DC: American Psychological Evaluation.
Epstein, E. S. (2017). *The Attorney-Client Privilege and the Work Product Doctrine* (6th ed., Vol. I). Chicago, IL: American Bar Association.
Fidler, B. J. et al. (2012). *Children Who Resist Postseparation Parental Contact: A Differential Approach for Legal and Mental Health Professionals*. New York, NY: Oxford University Press.
Gardner, R. A. (1998). *The Parental Alienation Syndrome: A Guide for Mental Health and Legal Professionals*. Cresskill, NJ: Creative Therapeutics.
Gardner, R. A., Sauber, S. R., & Lorandos, D. (2006). *The International Handbook of Parental Alienation Syndrome: Conceptual, Clinical and Legal Considerations*. Springfield, IL: Charles C. Thomas.
Goldstein, M. L., & Morewitz, S. J. (2013). *Handbook of Forensic Sociology and Psychology*. New York, NY: Springer.
Gottlieb, L. (2013). The Application of Structural Family Systems Therapy to the Treatment of Parental Alienation Syndrome. In Baker, A. J. L., & Sauber, S. R., (Eds.), *Working with Alienated Children and Families: A Clinical Guidebook*. New York, NY & Hove, East Sussex: Routledge, Taylor & Francis Group.
Gould, J. W., & Martindale, D. A. (2007). *The Art and Science of Child Custody Evaluations*. New York: The Guilford Press.
Harman, J., & Biringen, Z. (2016). *Parents Acting Badly: How Institutions and Societies Promote the Alienation of Children from their Loving Families*. Fort Collins, CO: The Colorado Parental Alienation Project.
Klika, J. B., & Conte, J. R. (2018). *The APSAC Handbook on Child Maltreatment* (4th ed.). Thousand Oaks, CA: SAGE Publications.
Lamb, M. E. (1987). *The Father's Role: Cross-Cultural Perspectives*. Hillsdale, NJ: Lawrence Erlbaum Associates.
Lorandos, D. (2013). Parental Alienation. In Goldstein, M. L., & Morewitz, S. J. (Eds.), *Handbook of Forensic Sociology and Psychology*. New York, NY: Springer.
Lorandos, D., & Bernet, W. (2020). *Parental Alienation: Science and Law*. Springfield, IL: Charles C. Thomas.
Lorandos, D., Bernet, W., & Sauber, S.R. (2013). *Parental Alienation: The Handbook for Mental Health and Legal Professionals*. Springfield, IL: Charles C. Thomas, Publisher.

Lorandos, D., & Campbell, T.W. (2005). *Benchbook in the Behavioral Sciences: Psychiatry—Psychology—Social Work*. Durham, NC: Carolina Academic Press.
Michalos, A. C. (2014). *Encyclopedia of Quality of Life and Well-Being Research*. Heidelberg, Germany: Springer Netherlands.
Reay, K. M. (2011). *Toxic Divorce: A Workbook for Alienated Parents*. Author.
Rosner, R., & Scott, C. L. (2017). *Principles and Practice of Forensic Psychiatry* (3rd ed.). Boca Raton, FL: Taylor & Francis Group.
Saini, M., Johnston, J. R., Fidler, B. J., & Bala, N. (2016). Empirical Studies of Alienation. In Drozd, L., Saini, M., & Olesen, N. (Eds.), *Parenting Plan Evaluation: Applied Research for the Family Court* (2nd ed.) (pp. 374–423). New York, NY: Oxford University Press.
Stahl, P. M., & Simon, R. A. (2013). *Forensic Psychology Consultation in Child Custody Litigation: A Handbook for Work Product Review, Case Preparation, and Expert Testimony*. Chicago, IL: American Bar Association.
Warshak, R. A. (1992). *The Custody Revolution: The Father Factor and the Motherhood Mystique*. New York, NY: Poseidon Press.
Warshak, R. A. (2009). *Divorce Poison: Protecting the Parent-Child Bond from a Vindictive Ex*. New York, NY: Regan Books.
Zervopoulus, J. A. (2008). *Confronting Mental Health Evidence: A Practical Guide to Reliability and Experts in Family Law*. Chicago, IL: American Bar Association.

APPENDIX B

Examples of Cases Documenting Alienating Strategies

1. Badmouthing
Weaver v. Weaver, 2019 WL 1504095 (Vt. Apr. 5, 2019). Because of M's persistent and unremitting effort to disparage F and undermine his relationship with child, no measure short of restricting M's contact with child's providers, school personnel, would prevent harm.
McNutt v. Yates, 2013 Ark. 427; 430 S.W.3d 91 (Ark. 2013). Court of appeals did not err in finding material change in circumstances existed so as to warrant modification of child custody where M accused F of sexual deviance, burglary, killing the children's dog (all without evidence); M made disparaging remarks about F in front of children, in public, and to people at the children's school; M made unproven accusations of sexual deviance of F in front of children.
In re Anya J.K., unreported, 2013 IL App (2d) 121194-U; 2013 WL 1932716 (Ill App. Ct. 2013). Factors, including M's efforts to destroy child and F relationship (M denigrates F in child's presence; M's words drive child from the chair to the floor, then under the chair, and finally under the table; child avoids any expression of affection for F in M's presence; child cannot give F a gift without hiding it from M) made the risk of alienating the child very real. For these reasons, it was not against manifest weight of the evidence to grant F sole custody.
J.F. v. D.F., 61 Misc.3d 1226(A) (NY Sup. Ct. 2018). Discussing badmouthing in the context of parental alienation, but not finding it in this case.
Brundage v. Brundage, unpublished, 68 N.E.3d 1130 (*Id.* Ct. App. 2016). M cheated on F. M asked for separation. F petitioned for dissolution of marriage. F told children about affair. Children indicated they hated M. F was awarded primary physical custody of the children. M contends that trial court abused its discretion in awarding primary physical custody to F. Although appellate court found F engaged in parental alienation, the children's relationship with M was so unworkable as to render it impossible for M have physical custody of the children.

McClain v. McClain, 539 S.W.3d 170 (Tenn. Ct. App. 2017). Affirmed trial court's determination that children's severe alienation from M was material change in circumstances and granting M exclusive custody and period of no contact with F was not precluded by expert testimony where, among other factors, (1) F denied M in-person and telephonic co-parenting time and (2) F severely alienated the children against M in violation of permanent parenting plan order. Regarding alienation, F "[acquiesced] to the boys' demands, endorsed the status quo (anti-M) and [accepted] the situation as is, with full custody to [F], no scheduled contacts with [M] and no other court-ordered intervention."
Noland-Vance v. Vance, 321 S.W.2d 398 (Mo. App. 2010). Held: evidence supported finding that M alienated children's affection toward F where M never said anything positive about F, incited fear about F, etc.
Fiala v. Fiala, unpublished Tenn. Ct. App. 2019, 2018 WL 4523206. Held: decision to change custody to F was not in error where, among other factors, M "engaged in a pattern of hostile behavior toward F often while the child was present. M's inappropriate behavior includes: (1) telling the child that F did not love him; (2) accusing F of kidnapping the child even though the child was returned to M on time; (3) telling the child that F "brainwash[ed]" the child; (4) calling Stepmother "whore," "bitch," and other names in the child's presence and encouraging the child to have nothing to do with Stepmother, including even hugging her; and (5) refusing to allow the child to participate in activities because Stepmother was present.
2. Limiting Contact
Sundstrom v. Sundstrom, 177 Vt. 577; 865 A.2d 358 (Vt. 2004). Obstruction of visitation and attempts at parental alienation are not in a child's best interests, and they may form the basis for a change in custody; cites other Vt. cases finding same.
Joy B. v. Everett B., 2019 WL 5656351, unreported case in Alaska Supreme Court (No. S-17129) (November 1, 2019). Held: (1) evidence supported finding that F rebutted the statutory presumption that a parent with a history of perpetrating domestic violence should not be awarded sole legal or sole physical custody of a child, and (2) evidence supported finding that it was in child's best interest to be in husband's sole custody where, among other factors, M had prevented and frustrated F's visitation and limited contact.
Mullins v. Mullins, 142 Ill.App.3d 57; 490 N.E.2d 1375 (Ill. App. Ct. 1986). Trial court's order transferring custody of minor children to F not contrary to the manifest weight of the evidence where (1) M deprived the children of F's surname, (2) forced children to address stepfather as "daddy"; (3) M removed the children from the jurisdiction, thereby depriving F and the children of any personal contact for several months; (4) M omitted F's name from their Florida school registration records "as if he didn't even exist."
In re Marriage of Divelbiss, 308 Ill.App.3d 198; 719 N.E.2d 375 (Ill. App. Ct. 1999). Among other issues, trial court found that M was unwilling to facilitate and encourage a close and continuing relationship between child and F; that M repeatedly denied visitations and her conduct generated problems with visitations. The trial court ordered a modification of residential custody and ongoing therapy in an attempt to break the cycle of parental alienation and to assist child in her adjustment.

In re Marriage of Debra N. and Michael S., 2013 IL App (1st) 122145. "Where, as here, the record supports the circuit court's finding that the custodial parent has made attempts to thwart the noncustodial parent's efforts to visit and maintain a close relationship with the child, the court's decision to modify the custody arrangement and transfer custody of the child to the noncustodial parent is not against the manifest weight of the evidence."
In re Marriage of Sheridan, unreported, 2013 IL App (4th) 130394-U; 2013 WL 5741858 (Ill App. Ct. 2013). Trial court decision to grant F sole custody of the children not against great weight of the evidence where, "the court seriously believes that if [F] is not awarded custody and if [M] is allowed to make all important life decisions, this [F] will have a difficult time ever maintaining a decent continuing relationship with these children. [M] has made it painfully obvious to the court the extent she would go . . . to limit the [F's] involvement with these children and downgrade the F's status with the children."
Ellis v. Ellis, 952 So.2d 982 (Miss. Ct. App. 2006). Trial court did not abuse its discretion in finding a material change in circumstances where child suffered from PAS with M and expert recommended a change in environment from M to F. M's actions included (1) M intentionally set up activities during the summer for child that would substantially interfere with F's visitation time, which the lower court specifically found was done to embarrass F; (2) M not allowing F any input in health, education, and welfare decisions; (3) child shows disregard for F while in the presence of M and family drawings by child exclude F.
Eisenlohr v. Eisenlohr, 135 Conn.App. 377; 43 A.3d 694 (Conn. App. Ct. 2012). The trial court ordered: "Because of the defendant's pattern and practice of interfering with the plaintiff's relationship with the minor child, the defendant's refusal to communicate appropriately with the minor child or the plaintiff, and, inter alia, her refusal to foster or support a relationship between the minor child and the plaintiff, sole physical and legal custody of the minor child is hereby vested in the plaintiff, post judgment." The appellate court did not find this to be an abuse of discretion because of the lengthy record on which the court based its change of custody.
Hibbard v. Hibbard, 139 Conn.App. 10; 55 A.3d 301 (Conn. App. Ct. 2012). The trial court found that the M aimed to "[eliminate the F] from their daughter's life" and that leaving the child with M would lead to the loss to the child of her F. The trial court awarded sole custody of the minor child to the F. The appellate court concluded that the record supports alienation (failure to deliver child for multiple visitations; unsupported allegations that F physically harmed child; unsupported allegations that child was afraid of F; erroneous statement to social worker that F had been arrested for child abuse before; unsupported allegation that child had been touched by F's friends) and the trial court did not err.
Hankey v. Hankey, 861 N.W.2d 479 (N.D. 2015). Held: F established prima facie case for modification of primary residential responsibility, entitling him to evidentiary hearing on his motion, where F alleged M's interference with parenting time (parental alienation), denial of right of first refusal for parenting time, and unilateral decision-making regarding enrolling child in occupational and play therapy without his knowledge or consent in derogation of terms of divorce judgment.

Maddux v. Maddux, 40 N.E.3d 971 (Ind. Ct. App. 2015). Appellate reversed trial court's denial of F's petition for custody modification because M's misconduct was so egregious as it placed child's mental welfare at stake where, among other things, (1) M denied F his parenting time, (2) M falsely accused F of abuse, (3) M relentlessly subjected children to her unsubstantiated opinions and accusations.
In re Paternity of N.W., unpublished, 35 N.E.3d 674 (Ind. Ct. App. 2015). Appellate court affirmed trial court's award of sole legal and primary physical custody of child to F as in the child's best interests and the only way to enable the child to restore his relationship with F with limited interference from M after her efforts that amounted to parental alienation. PA efforts included: M denying F parenting time; M alleging that F had abused the child; M stating that she will never do anything to help foster the F-child relationship; M registering child to camp under M's last name; M refusing to permit F to pick up child from school.
S.D. v. B.D., unpublished, 962 N.E.2d 702 (Ind. Ct. App. 2012). Isolated incidents not so egregious as to place child's welfare at stake where (1) M helped child make a family photograph collage that did not include photos of F but did include photos of M's new boyfriend and his three children; and (2) M enrolled child in day care during a summer when F was unemployed and available to watch the child.
3. Interfering with Communication
Eisenlohr v. Eisenlohr, 135 Conn.App. 377; 43 A.3d 694 (Conn. App. Ct. 2012). The trial court ordered: "Because of the defendant's pattern and practice of interfering with the plaintiff's relationship with the minor child, the defendant's refusal to communicate appropriately with the minor child or the plaintiff, and, inter alia, her refusal to foster or support a relationship between the minor child and the plaintiff, sole physical and legal custody of the minor child is hereby vested in the plaintiff, post judgment." The appellate court did not find this to be an abuse of discretion because of the lengthy record on which the court based its change of custody.
Shindell v. Shindell, 322 P.3d 1270 (Wyo. 2014). "Trial court did not abuse its discretion by finding M in indirect civil contempt of court for willfully violating divorce decree; . . . M engaged in a scheme of parental alienation since entry of the decree of divorce by interfering with F's efforts to communicate with parties' children, excluding F from decisions involving children, and failing to cooperate with GAL."
McClain v. McClain, 539 S.W.3d 170 (Tenn. Ct. App. 2017). Affirmed trial court's determination that children's severe alienation from M was material change in circumstances and granting M exclusive custody and period of no contact with F was not **precluded** by expert testimony where, among other factors, (1) F denied M in-person and telephonic co-parenting time and (2) F severely alienated the children against M in violation of permanent parenting plan order. Regarding alienation, F "[acquiesced] to the boys' demands, endorsed the status quo (anti-M) and [accepted] the situation as is, with full custody to [F], no scheduled contacts with [M] and no other court-ordered intervention."
Sundstrom v. Sundstrom, 177 Vt. 577; 865 A.2d 358 (Vt. 2004). Obstruction of visitation and attempts at parental alienation are not in a child's best interests, and they may form the **basis** for a change in custody; cites other Vt. cases finding same.

4. Interfering with Symbolic Communication
S.D. v. B.D., unpublished, 962 N.E.2d 702 (Ind. Ct. App. 2012). Isolated incidents not so egregious as to place child's welfare at stake where (1) M helped child make a family photograph collage that did not include photos of F but did include photos of M's new boyfriend and his three children; and (2) M enrolled child in day care during a summer when F was unemployed and available to watch the child.
Ellis v. Ellis, 952 So.2d 982 (Miss. Ct. App. 2006). Trial court did not abuse its discretion in finding a material change in circumstances where child suffered from PAS with M and expert recommended a change in environment from M to F. M's actions included (1) M intentionally set up activities during the summer for child that would substantially interfere with F's visitation time, which the lower court specifically found was done to embarrass F; (2) M not allowing F any input in health, education, and welfare decisions; (3) child shows disregard for F while in the presence of M and family drawings by child exclude F.
McClain v. McClain, 539 S.W.3d 170 (Tenn. Ct. App. 2017). Affirmed trial court's determination that children's severe alienation from M was material change in circumstances and granting M exclusive custody and period of no contact with F was not precluded by expert testimony where, among other factors, (1) F denied M in-person and telephonic co-parenting time and (2) F severely alienated the children against M in violation of permanent parenting plan order. Regarding alienation, F "[acquiesced] to the boys' demands, endorsed the status quo (anti-M) and [accepted] the situation as is, with full custody to [F], no scheduled contacts with [M] and no other court-ordered intervention." F did not share photos or information about important medical procedures. F said to M, "You're not even going to recognize your youngest son. He's grown so much you won't even recognize him."
5. Withholding Love and Approval
In re Anya J.K., unreported, 2013 IL App (2d) 121194-U; 2013 WL 1932716 (Ill App. Ct. 2013). Factors, including M's efforts to destroy child and F relationship (M denigrates F in child's presence; M's words drive child under the table and child avoids any expression of affection for F in M's presence; child cannot give F a gift without hiding it from M) made the risk of alienating the child very real. For these reasons, it was not against manifest weight of the evidence to grant F sole custody.
6. Telling Child the Other Parent Does Not Love Him or Her
Barnard v. Barnard, unreported Court of Appeals of Ohio, 1997 WL 379617 (July 3, 1997). The trial court did not abuse its discretion by modifying a prior custody order where, among other findings, the court found that "the F has not only failed to enhance and encourage the respect, love and affection of each child to the M, but has embarked upon a campaign to discredit the M in the eyes of the children, brainwashing them to believe the M is a liar and does not love them and that she steals their clothes."
Noland-Vance v. Vance, 321 S.W.2d 398 (Mo. App. 2010). Held: evidence supported finding that M alienated children's affection toward F where M never said anything positive about F, incited fear about F, etc.

Fiala v. Fiala, unpublished Tenn. Ct. App. 2019, 2018 WL 4523206. Held: decision to change custody to F was not in error where, among other factors, M "engaged in a pattern of hostile behavior toward F often while the child was present. M's inappropriate behavior includes: (1) telling the child that F did not love him; (2) accusing F of kidnapping the child even though the child was returned to M on time; (3) telling the child that F "brainwash[ed]" the child; (4) calling Stepmother "whore," "bitch," and other names in the child's presence and encouraging the child to have nothing to do with Stepmother, including even hugging her; and (5) refusing to allow the child to participate in activities because Stepmother was present.
7. Creating Impression That Other Parent Is Dangerous
McNutt v. Yates, 2013 Ark. 427; 430 S.W.3d 91 (Ark. 2013). Court of appeals did not err in finding material change in circumstances existed so as to warrant modification of child custody where M accused F of sexual deviance, burglary, killing the children's dog (all without evidence); M made disparaging remarks about F in front of children, in public, and to people at the children's school; M made unproven accusations of sexual deviance of F in front of children.
Stone v. Pellegrini-Stone, 2014 WL 1887606, unpublished decision in 2014 IL App (3d) 130977-U, (May 9, 2014). "*Held*: Trial court did not err in granting custody of children to F and ordering that M have supervised visitation where M made many unfounded allegations of abuse against F."
Hibbard v. Hibbard, 139 Conn.App. 10; 55 A.3d 301 (Conn. App. Ct. 2012). The trial court found that the M aimed to "[eliminate the F] from their daughter's life" and that leaving the child with M would lead to the loss to the child of her F. The trial court awarded sole custody of the minor child to the F. The appellate court concluded that the record supports alienation (failure to deliver child for multiple visitations; unsupported allegations that F physically harmed child; unsupported allegations that child was afraid of F; erroneous statement to social worker that F had been arrested for child abuse before; unsupported allegation that child had been touched by F's friends) and the trial court did not err.
Maddux v. Maddux, 40 N.E.3d 971 (Ind. Ct. App. 2015). Court of appeals reversed trial court's denial of F's petition for custody modification because M's misconduct was so egregious at it placed child's mental welfare at stake where, among other things, (1) M denied F his parenting time, (2) M falsely accused F of abuse, (3) M relentlessly subjected children to her unsubstantiated opinions and accusations.
In re Paternity of N.W., unpublished, 35 N.E.3d 674 (Ind. Ct. App. 2015). Appellate court affirmed trial court's award of sole legal and primary physical custody of child to F as in the child's best interests and the only way to enable the child to restore his relationship with F with limited interference from M after her efforts that amounted to parental alienation. PA efforts included: M denying F parenting time; M alleging that F had abused the child; M stating that she will never do anything to help foster the F-child relationship; M registering child to camp under M's last name; M refusing to permit F to pick up child from school.
Hanson v. Spolnik, 685 N.E.2d 71 (Ind. Ct. App. 1997). Trial court awarded sole custody to F because M "engaged in a concerted effort to destroy [the child's] relationship with [the F]." The actions the M took in the presence of child included accusing the F of sexually abusing the child.

Poag-Emery v. Emery, unpublished Court of Appeals of Michigan, 2014 WL 1618359, April 22, 2014. Trial court did not err by finding that granting F sole legal custody was in the child's best interest where, among other factors in the 12-factor test, M's alienation went against her moral fitness (factor f), her unwillingness and ability to encourage a parent-child relationship with the other parent (factor j), and her unwillingness to go to counseling (factor l).
Fortwengler v. Fortwengler, unreported Court of Appeals of Minnesota, 2017 WL 1053101 (March 20, 2017). District court did not err in granting sole physical and legal custody of children to F where "[therapist] opined that M has alienated [one child] from F and attempted to alienate [another child] from F. The GAL expressed similar concerns about M coaching the children and testified that [one child's] emotional status has declined. [Therapist] testified that she has no concerns about the children's safety with F but that M's refusal to bring the children to therapy has had a significant negative impact on their emotional well-being. F testified that M has not permitted him to care for the children when she is unavailable, instead sending them to her family members contrary to the district court's order."
Noland-Vance v. Vance, 321 S.W.2d 398 (Mo. App. 2010). Held: evidence supported finding that M alienated children's affection toward F where M never said anything positive about F, incited fear about F, etc.
Fiala v. Fiala, unpublished Tenn. Ct. App. 2019, 2018 WL 4523206. Held: decision to change custody to F was not in error where, among other factors, M "engaged in a pattern of hostile behavior toward F often while the child was present. M's inappropriate behavior includes: (1) telling the child that F did not love him; (2) accusing F of kidnapping the child even though the child was returned to M on time; (3) telling the child that F "brainwash[ed]" the child; (4) calling Stepmother "whore," "bitch," and other names in the child's presence and encouraging the child to have nothing to do with Stepmother, including even hugging her; and (5) refusing to allow the child to participate in activities because Stepmother was present.
Knutsen v. Cegalis, 201 Vt. 138; 137 A.3d 734 (Vt. 2016). Trial court acted within its discretion to disallow M to reestablish contact with child nor allow M any rights to contact until 08/2016 unless the trauma therapist recommended contact earlier where F so alienated their child from M (child thought M would kill child) that immediate concerns for child's psyche required slow reunification.
Ryder v. Mitchell, 54 P.3d 885 (Co. 2002). Distinguishes cases in which a therapist makes allegations of sexual abuse by a parent from cases in which the therapist misdiagnosis improper parenting skills or even parental alienation. Creating a duty to the parents could conflict with or disserve the primary duty.
Holmes v. Holmes, 436 W.E.3d 599 (Mo. Ct. App. 2014. Custody decision for F not against the weight of the evidence to grant F sole legal and physical custody where child was subjected to significant instability originating from M's household ("Child 'was subjected to two hot line calls, two Children's Division investigations, two psychological evaluations, two CAC interviews, and numerous visits to counselors and therapists,' was taken to St. Louis for a SAFE exam, and had even spent time in foster care," because of multiple unsubstantiated claims by M of F abuse of child.)

8. Confiding in the Child
McNutt v. Yates, 2013 Ark. 427; 430 S.W.3d 91 (Ark. 2013). Court of appeals did not err in finding material change in circumstances existed so as to warrant modification of child custody where M accused F of sexual deviance, burglary, killing the children's dog (all without evidence); M made disparaging remarks about F in front of children, in public, and to people at the children's school; M made unproven accusations of sexual deviance of F in front of children.
Eisenlohr v. Eisenlohr, 135 Conn.App. 377; 43 A.3d 694 (Conn. App. Ct. 2012). The trial court ordered: "Because of the defendant's pattern and practice of interfering with the plaintiff's relationship with the minor child, the defendant's refusal to communicate appropriately with the minor child or the plaintiff, and, inter alia, her refusal to foster or support a relationship between the minor child and the plaintiff, sole physical and legal custody of the minor child is hereby vested in the plaintiff, post judgment." The appellate court did not find this to be an abuse of discretion because of the lengthy record on which the court based its change of custody.
Maddux v. Maddux, 40 N.E.3d 971 (Ind. Ct. App. 2015). Court of appeals reversed trial court's denial of F's petition for custody modification because M's misconduct was so egregious at it placed child's mental welfare at stake where, among other things, (1) M denied F his parenting time, (2) M falsely accused F of abuse, (3) M relentlessly subjected children to her unsubstantiated opinions and accusations.
Brundage v. Brundage, unpublished, 68 N.E.3d 1130 (*Id.* Ct. App. 2016). M cheated on F. M asked for separation. F petitioned for dissolution of marriage. F told children about affair. Children indicated they hated M. F was awarded primary physical custody of the children. M contends that trial court abused its discretion in awarding primary physical custody to F. Although appellate court found F engaged in parental alienation, the children's relationship with M was so unworkable as to render it impossible for M have physical custody of the children.
9. Forcing Child to Reject Other Parent
Mullins v. Mullins, 142 Ill.App.3d 57; 490 N.E.2d 1375 (Ill. App. Ct. 1986). Trial court's order transferring custody of minor children to F not contrary to the manifest weight of the evidence where (1) M deprived the children of F's surname, (2) forced children to address stepfather as "daddy;" (3) M removed the children from the jurisdiction, thereby depriving F and the children of any personal contact for several months; (4) M omitted F's name from their Florida school registration records "as if he didn't even exist."
Ellis v. Ellis, 952 So.2d 982 (Miss. Ct. App. 2006) Trial court did not abuse its discretion in finding a material change in circumstances where child suffered from PAS with M and expert recommended a change in environment from M to F. M's actions included (1) M intentionally set up activities during the summer for child that would substantially interfere with F's visitation time, which the lower court specifically found was done to embarrass F; (2) M not allowing F any input in health, education, and welfare decisions; (3) child shows disregard for F while in the presence of M and family drawings by child exclude F.

Fortwengler v. Fortwengler, unreported Court of Appeals of Minnesota, 2017 WL 1053101 (March 20, 2017). District court did not err in granting sole physical and legal custody of children to F where "[therapist] opined that M has alienated [one child]. from F and attempted to alienate [another child] from F. The GAL expressed similar concerns about M coaching the children and testified that [one child's] emotional status has declined. [Therapist] testified that she has no concerns about the children's safety with F but that M's refusal to bring the children to therapy has had a significant negative impact on their emotional well-being. F testified that M has not permitted him to care for the children when she is unavailable, instead sending them to her family members contrary to the district court's order."
Fiala v. Fiala, unpublished Tenn. Ct. App. 2019, 2018 WL 4523206. Held: decision to change custody to F was not in error where, among other factors, M "engaged in a pattern of hostile behavior toward F often while the child was present. M's inappropriate behavior includes: (1) telling the child that F did not love him; (2) accusing F of kidnapping the child even though the child was returned to M on time; (3) telling the child that F "brainwash[ed]" the child; (4) calling Stepmother "whore," "bitch," and other names in the child's presence and encouraging the child to have nothing to do with Stepmother, including even hugging her; and (5) refusing to allow the child to participate in activities because Stepmother was present.
In re N.W., unreported Ct. App. Tx., 2013 WL 5302716. Trial court was within its discretion to follow the recommendations of expert testimony regarding psychological testing of M, F, and children; had sufficient information upon which to exercise its discretion; and did not err by determining child's best interests were for F as sole managing conservator with primary custody.
10. Asking Child to Spy on Other Parent
Horace P. v. Superior Court of Appeal, Second District, Division 2, California. January 04, 2012 Not Reported in Cal.Rptr.3d 2012 WL 11116 B236617. A noteworthy case that reminds the litigants to not make unfounded allegations of alienation. F argued that there was "no evidence that he was inappropriate in any way with the child during the visits." Not so. F referred to the child as a "spy" in her presence. Although F claimed that this comment was mere jest and that the child thought it was funny, the court was entitled to adopt a different interpretation and view the comment as needlessly placing the child in the middle of the feud that F had with M.
11. Asking Child to Keep Secrets from Other Parent
D.D. v. A.D., unreported supreme court of NY, 56 Misc.3d 1201(A)(2017). Sufficient evidence to suggest that if F were awarded sole custody, he would likely limit any meaningful relationship between M and children, where, among other things, M testified that the kids are being "encouraged to lie[,] hide things[,] and keep secrets they are traumatized." Given totality of circumstances, court awards sole custody to M.

12. Referring to Other Parent by First Name, Encouraging Same
In re Marriage of Divelbiss, 308 Ill.App.3d 198; 719 N.E.2d 375 (Ill. App. Ct. 1999). M was residential custodian of minor child. F noticed that child began to refer to F as "Rick," instead of "Dad," and F noticed that child's last name was written on some of her homework and a book as child's stepfather's name. F moved for sole custody of child. The court did not grant sole custody but found by clear and convincing evidence that there had been a change in circumstances and that modification was necessary to serve the best interest of the child. The trial court found evidence of substantial parental alienation, which would require that child to spend an extended period of time with F with less interference from M.
Russell v. Russell, Supreme Court, Appellate Division, Fourth Department, New York. June 07, 2019 173 A.D.3d 1607 105 N.Y.S.3d 626 18–00406, 32. M allowed the child to believe that the deceased fiancé was her actual father; M allowed the child to refer to the deceased fiancé as "dad" and to the father by his first name.
13. Referring to Stepparent as "Mom" or "Dad," Encouraging Same
Williams v. Ramsey, 101 Ark. App. 61; 270 S.W.3d 345 (Ark. Ct. App. 2007). F having child call stepmother "Mommy," among other issues, did not rise to the level of a change in circumstances sufficient to support reduction of F's child visitation rights.
Mullins v. Mullins, 142 Ill.App.3d 57; 490 N.E.2d 1375 (Ill. App. Ct. 1986). Trial court's order transferring custody of minor children to F not contrary to the manifest weight of the evidence where (1) M deprived the children of F's surname, (2) forced children to address stepfather as "daddy;" (3) M removed the children from the jurisdiction, thereby depriving F and the children of any personal contact for several months; (4) M omitted F's name from their Florida school registration records "as if he didn't even exist."
14. Withholding Important Information from Other Parent, Taking Name Off Records
Sharp v. Keeler, 99 Ark. App. 42; 256 S.W.3d 528 (Ark Ct. App. 2007). No error in trial court decision where record replete with M attempts to alienate F from his son, including M refusing to sign a medical release and instructing nurses not to give F any medical information, especially in light of son's serious medical conditions.
Mullins v. Mullins, 142 Ill.App.3d 57; 490 N.E.2d 1375 (Ill. App. Ct. 1986). Trial court's order transferring custody of minor children to F not contrary to the manifest weight of the evidence where (1) M deprived the children of F's surname, (2) forced children to address stepfather as "daddy;" (3) M removed the children from the jurisdiction, thereby depriving F and the children of any personal contact for several months; (4) M omitted F's name from their Florida school registration records "as if he didn't even exist."
Hankey v. Hankey, 861 N.W.2d 479 (N.D. 2015). Held: F established prima facie case for modification of primary residential responsibility, entitling him to evidentiary hearing on his motion, where F alleged M's interference with parenting time (parental alienation), denial of right of first refusal for parenting time, and unilateral decision-making regarding enrolling child in occupational and play therapy without his knowledge or consent in derogation of terms of divorce judgment.

Shindell v. Shindell, 322 P.3d 1270 (Wyo. 2014) "Trial court did not abuse its discretion by finding M in indirect civil contempt of court for willfully violating divorce decree; . . . M engaged in a scheme of parental alienation since entry of the decree of divorce by interfering with F's efforts to communicate with parties' children, excluding F from decisions involving children, and failing to cooperate with GAL."
Barnard v. Barnard, unreported Court of Appeals of Ohio, 1997 WL 379617 (July 3, 1997). The trial court did not abuse its discretion by modifying a prior custody order where, among other findings, the court found that "the F attempted to remove the M from 'the loop' as far as school activities were concerned, for example, notifying a school not to allow unrestricted contact between M and children, failing to notify the M of scheduled parent-teacher conferences, and removing the children from St. Patrick's school unilaterally and in retaliation for that school's failure to comply with the F's directives to not allow contact with the M."
Sundstrom v. Sundstrom, 177 Vt. 577; 865 A.2d 358 (Vt. 2004). Obstruction of visitation and attempts at parental alienation are not in a child's best interests, and they may form the basis for a change in custody; cites other Vt. cases finding same.
15. Changing Child's Name
Mullins v. Mullins, 142 Ill.App.3d 57; 490 N.E.2d 1375 (Ill. App. Ct. 1986). Trial court's order transferring custody of minor children to F not contrary to the manifest weight of the evidence where (1) M deprived the children of F's surname, (2) forced children to address stepfather as "daddy"; (3) M removed the children from the jurisdiction, thereby depriving F and the children of any personal contact for several months; (4) M omitted F's name from their Florida school registration records "as if he didn't even exist."
In re Paternity of N.W., unpublished, 35 N.E.3d 674 (Ind. Ct. App. 2015). Appellate court affirmed trial court's award of sole legal and primary physical custody of child to F as in the child's best interests and the only way to enable the child to restore his relationship with F with limited interference from M after her efforts that amounted to parental alienation. PA efforts included: M denying F parenting time; M alleging that F had abused the child; M stating that she will never do anything to help foster the F-child relationship; M registering child to camp under M's last name; M refusing to permit F to pick up child from school.
16. Undermining Authority of Disfavored Parent
McNutt v. Yates, 2013 Ark. 427; 430 S.W.3d 91 (Ark. 2013). Court of appeals did not err in finding material change in circumstances existed so as to warrant modification of child custody where M accused F of sexual deviance, burglary, killing the children's dog (all without evidence); M made disparaging remarks about F in front of children, in public, and to people at the children's school; M made unproven accusations of sexual deviance of F in front of children.
Hankey v. Hankey, 861 N.W.2d 479 (N.D. 2015). Held: F established prima facie case for modification of primary residential responsibility, entitling him to evidentiary hearing on his motion, where F alleged M's interference with parenting time (parental alienation), denial of right of first refusal for parenting time, and unilateral decision-making regarding enrolling child in occupational and play therapy without his knowledge or consent in derogation of terms of divorce judgment.

Shindell v. Shindell, 322 P.3d 1270 (Wyo. 2014). "Trial court did not abuse its discretion by finding M in indirect civil contempt of court for willfully violating divorce decree; . . . M engaged in a scheme of parental alienation since entry of the decree of divorce by interfering with F's efforts to communicate with parties' children, excluding F from decisions involving children, and failing to cooperate with GAL."
Fiala v. Fiala, unpublished Tenn. Ct. App. 2019, 2018 WL 4523206. Held: decision to change custody to F was not in error where, among other factors, M "engaged in a pattern of hostile behavior toward F often while the child was present. M's inappropriate behavior includes: (1) telling the child that F did not love him; (2) accusing F of kidnapping the child even though the child was returned to M on time; (3) telling the child that F "brainwash[ed]" the child; (4) calling Stepmother "whore," "bitch," and other names in the child's presence and encouraging the child to have nothing to do with Stepmother, including even hugging her; and (5) refusing to allow the child to participate in activities because Stepmother was present.
Chandler v. Bishop, 142 N.H. 404; 702 A.2d 813 (N.H. 1997). Ruling that non-custodial parent could not indoctrinate the child in his religion if doing so interfered with the custodial parent's right to determine the child's religious upbringing was in error. Vacated this religious restriction.
L.R. v. C.R., unreported Supreme Court of NY opinion, 44 Misc.3d 1208(A); 2014 WL 3376889 (July 9, 2014). Considering totality of the circumstances, including F's poor treatment of M in the presence of the children, which served to undermine her parental authority, M received sole legal and physical custody.

APPENDIX C

Examples of Cases Documenting Signs of Alienation in Children

1. Campaign of Denigration
Duke v. Duke, No. M2013-00624-COA-R3CV, 2014 WL 4966902 (Tenn. Ct. App. Oct. 3, 2014). The trial court reduced F's time with the parties' children to four hours of supervised time every other weekend as a result of F's intentional interference with the children's relationship with M. ". . . when reaching to a recommendation in the absence of parental alienation, I would give considerable attention to the children's preferences. However, if the children's strong opinions are simply the result of parental alienation—driven by the F's active indoctrination of the children against their M—I do not take the children's preferences literally . . ."
In re Marriage of Bates, 212 Ill. 2d 489, 819 N.E.2d 714 (Oct. 28, 2004). Section 506(a)(3) of the Act, as applied in this case, deprived M of procedural due process of law because her protected liberty interest in the care, custody, and control of her daughter was adversely affected by the statutory prohibition of calling the child's representative as a witness and cross-examining him. Nevertheless, in light of the overwhelming expert testimony supporting a modification of custody, and because the content of the representative's report was not inconsistent with the other evidence at trial, admission of the report was not prejudicial, and the error in failing to allow cross-examination was harmless. *In view of the sparse record challenging the general acceptance of the PAS principle, allowing Dr. Gardner's parental alienation syndrome testimony was not an abuse of discretion.*
Palazzolo v Mire, 2008-0075 (La. App. 4 Cir. 1/7/09), 10 So. 3d 748. AM (Ms. Palazzolo, adoptive mother) contends that, because I.P. is an "alienated child," the trial court erred in awarding sole custody to BM (Ms. Mire, birth mother). The judgment of the trial court terminating AM's visitation rights is reversed. This matter is remanded to the trial court for a hearing to determine the parameters of the visitation to which AM is entitled.

People v. Bimonte, 185 Misc. 2d 390, 712 N.Y.S.2d 829 (Crim. Ct. 2000) Criminal Court, City of New York, Queens County. August 1, 2000185 Misc.2d 390712 N.Y.S.2d 8292000 N.Y. Slip Op. 20416. Defendant pleads that PAS was introduced in 1985 by Richard A. Gardner, Ph.D., to cover a combination of factors which have evolved in the area of child custody disputes. According to defendant, Gardner defines PAS as a disorder that arises primarily in the context of child custody disputes. It's [sic] primary manifestation is the child's campaign of denigration against the parent, a campaign that has no justification. It results from a combination of a programming 'brainwashing' parent's indoctrinations of the child's own contributions to the nullification of the target parent. When true parental abuse and/or neglect is present, the child's animosity may be justified, and so the parental alienation syndrome explanation for the child's hostility is not applicable.
2. Weak, Frivolous, and Absurd Rationalizations for the Deprecation
Costley v Benjamin, No. M200400375COAR3CV, 2005 WL 1950114 (Tenn. Ct. App. Aug. 12, 2005). M was awarded primary custody of the parties' two young children. F petitioned the trial court for primary custody of both children twice in less than a year. The second time, the trial court granted the petition, reasoning that the F would never relent in his efforts to obtain primary residential placement and that the parents' continuing struggle was detrimental to the child's well-being. The Court of Appeals reversed the trial court, stating that F has not demonstrated a proper ground for modification of the prior parenting arrangement and because *the proof shows that the M is more inclined than the F to encourage the child's relationship with the other parent.*
Duke v Duke, No. M2013-00624-COA-R3CV, 2014 WL 4966902 (Tenn. Ct. App. Oct. 3, 2014). The trial court reduced F's time with the parties' children to four hours of supervised time every other weekend as a result of F's intentional interference with the children's relationship with M. ". . . when reaching to a recommendation in the absence of parental alienation, I would give considerable attention to the children's preferences. However, if the children's strong opinions are simply the result of parental alienation—driven by the F's active indoctrination of the children against their M—I do not take the children's preferences literally . . ."
Palazzolo v Mire, 2008-0075 (La. App. 4 Cir. 1/7/09), 10 So. 3d 748. AM (Ms. Palazzolo, adoptive mother) contends that, because I.P. is an "alienated child," the trial court erred in awarding sole custody to BM (Ms. Mire, birth mother). The judgment of the trial court terminating AM's visitation rights is reversed. This matter is remanded to the trial court for a hearing to determine the parameters of the visitation to which AM is entitled.
3. Lack of Ambivalence
Costley v Benjamin, No. M200400375COAR3CV, 2005 WL 1950114 (Tenn. Ct. App. Aug. 12, 2005). M was awarded primary custody of the parties' two young children. F petitioned the trial court for primary custody of both children twice in less than a year. The second time, the trial court granted the petition, reasoning that the F would never relent in his efforts to obtain primary residential placement and that the parents' continuing struggle was detrimental to the child's well-being. The Court of Appeals reversed the trial court, stating that F has not demonstrated a proper ground for modification of the prior parenting arrangement and because the proof shows that the M is more inclined than the F to encourage the child's relationship with the other parent.

Duke v Duke, No. M2013-00624-COA-R3CV, 2014 WL 4966902 (Tenn. Ct. App. Oct. 3, 2014). The trial court reduced F's time with the parties' children to four hours of supervised time every other weekend as a result of F's intentional interference with the children's relationship with M. ". . . when reaching to a recommendation in the absence of parental alienation, I would give considerable attention to the children's preferences. However, if the children's strong opinions are simply the result of parental alienation—driven by the F's active indoctrination of the children against their M—I do not take the children's preferences literally . . ."
Knutsen v Cegalis, 2016 VT 2, 201 Vt. 138, 137 A.3d 734 (2016). The Superior Court denied M's motion to modify and denied her any rights of parent-child contact unless the child's trauma therapist recommended contact. M appealed. The Supreme Court held that child's best interests superseded considerations of unfairness to M in being denied contact for years based on F's false allegations of abuse. In this case, the court focused its analysis on the child's best interests. It recognized that F and stepmother had alienated the child from M, but credited expert testimony that the child would be at significant risk of mental health problems if efforts at reunification with M continued.
Noland-Vance v Vance, 321 S.W.3d 398 (Mo. Ct. App. 2010). M alienated children from F, and the evidence supported finding, with respect to child custody determination.
Palazzolo v Mire, 2008-0075 (La. App. 4 Cir. 1/7/09), 10 So. 3d 748. AM (Ms. Palazzolo, adoptive mother) contends that, because I.P. is an "alienated child," the trial court erred in awarding sole custody to BM (Ms. Mire, birth mother). In this case, Dr. Pellegrin found the alienation to be severe and recommended the same remedy that Dr. Gardner recommended in cases of severe PAS—awarding sole custody to the alienated parent. Dr. Jordan agreed that I.P. is an "alienated child" in that she freely expresses hatred or intense dislike towards AM (the rejected parent) and shows a complete lack of ambivalence. The judgment of the trial court terminating AM's visitation rights is reversed. This matter is remanded to the trial court for a hearing to determine the parameters of the visitation to which AM is entitled.
4. The Independent Thinker Phenomenon
Costley v Benjamin, No. M200400375COAR3CV, 2005 WL 1950114 (Tenn. Ct. App. Aug. 12, 2005). M was awarded primary custody of the parties' two young children. F petitioned the trial court for primary custody of both children twice in less than a year. The second time, the trial court granted the petition, reasoning that the F would never relent in his efforts to obtain primary residential placement and that the parents' continuing struggle was detrimental to the child's well-being. The Court of Appeals reversed the trial court, stating that F has not demonstrated a proper ground for modification of the prior parenting arrangement and because the proof shows that the M is more inclined than the F to encourage the child's relationship with the other parent.
Duke v Duke, No. M2013-00624-COA-R3CV, 2014 WL 4966902 (Tenn. Ct. App. Oct. 3, 2014). The trial court reduced F's time with the parties' children to four hours of supervised time every other weekend as a result of F's intentional interference with the children's relationship with M. ". . . when reaching to a recommendation in the absence of parental alienation, I would give considerable attention to the children's preferences. However, if the children's strong opinions are simply the result of parental alienation—driven by the F's active indoctrination of the children against their M—I do not take the children's preferences literally . . ."

Palazzolo v Mire, 2008-0075 (La. App. 4 Cir. 1/7/09), 10 So. 3d 748. AM (Ms. Palazzolo, adoptive mother) contends that, because I.P. is an "alienated child," the trial court erred in awarding sole custody to BM (Ms. Mire, birth mother). The judgment of the trial court terminating AM's visitation rights is reversed. This matter is remanded to the trial court for a hearing to determine the parameters of the visitation to which AM is entitled.
5. Cruelty towards the Alienated Parent
Duke v Duke, No. M2013-00624-COA-R3CV, 2014 WL 4966902 (Tenn. Ct. App. Oct. 3, 2014). The trial court reduced F's time with the parties' children to four hours of supervised time every other weekend as a result of F's intentional interference with the children's relationship with M. ". . . when reaching to a recommendation in the absence of parental alienation, I would give considerable attention to the children's preferences. However, if the children's strong opinions are simply the result of parental alienation—driven by the F's active indoctrination of the children against their M—I do not take the children's preferences literally . . ."
Palazzolo v Mire, 2008-0075 (La. App. 4 Cir. 1/7/09), 10 So. 3d 748. AM (Ms. Palazzolo, adoptive mother) contends that, because I.P. is an "alienated child," the trial court erred in awarding sole custody to BM (Ms. Mire, birth mother). The judgment of the trial court terminating AM's visitation rights is reversed. This matter is remanded to the trial court for a hearing to determine the parameters of the visitation to which AM is entitled.
6. Reflexive Support of the Alienating Parent
Palazzolo v Mire, 2008-0075 (La. App. 4 Cir. 1/7/09), 10 So. 3d 748. AM (Ms. Palazzolo, adoptive mother) contends that, because I.P. is an "alienated child," the trial court erred in awarding sole custody to BM (Ms. Mire, birth mother). The judgment of the trial court terminating AM's visitation rights is reversed. This matter is remanded to the trial court for a hearing to determine the parameters of the visitation to which AM is entitled.
Knutsen v Cegalis, 2016 VT 2, 201 Vt. 138, 137 A.3d 734 (2016). The Superior Court denied M's motion to modify and denied her any rights of parent-child contact unless the child's trauma therapist recommended contact. M appealed. The Supreme Court held that child's best interests superseded considerations of unfairness to M in being denied contact for years based on F's false allegations of abuse. In this case, the court focused its analysis on the child's best interests. It recognized that F and stepmother had alienated the child from M but credited expert testimony that the child would be at significant risk of mental health problems if efforts at reunification with M continued.
Duke v Duke, No. M2013-00624-COA-R3CV, 2014 WL 4966902 (Tenn. Ct. App. Oct. 3, 2014). The trial court reduced F's time with the parties' children to four hours of supervised time every other weekend as a result of F's intentional interference with the children's relationship with M. ". . . when reaching to a recommendation in the absence of parental alienation, I would give considerable attention to the children's preferences. However, if the children's strong opinions are simply the result of parental alienation—driven by the F's active indoctrination of the children against their M—I do not take the children's preferences literally . . ."

7. Presence of Borrowed Scenarios
Duke v Duke, No. M2013-00624-COA-R3CV, 2014 WL 4966902 (Tenn. Ct. App. Oct. 3, 2014). The trial court reduced F's time with the parties' children to four hours of supervised time every other weekend as a result of F's intentional interference with the children's relationship with M. ". . . when reaching to a recommendation in the absence of parental alienation, I would give considerable attention to the children's preferences. However, if the children's strong opinions are simply the result of parental alienation-driven by the F's active indoctrination of the children against their M-I do not take the children's preferences literally . . ."
In re Marriage of Bates, 212 Ill. 2d 489, 819 N.E.2d 714 (Oct. 28, 2004). Section 506(a)(3) of the Act, as applied in this case, deprived M of procedural due process of law because her protected liberty interest in the care, custody, and control of her daughter was adversely affected by the statutory prohibition of calling the child's representative as a witness and cross-examining him. Nevertheless, in light of the overwhelming expert testimony supporting a modification of custody, and because the content of the representative's report was not inconsistent with the other evidence at trial, admission of the report was not prejudicial, and the error in failing to allow cross-examination was harmless. In view of the sparse record challenging the general acceptance of the PAS principle, allowing Dr. Gardner's parental alienation syndrome testimony was not an abuse of discretion.
Palazzolo v Mire, 2008-0075 (La. App. 4 Cir. 1/7/09), 10 So. 3d 748. AM (Ms. Palazzolo, adoptive mother) contends that, because I.P. is an "alienated child," the trial court erred in awarding sole custody to BM (Ms. Mire, birth mother). The judgment of the trial court terminating AM's visitation rights is reversed. This matter is remanded to the trial court for a hearing to determine the parameters of the visitation to which AM is entitled.
8. Spread of Animosity to Extended Family of the Alienated Parent
Costley v Benjamin, No. M200400375COAR3CV, 2005 WL 1950114 (Tenn. Ct. App. Aug. 12, 2005). M was awarded primary custody of the parties' two young children. F petitioned the trial court for primary custody of both children twice in less than a year. The second time, the trial court granted the petition, reasoning that the F would never relent in his efforts to obtain primary residential placement and that the parents' continuing struggle was detrimental to the child's well-being. The Court of Appeals reversed the trial court, stating that F has not demonstrated a proper ground for modification of the prior parenting arrangement and because the proof shows that the M is more inclined than the F to encourage the child's relationship with the other parent.
Duke v Duke, No. M2013-00624-COA-R3CV, 2014 WL 4966902 (Tenn. Ct. App. Oct. 3, 2014). The trial court reduced F's time with the parties' children to four hours of supervised time every other weekend as a result of F's intentional interference with the children's relationship with M. ". . . when reaching to a recommendation in the absence of parental alienation, I would give considerable attention to the children's preferences. However, if the children's strong opinions are simply the result of parental alienation—driven by the F's active indoctrination of the children against their M—I do not take the children's preferences literally . . ."

Palazzolo v Mire, 2008-0075 (La. App. 4 Cir. 1/7/09), 10 So. 3d 748. AM (Ms. Palazzolo, adoptive mother) contends that, because I.P. is an "alienated child," the trial court erred in awarding sole custody to BM (Ms. Mire, birth mother). The judgment of the trial court terminating AM's visitation rights is reversed. This matter is remanded to the trial court for a hearing to determine the parameters of the visitation to which AM is entitled.

APPENDIX D

Admissibility of Expert Evidence in Different States

State	Governing Case or Statute	Admissibility Standard
Alabama (AL)	Ala. Code § 12-21-160. Mazda Motor Corporation v. Hurst, Prod. Liab. Rep. (CCH) P 20106, 2017 WL 2888857 (Ala. 2017).	Daubert
Alaska (AK)	State v. Coon, 974 P.2d 386, 402-403, 95 A.L.R 5th 729 (Alaska 1999). Vent v. State, 67 P.3d 661, 668 (Alaska Ct. App. 2003). Guerre-Chaley v. State, 88 P.3d 539, 541, 544 (Alaska Ct. App. 2004). Marsingill v. O'Malley, 128 P.3d 151, 160 (Alaska 2006). Marron v. Stromstad, 123 P. 3d 992, 1001-1004, 1008 (Alaska 2005). South Anchorage Concerned Coalition, Inc. v. Municipality of Anchorage Bd. of Adjustment, 172 P.3d 774, 780-81 (Alaska 2007).	Daubert
Arizona (AZ)	"Arizona Supreme Court revised Ariz. R. Evid. 702. To adopt the restyled form of the Fed. R. Evid. 702, moving Arizona from the Frye standard to the Daubert standard for expert testimony. Effective as of January 1, 2012."	Daubert

Arkansas (AR)	Jones v. State, 314 Ark. 289, 289-94, 682 S.W.2d 242, 245 (1993). Farm Bureau Mut. Ins. Co. of Arkansas, Inc. v. Foote, 341 Ark. 105, 116, 14 S.W.3d 512 (2000). Flowers v. State, 373 Ak, 137, 132-33, 282 S.W.3d 767 (2008).	Daubert
California (CA)	People v. Leahy, 882 P.2d 321 (Cal. 1994). Rejected Daubert standard. Sargon Enterprises, Inc. V. University of Southern California, 55 Cal. 4th 747, 288 P.3d 1237 (Cal., 2012). People v. Superior Court, 40 Cal. 4th 999, 1013-14, 56 Cal. Rptr. 3d 851, 155 P.3d 259 (2007). People v. Alexander, 49 Cal. 4th 846, 882, 113 Cal. Rptr. 3d 190, 235 P.3d 873 (2010).	Frye
Colorado (CO)	People v. Shreck, 22 P.3d 68, 75, 90 A.L.R. 5th 765 (Colo. 2001). Masters v. People, 58 P.3d 979, 988 (Colo. 2002). People v. Rector, 226 P.3d 1170, 1174 (Colo. App. 2009)	Daubert
Connecticut (CT)	State v. Porter, 241 Conn. 57, 77, 698 A.2d 739 (1997). State v. Kirsch, 263 Conn. 390, 403, 820 A.2d 236 (2003). State v. Swinton, 268 Conn. 781, 933, 847 A.2d 921 (2004). State v. Outing, 298 Conn. 34, 3 A.3d 1 (2010).	Daubert
Delaware (DE)	Nelson v. State, 628 A. 2d 69, 73 (Del. 1993). M.G. Bancorporation, Inc. v. Le Beau, 737 A.2d 513, 522 (Del. 1999). Perry v. Berkley, 996 A.2d 1262, 1267 (Del. 2010).	Daubert
District of Columbia (DC)	Motorola Inc. v. Murray, 147 A.3d 751, Prod. Liab. Rep. (CCH) P 19931 (D.C. 2016).	Daubert

Florida (FL)	F.S.A. § 90.702. "Florida has gone back and forth on its position on Daubert, with the Florida Supreme Court finally adopting Chapter 2013-107, sections 1 and 2, Laws of Florida (Daubert amendments), which amended sections 90.702 (Testimony by Experts) and 90.704 (Basis of opinion testimony by experts), Florida statutes, of the Florida Evidence Code to replace the Frye standard for admitting certain expert evidence with the Daubert Standard."	Daubert
Georgia (GA)	Ga. Code Ann., §24-9-67. Moran v. Kia Motros America, Inc., 276 Ga. App. 96, 98, 622 S.E.2d 439, 60 U.C.C. Rep Serv. 2d 216 (2005). HNTB Georgia, Inc. v. Hamilton-King, 287 Ga. 641, 642-643, 697 S.E.2d 770 (2010).	Daubert
Hawaii (HI)	State v. Montalbo, 73 Haw. 130, 138, 828 P.2d 1274 (1992). State v. Vliet, 95 Haw. 94, 19 P.3d 42, 53 (2001) State v. Escobido-Ortiz, 109 Haw. 359, 410, 126 P.3d 402 (Ct. App. 2005).	Daubert
Idaho (ID)	State v. Trevino, 132 Idaho 888, 892, 980 P.2d 552 (1999). Carnell v. Barker Management, Inc., 137 Idaho 322, 328, 48 P.3d 651 (2002). Weeks v. Eastern Idaho Health Services, 143 Idaho 834, 838, 153 P.3d 1180 (Idaho 2007).	Daubert
Illinois (IL)	Turner v. Williams, 326 Ill. App. 3d 541, 260 Ill. Dec. 804, 762 N.E.2d 70, 81 (2nd Dist. 2001). In re K.T., 361 Ill. App. 3d 187, 202, 297 Ill. Dec. 38, 836 N.E.2d 769 (1st Dist. 2005). People v. Safford, 392 Ill. App. 3d 212, 230, 331 Ill. Dec. 70, 910 N.E.2d 143 (1st Dist. 2009). People v. McKown, 236 Ill. 2d 278, 282-283, 338 Ill. Dec. 415, 924 N.E.2d 941 (2010).	Frye

Indiana (IN)	Steward v. State, 652 N.E.2d 490, 498 (Ind. 1995) Smith v. Yang, 829 N.E.2d 624, 626-627 (Ind. Ct. App. 2005) Franciose v. Jones, 907 N.E.2d 139, 146 (Ind. Ct. App. 2009). Alsheik v. Guerrero, 956 N.E.2d 1115 (Ind. Ct. App. 2011).	Daubert
Iowa (IA)	Hutchinson v. American Family Mut. Ins. Co., 514 N.W.2d 882, 885-886, 72 A.L.R.5th 785 (Iowa 1994) Leaf v. Goodyear Tire & Rubber Co., 590 N.W.2d 525, 533, Prod. Liab. Rep. (CCH) P 15496 (Iowa 1999) Ranes v. Adams Laboratories, Inc. 778 N.W.2d 677, 686, Prod. Liab. Rep. (CCH) P 18363 (Iowa 2010).	Daubert
Kansas (KS)	K.S.A. 60-456 (Testimony in form of opinion or inferences). K.S.A. 60-457 (Preliminary examination for non-expert witness; pre-trial hearing for expert witness). K.S.A. 60-458 (Expert opinion or inference; facts or data relied upon, admissibility).	Daubert
Kentucky (KY)	Cecil v. Com., 888 S.W.2d 669, 675 (Ky. 1994). Dixon v. Com., 149 S.W.3d 426, 430 (Ky. 2004). Jenkins v. Com., 308 S.W.3d 704, 709 (Ky. 2010).	Daubert
Louisiana (LA)	State v. Foret, 628 So. 2d 1116, 1122-1123 (La. 1993). In re Alford, 977 So. 2d 811, 837 (La. 2008). State v. Young, 35 So. 3d 1042, 1045 (La. 2010).	Daubert
Maine (ME)	State v. Taylor, 1997 ME 81, 694 A.2d 907, 910 (Me. 1997). Searles v. Fleetwood Homes of Pennsylvania, Inc., 2005 ME 94, 878 A2d509, 516 (Me. 2005). State v. Bickart, 2009 ME 7, 963 A.2d 183, 189 (Me. 2009).	Daubert

Maryland (MD)	Burral v. State, 352 Md. 707, 724 A.2d 65-80 (1999). Bomas v. State, 412 Md. 392, 405 n.3, 987 A.2d 93 (2010). Montgomery Mut. Ins. Co. v. Chesson, 206 Md. App. 569, 51 A.3d 18 (2012). State v. Baby, 404 Md. 220, 270, 946 A.2d 463, 492-93 (2008). In Savage v. Savage, 455 Md. 138, 166 A.3d 183 (2017). In Sissoko v. State, 236 Md. App. 676, 182 A.3d 874 (2018).	Frye
Massachusetts (MA)	Com. v. Lanigan, 419 Mass. 15, 26, 641 N.E.2d 1342 (1994). Com. v. Patterson, 445 Mass. 626, 640-641, 840 N.E.2d 12 (2005). Com. v. Gambora, 457 Mass. 715, 720-721, 933 N.E.2d 50 (2010).	Daubert
Michigan (MI)	MRE 702 Gilbert v. DaimlerChrysler Corp., 470 Mich. 749, 781, 685 N.W.2d 391, 94 Fair Empl. Prac. Cas. (BNA) 315, 85 Empl. Prac. Dec. (CCH) P 41695, 14 A.L.R.6th 801 (2004). Edry v. Adelman, 486 Mich. 634, 639-640, 786 N.W.2d 567 (2010).	Daubert
Minnesota (MN)	Goeb v. Tharaldson, 615 N.W. 2d 800, 814, Prod. Liab. Rep. (CCH) P 15879, 31 Envtl. L Rep. 20101 (Minn. 2000). State v. Roman Nose, 649 N.W.2d 815, 818 (Minn. 2002). State v. MacLennan, 702 N.W.2d 219, 230 (Minn. 2005). State v, Hull, 788 N.W.2d 91, 103 (Minn. 2010).	Frye
Mississippi (MS)	Kansas City Southern Ry. Co., Inc. v. Johnson, 798 So. 2d 374, 382 (Miss. 2001). Mississippi Transp. Com'n v. McLemore, 863 So. 2d 31, 39 (Miss. 2003). Burnwatt v. Ear, Nose & Throat Consultations of North Mississippi, 47 So. 3d 109, 114 (Miss. 2010).	Daubert

Missouri (MO)	"In 2017, Missouri governor signed H.B. 153 repelling section MO. St. 490.065 replacing it with language mirroring the Daubert standard. The new law carved out some exceptions. The new law will go into effect August 17, 2017. It remains to be seen if the bill will apply retroactively."	Daubert
Montana (MT)	State v. Cline, 275 Mont. 46, 54, 909 P2d 1171 (1996). State v. Bowman, 2005 MT 119, 321 Mont. 176, 186, 89 P 3d 1194 (2005). Harris v. Hanson, 2009 MT 13, 349 Mont. 29, 37-38, 201 P3d 151 (2009).	Daubert
Nebraska (NE)	Schaferrman v. Agland Coop, 262 Neb. 215, 232, 631 N.W.2d 862 (2001). State v. Leibhart, 266 Neb. 133, 142, 662 N.W.2d 618, 626 (2003). State v. Casillas, 279 Neb. 820, 834, 782 N.W.2d 882 (2010).	Daubert
Nevada (NV)	Krause Inc. v. Little, 117 Nev. 929, 34 P.3d 566, 569, Prod. Liab. Rep. (CCH) P 16209 (2001). Higgs v. State, 222 P.3d 648, 650, 126 Nev. Adv. Op. No. 1 (Nev. 2010).	Frye
New Hampshire (NH)	State v. Vandebogart, 136 N.H. 365, 374, 616 A.2d 483 (1992). State v. Hungerford, 142 N.H. 110,121, 697 A.2d 916 (1997). State v. Pelletier, 149 N.H. 243, 252, 818 A.2d 292 (2003). State v. Pelletier, 149 N.H. 77, 88, 945 A.2d 1 (2008). State v. Shepherd, 159 N.H. 163, 168, 977 A.2d 1029 (2009).	Daubert
New Jersey (NJ)	N.J.R. Evid. 702 In re Accutane Litigation, 2018 WL 3636867 (N.J. 2018) (Adopting use of Daubert factors but stating that the Court stops short of declaring New Jersey as a Daubert jurisdiction, stating that we find the factors useful, but hesitate to embrace the full body of Daubert case law as applied by state and federal courts. . .)	Frye

New Mexico (NM)	State v. Alberico, 116 N.M. 156, 167, 861 P.2d 192 (1993). Banks v. IMC Kalium Carlbad Potash Co., 2003-NMSC-026, 134 N.M. 421, 428, 77 P.3d 1014 (2003). State v. Fry, 2006-NMSC-001, 138 N.M. 700, 724-25, 126 P.3d 516, 541 (2005). State v. Downey, 2008-NMSC-061, 145 N.M. 232, 239, 195 P.3d 1244 (2008). State v. Wilson, 2011-NMSC-001, 149 N.M. 273, 248 P.3d, 315, 323 (2010).	
New York (NY)	People v. Johnston, 273 A.D.2d 514, 709 N.Y.S. 230, 236 (3d Dep't 2000). People v. Kogut, 10 Misc. 3d 314, 377, 806, N.Y.S.2d 373 (Sup 2005). Giordano v. Market America, Inc., 15 N.Y.3d 590, 601, 915 N.Y.S.2d 884, 941 N.E.2d 727 (2010).	Frye
North Carolina (NC)	N.C.R. Evid. 702 State v. McGrady, 232 N.C. App. 95, 753 S.E. 2d 361 (2014).	Daubert
North Dakota (ND)	Howe v. Microsoft Corp., 2003 ND 12, 656 N.W.2d 285, 296 n.1, 2003-1 Trade Cas. (CCH) ¶ 73945 (N.D. 2003). State v. Hernandez, 2005 ND 214, 707 N.W.2d 449, 453 (N.D. 2005). State v. Paul, 2009 ND 120, 769 N.W..d 416 (N.D. 2009).	Other
Ohio (OH)	Miller v. Bike Athletic Co., 80 Ohio St. 3d 607, 611-12, 1995-Ohio, 178, 687 N.E.2d 735, Prod. Liab. Rep. (CCH) P 15161 (1998). Hess v. Norfolk S. Ry. Co., 153 Ohio App. 3d 565, 585, 2003-Ohio-4172, 795 N.E. 2d 378 (9th Dist. Summit County 2009).	Daubert

Oklahoma (OK)	Taylor v. State, 1995 OK CR 10, 889 P.2d 319, 328, 332, (Okla. Crim. App. 1995). Christian v. Gray, 2003 OK 10, 65 P.3d 591, 594 (Okla. 2003). Frasier, Frasier & Hickman, L.L.P. v. Flynn, 2005 OK CIV APP 33, 114 P.3d 1095, 1102 (Div. 4 2005). Howard v. ACI Distribution South, 2009 OK CIV APP 95, 229 P.3d 565, 569 (Div. 4 2009). In re BTW, 2010Ok 69, 241 P.3d 199, 211 n. 70 (Okla. 2010).	Daubert
Oregon (OR)	State v. O'Key, 321 Or. 285, 306, 899 P.2d 663, 680 (1995). State v. Southard, 347 Or. 127, 133-34, 218 P.3d 104(2009).	Daubert
Pennsylvania (PA)	P.a.R.E. 702(c). Thomas v. West Bend Co., 760 A.2d 1174, 1179, Prod. Liab. Rep. (CCH) P 15920 (Pa. Super Ct. 2000). Grady v. Frito-Lay, Inc., 576 Pa. 546, 839 A.2d 1038, 1044, Prod. Liab. Rep. (CCH) P 16870 (2003). Com. v. Smith, 606 Pa. 127, 995 A.24 1143, 1159 (2010).	Frye
Rhode Island (RI)	Raimbeault v. Takeuchi Mfg. (U.S.), Ltd., 772 A.2d 1056, 1061, Prod. Liab. Rep. (CCH) P 16113 (R.I. 2001). Owens v. Silvia, 838 A.2d 881, 890 (R.I. 2001). In re Mackenzie C., 877 A.2d 674, 683 (R.I. 2005).	Daubert
South Carolina (SC)	In re Robert R., 340 S.C. 242, 531 S.E.2d 301, 303 (Ct. App. 2000). State v. Jones, 383 S.C. 535, 681 S.E.2d 580 (2009). Graves v. CAS Medical Systems, Inc., 401 S.C. 63, 735 S.E.2d 650 (2012).	Frye
South Dakota (SD)	Department of Social Services of State ex rel. Wolf v. McCarty, 506 N.W.2d 144, 147 (S.D. 1993). Moeller v. Weber, 2004 SD 110, 689 N.W.2d 1, 13 (S.D. 2004). State v. Huber, 2010 SD 63, 789 N.W.2d 283, 289 (S.D. 2010).	Daubert

Tennessee (TN)	McDaniel v. CSX Transp., Inc., 955 S.W.2d 257, 265 (Tenn. 1997). Pullum v. Robinette, 174 S.W.3d 124, 137-38 (Tenn. Ct. App. 2004). State v. Kiser, 284 S.W.3d 227, 284-85 (Tenn. 2009).	Daubert
Texas (TX)	E.I. du Pont de Nemours and Co., Inc. v. Robinson, 923 S.W.2d 549, Prod. Liab. Rep. (CCH) P 14294 (Tex. 1995). Perez v. State, 113 S.W. 3d 819, 833 (Tex. App. Austin 2003). Taylor v. Texas Dept. of Protective and Regulatory Services, 160 S.W.3d 641 (Tex. App. Austin 2005). Lincoln v. Clark Freight Lines, Inc., 285 S.W.3d 79, 84 (Tex. App. Houston 1st Dist. 2009).	Daubert
Utah (UT)	Brewer v. Denver & Rio Grande Western Railroad, 2001 UT 77, 31 P.3d 557, 563 (Utah 2001).	Daubert
Vermont (VT)	State v. Brooks, 162 Vt. 26, 30-31, 643 A.2d 226(1993). State v. Kinney, 171 Vt. 239, 248, 762 A.2d 833 (2000). Estate of George v. Vermont league of Cities and Towns, 187 Vt. 229, 235, 2010 VT 1, 993 A.2d 367 (2010).	Daubert
Virginia (VA)	Cotton v. Com., 19 Va. App. 306, 451 S.E. 2d 675 (1994). John v. Im, 263 Va. App. 315, 559 S.E.2d 694, 698 (2002).	Other
Washington (WA)	State v. Copeland, 130 Wash. 2d 244, 922 P.d2 1304, 1315 (1996). State v. Phillips, 123 Wash. App. 761, 766, 98 P.3d 838 (Div. 2 2004). In re Detention of Hawkins, 169 Wash. 2d 798, 802, 809, 238 P.3d 1175 (2010). Anderson v. Azko Nobel Coating, Inc., 172 Wash. 2d 593, 260 P.3d 857 (2011).	Frye

West Virginia (WV)	Wilt. Buracker, 191 W. Va. 39, 46-47, 443 S.E.2d 196, 203 (1993). Watson v. Inco Alloys Intern., Inc., 209 W. Va. 234, 238, 545 S.E.2d 294, Prod. Liab. Rep. (CCH) P 16035 (2001). State v. Black, 708 S.E.2d 491, 494 (W. Va. 2010).	Daubert
Wisconsin (WI)	Wisc. Stat. §907.02 Commitment of Jones, 2018 WI 44, 381 Wis. 2d 284, 911 N.W.2d 97 (2018).	Daubert
Wyoming (WY)	Springfield v. State, 860 P.2d 435, 442-43 (Wyo. 1993). Bunting v. Jamieson, 984 P.2d 467, 471 (Wyo. 1999). Cooper v. State, 2008 Wy 5, 174 P.3d 726, 729 (Wyo. 2008). Rolle v. State, 2010 WT 100, 236 P.3d 259, 257 (Wyo. 2000).	Daubert

Source: Campbell, T. W., & Lorandos, D. (2019; original work published 2001). Chapter 1, Mental Health Experts: Science and the Law, §1:16.16 Law Updates. In *Cross Examining Experts in the Behavioral Sciences* (Vol. 1, pp. 3–50). Eagan, MN: Thomson Reuters.

APPENDIX E

Statutes and Cases Regarding Minors' Counsel

State	Relevant Statute	Best Interest of the Child and/or Child's Wishes
Alabama (AL)	ALA. Code § 26-2A-52 ALA. Code § 12-15-304 Ex parte J.G., 281 So. 3d 371 (Ala. 2019) Livengood v. Sechler, 382 So. 2d 567 (Ala. Civ. App. 1980)	Best interest of the child.
Alaska (AK)	Alaska Stat. Ann. § 47.10.050 Alaska Stat. Ann. § 25.24.310 Matter of C.L.T., 597 P.2d 518 (Alaska 1979) Veazey v. Veazey, 560 P.2d 382 (Alaska 1977)	Best interest of the child.
Arizona (AZ)	AZ ST RFLP Rule 10 AZ ST RFLP Rule 10.1 Aksamit v. Krahn, 224 Ariz. 68, 227 P.3d 475 (Ct. App. 2010)	Best interest of the child and/or child's wishes.
Arkansas (AR)	AR Code § 9-13-106 AR Code § 28-1-111 Tracy v. Dennie, 2012 Ark. 281, 411 S.W.3d 702 (2012)	Best interest of the child and/or child's wishes.

California (CA)	CA FAM Code § 7635 CA FAM Code § 3150 In re Cole C., 174 Cal. App. 4th 900, 95 Cal. Rptr. 3d 62 (2009)	Best interest of the child.
Colorado (CO)	Colo. Rev. Stat. Ann. § 19-1-111 Colo. Rev. Stat. Ann. § 19-3-203 Colo. Rev. Stat. Ann. § 14-10-116 In re Marriage of Hartley, 886 P.2d 665 (Colo. 1994) In re Marriage of Osborn, 35 Kan. App. 2d 853, 135 P.3d 199 (2006)	Best interest of the child.
Connecticut (CT)	CT Gen Stat § 46b-54 In re Tayquon H., 76 Conn. App. 693, 821 A.2d 796 (2003)	Best interest of the child.
Delaware (DE)	29 DE Code § 9007A In re Truselo, 846 A.2d 256 (Del. Fam. Ct. 2000) N.R.S. v. Div. of Family Servs., No. CS12-01506, 2013 WL 1858138 (Del. Fam. Ct. Mar. 6, 2013)	Best interest of the child.
District of Columbia (DC)	DC ST § 16-2304 DC ST § 21-2033 In re J.J.Z., 630 A.2d 186 (D.C. 1993)	Best interest of the child and/or child's wishes.
Florida (FL)	Fla. Stat. Ann. § 61.401 Attorney ad Litem for D.K. v. Parents of D.K., 780 So. 2d 301 (Fla. Dist. Ct. App. 2001)	Best interest of the child.
Georgia (GA)	GA Code § 15-11-104 (2014) Interest of N. T., 843 S.E.2d 877 (Ga. Ct. App. 2020)	Best interest of the child.
Hawaii (HI)	HI Rev Stat § 587A-16 In re K Children, 120 Haw. 116, 202 P.3d 577 (Ct. App. 2007)	Best interest of the child.

Idaho (ID)	Idaho Code Ann. § 16-1614 Idaho Code Ann. § 15-5-207 In Interest of Doe, 164 Idaho 84, 425 P.3d 285 (2018), reh'g denied (Aug. 22, 2018)	Best interest of the child and/or child's wishes.
Illinois (IL)	750 Ill. Comp. Stat. Ann. 5/506 Nichols v. Fahrenkamp, 2019 IL 123990, reh'g denied (Sept. 23, 2019)	Best interest of the child and/or child's wishes.
Indiana (IN)	Ind. Code Ann. § 31-17-6-5 Deasy-Leas v. Leas, 693 N.E.2d 90 (Ind. Ct. App. 1998), abrogated by Martin v. State, 774 N.E.2d 43 (Ind. 2002)	Best interest of the child.
Iowa (IA)	Iowa Code Ann. § 598.12 In re Marriage of Joens, 284 N.W.2d 326 (Iowa 1979)	Best interest of the child.
Kansas (KS)	Kan. Stat. Ann. § 38-2205 Interests of K.J.S., 462 P.3d 199 (Kan. Ct. App. 2020)	Best interest of the child and/or child's wishes.
Kentucky (KY)	Ky. Rev. Stat. Ann. § 403.270 (West) § 310. [Representation of Child]., Unif. Marriage & Divorce Act § 310 Morgan v. Getter, 441 S.W.3d 94 (Ky. 2014)	Best interest of the child and/or child's wishes.
Louisiana (LA)	La. Stat. Ann. § 9:345 La. Child. Code Ann. art. 607 State in Interest of L.P., 2019-1023 (La. App. 1 Cir. 7/8/20), reh'g denied (Aug. 12, 2020)	Best interest of the child.
Maine (ME)	Me. R. Civ. P. 17 Miller v. Miller, 677 A.2d 64 (Me. 1996)	Best interest of the child.

Maryland (MD)	Md. Code Ann., Fam. Law § 1-202 Md. Code Ann., Fam. Law § 9-103 McAllister v. McAllister, 218 Md. App. 386, 97 A.3d 227 (2014) In re J.W., No. 1163, SEPT.TERM,2019, 2020 WL 1488547 (Md. Ct. Spec. App. Mar. 26, 2020)	Best interest of the child and/or child's wishes.
Massachusetts (MA)	MA R PROB AND FAM CT Order 1-17 In re Georgette, 439 Mass. 28, 785 N.E.2d 356 (2003) Adoption of Erica, 426 Mass. 55, 686 N.E.2d 967 (1997)	Best interest of the child and/or child's wishes.
Michigan (MI)	Mich. Comp. Laws Ann. § 712A.17c In re Hubbell, No. 350963, 2020 WL 3396080 (Mich. Ct. App. June 18, 2020)	Best interest of the child and/or child's wishes.
Minnesota (MN)	Minn. Stat. Ann. § 260C.163 Matter of Welfare of Child of J. R. R., 943 N.W.2d 661 (Minn. Ct. App. 2020)	Best interest of the child and/or child's wishes.
Mississippi (MS)	Miss. Code. Ann. § 43-21-121 S.G. v. D.C., 13 So. 3d 269 (Miss. 2009)	Best interest of the child and/or child's wishes.
Missouri (MO)	Mo. Ann. Stat. § 507.184 Mo. Ann. Stat. § 475.602 Mo. Ann. Stat. § 452.423 Lechner v. Whitesell by Whitesell, 811 S.W.2d 859 (Mo. Ct. App. 1991)	Best interest of the child and/or child's wishes.
Montana (MT)	Mont. Code Ann. § 40-4-205 Mont. Code Ann. § 25-5-301 In re Marriage of Brown, 218 Mont. 14, 706 P.2d 116 (1985) In re Marriage of Rolfe, 216 Mont. 39, 699 P.2d 79 (1985) In re Marriage of Hickey, 213 Mont. 38, 689 P.2d 1222 (1984)	Best interest of the child and/or child's wishes.

Nebraska (NE)	Neb. Rev. Stat. Ann. § 42-358 Betz v. Betz, 254 Neb. 341, 575 N.W.2d 406 (1998)	Best interest of the child and/or child's wishes.
Nevada (NV)	Nev. Rev. Stat. Ann. § 432B.420 Nev. Rev. Stat. Ann. § 12.050 In re Guardianship of Walker, 74 Nev. 230, 327 P.2d 344 (1958)	Best interest of the child.
New Hampshire (NH)	N.H. Rev. Stat. Ann. § 169-C:10 In re Stapleford, 156 N.H. 260, 931 A.2d 1199 (2007) In re Lisa G., 127 N.H. 585, 504 A.2d 1 (1986)	Best interest of the child.
New Jersey (NJ)	N.J. Stat. Ann. § 9:6-8.23 In re Maraziti, 233 N.J. Super. 488, 559 A.2d 447 (App. Div. 1989)	Best interest of the child.
New Mexico (NM)	N.M. Stat. Ann. § 32A-1-6 N.M. Stat. Ann. § 40-4-8 NMRA, Rule 1-053.3 Kimbrell v. Kimbrell, 2014-NMSC-027, 331 P.3d 915	Best interest of the child.
New York (NY)	N.Y. Fam. Ct. Act § 241 (McKinney) Awan v. Awan, 75 A.D.3d 597, 906 N.Y.S.2d 70 (2010) Newton v. McFarlane, 174 A.D.3d 67, 103 N.Y.S.3d 445 (2019)	Best interest of the child and/or child's wishes.
North Carolina (NC)	N.C. Gen. Stat. Ann. § 7B-601 (GAL) Matter of C.J.C., 374 N.C. 42, 839 S.E.2d 742 (2020)	Best interest of the child.
North Dakota (ND)	N.D. Cent. Code Ann. § 14-07.1-05.1 (GAL)	Best interest of the child.
Ohio (OH)	Ohio Rev. Code Ann. § 2151.352 In re Julius H., 2002-Ohio-394 In re Hilyard, 2006-Ohio-1965	Best interest of the child and/or child's wishes.

Oklahoma (OK)	Okla. Stat. Ann. tit. 10A, § 1-4-306 Okla. Stat. Ann. tit. 10, § 7505-1.2 In re N.L., 2015 OK CIV APP 24, 347 P.3d 301	Best interest of the child and/or child's wishes.
Oregon (OR)	Or. Rev. Stat. Ann. § 419B.195 Or. Rev. Stat. Ann. § 419B.231 (GAL) Caldwell v. Lucas, 170 Or. App. 587, 13 P.3d 560 (2000)	Best interest of the child and/or child's wishes.
Pennsylvania (PA)	23 Pa. Stat. and Cons. Stat. Ann. § 2313 Pa.R.C.P. No. 1915.11 R.S. v. J.M., No. 126 WDA 2020, 2020 WL 3639931 (Pa. Super. Ct. July 6, 2020) In re S.R.H., No. 333 MDA 2020, 2020 WL 4646177 (Pa. Super. Ct. Aug. 11, 2020)	Best interest of the child and/or child's wishes.
Rhode Island (RI)	15 R.I. Gen. Laws Ann. § 15-5-16.2 (West) Kenney v. Hickey, 486 A.2d 1079 (R.I. 1985)	Best interest of the child and/or child's wishes.
South Carolina (SC)	S.C. Code Ann. § 63-3-830 (GAL) S.C. Code Ann. § 63-3-810 (GAL) Loe v. Mother, Father, & Berkeley Cty. Dep't of Soc. Servs., 382 S.C. 457, 675 S.E.2d 807 (Ct. App. 2009)	Best interest of the child and/or child's wishes.
South Dakota (SD)	S.D. Codified Laws § 15-6-17(c) (GAL)	Best interest of the child and/or child's wishes.
Tennessee (TN)	Tenn. Code Ann. § 33-8-310 Tenn. Code Ann. § 36-4-132 Toms v. Toms, 209 S.W.3d 76 (Tenn. Ct. App. 2005)	Best interest of the child and/or child's wishes.
Texas (TX)	Tex. Fam. Code Ann. § 107.003 In Interest of D.M.O., No. 04-17-00290-CV, 2018 WL 1402030 (Tex. App. Mar. 21, 2018), reh'g denied (May 2, 2018)	Best interest of the child and/or child's wishes.

Utah (UT)	Utah Code Ann. § 78A-6-902 K.P.S. v. E.J.P., 2018 UT App 5, 414 P.3d 933	Best interest of the child and/or child's wishes.
Vermont (VT)	Vt. Stat. Ann. tit. 15, § 594 Va. Code Ann. § 16.1-266 Wright v. Kemp, 2019 VT 11, 209 Vt. 476, 207 A.3d 1021 (2019)	Best interest of the child and/or child's wishes.
Virginia (VA)	Va. Code Ann. § 16.1-266 Va. Code Ann. § 16.1-266.1 Ferguson v. Grubb, 39 Va. App. 549, 574 S.E.2d 769 (2003)	Best interest of the child and/or child's wishes.
Washington (WA)	Wash. Rev. Code Ann. § 13.34.100 Wash. Rev. Code Ann. § 26.09.110 Matter of Dependency of E.M., 12 Wash. App. 2d 510, 458 P.3d 810 Matter of Dependency of E.H., 191 Wash. 2d 872, 427 P.3d 587 (2018)	Best interest of the child and/or child's wishes.
West Virginia (WV)	W. Va. Code Ann. § 49-4-601 In re Jeffrey R.L., 190 W. Va. 24, 435 S.E.2d 162 (1993)	Best interest of the child and/or child's wishes.
Wisconsin (WI)	Wis. Stat. Ann. § 767.407	Best interest of the child and/or child's wishes.
Wyoming (WY)	Wyo. Stat. Ann. § 14-3-211 In re ""H" Children, 2003 WY 155, 79 P.3d 997 (Wyo. 2003) Clark v. Alexander, 953 P.2d 145 (Wyo. 1998)	Best interest of the child and/or child's wishes.

TABLE OF CASES

INDEX